Nutrition

A health promotion approach

on or before

Nutrition

A health promotion approach

3rd Edition

Geoffrey P Webb BSC, MSC, PHD
Senior Lecturer in Nutrition and Physiology, University of
East London, London, UK

Hodder Arnold

www.hoddereducation.com

First published in Great Britian in 1994 by Butterworth Heinemann
Second edition 2002 by Hodder Arnold, an imprint of Hodder Education

This third edition published in 2008 by
Hodder Arnold, an imprint of Hodder Education, part of Hachette Livre UK,
338 Euston Road, London NW1 3BH

http://www.hoddereducation.com

*Hodder Headline's policy is to use papers that are natural, renewable and recycla-
ble products and made from wood grown in sustainable forests. The logging and
manufacturing processes are expected to conform to the environmental regulations
of the country of origin*

Whilst the advice and information in this book are believed to be true and
accurate at the date of going to press, neither the author[s] nor the publisher
can accept any legal responsibility or liability for any errors or omissions that
may be made. In particular (but without limiting the generality of the preced-
ing disclaimer) every effort has been made to check drug dosages; however it
is still possible that errors have been missed. Furthermore, dosage schedules
are constantly being revised and new side-effects recognized. For these reasons
the reader is strongly urged to consult the drug companies' printed instruc-
tions before administering any of the drugs recommended in this book.

British Library Cataloguing in Publication Data
A catalogue record for this book is available from the British Library

Library of Congress Cataloging-in-Publication Data
A catalog record for this book is available from the Library of Congress

ISBN-13   978-0-340-93882-9

1 2 3 4 5 6 7 8 9 10

Commissioning Editor: Jo Koster/Naomi Wilkinson
Project Editor: Clare Patterson
Production Controller: Andre Sim
Cover Designer: Helen Townson

Typeset in 9.5/12 Berling Roman by Charon Tec Ltd (A Macmillan Company)
www.charontec.com
Printed and bound in Spain

For my parents Maisie and William who made many personal sacrifices to
ensure my education and for daughter Katherine and my wife Susan for their
patience and support during the writing of this book.

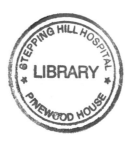

Contents

Preface

It is now 6 years since I sat down to write the preface for the second edition of this book. The aims that I listed in the first two editions are still the aims for this edition. I have tried to produce a book with the following characteristics. It is comprehensive in its range of coverage of the various aspects of nutrition. It is designed to be flexible enough to be used at different academic levels by students who are new to the subject of nutrition. I have tried to make it accessible to students with limited mathematical and biochemical background. Finally, I have focused on nutritional priorities in industrialized countries and more specifically on the role of diet and lifestyle in the prevention of chronic disease and the promotion of long-term health.

Most of the chapters are recognizable updates and revisions of chapters in the previous edition. I have incorporated new statistical data and research output that has been published in the past 6 years. Where recent research has confirmed and reinforced what was written in previous editions, I have added a review of this new confirmatory evidence to descriptions of the earlier work; this should indicate to the reader that earlier conclusions have now withstood the test of time.

The biggest changes since the second edition have occurred in the section dealing with the micronutrients, which has been expanded from two to three chapters, one each covering the individual vitamins and minerals and a new one which introduces and overviews the micronutrients including their use as dietary supplements. This new chapter (Chapter 12) discusses issues such as general levels of micronutrient adequacy, the uses and hazards of dietary supplements, and conditionally essential nutrients. Many substances that are not strictly nutrients but which may have nutritional implications and may be widely used as dietary supplements are overviewed in this chapter – for example, several natural metabolites which are endogenously produced and so not considered to be essential in the diet and the many thousands of so-called plant secondary metabolites found in natural plant extracts, which are taken as supplements as well as being eaten in plant foods. A third of

adults in Britain take a dietary supplement, so supplements is a topic that cannot be ignored in any nutrition text that aims to be comprehensive. The section dealing with free radicals and antioxidants has also been moved into the new Chapter 12. The chapters dealing with the individual vitamins and minerals (Chapters 13 and 14) now have a summary of key facts about each micronutrient at the start of the section dealing with it. The chapter on minerals has been expanded to include some discussion of each mineral and trace element accepted to be 'essential'. I have spent much of the time since the last edition researching and writing about dietary supplements and functional foods, which has obviously influenced my decision to expand the coverage of supplements in this book. The section on functional foods in Chapter 18 has also been expanded to reflect current interest in this area.

Food safety issues and particularly the bovine spongiform encephalopathy (BSE) crisis were at the forefront of nutritional concerns when the second edition was being written. Thankfully, it now seems almost certain that the epidemic of the human form of BSE (variant Creutzfeldt–Jakob disease (vCJD)) caused by eating contaminated beef will be at the very lowest end of projections; 160 deaths to date and maybe less than 200 deaths in total. Two of the biggest issues in nutrition currently are obesity and its implications for health and the health benefits of foods and supplements rich in antioxidants. Obesity and weight control continues to receive extensive coverage in this edition and there is increased focus on childhood obesity and the assessment of overweight and obesity in children. Few days go by without some new food or supplement being touted in the media as having the potential to prevent cancer or heart disease on the basis of its antioxidant content e.g. tea, red wines, watercress and even chocolate. I have tried to give a realistic appraisal of the benefits and hazards of our current preoccupation with antioxidants, many of which do not even classify as nutrients. A recurring theme throughout all three editions of this book has been that dietary change should not be promoted unless there is some substantial evidence that it will yield tangible and holistic benefits and that we are confident that any changes we encourage will not do more harm than good. Those encouraging the use of concentrated supplements or even the consumption of individual foods in much greater than normal amounts for highly speculative long-term benefits need to be particularly careful in this respect. Several examples of past dietary and lifestyle advice or policies that are now discredited are discussed in the first chapter as a warning that ill-considered health promotion may not always promote health and may instead have undesirable consequences. Some research into the nutritional benefits of individual foods seems to be primarily geared towards gaining publicity that will be in the commercial interests of the research sponsor.

Good nutrition education and good health promotion offers simple, clear, broad and realistic guidelines.

It is not about promotion of individual superfoods based on very limited evidence that they may prevent individual diseases. I have avoided recommending single foods in this book and have generally not discussed any of the hundreds of reductionist studies linking consumption of large amounts of specific foods to prevention of individual diseases on the basis of very tenuous evidence. I believe that many of these studies are logically flawed even if their technical execution is good. I encourage people to eat good amounts of a variety of fruits and vegetables and strongly believe that this will improve long-term health, but I would not encourage people to force down large amounts of broccoli or watercress or pumpkin or bananas if they dislike them.

PART ONE

CONCEPTS AND PRINCIPLES

1

Changing priorities for nutrition education

IDENTIFICATION OF THE ESSENTIAL NUTRIENTS

Scientific research into food and nutrition was initially directed towards identifying the essential nutrients and quantifying our requirement for them. All of the essential nutrients must be present in our diet in certain minimum quantities if we are to remain healthy. These essential nutrients can be broadly divided into two categories.

- *The macronutrients* – carbohydrates, fats and protein. These are required in relatively large quantities and can act as dietary sources of energy.
- *The micronutrients* – vitamins and minerals. These are required in only small amounts (milligram or microgram quantities) and do not act as sources of energy.

A shortage of one of the essential micronutrients leads to adverse symptoms, often to a characteristic **deficiency disease**. In the first half of the twentieth century, many essential nutrients were identified, and their ability to cure these deficiency diseases was recognized. Some examples are given below.

- Niacin (vitamin B_3) was shown to cure the deficiency disease **pellagra**. This often fatal disease was so prevalent in some southern states of the USA in the early decades of the twentieth century that it was thought to be an infectious disease. Pellagra remained a problem in several southern states of America until the 1940s.

- In the late nineteenth and early twentieth centuries up to 75 per cent of children in some British industrial cities had **rickets**, a disease which was shown to be due to lack of vitamin D. Again, it was not until the 1940s that this disease was largely eradicated in British children. Rickets can be cured either by consuming vitamin D or by exposing the skin to summer sunlight, which enables us to make our own vitamin D.

- The disease **beriberi** exacted a heavy toll of death and misery in the rice-eating countries of the Far East well into the third quarter of the twentieth century. Thiamin (vitamin B_1), a vitamin that is largely removed from white rice during the milling process, cured it.

Several of the Nobel prizes in physiology and medicine in this era were awarded for work on the vitamins – the prizes of 1929, 1934 and 1943. It was for the work on thiamin and beriberi, mentioned above, that Christiaan Eijkman received the 1929 prize.

Such spectacular successes may have encouraged a 'magic bullet' image of nutrition – the expectation that simple dietary changes may be able to prevent or cure diseases other than those due to dietary inadequacy. This expectation is generally misplaced although there is no doubt that poor nutritional status can adversely affect the course of all illnesses, and some conditions do respond to restriction or extra supply of some dietary components. For example, the symptoms and the progression of both

diabetes mellitus and **chronic renal failure** can be controlled to a degree by diet (see Chapter 16). There are even a few, relatively uncommon diseases whose symptoms are due to an inborn or acquired intolerance to a specific component of food. In these cases, although diet does not strictly cure the condition, the symptoms can be controlled by preventing or limiting intake of the offending substance, e.g.:

- *phenylketonuria* (intolerance to the essential amino acid phenylalanine)
- *galactosaemia* (intolerance to one of the components of milk sugar – galactose)
- *coeliac disease* (intolerance/delayed hypersensitivity to the wheat protein, gluten)
- *acute hypersensitivity* (an acute allergic response to a particular food or ingredient).

There are also a few conditions in which the symptoms are alleviated by increased intake of a nutrient. For example, **pernicious anaemia** is an autoimmune condition that results in an inability to absorb vitamin B_{12} and is relieved by injections of the vitamin.

Harper (1999) provided the following criteria for establishing that a nutrient is essential.

- The substance is essential for growth, health and survival.
- Characteristic signs of deficiency result from inadequate intakes and these are only cured by the administration of the nutrient or a known precursor.
- The severity of the deficiency symptoms is dose dependent; they get worse as the intake of nutrient decreases.
- The substance is not synthesized in the body (or only synthesized from a specific dietary precursor) and so is required throughout life. (Note that a strict application of this rule would eliminate vitamin D which can be synthesized in the skin in sufficient amounts to meet our needs provided the skin is regularly exposed to summer sunlight.)

Around 40 essential nutrients have now been identified, namely:

- water
- energy sources
- protein and the nine essential amino acids
- essential fatty acids
- the vitamins A, C, D, E and K

- eight substances that make up the B group of vitamins
- around 15 minerals and trace minerals.

In most cases, these nutrients have not only been identified but good estimates of average requirements have also been made. Many governments and international agencies use these estimates of requirements to publish lists of dietary standards that can be used as yardsticks to test the adequacy of diets or food supplies. These standards are variously termed **recommended dietary/daily allowances (RDA)** or **dietary reference values (DRV)**. They are discussed fully in Chapter 3.

Conditionally essential nutrients

Some substances may be required in the diet only under particular circumstances or by particular groups of people, e.g. premature babies, and people with genetic defects or other pathological conditions. Harper (1999) designated these as **conditionally essential nutrients** and defined these as substances that are 'not ordinarily required in the diet but which must be supplied exogenously to specific groups that do not synthesise them in adequate amounts', e.g.:

- L-carnitine may be essential in people with rare inherited disorders of fatty acid metabolism
- the amino acid glutamine may become essential in people with serious illness or injury because they cannot synthesize it fast enough to meet their increased needs
- the amino acids cysteine and tyrosine may be conditionally essential for premature babies who have not yet developed the enzymes necessary for their synthesis
- tyrosine also becomes an essential amino acid in people with the inherited disease phenylketonuria mentioned in the previous section.

Conditionally essential nutrients are discussed further in Chapter 12.

Some substances which have vitamin-like functions in the body, but which are not considered to be essential, are frequently taken as dietary supplements; these include carnitine, **creatine, glucosamine, coenzyme** Q_{10} and **s-adenosyl methionine**. The implication underpinning their use as supplements is that endogenous synthesis may not always ensure optimal health or may become insufficient in certain pathological states. In effect it is being implied that they can become conditionally essential nutrients. Several of these substances are briefly overviewed in Chapter 12 and discussed in greater depth in Webb (2006).

Some other substances may be desirable for health even though they do not meet the criteria for essentiality, e.g. fluoride for its beneficial effects on teeth and **dietary fibre** for its effects on gut function. Some nutrients may also be used in doses that greatly exceed those that would be obtained from food to produce a pharmacological effect (i.e. they are used as drugs).

There are also tens of thousands of substances termed **secondary plant metabolites** that are present in the plant foods we eat and, although they are not essential or even conditionally essential nutrients, many of these may have beneficial (or deleterious) effects on health. Plant preparations and extracts have been used as herbal medicines throughout human history, and many of them are now marketed and promoted as dietary supplements useful for maintaining or restoring health. Many of these secondary plant metabolites are popular and effective drugs and several are potent poisons. These secondary metabolites are classified and briefly overviewed in Chapter 13 and are discussed at greater length in Webb (2006).

Key points

- In the first half of the twentieth century most of the vitamins were discovered and the ability of vitamin and mineral supplements to cure deficiency diseases was recognized.
- These discoveries may have encouraged the illusion that dietary change could cure many other diseases.
- A nutrient is classified as essential if it is needed for growth and survival, if deprivation leads to dose-dependent symptoms of deficiency, and if the substance is not synthesized in sufficient quantities to meet physiological needs.
- Some nutrients are classified as conditionally essential because they are only essential in some circumstances or for some people.
- Some endogenously produced substances with vitamin-like functions are promoted as dietary supplements with the implication that they become conditionally essential under some circumstances.

- Although dietary change can rarely cure or remove the symptoms of a disease, the progress of all diseases will be affected by poor nutritional status.
- In a few fairly uncommon conditions, diet may be the sole treatment, usually because the symptoms are due to intolerance to a component of food.
- Some nutrients may be used in pharmacological quantities, i.e. used as drugs.
- Intakes of some 'nutrients' may be desirable for health while not being strictly essential.
- Plants produce thousands of so-called secondary metabolites that may have beneficial or deleterious effects on health; some of these have been developed into effective drugs and some are potent poisons.
- Around 40 essential nutrients have been identified and estimates of average requirements have been made and published as recommended dietary/daily allowances or dietary reference values in the UK.

ADEQUACY: THE TRADITIONAL PRIORITY IN NUTRITION

The traditional priority in nutrition has been to ensure nutritional **adequacy**; to ensure that diets contain adequate amounts of energy and all of the essential nutrients. Adequacy was the traditional priority in all countries, and it remains the nutritional priority for the majority of the world population. Even today, dietary inadequacy is prevalent in many countries as illustrated by the examples below.

- Large sections of the world population still suffer from overt starvation.
- Several vitamin and mineral deficiency diseases are still prevalent in many parts of the world. Vitamin A deficiency causes hundreds of thousands of children to go blind each year and is a contributory factor in the deaths of millions of infants and children in developing countries. Iodine deficiency is endemic in many parts of the world and retards the mental and physical development of tens of millions of children.
- Many more people in developing countries, especially children, suffer more subtle consequences of suboptimal nutrition (Box 1.1).

Box 1.1	Some adverse consequences of inadequate food intake

- Increased probability of developing a specific nutrient deficiency disease
- Reduced growth and reduced mental and physical development in children
- Wasting of muscles and essential organs; wasting of the heart muscle leads to abnormal cardiac rhythms and risk of heart failure
- Reduced capacity of the gut for digestion and absorption. An inability to digest lactose (milk sugar) and diarrhoea are both common features of malnutrition
- Impaired functioning of the immune system leading to increased risk of infection as well as more prolonged and severe symptoms of infection
- Slow healing of wounds
- Reduced strength and physical capacity that may impair the ability to earn an adequate income or cultivate food
- Changes in personality and other adverse psychological effects

In the first half of the twentieth century, even in developed countries, the quality of a diet would thus have been judged by its ability to supply all of the essential nutrients and to prevent nutritional inadequacy. The official priorities for improving the nutritional health of the British population during the 1930s were:

- to reduce the consumption of bread and starchy foods
- to increase the consumption of nutrient-rich, so-called 'protective foods', such as milk, cheese, eggs and green vegetables.

The following benefits were expected to result from these changes:

- a taller, more active and mentally alert population
- decreased incidence of the deficiency diseases such as **goitre**, rickets and **anaemia**
- a reduced toll of death and incapacity due to infectious diseases such as pneumonia, tuberculosis and rheumatic fever.

Britons are indeed much taller now than they were in the first half of the twentieth century and occurrences of overt deficiency diseases are rare and usually confined to particular high-risk sectors of the population. Children now mature faster and reach puberty earlier. The potential physical capability of the population has probably increased even though many of us now accept the opportunity to lead very inactive lives that mechanization has given us. Infectious diseases now account for less than 1 per cent of deaths in Britain.

In the affluent industrialized countries of North America, western Europe and Australasia, nutritional adequacy has in recent years been almost taken for granted. Nutrient deficiencies become likely only if total food intake is low or restricted or if the range of foods that are available or acceptable is narrowed. In these industrialized countries, there is an almost limitless abundance of food and a year-round variety that would have astounded our ancestors. One would expect therefore that even the poor in these countries should usually be able to obtain at least their minimum needs of energy and the essential nutrients. Overt deficiency diseases are uncommon among most sections of these populations. Over-nutrition, manifested most obviously by obesity, is far more common in such countries than all of the diseases of under-nutrition. Overt malnutrition and deficiency diseases in the industrialized countries are usually concentrated in groups such as:

- those who suffer chronic ill health or some medical condition that specifically predisposes to nutrient deficiency (a high proportion of patients admitted to hospital are malnourished on admission – see Chapter 16)
- alcoholics and drug addicts
- those at the extremes of social and economic disadvantage
- the very elderly (see Chapter 15).

War or severe economic dislocation can rapidly undermine this assumption of even minimal adequacy in developed countries as witnessed by events in parts of the former Soviet Union and former Yugoslavia during the 1980s and 1990s. Wartime mass starvation in the Netherlands and Germany are still recent enough to be just within living memory. In Britain, during World War II considerable constraints were placed on the food supply by attacks on merchant shipping. This certainly led to shortages of certain foods and a more austere and less palatable diet. However, because of very effective food policy measures and strict rationing it also paradoxically led to an apparent improvement in the nutritional health of the British population.

In the both the UK and USA, average energy intakes of the population have fallen substantially in recent decades; a reflection of reduced energy expenditure caused by our increasingly sedentary lifestyle. This trend towards reduced energy intake (i.e. total food intake) coupled with a high proportion of energy being obtained from nutrient-depleted sugars, fats and alcoholic drinks may increase the likelihood of suboptimal nutrient intakes. It may even precipitate overt nutrient deficiencies in some groups such as the elderly or those on prolonged weight-reducing diets. In Chapter 13 there is a discussion of disturbing evidence that substantial numbers of individuals in all age groups in the UK have intakes of one or more essential nutrients that is considered to be inadequate even where average population intakes of these nutrients seem to be satisfactory. In the case of a few nutrients even average intakes seem to be less than satisfactory and millions of individuals show biochemical indications of an unsatisfactory vitamin or mineral status.

Key points

- Ensuring adequate intakes of energy and essential nutrients has been the traditional priority in nutrition and it remains the priority for most of the world population.
- Dietary inadequacy results in a number of adverse consequences (see Box 1.1).
- In the 1930s, the dietary priorities for improving health in Britain were to reduce the consumption of starchy foods and to increase the consumption of so-called protective foods like milk, cheese, eggs and green vegetables.
- These changes to the 1930s British diet were expected to lead to a taller, more active and mentally alert population, elimination of the deficiency diseases and a reduced toll from many infectious diseases. These objectives have been largely achieved.
- In the industrialized countries, deficiency diseases are largely confined to the very elderly, the infirm, alcoholics and drug addicts, or those at the extremes of social and economic deprivation.
- War and economic disruption can lead to a rapid re-emergence of the deficiency diseases in a previously affluent country.

- Evidence from major dietary and nutritional surveys in the UK suggests that millions of individuals may have less than satisfactory status for one or more vitamins or minerals.

THE NEW PRIORITY: DIET AS A MEANS TO HEALTH PROMOTION OR DISEASE PREVENTION

The priority of health promotion and nutrition education in industrialized countries is now directed towards changing the 'Western diet and lifestyle', with the aim of reducing the toll of chronic diseases such as cardiovascular disease, cancer, maturity-onset diabetes, osteoporosis and dental disease. These diseases are variously known as the 'Western diseases' or the 'diseases of affluence/civilization/ industrialization'. As a population becomes more affluent, its life expectancy tends to increase and mortality, particularly among children and younger adults, falls. However these chronic, degenerative 'diseases of industrialization' become more prevalent in middle-aged and older adults, and so account for an increasing proportion of death and disability.

There is no doubt that people in industrialized countries live much longer and die of different things than they did a century ago. In 1901, average life expectancy was around 47 years in both Britain and the USA. It is now well over 75 years in both countries. In 1901, less than half of British people survived to reach 65 years but now around 95 per cent do. In 1901, only 4 per cent of the population of Britain was over 65 years but now they make up 16 per cent of the population. These dramatic increases in life expectancy have been largely the result of reducing deaths, particularly in children and younger adults, from acute causes such as infection, complications of childbirth, accidents and appendicitis. Life expectancy has increased substantially for all age groups over this period; even older people have an increased expectancy of further years (Webb and Copeman, 1996). This inevitably means that there have been big increases in the proportion of deaths attributable to the chronic, degenerative diseases of industrialization that affect mainly middle-aged and elderly people. Infectious diseases were the major cause of death in Britain in the nineteenth century, but now it is the cardiovascular diseases (heart disease and strokes). Infectious diseases accounted for 1 in 3 deaths in Britain in 1850, about 1 in 5 deaths in 1900, but today this figure is well under 1 per cent. At the turn of the twentieth century probably less than a quarter of all deaths were attributed to cardiovascular disease and cancer but now it is three quarters. In the period 1931 to 1991, cardiovascular diseases rose from causing 26 per cent of all deaths to 46 per cent.

There is an almost unanimous assumption that the diseases of industrialization are environmentally triggered, i.e. due to the 'Western lifestyle'. This assumption leads to the widespread belief that major improvements in health and longevity can be achieved by simple modifications of lifestyle. Diet is one of the environmental variables that has received much attention in recent years, and poor diet has been blamed for contributing to the relatively poor health record of some affluent groups. Of the top 10 leading causes of death in the USA, eight have been associated with nutritional causes or excessive alcohol consumption. Numerous expert committees in the industrialized countries have suggested dietary modifications that they consider would reduce or delay mortality and morbidity from these diseases of industrialization and thus ultimately lead to increases in life expectancy and improved health. These recommendations usually include advice to reduce consumption of fats, sugar, alcohol and salt, and to replace them with starchy foods and more fruits and vegetables. Consumers are being advised to eat less meat, milk, eggs and dairy produce, but more bread and starchy foods and more fruits and vegetables. Compare these recommendations with the British priorities for nutrition in the 1930s when Britons were being advised to eat less starchy foods and more milk, cheese and eggs. A good diet today is not just one that is nutritionally adequate but one that is also considered likely to reduce morbidity and mortality from the diseases of industrialization.

Risk factors

Certain measured parameters and lifestyle characteristics partially predict an individual's likelihood of developing or dying of a particular disease, e.g.:

- a high plasma cholesterol concentration indicates an increased risk of developing coronary heart disease

- high blood pressure is associated with increased risk of renal failure, heart disease and stroke
- obesity is associated with increased likelihood of developing **type 2 diabetes**.

Many of these 'risk markers' are thought to be a contributory cause of the disease, i.e. they are not just markers for those at risk but are true **risk factors** that directly contribute to the development of the disease. For example, raised plasma cholesterol concentration is generally believed to accelerate the lipid deposition and fibrosis of artery walls (**atherosclerosis**) that leads to increase risk of coronary heart disease. Such an assumption of cause and effect would suggest that altering the risk factor, e.g. lowering plasma cholesterol, should also reduce the risk of the disease provided such changes occur before there is irreversible damage. Much of current health promotion, nutrition education and preventive medicine are based on such assumptions. Dietary variables can be direct risk factors for disease as in the examples below:

- a diet that is low in fruits and vegetables is associated with increased risk of several types of cancer
- high sugar consumption is strongly implicated as a cause of tooth decay whereas high fluoride intake seems to prevent it.

Dietary variables can also have a major influence on some of the other well-established risk factors, particularly the cardiovascular risk factors. Some examples are:

- a high population salt intake is associated with high average blood pressure and increased prevalence of **hypertension**
- changes in the types of fat eaten can have readily demonstrable effects on plasma cholesterol concentration; a high proportion of saturated fat raises plasma cholesterol but replacing saturated with unsaturated fat lowers it.

Much current nutrition research is focused on these risk factors. Individual components of the diet are related to individual diseases or even to other risk factors such as high plasma cholesterol and high blood pressure. The identification of dietary and other environmental risk factors should enable health educators to promote changes in behaviour that will lessen exposure to the risk factor, prevent the disease and so eventually improve health and longevity. However, one practical result of this approach is a profusion of papers in the medical and scientific literature cataloguing a series of suggested associations between individual dietary variables and individual diseases and risk factors. The sheer number of such reported associations is sometimes bewildering, and this may be compounded because there are, more often than not, contradictory reports. As an extreme example, McCormick and Skrabanek (1988) suggested that a staggering 250 risk markers had been reported for coronary heart disease.

A major problem that will inevitably confront those involved in health promotion will be to decide whether and how to act on the latest reported association between a lifestyle variable and a disease. These associations will often be relayed to the general public through brief summaries in the media that may be distorted and sensationalized. Health conscious members of the public may then try to decide on the optimal diet and lifestyle on the basis of such snippets – this is rather like trying to work out the picture on a huge jigsaw puzzle by reading inaccurate and incomplete descriptions of some of the individual pieces. All too often the initial research on which these health stories are based is sponsored by those with commercial interests in the product and so researchers may, perhaps unconsciously, be complicit in this sensationalization because it keeps their sponsors happy and raises their own profile.

Several of these individual associations are discussed and evaluated in this book. These discussions have two broad aims:

- to indicate not only where the current consensus of scientific opinion lies but also to give a flavour of the reasoning and evidence underpinning that position and to highlight unresolved issues and/or alternative opinions
- to indicate diet and lifestyle patterns or modifications that are realistic, low risk, consistent and likely to produce overall health benefits.

Are recommendations to alter diet and lifestyle offered too freely?

A drug or a food additive intended for use by vast numbers of apparently healthy people would be subject to an extremely rigorous and highly structured evaluation of both its efficacy and safety. A drug is not licensed until the Medicines and Healthcare products Regulatory Authority (MHRA) in the UK or Food and Drug Administration (FDA) in the USA have been satisfied that it is both safe and effective. Despite this, mistakes still occur and drugs or additives have to be withdrawn after sometimes many years of use. Compared with this rigorous approval procedure, some dietary and lifestyle interventions (including some dietary supplements and unlicensed drugs masquerading as dietary supplements) seem to be advocated on the basis of incomplete appraisal of either efficacy or safety – perhaps, on occasion, almost recklessly. Even properly constituted expert committees may make premature judgements based on incomplete or incorrect evidence. There will also be a plethora of advice from those whose actions are prompted by belief in an untenable theory or myth (quackery), by political or ethical prejudice or even by economic or other self-interest. One would not take seriously a book on brain surgery or nuclear physics by an unqualified celebrity but celebrities, self-proclaimed experts in alternative treatments and professional journalists are deemed suitable to give their advice on diet and health in the media and in diet books.

There are clear legal frameworks regulating the licensing of drugs and food additives, yet there is not, nor can there realistically be, any restrictions on the offering of dietary or lifestyle advice. All that governments and professional bodies can do is to try to ensure that there is some system of registration or accreditation, so that those seeking or offered advice have some means of checking the credentials of the would-be adviser. One can only hope that the responsible sections of the media will be more discerning about what they are prepared to publish, and perhaps choose their diet and health contributors on the basis of their knowledge and understanding rather than solely on their celebrity status and media appeal. Regulators can be more proactive in the control and advertising of 'dietary supplements'.

The author's perception is thus that there is a tendency for dietary or lifestyle intervention to be advocated before rigorous appraisal has been satisfactorily completed or sometimes before it has even been really started. Dietary supplements, even plant extracts and preparations that have no remarkable culinary use, can be sold freely and with little regulation provided they do not produce obvious acute toxic effects and provided the supplier is careful with the wording of any promotional material. This is probably because of the implicit assumption that simple changes in diet and behaviour and 'natural supplements' are innocuous and that even if they do no good, then neither will they do any harm. Intervention, rather than non-intervention, therefore becomes almost automatically regarded as the safer option – 'If dietary change can't hurt and might help, why not make it?' Hamilton *et al.* (1991). This means that even if dietary and lifestyle advice is offered recklessly or by those with no credible expertise then it is assumed at worst to be just harmless nonsense.

Simple changes in diet or lifestyle can't do any harm?

This assumption that simple dietary and lifestyle changes are innocuous seems logically inconsistent with the clear evidence that diet, lifestyle and environment are major determinants of health and longevity. This not only means that appropriate changes in diet and lifestyle can improve health and longevity (the theoretical justification for health promotion) but it also inevitably means that inappropriate changes can worsen health and longevity. Dietary and lifestyle changes have the potential to do harm as well as great good (see possible examples in the next section). The fact that some 'natural extracts' are potent poisons clearly means that they cannot be assumed to be safe by default.

Even if unjustified intervention does not do direct physiological harm, it may have important social, psychological or economic repercussions. Social and psychological factors have traditionally been the dominant influences on food selection and any ill-considered intervention risks causing anxiety, cultural impoverishment and social and family tensions. It has been suggested that the resources spent on unjustified health education interventions may serve only to induce a morbid preoccupation with death (McCormick and Skrabanek, 1988). Major changes in food selection practices will also have economic repercussions, perhaps disrupting the livelihoods of many people and reducing their quality of life.

Repeated changes of mind and shifts of emphasis by health educators are also liable to undermine their credibility and thereby increase public resistance to future campaigns. We saw earlier in the chapter how dietary advice changed as the nutritional priority changed away from trying to ensure adequacy and towards using diet as a means of preventing chronic disease. These changes in emphasis often reflect changing social conditions and consumption patterns but some may be justifiably perceived as evidence of the inconsistency and thus unreliability of expert advice. The following two examples may serve to illustrate this latter point.

Obesity was once blamed on excessive consumption of high-carbohydrate foods, such as bread and potatoes. These foods would have been strictly regulated in many reducing diets (e.g. Yudkin, 1958). Nutritionists now view bread and potatoes much more positively. They are high in starch and fibre and consumers are recommended to incorporate more of them into their diets to make them bulkier (i.e. to reduce the **energy density**). This bulkier diet may in turn reduce the likelihood of excessive energy intake and obesity. These low-carbohydrate diets became fashionable again a few years ago – their popularity driven by popular diet books and celebrity endorsements.

Scientific support for nutritional guidelines aimed at lowering plasma cholesterol concentrations has now been increasing for almost 50 years. Although this cholesterol-lowering objective may have remained constant, there have been several subtle shifts of opinion on the best dietary means to achieve this goal.

- Reducing dietary cholesterol was once considered an important factor in lowering plasma cholesterol; it is now usually given low priority.
- A wholesale switch from saturated to the **n-6 (ω-6) type of polyunsaturated fatty acids** prevalent in many vegetable oils was once advocated, but very high intakes of these polyunsaturated fats is now considered undesirable.
- Monounsaturated fats were once considered neutral in their effects on plasma cholesterol but are now much more positively regarded. This accounts for the current healthy image of olive oil and rapeseed (canola) oil.
- The **n-3 (ω-3) polyunsaturated fatty acids** have also been viewed much more positively in recent years, especially the long chain acids found predominantly in fish oils.
- The current emphasis of both UK and US recommendations is reduction in total fat intake with a proportionately greater reduction in the saturated fraction of dietary fat.

Table 1.1 Rank orders by different fat-related criteria of some foods. Ranks are from 1 'worst' to 14 'best'*

Food	% Energy as fat	% Energy saturated fat	Cholesterol content	P:S ratio
Liver	11	8	2	8
Lean steak	12	9=	6	4
Cheddar cheese	7	2	7	2=
Butter	1=	1	3	2=
Polyunsaturated margarine	1=	6	10=	13
Low fat spread	1=	4	10=	10
Sunflower oil	1=	11	10=	14
Milk	9=	3	9	1
Human milk	9=	5	8	5
Chicken meat	13	12=	5	7
Avocado	5	12=	10=	9
Peanuts	6	9=	10=	11
Egg	8	7	1	6
Prawns	14	14	4	12

*After Webb (1992a).
P:S ratio, ratio of polyunsaturated to saturated fatty acids.

Attitudes to some individual foods could be strongly affected by such changes of emphasis. This is illustrated in Table 1.1; certain fatty foods come out very differently in a 'worst' to 'best' rank order when cholesterol content, total fat content, saturated fat content or ratio of polyunsaturated to saturated fatty acids (**P:S ratio**) is used as the criterion. Sunflower oil comes out at the 'worst' end of the rankings if total fat content is the criterion but at or near the 'best' end if cholesterol content, P:S ratio or saturated fat content is used. Eggs and liver are worst by the cholesterol criterion but around half way down by all other criteria; prawns are at or near the best rank for all criteria except cholesterol content, they are also relatively rich in the now positively regarded long chain, n-3 (ω-3)polyunsaturated fatty acids.

Promoting ineffective behaviour changes will also dilute the impact of campaigns to promote effective changes. If the ineffective changes are easier to adopt than the effective ones then they may actually inhibit effective change, e.g.:

- taking β-carotene supplements to lessen the damage done by cigarette smoke rather than giving up smoking
- taking an antioxidant supplement rather than eating five portions of fruit and vegetables each day
- taking supplements of milk thistle to protect the liver rather than moderating alcohol consumption.

Does health promotion always promote health? Examples of past interventions that are now viewed less positively

It would seem prudent to regard any dietary or lifestyle changes considered for health promotion as potentially harmful until this possibility has been actively considered and, as far as possible, eliminated. Some of the examples below may serve to demonstrate that this is a real possibility rather than just a theoretical one.

Sleeping position and cot death

In 1991 a campaign called 'Back to Sleep' was launched in the UK that advised parents not to lay babies down to sleep on their fronts, i.e. to avoid the prone sleeping position. This campaign was launched because of a substantial body of evidence which suggested that babies who slept on their fronts were up to eight times more likely to suffer a cot death than those laid on their backs. The following year the rate of cot death was halved. It has continued to decline since then and now is just a quarter of the peak rate seen in the late 1980s. The Foundation for the Study of Infant Deaths (FSID, 2007) estimated that 15 000 babies' lives had been saved by this 'Back to Sleep' campaign. In 1993 when the cot death figures for the first year after the launch of this campaign were released, the Secretary of State for Health was quoted as saying that the sharp drop in cot deaths illustrated the benefits of health education:

> The figures on cot deaths show that behaviour change can work, can save lives.
>
> *Daily Telegraph*, 30 May 1993

This campaign is frequently mentioned in the media and is almost always presented in a very positive light. It is used in health promotion courses as an example of what effective health promotion can achieve.

Figure 1.1 shows the trend in cot death prevalence in England and Wales between 1971 and 2004. The graph shows that rates of cot death in 1971 were very similar to current low rates but rose steeply during the 1970s and 1980s to reach a peak of four times current levels in the late 1980s. What the figure suggests is that we had a 20-year epidemic of extra cot deaths that cost the lives of thousands of British babies and similar epidemics were seen in many other industrialized countries which killed tens of thousands more babies. The key question therefore is what caused these epidemics of extra cot deaths in so many countries?

In the 1950s and 1960s very few British babies (about 4 per cent) slept on their fronts. During the 1970s and much of the 1980s health professionals and childcare writers in the UK advised parents to put babies down to sleep on their front (prone) rather than on their back (supine) as they had traditionally done. This advice to use the front sleeping position first began because premature babies were reported to have less respiratory distress in the prone position and babies with severe gastro-oesophageal reflux were less likely to choke on regurgitated milk. This front sleeping position then became widely used in special care baby units, and very soon it became usual for midwives, doctors, other healthcare professionals and baby care writers to advise all parents to use the front sleeping position. This decreased risk of choking was thought to be important for all babies, and the back sleeping position came to be regarded as unsafe. In a survey of baby care books published before 1991, Webb (1995) found an almost unanimous recommendation to use front sleeping:

> For the first two months or so, the safest way for babies to sleep is on their fronts, head to one side, or else curled up on one side. Then if they are sick, there is no chance that they will choke.
>
> *Pregnancy Book*, Health Education Council, 1984

> A young baby is best not left alone lying on his back. Because he cannot move very much he might choke if he were sick. Lie the baby in the cot on his front with his head to one side, or on his side.
>
> *Reader's Digest*, family medical adviser, 1986

Compare the quote below which comes from the 1993 edition of the Health Education Council's

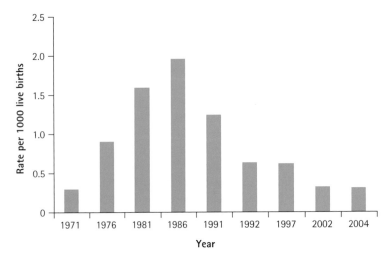

Figure 1.1 *Trends in cot death rates in England and Wales (1971–2004).*

Pregnancy Book with that from the 1984 version above:

> Babies laid to sleep on their tummies are more at risk of cot death than babies laid down to sleep on their backs or sides ... . Only lay your baby down to sleep on his or her front if your doctor advises it.

Given the weight of advice from healthcare professionals and baby care writers to use the 'safer' front sleeping position it is not surprising that most parents had adopted this position by the late 1980s. This epidemic of cot deaths was therefore caused by 'experts' persuading parents to use the front sleeping position. The 15 000 babies saved by 'Back to Sleep' are the babies who might have also died if 'the experts' had continued to promote front sleeping. Looking back one can now see that there was never any real evidence that front sleeping would benefit more than a handful of high-risk babies but 'What harm could a simple change of sleeping position do?'. Further discussion of this example can be found in Webb (1995). As well as illustrating the benefits of effective health promotion this example also provides a quantitative demonstration of the dangers of recklessly promoting untested behaviour changes. This latter point is seldom mentioned in the media and many people including many health promotion academics are unaware of this negative aspect. It is important that we examine, analyse and fully acknowledge such 'mistakes' so that we can learn not to continue to make the same mistakes.

If one is seeking to justify intervention for a whole population then it is not enough merely to show that a specific group will benefit from the proposed change. Intervention with a relatively small sample of 'high-risk' subjects is likely to exaggerate the benefits of intervention for the population as a whole. Such small-scale intervention will also only show up the grossest of harmful effects. It may thus fail to show up harmful effects that could be very important for indiscriminate intervention and which might cancel out or even exceed any benefits of the intervention.

Some cholesterol-lowering interventions

As noted earlier, diets containing very large amounts of polyunsaturated fatty acids were widely advocated as a means of lowering plasma cholesterol concentrations. Short-term experiments had showed very convincingly that switching from high-saturated to high-polyunsaturated-fat diets could reduce serum cholesterol concentrations in young men (e.g. Keys *et al.*, 1959). However, there was no convincing evidence that, in the long term, such a wholesale switch from saturated to polyunsaturated fat produced any increase in life expectancy even in studies using 'high-risk' subjects. Concerns have been raised about the long-term safety of diets that are very high in polyunsaturated fat. Britons have been advised to limit their individual intakes of n-6 (ω-6) polyunsaturated fatty acids to no more than 10 per cent of energy with a population average of 6 per cent (COMA, 1991). Concerns have also been raised about the large rise in the ratio ω-6 to ω-3 polyunsaturated fatty acids that will affect ω-3 metabolism and the production of the long-chain ω-3 fatty acids (see Chapter 11 for details). Some of the early cholesterol-lowering drugs (before the widespread use of statin-type drugs) led to increased total mortality despite lowering blood cholesterol levels. Smith *et al.* (1993) in a review of pre-1993 cholesterol-lowering trials (about two-thirds of which involved cholesterol-lowering drugs) suggested that only those at very high risk of death from coronary heart disease showed any improved mortality risk from taking these drugs and that they should be only prescribed to very-high-risk patients.

Reducing an asymptomatic risk factor, such as plasma cholesterol concentration, cannot, in itself, be taken as evidence of benefit. There must be evidence that it will lead to the predicted decrease in disease risk and also that there will not be an accompanying increase in some other risk.

'The world protein crisis'

In the 1950s and 1960s, protein deficiency was thought to be the most prevalent and serious form of worldwide malnutrition. It was considered likely that 'in many parts of the world the majority of young children suffer some protein malnutrition' (Trowell, 1954). Considerable efforts and resources were committed to alleviating this perceived problem (amounting to many hundreds of millions of pounds/dollars). However, as estimates of human protein requirements were revised downwards, it seemed probable that primary protein deficiency was probably uncommon and thus that the resources committed to alleviating widespread protein deficiency were largely wasted (Webb, 1989). See Chapter 10 for further discussion.

There is no compelling evidence that provision of extra protein was directly harmful. Nevertheless, scarce resources were committed to a non-beneficial measure and other, more real, problems deprived of resources. Research and teaching in nutrition were unreasonably distorted towards protein nutrition for at least a generation. In the USA (National Research Council (NRC), 1989a), and in the current UK dietary standards (COMA, 1991), the possibility that high intakes of protein might even be directly harmful is acknowledged and an upper limit of twice the dietary standard has been advised. There is growing evidence that high intakes of animal protein, in particular, may be associated with increased risk of some cancers.

Resources for research, development, international aid and educational programmes are always finite. If these resources are diverted into unnecessary measures or programmes based on false theories, then inevitably worthwhile projects will be deprived of funding.

Routine iron supplementation during pregnancy

Iron supplements were once routinely and almost universally prescribed for pregnant women in the UK. These supplements were considered necessary because of the perception that the risks of anaemia in pregnancy were very high, a perception that was compounded by the misinterpretation of the normal decline in blood haemoglobin concentration during pregnancy as pathological. This decline is caused by increased plasma volume and occurs despite increased total amounts of circulating haemoglobin. In the UK, routine iron supplements in pregnancy are now thought to be unnecessary. The UK panel on dietary reference values (COMA, 1991) suggested that, for most women, the extra iron demands of pregnancy can be met by utilization of maternal stores and physiological adaptation. Note that in the USA a different view is taken and universal iron supplementation is still recommended for pregnant women. A similar natural decline in haemoglobin concentration caused by 'haemodilution' can also occur in endurance, and this has probably exaggerated the risk of anaemia in athletes, especially female athletes.

Use of β-carotene supplements

There is overwhelming evidence that diets high in fruits and vegetables are associated with reduced risk of several cancers. There have been active campaigns in both the UK and USA to increase fruit and vegetable consumption and to persuade people to consume at least five portions a day.

β-Carotene is a plant pigment found in green and brightly coloured fruits and vegetables. It acts as a source of vitamin A and is the usual source of vitamin A used in so-called ACE vitamin supplements. It is also one of a group of antioxidant substances that might protect the body from oxidative damage by **free radicals** and perhaps lessen the risks of cancer and atherosclerosis (see Chapter 13). This means that diets high in coloured fruits and vegetables also tend to be high in β-carotene and that high carotene intakes are associated with reduced cancer risk. Low blood carotenoid levels are, as one might expect, often associated with increased cancer risk. A number of trials of β-carotene supplementation have paradoxically found higher rates of cancer in the supplemented group than in the non-supplemented controls (e.g. Group, 1994; Omenn et al., 1996). Particularly in heavy smokers and asbestos workers there is evidence that large β-carotene supplements may increase the risk of lung cancer. β-Carotene does not produce symptoms immediately after consumption even when very large amounts are taken (i.e. it has very low acute toxicity). More recently Vivekanathan et al. (2003) in a meta-analysis of published trials recorded a small but marked increase in both cardiovascular and all-cause mortality in those receiving the β-carotene supplements compared with those receiving the placebo. In 1998 an expert panel in the UK counselled against the taking of large doses of β-carotene supplements (COMA, 1998) and in 2003 the Food Standards Agency (FSA, 2003) suggested a safe upper limit of 7 mg/day for supplements of β-carotene. Despite this, supplements containing at least 15 mg/day continue to be advertised and sold; so a dietary supplement that seems to be at best ineffective and probably does net long-term harm is still sold in amounts that are way beyond the advised safe limits. Compare this with the case of a new drug which must convince the regulators that it is both effective and safe before it is approved for sale. Major reviews commissioned by the Agency for Healthcare Research and Quality (AHRQ) in the USA have concluded that neither vitamin E nor vitamin C supplements (the two other so-called ACE vitamins) reduces heart disease, cancer or all-cause mortality, and nor do they reduce non-fatal cardiac events or have any value in the treatment of cancer (Coulter *et al.*, 2003; Shekelle *et al.*, 2003).

The five examples described above were selected to try to illustrate that once very popular dietary or lifestyle interventions may in later years become regarded as unnecessary or perhaps even harmful. The eventual outcome of each debate will not alter their demonstration of how scientific opinion about the value and safety of such interventions fluctuates.

If a holistic view is taken then it is likely that any intervention that produces no benefits will have some detrimental effects even though this may not always involve direct physiological harm. Majority support among scientists and health professionals for intervention based on a particular theory is no guarantee that it will continue to be regarded as useful or even safe.

Those involved in health promotion and nutrition education need to be constructively critical of current fashions. They need to be receptive to criticism of current wisdom and objective in their evaluation of such criticism. They need to be cautious about advocating mass intervention, especially if there is no convincing, direct evidence of overall long-term benefit or where evidence of benefit is restricted to a relatively small 'high-risk' group. Any non-beneficial intervention should be regarded as almost inevitably detrimental in some way.

Key points

- Average life expectancy in Britain and the USA increased by more than 50 per cent during the twentieth century and this has led to a large increase in the proportion of elderly people.

- This increased life expectancy means that most deaths and much of the chronic illness and disability are now due to the chronic diseases of industrialization that affect mainly middle-aged and elderly people, i.e. cardiovascular disease, cancer, diabetes, osteoporosis.

- Reducing mortality and morbidity from these chronic diseases is now seen as the priority for nutrition education and health promotion in the industrialized nations.

- The new dietary recommendations to achieve this objective are in some ways almost the opposite of those of the 1930s, e.g. to moderate consumption of meat, eggs and dairy produce but to increase consumption of starchy foods, fruits and vegetables.

- A risk factor is some parameter that partially predicts one's risk of developing a disease and that is causally linked to the onset of the disease.

- Dietary factors can be direct risk factors or they can influence the level of others such as plasma cholesterol, blood pressure or glucose tolerance.

- Much modern health promotion is focused on identifying and reducing these risk factors and the sheer number of such risk factors can cause confusion and increase the possibility of conflicting advice.

- Recommendations to alter diet and lifestyle are sometimes not fully underpinned by adequate supporting evidence. There seems to be an implicit but illogical assumption that simple changes in diet and lifestyle have the potential to do good but not harm.

- There are examples of dietary or lifestyle changes based on past health promotion that seem to have done net harm:
  - past recommendations to put babies to sleep in the prone position seem to have increased the risk of cot death
  - β-carotene supplements have actually increased the rate of deaths in several controlled trials.

- Even where a non-beneficial dietary or lifestyle change does no direct physiological harm, it may have less obvious adverse consequences, e.g. the resources wasted in trying to solve the illusory crisis in world protein supplies.

- Promoting ineffective behaviour change will deflect attention away from more effective measures especially where they offer an easy alternative to making effective changes, e.g. taking an antioxidant pill rather than eating more fruit and vegetables.

- At the very least, recommendations that are changed or withdrawn will undermine confidence in nutrition education and increase resistance to future advice.

- It is particularly illogical to assume that 'natural supplements' are inevitably safe; many potent poisons are natural extracts and even some essential nutrients are very toxic in high doses.

IS INTERVENTION TO INDUCE DIETARY CHANGE JUSTIFIED? (AFTER WEBB, 1992A)

Evidence linking diet and disease seldom materializes in complete and unequivocal form overnight. More usually, it accumulates gradually over a period of years with a high probability that some of the evidence will be conflicting. The problem of deciding when evidence is sufficient to warrant issuing advice or some other intervention is thus one that will frequently need to be faced. If action is initiated too soon then there is a risk of costly and potentially harmful errors. If action is too slow then the potential benefits of change may be unduly delayed.

There is likely to be intense pressure to take action or to issue guidelines in the light of the latest highly publicized research findings. Box 1.2 lists a set of criteria that might be used to decide whether any particular intervention is justified by available knowledge.

Intervention that precedes satisfactory consideration of the likely risks and benefits is experimentation and not health promotion.

Such criteria are probably not, in themselves, controversial; it is in deciding when these criteria have been satisfactorily fulfilled or even whether they have been properly considered that the controversy arises.

Judging whether the intervention criteria have been fulfilled

Many practical questions such as those listed below need to be satisfactorily answered before any apparent association between a dietary variable and a disease or risk factor is translated into practical health promotion advice.

- Is the reported association likely to be genuine?
- Is the association likely to represent cause and effect?
- What change in dietary composition is realistically achievable and what magnitude of benefit is this predicted to produce?
- Is this predicted benefit sufficient to warrant intervention – at the population level – at the individual level?
- Are there any foreseeable risks from the proposed compositional change for any group within the target population?
- Are there any foreseeable non-nutritional adverse consequences of these changes?
- What changes in other nutrient intakes are likely to occur as a result of the proposed advice?
- Are there any foreseeable risks from these consequential changes?
- How can the desired compositional change be brought about?

Box 1.2   Criteria for deciding whether an intervention is justified

- Have clear and realistic dietary objectives been set and all foreseeable aspects of their likely impact considered?
- Is there strong evidence that a large proportion of the population or target group will gain significant benefits from the proposed intervention?
- Has there been active and adequate consideration of whether the promoted action, or any consequential change, may have adverse effects in a significant number of people?
- Have the evaluations of risk and benefit been made holistically? A reduction in a disease risk marker, or even reduced incidence of a particular disease, are not ends in themselves; the ultimate criterion of success must be an increase in life expectancy or a net improvement in quality of life. Likewise the evaluation of risks should not be confined to possible direct physiological harm but should also include, for example, economic, psychological or social repercussions. It should also include the possibly harmful effects of any consequential changes and consider the damage ineffective intervention might have on the future credibility of health educators.
- Has the possibility of targeting intervention to likely gainers been fully explored to maximize the benefits to risks ratio?
- Has consideration been given to how the desired change can be implemented with the minimum intrusion into the chosen lifestyle and cuisine of the target group?

Is the association genuine?

It is quite possible that an apparent association between diet and a disease may have arisen because of bias in the study or simply by chance. There is often a range of papers reporting conflicting findings; these need to be evaluated and weighted rather than the latest or the majority view being mechanically accepted. It is quite possible that a common logical flaw, incorrect assumption or methodological error is present in all of the papers supporting one side of an argument.

Easterbrook *et al.* (1992) reported that, in clinical research, positive results are more likely to be published than negative ones. This not only means that the literature may give an unbalanced view of total research findings, but also encourages authors to highlight positive findings. In another analysis Ravnskov (1992) reported that when citation rates were determined for papers dealing with cholesterol-lowering trials, then those with positive outcomes (i.e. suggesting a beneficial effect on coronary heart disease) were cited six times more frequently than those with negative outcomes. Thus at the author, peer review, editorial selection and citation level there may be bias towards positive over negative findings.

Statistical significance at, or below, the 5 per cent level (i.e. $P < 0.05$) is, by convention, taken as the point at which a scientist can claim that a correlation or a difference between two means is 'statistically significant'. It means that there is less than a 1 in 20 likelihood that the correlation or difference between the means has arisen simply by chance. This statistical significance may simply reflect flaws or bias in the design of the study, in the allocation of subjects or in the measurement of variables. With numerous investigators all correlating numerous dietary variables with health indicators it is inevitable that some statistically significant associations will arise simply by chance. Significance at the 5 per cent level is not proof of the underlying theory, merely an indication that any difference or association is unlikely to be due to pure chance. This should be borne in mind when evaluating isolated reports of improbable sounding associations. Given the perceived onus on authors to highlight positive results, they may be tempted to highlight the one barely significant correlation in a whole battery of otherwise insignificant tests.

Dietary guidelines often stem from reviews of the scientific literature or the conclusions of expert committees, but we have already seen that even apparent consensus among experts does not guarantee the long-term future of a particular position or theory. There was once an almost unanimous belief in a crisis of world protein supply but few would support this view today. Scientists are trained to make objective judgements based solely on scientific evidence but they are also fallible human beings whose judgements may, perhaps unwittingly, be affected by prejudice, political or peer pressure and self-interest. Reviewers and committee members will often be selected because of their active involvement and expertise in a particular field of study. This may sometimes hamper their objectivity especially when they are required to evaluate material that may undermine or support their own work and reputation, or to evaluate material that might even jeopardize their own career or research funding. McLaren (1974) tried to identify some of the reasons for the now discredited concept of a world protein crisis or protein gap and for its persistence (see Chapter 10). He suggested that even in 1966, when this theory was still at its height, many scientists had privately expressed sympathy with his opposition to the theory and some of the consequential measures designed to alleviate the perceived crisis. He also claims that they were unwilling to publicly support him for fear of having their research funding withdrawn. He even suggests that critical discussion of the issues was suppressed.

I have made a conscious decision to include in this book a substantial section on nutrition research methods even though many readers may not be aiming for research careers in nutrition. Those readers who are primarily interested in the practice of promoting health and healthy eating and are unlikely to participate in research projects may be tempted to disregard much of this section as superfluous to their needs. I think that this would be a narrow and short-sighted decision. Some general appreciation of the research methodology, especially the strengths, limitations and weaknesses of the various methods, is essential for any critical reading and evaluation of the literature. Anyone who wishes to keep up to date with the literature and be able to make quality judgements about conflicting evidence, or controversial new reports, will need some basic understanding of the methodology.

Is the association causal?

Epidemiological methods produce evidence of associations between diseases and suggested causes but even a strong association does not necessarily mean that there is a cause and effect relationship. It is quite probable that the statistical link between a risk marker and a disease may have arisen because both are associated with a third, **confounding variable**. For example, even though alcohol may not directly contribute to causing lung cancer, a statistical association between alcohol consumption and lung cancer might arise if heavy drinkers also tend to be heavy smokers. Earlier in this chapter it was noted that high fruit and vegetable consumption is associated with reduced cancer risk. This also means that high β-carotene intake is likely to be associated with lowered cancer risk but does not necessarily mean that high β-carotene intake prevents cancer. There are several other explanations for this finding such as:

- people who eat lots of fruits and vegetables may have other lifestyle characteristics that help to reduce their cancer risk, e.g. different smoking, drinking and exercise habits
- high fruit and vegetable consumption may be a marker for a diet that is healthier in other respects, e.g. lower in fat
- even if high fruit and vegetables are directly protecting against cancer then it may be some component(s) other than β-carotene that is/are exerting the protective effect.

As we saw earlier, several controlled trials have found that β-carotene supplements appear to increase mortality compared with placebos.

Epidemiologists almost always try to correct their results for the effects of confounding variables when aiming to establish a causal link between diet and disease. There is, however, no statistical magic wand that unerringly and accurately corrects for all confounding variables; it is a matter of judgement what the likely confounders are and the process of correction itself may be imprecise, particularly if there is imprecise or limited measurement of the confounding variable (Leon, 1993). Take the examples of smoking and exercise as possible confounding variables in epidemiological studies of relationship between diet and heart disease. Apparently reliable information on smoking habits is usually obtained in such studies and one has confidence that a reasonable correction of the results for the effects of smoking has been made. On the other hand, it is notoriously difficult to make accurate assessment of activity level and so in many of these studies there is little or no attempt to correct for the effects of variation in activity levels. This problem of confounding variables is discussed more fully in Chapter 3 along with some tests that may be applied to help decide whether any particular association is causal.

In some cases it may be that the disease itself leads to the measured changes in diet or behaviour, i.e. an effect and cause relationship. It is particularly important to consider this possibility when one is comparing the current behaviour of those who have or may have the disease with those who do not. Obese people are less active than lean people, is this a cause or an effect of their obesity? A low serum vitamin A concentration may be associated with an increased risk of developing symptomatic cancer within a few years but is this a cause of the cancer or an early symptom of it?

Dietary and lifestyle changes tend not to occur in isolation, often many changes occur simultaneously. Increasing affluence and industrialization tends to bring with it numerous changes in diet and lifestyle as well as major changes in the causes of death and disease. This means that an association between one of the 'diseases of industrialization' and one of the wealth-related environmental variables needs to be treated with extreme caution until there is substantial evidence to support this association being causal.

Realistically achievable change – magnitude of benefit?

If a cause and effect relationship is established between a dietary factor and a disease then one should be able to predict the magnitude of benefit that is likely to result from a given change in diet. For example, if there is a linear relationship between the average blood pressure of adult populations and their average daily salt consumption then one can attempt to predict the reduction in average blood pressure that would result from a reduction average salt consumption (e.g. Law *et al.*, 1991a). Then, making certain assumptions, one can go on to predict by how much the incidence of hypertension will fall and thence the beneficial effect on mortality from the hypertension-related diseases (see Chapter 14 for further discussion of this example). One must then decide what degree of change is realistically achievable and what the benefits of change on this scale are likely to be. It is unhelpful to predict the huge health gains that might result from a degree of change that is impractical or unrealistic. A reduction in average UK daily salt consumption from around 10 g to less than 1 g as seen in some populations such as the Yanomamo Indians of Brazil might eradicate hypertension and produce major reductions in mortality from hypertension-related diseases. There is, however, no chance that a change of this magnitude can be achieved.

In a major review of the effects of garlic on the cardiovascular system and cancer, commissioned by the Agency for Healthcare Research and Quality, Mulrow *et al.* (2000) found no evidence of substantial benefit from taking garlic supplements. They found 37 trials that had investigated the effects of garlic supplements on plasma cholesterol. These trials consistently found a small but statistically significant reduction in the garlic group at 1 month and 3 months but those that continued to 6 months found no effect. What these findings suggest is that garlic supplements probably have a small and transient effect on this risk factor but that this would have no clinical benefit to those taking the supplements. The effect is statistically significant but too small to have any real clinical importance, and even this small effect is probably not sustained beyond the first few months of taking the supplement.

At what level is intervention justified?

Even when there is clear evidence of a causal association between a dietary factor and a disease then it may still be difficult to decide whether this justifies intervention at the population level. The extreme scenarios are:

- if a minor dietary change could produce a major reduction in the risk of a common fatal disease then the case for intervention would appear strong
- if a major dietary change were only predicted to marginally reduce the risk of a relatively uncommon disease then clearly population level intervention would not be justified.

In between these extremes, the significance or 'cost' of the proposed change will need to be balanced against the predicted reduction in population risk. Even where likely benefit cannot justify intervention

at the population level, if those who are particularly 'at risk' or who are particularly susceptible to the causal factor can be identified then this may justify intervention for those high-risk groups. There are, therefore, essentially two strategies to choose from when designing a health promotion campaign aimed at risk reduction.

- *The population approach.* Advice is directed at the whole population, or large sections of it, with the aim of reducing average population exposure to the risk.
- *The individual approach.* Efforts are made to identify those most at risk from the risk factor and intervention is targeted specifically at these 'high-risk' individuals.

In a programme aimed at lowering plasma cholesterol to reduce the risk of coronary heart disease (CHD), one could choose either of the following options.

- *The population approach.* Direct the message at the whole adult population; if successful this would be expected to lower average plasma cholesterol concentrations and shift the whole population distribution of plasma cholesterol concentrations downwards.
- *The individual approach.* One could seek to identify those with the highest cholesterol concentrations and most 'at risk' from CHD and target the advice specifically at these 'high-risk' individuals.

Much health promotion/nutrition education in the UK has tended to use the population approach. If one is seeking to make major impact on population mortality/morbidity from a disease then the population approach appears to offer the greatest probability of success. Consider the example of the relationship between plasma cholesterol concentration and CHD. It is generally accepted that at least for young and middle-aged men, high plasma cholesterol concentrations predict an increased risk of premature death from CHD. For example, Figure 1.2 shows that for one population of American men, mortality risk for CHD approximately doubled as the plasma cholesterol concentration doubled. It is assumed that lowering of serum cholesterol will result in a corresponding reduction in CHD risk. Figure 1.3 shows that there were relatively few men in this population with very high plasma cholesterol levels (say over 7.8 mmol/L) and so restricting

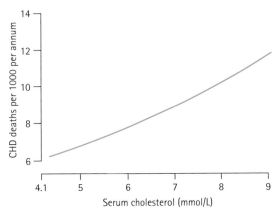

Figure 1.2 *The relationship between serum cholesterol concentration and subsequent death rate from coronary heart disease in a sample of American men. Source: Webb (1992a). After NACNE (1983).*

cholesterol-lowering efforts to these high-risk subjects can only have limited impact. Even a substantial reduction of risk in this small group will do little to affect population mortality from CHD. The majority of the population in Figures 1.2 and 1.3 (and the current population of the UK) have plasma cholesterol concentrations that are regarded as slightly or moderately elevated (say 5.2–7.8 mmol/L). Even a small reduction in individual risks for this very large group will have a marked effect on total population mortality. Some of the advantages and disadvantages of these two approaches are (after Webb and Copeman, 1996) listed below.

- If everyone is advised to change then the promoted behaviour may become the norm and may create conditions that make it easier for any

individual to change. For example, if everyone is urged to reduce their fat and saturated fat intake, then this increases the incentive for the food industry to develop and market products that are low in fat and/or saturated fat, such as: low-fat spreads; margarine and oils that are low in saturated fat; lower fat milks; and reduced fat processed foods. The ready availability of such foods makes it easier to adopt a low-fat diet and low-fat choices may come to be perceived as the norm.

- The population approach removes the need to identify the 'high-risk' subjects and mark them out as 'victims' of a particular condition. The individual approach may require a mass screening programme, e.g. to identify those above some arbitrary cut-off point for plasma cholesterol; if screening is not universal then some 'high-risk' individuals may not be identified. Once identified, 'high-risk' individuals would probably feel threatened by their 'high-risk' classification and change might be more difficult for them to implement because the changes in product availability and social norms discussed above would be unlikely to occur.
- The population approach requires mass change and, for many, that change will offer only a small reduction in individual risk and thus the motivation to change may be low.
- If mass change is induced, then there is increased likelihood that some currently 'low-risk' individuals may be harmed by the change, it may create norms of behaviour and perhaps even changes in the range and pricing of foods that are not universally beneficial. We saw earlier that increased use of the front sleeping position for babies in

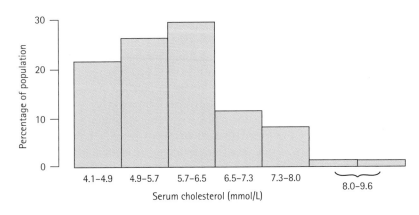

Figure 1.3 *Distribution of serum cholesterol concentrations in the sample of men in Figure 1.2. Source: Webb (1992a). After NACNE (1983).*

the 1970s and 1980s may have helped some premature babies and some babies with particular conditions but for the majority it increased the risk of cot death.

- The population approach may create an unhealthy preoccupation with death and disease in the whole population (McCormick and Skrabanek, 1988), e.g. even people at very low risk of CHD may be made extremely fearful of this condition. This would be particularly true if health promotion focused on the negative aspects of not accepting the message, i.e. if it used fear of death and disease and the threat of social isolation as the levers for effecting behaviour change.
- The population approach may lead to people being blamed for their condition and perhaps used by doctors and politicians to justify the withholding of expensive treatments: 'It is your fault that you have heart disease/cancer because you smoke/eat badly/do not take enough exercise.'

The debate about whether to fortify bread with folic acid is a good example of a difficult choice between whether to adopt a population or an individual approach. Clear evidence became available in the early 1990s that folic acid supplements given before conception and in the early weeks of pregnancy reduced the incidence of **neural tube defects** in babies (see Chapter 15 for details and references). Since that time, women in the UK and elsewhere have been advised to take supplements of 400 µg/day of folic acid when planning to become pregnant and in early pregnancy. The advice in the UK at the end of 2006 was that all women of childbearing age who might become pregnant should take this supplement because most pregnancies are not planned and the supplements are only effective at the start of the pregnancy. Almost immediately after confirmation of the benefits of folic acid, a campaign to make the fortification of bread with folic acid mandatory started to gain momentum in the UK. In the first edition of this book, written in 1993/4, I was very cautious about this mandatory fortification and suggested that if this happened there should be a number of conditions and safeguards and careful monitoring of the impact. I was already convinced that folic acid would benefit a small group of women whose babies were at risk of being born with a neural tube defect but not wholly convinced that this justified the whole population

being given supplemental folic acid. There were concerns that extra folic acid might:

- mask the anaemia caused by vitamin B_{12} deficiency in some older people and thus lead to increased risk of the neurological complications of B_{12} deficiency
- that it might interfere with actions of some drugs that work by affecting folate metabolism
- have other unexpected untoward effects.

By the time the second edition was written in 2001, concerns about the safety of modest supplemental doses had eased and there was some evidence that it might have wider benefits in reducing the risk of heart disease and my reservations about mandatory fortification were removed. Several countries have now introduced widespread fortification of bread/flour and have seen the expected drop in incidence of neural tube defects with no apparent adverse consequences. However in countries such as the UK, the rate has remained unaltered since 1991; despite a sustained campaign to increase supplement use in premenopausal women there has been no measurable reduction in the prevalence of neural tube defects (Botto *et al.*, 2005). In this edition, I am fully supporting folic acid fortification; it may reduce the risk of other congenital malformations such as cleft palate and cleft lip, and the evidence of wider benefits for the population at large has also strengthened. It seems probable that mandatory fortification will be introduced in the UK during the lifetime of this edition.

Harmful effects of intervention?

First do no harm.

Health promotion should increase life expectancy and reduce ill health. It is illogical to assume that dietary or lifestyle changes are an inevitable 'one way bet' and can only be beneficial. The possibility of harmful effects must be actively considered and tested. Several possible examples of simple dietary or lifestyle interventions having unexpected harmful effects have been discussed earlier in the chapter. Harmful social, psychological, economic or cultural repercussions are likely even where no direct physiological harm results from unjustified intervention. Non-beneficial intervention will, at the very least, ultimately undermine the credibility of future programmes.

What are the secondary consequences of change?

Dietary changes almost never occur in isolation. Changing the diet to produce an intended change will almost inevitably affect the intake of other nutrients. When dietary changes are to be advocated then the likely impact of the intended change on the total diet should be considered. If reduced intake of a particular food or nutrient is advised then how are the intakes of other nutrients likely to be affected and what is likely to replace the missing food? If people are advised to increase their intake of particular foods then what will they displace from the existing diet?

For example, if food manufacturers are persuaded to use less salt in processing then what effect will this have on shelf-life and therefore on cost and availability of foods? Will it compromise the microbiological safety of some foods? Or will it lead to increased reliance on other preservatives whose long-term safety may also be questioned? In Chapter 9 there is a brief discussion of the likely effects of using artificial sweeteners. Do they reduce total energy intake by reducing sugar consumption or is the lost sugar energy simply replaced by other foods leading to increases in total fat consumption?

effect relationship. It may arise because both the disease risk and dietary factor are linked to other confounding variables.

- Health promotion intervention may be directed at the whole population with the aim of inducing mass change (the population approach) or it may be targeted at those individuals regarded as at higher risk of the particular disease (the individual approach).

- Even if an intervention produces a statistically significant change in a risk factor in short-term trials, this change may be not be clinically significant and/or may only be transitory.

- The population approach may create a climate and conditions that facilitate individual change. It removes the need to identify and mark out those at high risk of the disease.

- On the other hand, mass change may only offer many people a small likelihood of benefit and it increases the probability that some will be harmed by the change. This approach may frighten even those who are at low risk of the disease, and it may foster an unhealthy preoccupation with death and disease.

- Any recommended dietary change will result in other consequential changes in diet composition that need to be considered before mass change is advocated.

Key points

- Dietary change should only be recommended if there is clear evidence that it will yield net holistic benefit.

- The possibility that change may have adverse direct or indirect effects should be considered and tested.

- Premature action based on insufficient evidence runs the risk of doing net harm but undue delay means that any benefits of the intervention will also be delayed.

- Some apparent links between diet and disease may arise because of statistical freaks or reflect bias in the study design.

- Trying to obtain a consensus view from published reports will be hampered because negative results are less likely to be published and cited than studies with positive outcomes.

- Association between diet and disease does not necessarily mean that there is a cause and

EFFECTING DIETARY CHANGE

It is easy to devise diets or plan menus that meet any particular set of compositional criteria but much more difficult to make them acceptable to the client. For example, it is easy to produce nutritionally adequate reducing diets but the long-term dietary treatment of obesity is notoriously unsuccessful. Diets or dietary recommendations that are sympathetic to the beliefs, preferences and usual selection practices of the recipients will probably fare better than those that ignore the non-nutritional influences on food selection or try to impose the prejudices and preferences of the adviser.

Food has a host of cultural, psychological and social functions in addition to its biological function. It is these non-nutritional uses that have traditionally been the dominant influences on our food selection. If we lose sight of these functions in the perhaps fruitless pursuit of the optimal chemical diet, then any technical improvements in our nutrition may be outweighed, or at least reduced, by damage to the general emotional health of the population. Miserable, anxious people will probably suffer more illnesses and die younger than happy contented people.

Some of these non-nutritional influences on food selection are discussed in Chapter 2. If health promoters want to effect changes in eating behaviour, they must have some appreciation of the determinants of food selection practices. They can then offer practical advice that will bring about any desired changes in diet in ways that are compatible with the overall cultural milieu of the target group. Nutrition educators should try to effect compositional changes in the desired direction with the least interference in current cultural practices, i.e. a cultural conservationist approach. This is the most ethical approach as well as the most likely to succeed.

Some factors influencing the likelihood of dietary change

Fieldhouse (1998) listed certain parameters that will particularly influence the likelihood of dietary change occurring.

- *The advantage of change and the observability of that advantage.* If a relatively minor dietary change results in immediate and apparent benefits then this increases the likelihood of permanent adoption. However, if the benefits of change are not immediately apparent or speculative or if the change itself is seen as having a major disadvantages (e.g. restricting favoured foods, increased cost or increased preparation time) then this will decrease the chances of its adoption.
- *Its compatibility with existing beliefs, cultural values and culinary style.* Advice that is compatible with existing beliefs and behaviour is more likely to be implemented than that which is contrary to these beliefs and behaviours (e.g. advising a pious person to break the dietary rules of their religion or advising a committed vegetarian to eat meat has a low probability of success).
- *Its complexity.* The more difficult it is to implement or understand any change, the less chance there is that it will be made. Advice aimed at lowering plasma cholesterol is often perceived as requiring major reductions in the consumption of meat and dairy produce. These high prestige and high flavour foods are central to the culinary practices and the food ideology of many Western consumers. Such changes may therefore be seen as requiring a complete re-structuring of the diet. Promoting simple modifications of existing practices that involve relatively little 'cost' for the consumer may produce more real change than advocating much more ambitious and drastic changes that will be implemented by relatively few people. Simple suggestions such as: buy leaner cuts of meat; trim off visible fat; grill (broil) rather than fry; use lower fat milk; use a spreading fat that is lower in saturated fat.

- *Its trialability.* If advice is easy to try out on a 'one-off' basis then people are more likely to try it out than if it requires more commitment such as the learning of a new preparation method or buying new catering equipment. Getting people to try out a dietary change is the first step towards adoption of the change. Switching from butter to margarine and cooking with vegetable oil rather than animal fats seem like readily trialable changes. Fluoridation of water supplies is an example of a change that is not readily trialable. If a change requires a period of adjustment this would reduce its trialability. People may, for example, get used to food cooked without added salt but to adjust to the change they may need an extended trial period. Increasing fibre intake by switching from white to wholemeal bread may seem eminently trialable. However, sudden increases in fibre intake may produce transient diarrhoea, flatulence and abdominal discomfort and it may require some time to adapt to the higher fibre intake.

Advice to make a dietary change that is aimed at curing a deficiency disease has a good chance of being accepted. The major advantages of such a change are usually readily apparent within a short period of time and can often be observed in others who have already done it. The disadvantages of changing may be small, e.g. incorporation of a nutrient-rich or fortified food into the diet or even the consumption of a nutrient supplement. This sort of dietary modification is also easy to understand and implement. It can usually be tried out without any long-term commitment, and the rapid and obvious benefits encourage people to continue with the change in diet.

Similarly, when a therapeutic diet gives rapid symptomatic relief then this will also act as powerful, positive reinforcement and encourage clients to stick with the diet and perhaps even to stick to it more rigorously, e.g. if adoption of a low-protein diet gives symptomatic relief to patients with chronic renal failure. This may well encourage them to persevere with this diet despite its relative complexity and restrictiveness and irrespective of any possible long-term benefits on the course of the disease (see Chapter 16 for more details). Increased fibre and water intakes will often relieve constipation or give symptomatic relief from other minor bowel disorders (e.g. diverticulosis or haemorrhoids). These benefits will act as a positive reinforcement for people with these conditions.

It may be much more difficult to persuade healthy people to make changes that are aimed at reducing the long-term risk of chronic disease. The benefits of many of the health-promoting dietary changes currently recommended by expert committees are often difficult to demonstrate at the individual level and in the short term. The benefits are often only expected to accrue some time after introduction of the change; they are often perceived as speculative with some expert opinion arguing against even the long-term benefits of change. These measures are designed to produce significant long-term reductions in the population risk of death and disease and the individual may only be offered a relatively small reduction in his or her individual risk of suffering from some disease at some seemingly distant date. A good part of any individual's risk of developing or dying of a particular disease is inherited. This means that anecdotal observations may often confound the predictions of the experts; there will be examples of 'healthy eaters' who nevertheless develop diet-related diseases and those who ignore dietary guidelines but remain healthy well into old age. This anecdotal tendency may be compounded by the tendency of people to adopt practices they perceive as healthful when they start to become concerned about their health, i.e. adoption of a healthy diet may apparently immediately precede the onset of overt symptoms and so may even seem causative.

The dietary changes required to meet current nutrition education guidelines may be perceived as having immediate and major disadvantages, i.e. the restriction of highly palatable sugary, salty and fatty foods and their partial replacement with bland, starchy and fibre-rich foods. Increasing fear and guilt about 'inappropriate' eating behaviours may be one way of altering the balance of advantage towards implementing change. Thus a first heart attack can persuade people to adopt strict cholesterol-lowering diets and the onset of serious lung disease may persuade people to give up smoking. However, health promotion that tries to harness such fear of death and disease as a means of inducing dietary/lifestyle change in healthy people serves to focus people's attention on death and disease. It may have some negative impact on quality of life. If such 'health promotion' succeeds in generating fear and guilt without changing behaviour, or results in changes that are ultimately proved not to be beneficial, then its impact will be totally negative. What is the effect of anti-smoking campaigns using graphic images and interviews of those dying from smoking-related disease on people who continue to smoke and on their children or others who care about them? Similarly, increased feedback by regular monitoring of risk factors such as plasma cholesterol may improve compliance but McCormick and Skrabanek (1988) argue that such focusing on symptomless risk markers may serve only to induce an unjustified and morbid preoccupation with death. Health and wellness promotion is a very positive sounding objective, death delaying has a much more negative ring to it; nutrition education must be presented and implemented in ways that emphasize the former objectives rather than unnecessarily increasing fear of, and preoccupation with, death and disease.

Barriers to successful health promotion

Figure 1.4 summarizes some of the stages in the process of a nutrition education or health promotion message leading to changes in behaviour that benefit health. There are potential barriers or blockages to successful health promotion at each of these stages and these blockage points on Figure 1.4 are discussed below.

Blockage point 1

The receiver fails to see or hear the message. An inappropriate channel may have been chosen for the message. The channel is the vehicle for transmitting the message, e.g. radio, television, newspaper or poster advertisements, leaflets provided at a doctor's surgery or community centre, speakers

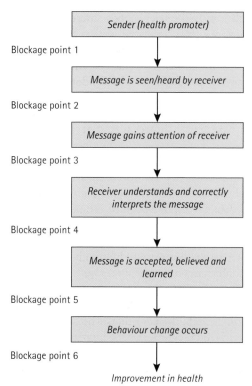

Figure 1.4 *Steps in the process by which a health promotion message leads to beneficial change in behaviour and potential barriers to change (modified from Webb and Copeman, 1996)*

addressing groups or one-to-one counselling. Those initiating the health promotion campaign should consider what channel is most likely to reach the target group and to influence their behaviour. They would also have to consider what will be the most cost-effective vehicle for transmitting the message to the target group. One would choose different television or radio slots and different newspapers and periodicals for targeting teenagers than if elderly people were the primary target group. Some simple market research may need to be done to ensure that the message will reach the receiver.

Blockage point 2

The message may not gain the attention of the target group. A poster or television advert may not attract or interest the target group – images of teenage pop stars are more likely to interest teenagers than elderly people. Programmes, posters, oral presentations and leaflets must be attractive and interesting; they must be appropriate for the target group.

Blockage point 3

The message may not be understood by the receiver. This may result in a blockage at this stage or if the message is misinterpreted it may result in an inappropriate behaviour change. For example, a message to increase dietary fibre may result in an inappropriate behaviour change if the nature and sources of dietary fibre are misunderstood. The health promoter must ensure that their message is clear, correct, believable and realistic. They must consider the standards of education and literacy of the target group and make special provision for groups where English is not their first language. If illiteracy is common then a written message is of little value. Ideally, any promotional material should be piloted to identify potential problems with terminology, understanding or interpretation.

Blockage point 4

The message may not be believed or, if it is too complex and not reinforced, then it may be forgotten. The source may be seen as biased or may lack credibility with the receiver. An elderly male speaker perceived as conservative might lack credibility with an audience of streetwise teenage girls. Promotional leaflets sponsored by a commercial company and bearing the company logo may be viewed as biased. The message may be inconsistent with existing scientific beliefs, e.g. advice to increase starchy foods may be inconsistent with the belief that they are fattening. It may be inconsistent with traditional cultural beliefs about diet such as the need of Chinese people to balance foods classified as **hot and cold** in their cultural food classification system (see Chapter 2 for details of this example).

Blockage point 5

Behaviour change does not occur despite the message being received and understood. The required change of behaviour may be difficult or impossible for the receiver to implement. Dietary changes that increase the cost of the diet may be beyond the economic means of some groups. Some groups who are largely reliant on others to provide their food may find it impossible to implement the change, e.g. children who rely on their parents to provide food or those living in residential homes for the elderly or other institutions.

Blockage point 6

Behaviour change occurs but does not result in improved health. The message may be wrong or inappropriately targeted (see earlier in the chapter) or it may be misunderstood and result in an inappropriate behaviour change (see blockage point 3). Those designing nutrition education or other health promotion campaigns must:

- ensure that *the source* of the message will be seen by the receivers as credible and reliable
- make sure that *the message* itself is clear, correct, realistic and appropriately targeted
- ensure that *the channel(s)* chosen for disseminating the message are likely to reach the target group, attract their attention and be likely to influence their behaviour
- consider the particular characteristics of *the receivers* or target group before they can design an appropriate strategy. What is their level of education and literacy? What is their first language? What are their recreational interests, cultural beliefs and media habits?

The BASNEF model (Figure 1.5)

- B – beliefs
- A – attitudes
- SN – subjective norm
- EF – enabling factors

An individual's beliefs about diet and health will clearly influence their judgement about whether a suggested change is beneficial. If one is seeking to persuade someone to modify their behaviour to reduce the risk of a particular disease, then first they must believe that they are susceptible to the disease, second that the consequences are serious, and finally that it can be prevented (Becker, 1984). Let us take heart disease as a specific example. To make a judgement to modify their behaviour to avoid heart disease, a person must believe that:

- they are at risk from heart disease (i.e. susceptible)
- heart disease can kill or disable (the consequences are serious)
- if they change their diet and behaviour (e.g. stop smoking), the risk is reduced (prevention is possible).

It is not only the beliefs of the person themselves that will influence their judgements but they will also be influenced by the beliefs of their family, friends, colleagues, teachers, religious leaders, health workers, etc. Ajzen and Fishbein (1980) described these influences from the beliefs and attitudes of others as the perceived social pressure or the **subjective norm**. Health promotion has succeeded in changing several norms of behaviour (see examples below).

Forty years ago, butter would have been regarded by most UK consumers as the most natural, palatable spreading fat and margarine a cheap and inferior substitute. Those who could afford it would usually have chosen butter and serving margarine to guests may well have been regarded as showing low esteem for them or meanness. Butter is now regarded as the least healthy of the spreading fats; it is seen as high in saturated fat. The majority of UK consumers now choose either soft margarine or a low-fat spread as their everyday spreading fat and often use them for social occasions as well.

In the 1950s, smoking was the norm in most sectors of British society and the non-smoker was often the odd one out. Now the opposite is often true, smokers are in a minority in many sectors of society, and in the UK and several other countries, smoking is no longer allowed in public places or considered acceptable in many social situations. Smokers are often made to feel ostracized because of their habit.

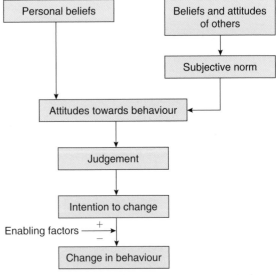

Figure 1.5 *A scheme to illustrate how beliefs, attitudes, the subjective norm and enabling factors (BASNEF) interact to determine whether health promotion recommendations result in actual behaviour change. After Hubley (1993).*

Changing the subjective norm can encourage others to follow the change and may even make it easier for people to adopt the promoted behaviour, e.g. the greater range, availability and acceptance of alternative spreading fats to butter. There are sound health reasons for trying to reduce the number of people who are overweight and obese. Nevertheless creating a climate (subjective norm) where fat is regarded as bad and lean as good may not be a helpful health promotion approach. Most people already desperately want to become or remain lean. By focusing on body weight *per se* health promoters may simply increase the unhappiness and discrimination already experienced by obese people. It may also encourage some normal or even underweight young women to try to become even leaner and adopt unhealthy dietary lifestyle practices to achieve this. Health promoters will instead need to promote dietary and lifestyle practices that encourage better weight control (see Chapter 8 for further discussion of this example).

Individual beliefs and the subjective norm will affect a person's judgement of any particular recommendation and thus affect their behaviour intentions. A host of 'enabling factors' will influence whether or not any intention or wish to change behaviour is translated into actual behaviour change. These enabling factors may come under a variety of headings such as those given below.

- *Physical resources.* Is the change physically possible for the person? Can they obtain the recommended foods? Have they the facilities necessary for their preparation? For example the range and quality of fresh fruit and vegetables available in some rural areas may be limited. If low-income groups are temporarily housed in accommodation without cooking facilities this may severely limit their dietary choices.
- *Financial resources.* Can they afford to make the recommended changes? Fruit and vegetables provide few calories per penny and so may be uneconomic choices for those seeking to satisfy appetites with a very low income.
- *Personal resources.* Have they the skills and mobility necessary to implement the recommended changes? Many frail elderly people have mobility problems that will restrict their shopping and cooking capabilities. Some widowed elderly men or students living away from home for the first

time may have had little experience of preparing food for themselves.

In Chapter 2 many of these enabling factors will be discussed using the 'hierarchy of availabilities' model of food selection (see Figure 2.2, p. 40). In this model it is assumed that a host of factors, at several levels, limit any individual's practical freedom of dietary choice and thus limit their ability to implement any recommended change.

People may be convinced that a health promotion message is applicable to them, the subjective norm may favour change and the enabling factors may permit them to make the recommended change. Despite this, change may still not occur; they may make a decision (judgement) to accept the risks associated with current behaviour, perhaps because of the perceived adverse effect of change on their quality of life. In younger men, for example, the acceptance of risks associated with dangerous or unhealthy practices may be seen as an expression of their virility.

Key points

- It is relatively easy to devise diets that meet any given set of scientific criteria but much more difficult to produce such a diet that will be complied with by the client.

- A dietary change is more likely to be implemented if there are clear and rapidly discernible benefits, if the change is consistent with existing beliefs and practices and if it is easy to understand, try out and incorporate.

- A dietary change that cures a deficiency disease produces clear and apparent benefits, and often involves changes that are easily understood and implemented.

- A dietary change to reduce the risk of chronic disease:
  - usually produces no immediate benefits
  - even the long-term benefits may be small and speculative for any individual
  - considerable and complex change may be required
  - the change may markedly reduce the desirability of the diet.

- Health promotion will be ineffective if:
  - the message is wrong

- the message is not seen and correctly assimilated by the client
- the message does not convince the client that change is desirable
- the client is unable or unwilling to make the recommended changes in behaviour.

● The BASNEF model suggests that beliefs, attitudes, the subjective norm and a range of enabling factors are the determinants of whether a health promotion message results in actual change.

● People must believe that the recommended change will benefit them.

● They must be of a mind to make changes for the benefit of their long-term health.

● The subjective norm is the beliefs and attitudes of those people who influence the client and perhaps of society as a whole.

● Enabling factors are a range of practical things like resources, skills, mobility and knowledge that can determine the extent to which the client can change.

CONCLUDING REMARKS

If the questions posed in this chapter are fully considered by those making nutrition or other health education recommendations then the likelihood of making changes that ultimately prove to be non-beneficial or harmful will be minimized. If a totally holistic view is taken then any intervention that is non-beneficial can probably be regarded as harmful. Observations in migrant populations show that in general they tend to progressively assume the mortality and morbidity patterns that are characteristic of their new homeland (Barker *et al.*, 1998).

This reaffirms the belief that many of the health differences between populations are due to environment rather than genetics and therefore also confirms that there is considerable potential for promoting health by lifestyle intervention. Paradoxically, as each population tends to have its own problem diseases, it also underlines the potential for harm from ill-considered and insufficiently tested interventions. A narrow preoccupation with changing diets to reduce the risk of one disease may simply lead to an increase in the risk of another.

2

Food selection

INTRODUCTION AND AIMS OF THE CHAPTER

Most of this book focuses on food as a source of energy and nutrients, e.g. which nutrients are essential and why; how much of these nutrients people need at various times of their lives; and how changing the balance of nutrients eaten can affect long-term health. This chapter is in some small way intended to be an antidote to the necessary scientific reductionism of much of the rest of the book. The general aim of the chapter is to remind readers that 'people eat food and not nutrients' and that nutrient content has only relatively recently become a significant factor in the making of food choices. Only in the latter part of the twentieth century did our knowledge of nutrient needs and the chemical composition of food become sufficient to allow them to be major influences on food selection.

A host of seasonal, geographical, social and economic factors determine the availability of different foods to any individual or group, whereas cultural and preference factors affect its acceptability. Some of these influences are listed in Box 2.1.

If the promotion of health requires one to try to influence people's food choices then some understanding of the non-nutritional uses of food, and of the way non-nutritional factors interact to influence food choices is essential. It is no use devising an excellent diet plan or drawing up detailed dietary guidelines unless they are actually implemented.

Box 2.1	Some factors affecting food choice and eating patterns

- Availability of foods in the local environment. This is in turn influenced by several factors such as climate, soil type, transportation links, rationing, shopping facilities
- Nutrition knowledge and/or food beliefs. This is in turn influenced by such things as cultural traditions, education and religious/ethical beliefs
- Habit and previous food experience
- Individual likes and dislikes
- Facilities for storing, preparing and cooking
- Cooking just for oneself or eating with and/or cooking for others
- Skills in food preparation and willingness to experiment and develop new skills
- Financial resources, budgeting skills and the cost of foods. These may be affected by political decisions about taxation, subsidy and welfare payments
- Time available and the time needed to prepare and eat foods
- State of health and appetite

After Webb and Copeman (1996)

Diets or dietary recommendations that may seem ideal from a reductionist biological viewpoint may have little impact on actual food choices. Some people may have very limited freedom to make food choices, e.g. those living in institutions where all of their food is provided by a caterer. There will be some restraints upon the food choices of everyone. Dietary recommendations will almost certainly be ineffective if they are culturally unacceptable to the clients, incompatible with their personal preferences or beliefs, beyond their economic means or incompatible with what is provided by their caterer or parent.

When making dietary recommendations (or devising therapeutic diets), advisers need to consider various questions.

- Can the clients obtain the ingredients of the recommended diet?
- Can they prepare it?
- Can they afford to implement the recommendations?
- Are the recommendations compatible with their cultural beliefs and practices?
- Will their caterer or parent provide a diet that complies with the recommendations?
- Will they find the recommended diet palatable?
- Can they tolerate the recommended foods?
- Are the recommendations environmentally sustainable if widely implemented? (Also discussed briefly in Chapter 4.)

An appreciation of the non-nutritional roles of food and the non-nutritional influences on food selection should enable health educators to give advice that is more acceptable to clients and easier for them to act upon. Dietary recommendations that are in sympathy with existing beliefs, preferences and selection practices will fare better than those that try to impose the prejudices and preferences of the adviser. This culturally sensitive approach should also reduce the likelihood that the cost of scientifically better nutrition will increase anxiety, social tension and cultural impoverishment. Readers who wish to explore the social and cultural determinants of food choice and the non-nutritional roles of food are recommended to see Fieldhouse (1998).

Key points

- Nutrient content has not traditionally been a significant influence on food selection; 'people eat food not nutrients'.

- Social, economic and geographical factors influence availability of food, whereas cultural and preference factors determine its acceptability.
- Dietary guidelines or prescribed diets are more likely to be complied with if they allow for and are sympathetic to the non-nutritional factors that influence or limit food choices of an individual or group.

THE BIOLOGICAL MODEL OF FOOD

The primary biological function of food is to provide the body with a sufficient supply of energy and essential nutrients to meet current physiological needs. Diet composition also influences long-term risk of chronic disease. The reductionist scientific model of food is that it is merely a complex mixture of nutrients that should be combined in optimal proportions to meet both current needs and to maximize health and longevity in the longer term. Eating could then be seen simply as a flawed and inefficient behavioural mechanism used to select and consume this mixture.

Such paradigms of food and of eating might tempt one to believe that if consumers are given extensive advice about optimal nutrient intakes coupled with full nutritional labelling of food then they will be enabled to select the ideal diet. Increasing information about healthy eating and food composition might be expected to lead to rapid and major 'improvements' in the diet of the population (see Chapter 4 for evidence of the effect of health promotion on 'the national diet').

It is quite obvious that most people do not select their food solely according to such biological criteria. In the past, selection on this basis would not have been possible because public awareness of nutrition and food composition is comparatively recent. Even today, few people would have the skills and knowledge to select food solely on a compositional basis. It has been suggested that biological mechanisms akin to thirst or salt hunger operate for some important nutrients enabling people to intuitively select a balanced diet. There is little evidence to support such mechanisms, but there is evidence that satiation tends to be food specific. Satiation for a particular food develops as that food is consumed, but satiation towards other foods is less affected. Such a mechanism would tend to increase the range of foods consumed and dietary deficiencies become less likely if energy needs are fully met and a wide variety of foods consumed. In the circumstances of almost limitless abundance and variety experienced by those in the industrialized countries, such a mechanism might also tend to encourage overeating and obesity (see **sensory specific satiety** in Chapter 8).

Much current food evangelism seems to be encouraging a trend towards the reductionist scientific models of food and eating. This could greatly impoverish human existence without necessarily extending its duration because food has numerous social, psychological and cultural functions in addition to its biological role of supplying nutrients.

> ## Key points
>
> - Scientists may see food as no more than a mixture of nutrients that need to be consumed in the correct proportions and eating as merely the process by which these nutrients are selected and eaten.
> - If food and eating fulfilled no other functions then one would expect scientific guidance to lead to rapid improvements in this selection process.
> - But food does have many other functions and food choices are influenced by many factors which may make it difficult to persuade people to make changes in their diet that seem rational from the purely scientific viewpoint.

DIETARY AND CULTURAL PREJUDICE

There is an almost inevitable tendency to regard one's own beliefs and patterns of behaviour as the norm and so preferable to those of other cultures. Foreign or unusual cultural practices tend to be regarded as wrong, irrational or misguided. The term **ethnocentrism** has been used to describe this tendency. Ethnocentrism is apparent in reactions to alien food habits. There is a widespread tendency to ridicule or even to abhor the food choices or eating habits of others. The intrepid explorer patronizingly accepting some revolting native delicacy to avoid offending his host is a Hollywood cliché. One manifestation of this phenomenon is in the slightly derogatory names used for other races that have their origins in food habits, such as those listed below.

- *Frogs*, because frog legs are a French delicacy.
- *Kraut*, from the traditional fermented cabbage (sauerkraut) associated with German cuisine.
- *Limey*, because of the past practice of providing lime juice to British sailors to prevent scurvy.
- The term *Eskimo* originates from a disparaging Indian term meaning 'eaters of raw flesh' and so the alternative name *Inuit* is now favoured.

Ethnocentric-type attitudes need not be confined to 'between culture' judgements. It is not uncommon to hear haughty disapproval and caricaturization of the dietary practices of other regions of one's own country, of other social or religious groups or indeed of anyone who does not share a particular food ideology, e.g.:

- within England, it is not uncommon to hear disparaging comments made about the diets of 'northerners' which often implicitly blame northerners for the relatively poor health statistics of the north compared to the south
- vegetarianism is frequently denigrated and ridiculed by meat eaters and conversely some vegetarian propaganda makes very hostile comments about meat eaters
- it is not uncommon to hear disparaging comments exchanged between those who do and those do not consciously attempt to practise healthy eating.

Criticisms of other dietary and cultural practices are often based on a prejudiced, narrow and inaccurate view of the other peoples' beliefs and behaviour. Nutritionists and dieticians are not immune to ethnocentrism but hopefully most would be aware of this tendency and consciously try to avoid it when dealing with an alien culture. They might, however, be more unsuspecting and thus inclined to behave ethnocentrically when dealing with the more familiar behaviour patterns of other groups within their own culture. Although these behaviour patterns may be familiar, they may nonetheless be quite different from their own. For example, it must be very difficult for a dietician who is a committed vegetarian to give advice to a meat eater that is totally uninfluenced by their own beliefs and, vice versa if the client is vegetarian and the dietician a meat eater.

The opposite of ethnocentrism is **cultural relativism**. The cultural relativist tries to understand and respect other cultural practices and to accept them as normal no matter how bizarre they may at first seem or how different they are from their own. Only if practices are clearly and demonstrably dysfunctional does one try to change them. There would be little argument that such an approach was correct if one were dealing with an unique alien culture but more familiar cultural practices may be handled with less sensitivity. The American's hamburger, the Briton's fish and chips and even children's sweets or candies have real cultural significance. Nutrition education need not try to totally forbid or blacken the image of such foods but should rather attempt to use them within a diet that, in its entirety, complies with reasonable nutritional guidelines.

It is likely that many practices that are strongly and acutely dysfunctional to a group will have been selected out during the cultural evolution of the group. Changing social or environmental conditions, or simply increased longevity and consequent changes in health priorities may cause traditional practices to become regarded as dysfunctional. The aim of nutrition education, under such circumstances, should be to minimize or avoid the dysfunction with the least possible cultural interference – the *cultural conservationist* approach. This is likely to be the most successful as well as the most ethical strategy.

> ## Key points
>
> - Ethnocentrism describes the tendency to regard one's own beliefs and practices as the norm and those of other cultures as wrong or abnormal.
> - Ethnocentric-type attitudes can also exist within cultures and in these circumstances they may be less obvious and harder to correct.
> - Cultural relativism is the acceptance of other cultural practices as normal even if they are very different from one's own.
> - No matter how strange they may seem, one should only try to change other dietary practices if they are clearly dysfunctional and then by the minimum amount to avoid the dysfunction – the cultural conservationist approach.

FOOD CLASSIFICATION SYSTEMS

Nutritionists, consumers and anthropologists all categorize foods but they use different criteria for their classification. These categorizations may be a formal and explicit classification system or a largely subconscious, practical classification.

Nutritional classification of food – food groups, plates and pyramids

Nutritionists classify foods according to the nutrients that they contain and these classifications are used to advise and guide consumers towards a healthy diet. Foods were initially classified into food groups according to their nutrient profiles and consumers advised to eat specified minimum amounts from each food group to ensure that their diet had adequate quantities of all the essential nutrients. As the priorities of nutrition education were widened to include the prevention of chronic disease, so new consumer guides were developed. These new guidance systems needed to indicate not just the minimum amounts needed for adequacy but also the balance between the various food groups that would minimize the risk of chronic disease. In the UK, a tilted plate model is used, and a food guide pyramid is used in the USA. Food group systems and these newer food guides are discussed more fully in Chapter 4.

> ## Key point
>
> Nutritionists classify foods according to their nutrient profiles. Food groups and food guide plates or pyramids are examples of nutritional classifications of food.

Consumer classifications of food

Consumers also classify foods but such classification systems have not traditionally had any theoretical basis in scientific nutrition. Despite this, such classification systems may have evolved rules that produce good practical diets even though they may have a theoretical framework that seems incompatible with scientific nutrition theory. Nutritionists and dieticians should try to understand such classification systems and to offer advice that is consistent with them.

One of the best known and most widespread of the traditional and formal classification systems is the **hot and cold** classification that is found in various forms in Latin America, India and China. The general principle is that good health results from a state of balance and thus to maintain or restore good health there must be a balance between hot and cold. Foods are classified as hot or cold and foods should be selected and mixed to produce or maintain the balanced state. Disease results from an imbalance. Certain diseases and phases of the reproductive cycle are also regarded as hot or cold states and so certain foods will be more or less appropriate in these different circumstances. As an example, in the Chinese system a sore throat is a hot disease and might be treated by a cold food such as watermelon to try and restore balance. Hot foods, such as beef, dates or chilli are considered detrimental in such hot conditions. Past surveys of Chinese families living in London (Wheeler and Tan, 1983) and Toronto (Yeung *et al.*, 1973) both found that at that time the traditional hot and cold system was still widely adhered to and practised despite Western cultural influences. Wheeler and Tan (1983) concluded that despite the use of such a non-science-based food classification system, the dietary pattern of the London Chinese families in their survey was varied and nutritionally excellent. Any programme designed to increase the science-based nutrition and food composition knowledge of the '**gatekeepers**' in these Chinese families runs the risk of undermining confidence in the traditional system and perhaps even worsening their diets. The 'gatekeepers' in English families living in the same area would probably have had more science-based nutrition knowledge but these authors would probably have judged that, by their criteria, the English diet was inferior to that of the Chinese. Knowledge of food and nutrition is perhaps more loosely correlated with good dietetic practice than many nutritionists would like to think.

Most Western consumers do not use such a formal and overtly structured classification system but they do classify foods. In any cultural group there is clearly a classification of potentially edible material into food and non-food. Except under conditions of extreme deprivation, any cultural group will only eat some of the substances around them that would comply with any biological definition of potential food. In the UK, there are numerous plants, animals, birds, fish and insects that are edible but are rarely if ever eaten by Britons. They are simply not viewed as potential foods and are classified as non-food. In many cases, the idea of eating such items would be repellent to most Britons. For example, cows,

chickens, cabbages and crabs are seen as potential food but not horses, dogs, crows, nettles or frogs.

The traditional main course of a British dinner (or lunch if that is the main meal of the day) consists of a meat or meat product, potatoes, one or more extra vegetables with sauce or gravy. Very few Britons would, however, consider eating such a meal or even some of the individual foods for breakfast. A 'cheeseburger and fries' is not (yet) on the breakfast menus of restaurant chains that have built their global empires on such fare. Clearly some foods are seen, or classified, as more appropriate for particular meals. These classifications of edible material into food or non-food and into foods appropriate for particular meals or occasions vary considerably even within the peoples of western Europe. In Britain, horsemeat is not classified as food and yet it has traditionally been eaten in France. Many Britons would not consider cheese and spicy cold meats as suitable breakfast foods yet in some other European countries they would be typical breakfast fare.

Schutz *et al.* (1975) conducted a survey of 200 female, mainly white and mainly middle class consumers distributed in four American cities. They used a questionnaire in which these consumers were asked to rate 56 different foods in terms of their appropriateness for a total of 48 food-use situations; they used a seven-point scale from 1 'never appropriate' to 7 'always appropriate'. Their aim was to allow the respondents to generate classifications of foods based on their appropriateness ratings. On the basis of consumer usage rather than on biological criteria, the authors identified the following five food categories.

- *High-calorie treats* such as wine, cakes and pies. These were considered especially suitable for social occasions and for offering to guests. The foods in this category tended to be rated towards the inappropriate end of the scale for questions relating to healthfulness, e.g. inappropriate when 'needing to lose weight' or when 'not feeling well'. Healthy, wholesome foods seemed to be considered more suitable for everyday eating and eating alone than for parties and entertaining.
- *Speciality meal items* were considered suitable only for special occasions and circumstances. The authors offered liver and chilli as examples. The foods in this category were notable for the number of food-use situations for which they were rated as never appropriate.

- *Common meal items* were considered suitable for all occasions and all ages and would be served at main meals, e.g. meats, fish and some vegetable items. They were generally rated as inappropriate 'for breakfast' and not surprisingly 'for dessert'.
- *Refreshing healthy foods* such as milk, orange juice and cottage cheese were considered to be nutritious but not viewed as suitable for a main course. These scored highly on the healthfulness questions 'nutritious' 'easy to digest' but were rated low as to spiciness. Perhaps spiciness/flavour and healthfulness were not seen as compatible.
- *Inexpensive filling foods* were considered cheap and filling as well as fattening, e.g. bread, peanut butter, potato chips (crisps) and candy bars. These were not considered appropriate for those trying to lose weight but were seen be useful to assuage hunger between meals and appropriate for hungry teenagers.

This is, of course, just one group of investigators' interpretation of the comments expressed by one group of consumers more than 30 years ago. It does, however, highlight how even Western consumers, despite not having a formal cultural food classification system like the Chinese hot and cold system, do nonetheless have clear and, within a group, fairly consistent views on the appropriateness of different foods in different situations. They may use quite elaborate classification systems for food, even though such classification may be informal or even subconscious.

If it is to be effective, then clearly any dietary advice or any prescribed diet must recognize such views on the appropriateness of particular foods for particular occasions and situations. It will also be more likely to succeed if it uses foods that are classified as appropriate for the individual. Many cultural groups might classify milk as a food for babies and therefore not suitable for adults, some Western consumers might only grudgingly concede that some pulses or salads are suitable for working men.

Key points

- Consumers classify foods according to the ways in which they are used.
- The hot and cold system is an example of a formal classification system in which foods are classified as hot or cold and selected to maintain or restore the body's hot–cold balance.

- Even where there is no overt classification, all consumers divide potentially edible material into food and non-food. They also regard different foods as more or less appropriate for particular uses, occasions or people. These classifications are culture specific.
- Dietary advisers must be aware of these cultural classifications and make sure that their recommendations are consistent with them.

Anthropological classification of foods

Several attempts have been made to devise food categorization systems that could be used across cultures. These are useful not only for the anthropologist seeking to describe the diets and the uses made of foods in particular cultures but they could also be of great use to the nutrition educator seeking to identify the most appropriate and effective ways of trying to bring about nutritional improvement. One of the earliest and simplest of these systems is that of Passim and Bennet (1943) who divided foods into three categories.

- *Core foods* are those that are regularly and universally consumed within the society. In developing countries, these are likely to be starchy staple foods (e.g. bread, rice, millet or cassava). In industrialized countries, such as Britain and the USA, milk, potatoes, bread and meats would probably fit into this category.
- *Secondary foods* are those that have widespread but not universal use. Most fruits and vegetables would probably be classified as secondary foods in the UK.
- *Peripheral foods* are the least widely and frequently used foods. It is in this category that the most individual variation would be expected. Most shellfish and most species of fish would probably be in this category in the UK.

Such categorization would almost certainly be easier to make in societies whose range of available foods is relatively restricted and most difficult in societies such as those in Europe and North America which have a vast array of foods available to an affluent population. Affluent consumers are able to express much more individuality in their diet structure.

Any particular food may be classified differently for different cultures, it may be classified differently for different social classes within a culture and foods may change categories over time. Rice is clearly a core food for the Japanese but for most British groups would probably be classified as secondary. A few decades ago, rice (except pudding rice) would probably have been classified as peripheral for most social groups in Britain. Prior to 1960 many working class Britons would almost never eat a savoury rice dish. Chinese and Indian restaurants and takeaway outlets and foreign holidays have transformed this situation so that there may now be some groups, even within the indigenous population, for whom rice might be approaching the status of a core food. The growth of vegetarianism and meat-restricted diets in Britain might lead some readers to question whether meat should still be regarded as a core food.

A nutritionist trying to effect change in the diet of any community might expect to find most resistance to change in the core foods, more ready acceptance in the secondary foods and the most flexibility in the peripheral foods. Some foods have acquired a cultural status beyond their purely dietary and nutritional significance; they play an integral part in the cultural life of the community and they have been termed **cultural superfoods**, e.g. rice in Japan and bread in many European cultures. Rice has maintained a particular emotional and cultural status for the Japanese despite a marked fall in consumption since World War II and a corresponding increase in bread consumption.

- The emperor still cultivates a symbolic crop of rice.
- In the Japanese language, the same word can mean either food or rice.
- Rice plays a part in Japanese cultural and religious rituals.
- In the past, the Japanese calendar was geared to the cycle of rice production, rice was used as a medium for taxation and some units of measurement were based on the amount of rice necessary to feed a man for a year.

Bread has declined in its cultural significance in some European countries but television scenes of people in war-ravaged areas of eastern Europe queuing for bread still strike a particularly poignant chord. If the bread supply is threatened, then the situation is perceived as that much more desperate than if other foods are in short supply. The arrival of bread is often seen as a symbol of hope for these people. There are numerous reminders of the past importance of bread in the UK, e.g.:

- bread and dough are both used as slang terms for money
- in Christian communion, bread is used to symbolically represent the body of Christ
- in the Lord's Prayer, Christians pray for their daily bread.

Nutrition educators need to understand and respect the cultural significance of such foods if they want their dietary advice and guidance to be effective. Insensitive denigration of a cultural superfood may provoke incredulity or even hostility and so reduce the chances of any of the advice being taken seriously. Meat has had a particular cultural importance to many Western men which may even have been reinforced in the past by nutrition education that presented meat as a good source of the high-quality protein that was seen as a key requirement of good nutrition. If nutrition educators now try to persuade such men that red meat and a healthy diet are incompatible then they may simply persuade them that the price for a healthy diet is too high and make them ignore all dietary advice. In a previous edition of a classic British nutrition text, Passmore and Eastwood (1986) quoted a passage which describes the African's craving for meat as:

> the strongest and most fraternal bond that the continent had in common. It was a dream, a longing, an aspiration that never ceased, a physiological cry of the body, stronger and more torturing than the sexual instinct.
>
> *Gary, R. 1958* The roots of heaven. *London: Michael Joseph*

The speaker goes on to assume that this need for meat is a universal craving for all men. If there is even a grain of truth in this assertion then nutrition education must not suggest that the only option for healthy eating is one that would require unreasonable sacrifice. To use a slightly more recent example, chips (French fries) are a traditional and important element in British cuisine and culture. The following quotation from a serious national newspaper emphasizes the importance that some Britons attach to their chips:

> According to the Chip Census, one person in 10 would rather give up sex, alcohol and smoking than chips!
>
> *Independent*, 2 March 1994

Once again if healthy eating appears to require total avoidance of chips then the chances of acceptance by a high proportion of the British population is probably doomed. Moderate amounts of chips can be included in a diet that meets current nutritional guidelines, especially if attention is paid to advice about their method of preparation and the foods that they most appropriately complement.

Cultural superfood is just one of five food categories described by Jelliffe (1967) in a food classification system that he thought had universal application, both in developing and industrialized countries. The five categories in this system are given below.

- *Cultural superfood* as discussed above. Considered by Schutz *et al.* (1975) to correspond to 'common meal item' in their consumer classification.
- *Prestige foods* are reserved for important occasions or important people. According to Jelliffe, foods in this category are usually high in protein, which is often animal protein. They are also usually difficult to obtain because of their scarcity, high cost or difficult preparation. Truffles, lobster and caviar might fall into this category in the UK. In past decades, salmon would have been in this category until the ready availability of cheaper, farmed salmon reduced its scarcity and price.
- *Body image foods* are those that are thought to promote wellness. Jelliffe lists foods that contribute to maintaining or restoring hot–cold balance as an example from developing countries. High-fibre foods or dairy products that contain **probiotic** (see Chapter 18) or good bacteria would be an example in the UK.
- *Sympathetic magic foods* are thought to have some special properties that they impart to the consumer. An example given by Jelliffe is the avoidance of eggs by many women in East African countries because they believe that they cause infertility. As another examples he uses underdone steak used in the training of athletes (in 1967) because it symbolized vigour, masculinity and energy.

- *Physiologic group foods* are foods reserved for or forbidden to certain physiologic groups. Taboos against certain foods for pregnant and lactating women or for young children are examples. Breast milk, infant formula and certain cereal preparations that are normally only consumed by infants and young children are obvious examples of this category.

Key points

- Anthropologists classify foods according to their importance to a culture and the roles they have within the culture's diet.
- The simplest anthropological classification divides foods into three categories: core foods, secondary foods and peripheral foods.
- The same foods may be used differently and be in a different categories in different cultural groups and a food may change categories within a group over time.
- A cultural superfood is one that plays an important part in the cultural life and identity of the group and has acquired a cultural significance that transcends its purely nutritional one, e.g. rice in Japan, maize among the Hopi Indians, and bread in some European societies.
- Jelliffe classified foods into five categories:
  - cultural superfoods – usually the starchy staple of the group
  - prestige foods – reserved for special occasions or important people
  - body image foods – foods thought to contribute to good health
  - sympathetic magic foods – foods that impart some special property to the consumer
  - Physiologic group foods – foods considered suitable for particular groups.

NON–NUTRITIONAL USES OF FOOD

The primary biological role of food is to provide an adequate supply of energy and essential nutrients but food also has many non-nutritional functions and several examples are listed below. This list is not definitive. It is merely intended to illustrate the enormous diversity and range of potential non-nutritional uses of food.

Religion, morality and ethics

- Food and drink are used symbolically in the rituals and ceremonies of many religions. For example, the use of bread and wine in Christian communion to symbolize the body and blood of Christ.
- Adherence to the dietary rules of a religion acts as a common bond for adherents and serves to differentiate them from non-believers. For example, adherence to the dietary rules and customs of the Torah helps to bond orthodox Jewish families and to set them apart from gentiles.
- Adhering to dietary rules is an outward symbol of a person's piety and self-discipline, e.g. the dawn to dusk fasting undertaken by Muslims during Ramadan.
- Policing of dietary rules provides a mechanism for religious leaders to exert control over their followers and to demonstrate their authority, e.g. the severe penalties for alcohol consumption, even for non-believers, underlines the primacy of Islam and the mullahs in some countries.
- People may avoid certain foods to demonstrate their disapproval of animal cruelty or their ecological awareness, e.g. the avoidance of veal raised in crates or tuna caught in drift nets.
- People may boycott food from particular countries or companies to express their moral disapproval of human rights abuses, exploitation of workers or other perceived moral transgressions, e.g. boycotts of South African produce during the apartheid era and boycotts of food companies that are accused of 'pushing' powdered infant formulae in developing countries.

Status and wealth

- Expensive and exotic foods can be used to demonstrate one's wealth and sophistication, e.g. serving expensive, but essentially rather bland, caviar as a snack with champagne.
- Serving elaborate and expensive meals can be used to demonstrate esteem for guests as in traditional feasts of welcome and the Western dinner party.
- A person's social status may be defined by whom they eat with and where they eat, e.g. it was common practice for large companies to have different dining areas for workers of different status

and different Hindu castes have not traditionally eaten together.
- Unusual food choices may be used to express a person's individuality, e.g. serving foods associated with one's distant ethnic roots.

Interpersonal relationships

- Offerings of food and drink are commonly used to initiate and maintain personal and business relationships. Offering new neighbours a drink or food is primarily a gesture of welcome and warmth rather than an attempt to satisfy any perceived nutritional need.
- Giving of food can be a demonstration of love and withdrawal or failure to offer food can be used to signal disapproval or even to punish, e.g. use of bread and water punishment for prisoners. A gift of chocolate can be used as a reward, a gesture of affection or apology; any nutritional impact of the chocolate is incidental.
- Food and drink may provide a focus for social gatherings.

Political

Control of the food supply and the price of food can be a very potent method of exerting political control or of gaining political favour. Some would argue that food aid has purposes or effects beyond its obvious humanitarian one. It may salve the consciences of wealthy donor nations, foster dependence and subservience in the recipients or help to bolster the political and diplomatic fortunes of the donor government.

Folk medicine

Diet is an element in many traditional treatments for disease. In the traditional hot and cold system, cold foods may be used to treat hot diseases. In many Western countries the boundaries between food as a source of sustenance and as a medicine are becoming increasingly blurred. There is widespread use of dietary supplements which are taken not just to ensure adequacy but also to prevent or treat diseases and doses of nutrients consumed in this form may be much greater than those obtained from any normal diet. Some substances that should logically be classified as medicines are marketed as dietary supplements to avoid the costly process of demonstrating their safety and efficacy and obtaining a medicinal licence. In recent years there has been a huge growth in the sale of so-called **functional foods** (see Chapter 18) that are marketed on their potential to maintain or restore health.

Key points

- Food has many functions over and above its purely nutritional purpose.
- Dietary rules and traditions can be an important part of religious life and cultural identity.
- Food selection can be used to make ethical and political statements.
- Eating habits and food choices can be used to indicate a person's social status, wealth or uniqueness as an individual.
- Food can be used to initiate and foster interpersonal and business relationships.
- Control of the food supply can be used as a means of political control.
- Food can be used to reward or to punish.
- Foods can be used as medicines in traditional medicine and substances legally classified as food (dietary supplements and functional foods) are widely used for quasi-medical purposes in industrialized countries.

THE HIERARCHY OF HUMAN NEEDS

The relative importance of any particular influence on diet may be quite different in different groups, even within the same local environment. Take, for example, the influence of religion on food choice in the UK or USA. Religion would have a major influence on food choices of strictly orthodox Jews or Seventh Day Adventists but minimal influence on those of equally devout Anglicans or Episcopalians. For example, an orthodox Jew would:

- avoid all pig meat and meat from any animal that does not have cloven hooves and chew the cud
- not eat the hind quarters of animals or unbled meat

- not eat flightless birds, shellfish or other fish without fins and scales
- not eat meat and dairy produce together
- not prepare food on Sabbath.

It would be difficult to identify any specifically religious influences on the diets of the two Protestant groups except, perhaps, the occasional communion bread and wine or voluntary and self-selected abstinence during Lent.

The priorities attached to the various biological and non-biological factors influencing food selection are likely to change as one moves from a situation of gross deprivation or scarcity to one of almost limitless abundance. Maslow (1943) suggested that human needs could be arranged into a hierarchy of motivation (summarized in Figure 2.1). In this very well-known theory of motivation, needs that are lower down the hierarchy must be at least partially satisfied before the higher-up needs can become significant motivating factors. In Maslow's theory, the basic biological and emotional needs come at the base of the hierarchy and only once there has been reasonable satisfaction of these needs do the more aesthetic and esoteric needs become significantly motivating.

Maslow's hierarchy of needs can be applied to food selection. In conditions of extreme deprivation survival is the priority and people may resort to eating almost anything that is remotely edible, perhaps

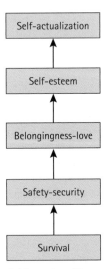

Figure 2.1 *Maslow's hierarchy of human needs. After Maslow (1943).*

even breaking one of the strongest and most wide-spread of all dietary taboos – that against the consumption of human flesh. After survival, the need to ensure future security and safety becomes motivating. Potentially edible material is classified into food and non-food and ensuring that future needs are met becomes a priority. Food hoarding, perhaps even obesity, might be outward manifestations of this desire for security. Obesity in some cultures has been sought after and admired rather than dreaded and despised as it usually is in the UK and USA. Once security of food supply is relatively assured, the need for love and belongingness becomes a motivating influence on food selection. This could be manifested in the extensive use of food to demonstrate group membership and affection. Then comes the need for self-esteem. This might be manifested in the selection of high cost, prestige foods to demonstrate one's wealth and success. At the pinnacle of Maslow's hierarchy the need for self-actualization becomes motivating. Selection of food to demonstrate one's individuality or uniqueness becomes prominent and this may be manifested in experimentation with new foods, new recipes and non-conforming patterns of selection.

The current penchant for the simple peasant foods of the East by some educated, affluent 'Westerners' may be one manifestation of the need for self-actualization. The partial replacement of these traditional foods with a more 'Western diet' by some in the East may be symbolizing their need to demonstrate their new wealth, i.e. to improve their self-esteem. In many developing countries bottle feeds for infants are promoted as the modern and sophisticated Western alternative to 'primitive' breast-feeding. In many affluent countries, like the USA and UK, breastfeeding predominates in the upper social classes (e.g. Hamlyn et al., 2002).

There may be some disagreement over the details of Maslow's hierarchy, as it has been applied to food selection, but the underlying principle seems unquestionable, i.e. that the priority attached to different influences will change with increasing affluence and food availability. The range of factors influencing selection will tend to be greater in affluent than in poor populations and the relative prominence of these different factors will also change with increasing affluence. The more physiological, biological drives tend to become less important in the affluent.

Key points

- The importance of any influence on food selection and eating behaviour will vary from group to group.
- Religion would be a major influence on the food choices of orthodox Jews but not Protestants.
- In situations of shortage or deprivation, survival and security would be dominant influences on food choices.
- In situations of abundance, prestige and aesthetic factors would come into play.
- Maslow devised a theory of human motivation that envisaged a hierarchy of human needs (see Figure 2.1), which can be applied to food selection.
- In Maslow's scheme there has to be some minimum satisfaction of a need lower down in the hierarchy before the next need becomes a significant motivating influence.

A MODEL OF FOOD SELECTION: THE HIERARCHY OF AVAILABILITIES MODEL

Several workers have attempted to organize and integrate the various and disparate factors influencing food selection into a unified model. Without such a model, any discussion of the vast array of factors that can influence food choices can end up being an amorphous jumble of ideas and facts. Such a model should be simple but comprehensive and provide a useful framework for consideration of the factors that affect food choices. Availability of a food is clearly a prerequisite for selection. Wheeler (1992) suggested that various constraints act to limit the range of foods that are, in practice, available to the individual; in effect, that the image of the affluent Western consumer having almost limitless theoretical choice of food is partly an illusion. Practical limits upon the range of foods that are really available to different individuals may greatly limit the scope of the nutrition educator for effecting change. Even if an individual understands and accepts dietary advice there may still be barriers, sometimes beyond their control, that prevent or limit the implementation of change.

Figure 2.2 shows a simple model for food selection. This 'hierarchy of availabilities' model assumes that many different types of factors will limit the practical availability of foods to an individual and thus the chances of different foods being eaten. As with Maslow's hierarchy of human needs, it is envisaged that some minimum availability at lower levels in the hierarchy must be achieved before the next level becomes a significant influence on selection. These influences at each level can be absolute, i.e. complete unavailability to sole availability. More often in Western countries they will be more subtle variations in the practical availability of different foods.

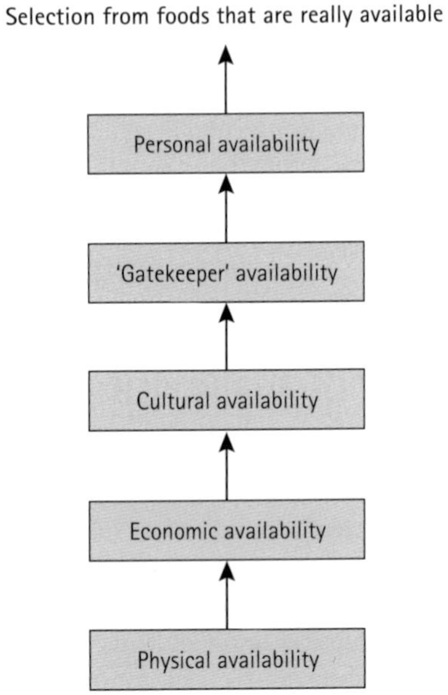

Selection from foods that are really available

```
          ↑
┌─────────────────────────┐
│   Personal availability  │
└─────────────────────────┘
          ↑
┌─────────────────────────┐
│  'Gatekeeper' availability │
└─────────────────────────┘
          ↑
┌─────────────────────────┐
│   Cultural availability  │
└─────────────────────────┘
          ↑
┌─────────────────────────┐
│   Economic availability  │
└─────────────────────────┘
          ↑
┌─────────────────────────┐
│   Physical availability  │
└─────────────────────────┘
```

Figure 2.2 *The 'hierarchy of availabilities' model of food selection.*

- *Physical availability.* A food can only be eaten if it is physically present in the local environment.
- *Economic availability.* People can only eat the foods that they can afford to buy. If a food is available locally but they cannot afford to buy it then it is economically unavailable to them.
- *Cultural availability.* People will normally only eat things that they recognize as food and which are culturally acceptable to them. Foods that are present and affordable but culturally unacceptable to them are culturally unavailable.

- *'Gatekeeper' availability.* A gatekeeper is someone who controls the supply of food to others. A mother may regulate what her family eats and a catering manager may regulate what the residents of an institution eat. What the gatekeeper provides may limit the supply of particular foods even though they may be physically, economically and culturally available to the consumer.
- *Personal availability.* Even foods that have overcome all of the previous barriers to their availability may still not be consumed. Individual dislike of a food, avoidance for reasons of individual belief or because of physiological intolerance may make it personally unavailable. Someone who is, or who believes that they are, allergic to fish will be effectively prevented from consuming fish. Someone revolted by the taste or texture of broccoli will not eat it and meat will not be available to someone revolted by the idea of eating the flesh of dead animals. Someone who relies on poorly fitting dentures may be discouraged from eating foods that require a strong bite and lots of chewing.

These availabilities are not usually absolute 'all or nothing' phenomena but a continuum varying from absolute unavailability to high desirability and availability. There can be both positive and negative influences on the availability of foods at each level of the hierarchy, e.g.:

- the number and locations of retail outlets stocking a food would influence its physical availability
- subsidy increases economic availability of a food but a tax reduces it
- clever advertising that raised the prestige of a food might increase its cultural availability
- increased menu choice in an institution might lessen the impact of the gatekeeper
- an 'acquired taste' might increase the personal availability of a food.

Much current nutrition education is geared towards partly reversing some of the dietary changes that accompany affluence. In many populations lack of physical or economic availability limits consumption of sugars, fats and animal foods but affluence removes these constraints. These foods often have high prestige and palatability, which increases their cultural, gatekeeper and personal availability. Nutrition education in affluent countries may be seen as trying to introduce constraints higher up the hierarchy in Figure 2.2 to compensate for the lessening of economic and physical restraints at the base of the hierarchy.

Key points

- A model of food selection should provide a framework for organizing and discussing the many disparate influences upon food selection and eating.
- The 'hierarchy of availabilities' model is based on Maslow's hierarchy of human needs. It envisages a hierarchy of factors that will limit the practical availability of foods to any individual.
- As with Maslow's hierarchy, there must be minimum availability at a lower level in the hierarchy before influences at the next level start to come into play.
- A continuum of availability is envisaged from absolute unavailability to limitless abundance and easy access.
- The five levels of this hierarchy of availability are:
  - physical (can the food be obtained?)
  - economic (can it be afforded?)
  - cultural (is it culturally recognized as food and culturally acceptable?)
  - 'gatekeeper' (is it provided by the parent, caterer or other gatekeeper?)
  - personal (does the person like the food, can they eat it and is it personally acceptable to them?).

PHYSICAL AVAILABILITY

There will be absolute limitations on the range of potentially edible materials that are available in any particular local environment. Physical and geographical factors are key determinants of food availability, factors such as climate, soil type, storage facilities, water supply, and quality of transportation links. The range and amounts of food available in an isolated and arid region may be severely limited by such factors. During severe famines, physical availability may be an absolute limitation on what food most people can eat.

Even within affluent countries, some foods will only be available seasonally. In fact, many seasonal foods are now imported and available all year round although the price will often vary considerably in and out of the local season. Some foods may be unavailable locally because of lack of sufficient demand. Shops will only stock foods that they expect to sell, e.g. kosher foods may be difficult to obtain in areas where few Jews live. Small local stores will inevitably stock a more limited range than large supermarkets and there may even be quite marked differences in the range of products stocked by shops in poor and affluent areas.

According to Henson (1992), the number of retail food outlets in Britain fell by a third between 1976 and 1987. There was a marked trend towards fewer but larger shops. The great majority of new superstores that have opened in recent years in Britain are located on the outskirts of towns and relatively few are being opened in shopping centres and high streets. These trends inevitably meant that people on average had to travel further for their shopping. Around three-quarters of households in Britain now use a car to make their shopping trips. These new superstores have wider choice and lower prices than local shops which means that they also reduce the viability of these smaller shops and may result in their closure. To take full advantage of them, consumers need good mobility (preferably access to a car), the financial resources to allow them to buy in larger quantities and adequate storage facilities (including access to a freezer). These retailing trends may be to the disadvantage of some groups and severely affect their access to a varied and inexpensive diet. Some examples are:

- people who do not have access to a car especially if they live in rural areas where local shops have all but disappeared. In some rural areas, it may be difficult to obtain a reasonable variety of fresh fruits and vegetables
- elderly and disabled people whose mobility is limited
- those living in accommodation without a freezer, little or no cooking facilities and no space for storing food.

In the past few years we have seen the major food retailers moving back into the high street by opening up smaller convenience-type stores and this may improve access to affordable food for people in these disadvantaged groups who live in urban areas. Most of the large supermarket chains also have facilities for online ordering and home delivery (at a cost) which may help those with limited mobility, but to make use of such facilities, consumers need computer literacy, internet access and the financial resources to afford delivery charges.

Key points

- People can only eat food that is physically accessible to them.
- During famines, physical absence of food may be an absolute limitation on food choice.
- A range of physical and geographical factors can affect what foods are available at any time and place. Many seasonal foods are, however, now available all year round at a price.
- The trend in Britain during the last 30 years of the twentieth century was for fewer, larger food shops often located on the edge of town. People must therefore travel further to do their shopping.
- These large superstores offer great variety at relatively low prices but those with limited mobility or no car may not be able to take full advantage of them.
- There has been some move back to the high street by the larger retail chains through the opening of smaller neighbourhood supermarkets.
- Online ordering and home delivery may help those with limited mobility but only if they have internet access and can afford the delivery charges.
- People who live in rural areas without a car may have limited access to some foods, especially perishable foods such as fresh fruit and vegetables.

ECONOMIC AVAILABILITY

Availability of money exerts a variable limiting influence on the availability of foods. In some circumstances, lack of money may have an absolute effect in limiting availability of particular foods or even of food in general. This is very clear in some developing countries where having enough money may mean the difference between relative comfort and starvation. Excepting times of acute famine, it is poverty rather than inadequate physical availability of food that is the dominant cause of malnutrition.

Wealthy countries with inadequate indigenous agriculture do not go hungry and wealthy people within poor countries do not usually go hungry either. People may go hungry even where food supplies are comparatively plentiful if they do not have the money to pay for food.

Even in affluent countries, financial constraints can have a marked effect upon dietary freedom of choice. In the UK and USA, there are quite marked differences between the food choices of the richest and poorest and this is partly due to differences in purchasing power. In these countries, health and longevity are strongly and positively correlated with higher socioeconomic status and diet is probably one of the factors contributing to these inequalities in health. It is ironic that the chronic diseases of industrialization that are internationally strongly and positively correlated with increasing affluence, are within the industrialized countries, associated with relative poverty.

Key points

- Poverty is the major cause of malnutrition in the world. People usually go hungry because they do not have the money to buy food.
- In affluent countries there are marked differences between the diets of the richest and the poorest, and there are also major inequalities in health.

International trends

If one looks worldwide at the influence of economic status on food 'selection', then some very general trends emerge. Increasing affluence leads initially to increases in total energy intake, followed by a switch away from starchy staples to other higher prestige and more palatable foods including fats, meats, dairy produce and sugars. Poleman (1975) suggested that the percentage of dietary energy that is provided by starchy staples provided a very simple economic ranking of diets. In 1875 starchy staples made up 55 per cent of total energy intake in the USA. A century later this figure had dropped to around 20 per cent. In the early decades of the twentieth century, maize was a sufficiently dominant component of the diets of poor farmers in some southern US states to trigger epidemics of pellagra (see Chapter 13).

At very low incomes, increased wealth leads to increases in energy intake, usually based on local starchy staples. Only when income level has risen beyond the point where energy needs are satisfied does increasing affluence lead to changes in the nature and quality of the diet. The local starchy staple is partly replaced by higher prestige rice or wheat. This is followed by a reduced consumption of starchy staples and replacement with foods of animal origin, fattier foods and simple sugars. In some developing countries, fat accounts for less than 10 per cent of total energy intake and carbohydrate more than 75 per cent. In the UK, fat accounts for around 36 per cent of food energy and carbohydrate only 48 per cent. In the poorer countries almost all of the carbohydrate calories are likely to be starches whereas in some richer countries a third or more of the carbohydrate calories may be in the form of simple sugars. Improved palatability, higher prestige and simple increases in physical availability all compound to persuade those with the economic means to make changes in this general direction.

Paralleling these changes in food selection practices there will be changes in the general pattern of mortality and disease. Child mortality will fall due largely to a general reduction in mortality from infectious diseases. Malnutrition and the deficiency diseases will all but disappear, life expectancy will increase but the chronic degenerative diseases will account for an increasing proportion of deaths and will be an increasing cause of illness and disability. The nutritional guidelines aimed at reducing the prevalence of these chronic diseases (discussed in Chapter 4) would partly reverse these wealth-related changes in dietary habits.

Key points

- As populations become more affluent their diet changes. First there is an increase in energy consumption as starchy staple but then the starchy food is partly replaced by animal produce, fatty foods and sugars.
- The proportion of dietary energy derived from starchy foods decreases with affluence and provides a simple economic ranking of diets.

- In some developing countries fats account for less than 10 per cent of dietary energy and starches as much as 75 per cent.
- In some affluent countries fats may provide 40 per cent of the energy and starches not much more than a quarter.
- Life expectancy increases with affluence, child mortality falls, deficiency diseases largely disappear and deaths from acute causes such as infection fall.
- The chronic diseases of industrialization account for most deaths among affluent populations.

The problem of feeding the world

In 1798, Thomas Malthus published his now infamous *Essay on the principle of population*. In this treatise he predicted that unless steps were taken to regulate the family size of the poor, population growth would outstrip growth in the food supply leading to global famine and epidemics. In the early 1960s, when world population was growing at an annual rate of around 2 per cent, a spate of Malthusian-type predictions of impending population disaster were also published.

Two hundred years ago when Malthus published his essay, the world population was less than 1 billion and in 2005 it reached 6.5 billion (Table 2.1). This rate of growth would have astounded even the most ardent Malthusian. There has, however, been a distinct slowing in the rate of population growth since the 1960s. In 1965–70 growth rate peaked at 2 per cent per year but by 2000 was down to 1.3 per cent (still a net addition of 76 million people each year). The deceleration in the rate of population growth has been sharper than was predicted even a few years ago. Table 2.1 shows the United Nations (UN) population estimates and projections for the period 0–2050 made in 2004 (UN, 2005). In brackets in this table are the projections made in this biennial UN publication in 1994. The projected population in 2050 has fallen from over 10 billion predicted in 1994 to the 9.01 billion predicted in 2004. Almost all of the predicted growth in population by 2050 will take place in the less developed regions whereas the population of the developed regions will remain largely unchanged at around 1.2 billion. In some countries such as Germany,

Table 2.1 The growth in world population from year 0 to 2050. Data from United Nations biennial estimates. The figures from 1950 onwards are from the 2004 estimates (UN, 2005) and in brackets are the predictions made by the UN in 1994

Year	Population in billions
0	0.30
1000	0.31
1250	0.40
1500	0.50
1750	0.79
1800	0.98
1850	1.26
1900	1.65
1920	1.86
1940	2.30
1950	2.52
1960	3.02
1970	3.70
1980	4.44
1990	5.27
1998	5.90
2000	6.09 (6.23)
2010	6.84
2020	7.58
2030	8.20
2040	8.70
2050	9.01 (10.02)

Japan, Italy, and the former Soviet Union the population is predicted to fall by 2050 but in some of the least developed countries it is expected to at least triple, e.g. in Afghanistan, Burundi, Chad, Congo, Democratic Republic of the Congo, Liberia, Mali, Niger and Uganda.

The projected changes in world population by 2050 are highly dependent on what happens to human fertility over this period. The projection in Table 2.1 is based upon the medium variant, i.e. that it will fall from 2.65 children per woman in 2000–05 to just 2.05 children per woman by 2050. The current fertility rate is just over half that in the early 1950s when it stood at 5 children per woman. Although average fertility has fallen sharply over the past 50 years and is projected to continue falling slowly over the next 50 years, there is marked regional variation across the world. In the developed countries fertility is just 1.56 children per woman but in the very least developed countries it is still 5 children per woman. Just eight countries are expected to account for half of the increase in world population by 2050, namely: India, Pakistan, Nigeria, Democratic Republic of the Congo, Bangladesh, Uganda, USA, Ethiopia and China.

Despite the massive increase in the world's population, calculations of worldwide production of primary foods (mainly cereals) indicate that sufficient is produced to meet the estimated nutritional needs of the world population. Yet in some poor countries there is starvation and in other richer countries there are 'mountains' and 'lakes' of surplus food. Poleman (1975) estimated that in the USA, per capita grain consumption was 1800 lb (816.5 kg) per year but less than 100 lb (45 kg) of this was directly consumed with almost all of the rest being used as animal feed. An animal consumes between 3 lb (1.4 kg) and 10 lb (4.5 kg) of grain to produce 1 lb (450 g) of meat. In 1995, per capita grain consumption was 250 kg per year in the developing world but 665 kg per year in the industrialized nations. The USA is the world's largest producer of surplus grain. The primary cause of worldwide malnutrition is not inadequate food production per se but an imbalance in the way this food is distributed between the peoples of the world. Differences in wealth are the key determinant of this uneven distribution.

The image of rapid world population growth outstripping growth in food production and being entirely responsible for creating current food shortages is not borne out by the statistics. Wortman (1976) estimated that, in developed countries, rates of food production between 1961 and 1975 rose by almost 40 per cent on a per capita basis. Even in developing countries, population growth did not entirely negate the substantial increases in absolute food production when they were expressed on a per capita basis. Sanderson (1975) suggested that even though population growth had exceeded even the most pessimistic forecasts, worldwide grain production had increased by enough to theoretically allow a 1 per cent annual improvement in world wide per capita consumption. Wortman (1976) predicted that world food production was likely to keep up with population growth for some time to come. A report in 1995 by the International Food Policy Research Institute (see IFPRI, 1996) confirmed that this trend of increasing per capita grain production also continued over the period 1970–95. The world population grew by around 2 billion (55 per cent) over this period but was offset by a 64 per cent increase in world cereal production. In developing countries, *per capita* grain production increased by 15 per cent and by 10 per cent in industrialized countries. The *per capita* availability of food calories was also higher in the early 1990s than the early 1970s in all of the major developing regions of the world. Over the 20 year period from 1970 to 1990 the number of chronically undernourished people in the world fell by 17 per cent but still amounted to 780 million people. This global improvement masks some regional disparities; the number of undernourished people rose slightly in south Asia and almost doubled in sub-Saharan Africa where over 20 per cent of the world's malnourished people now live. The absolute number of pre-school children who were malnourished actually rose over this 20-year period (to 184 million) although the proportion of malnourished children fell because of the increase in the population. Any encouraging aspects of the figures in the IFPRI report should not mask the massive scale of malnutrition and food insecurity that still afflicts the developing world. In a more recent overview of the world food situation, von Braun (2005) made the following estimates of the prevalence of worldwide nutrition problems:

- 0.9 billion people suffering from hunger, i.e. a deficiency of calories and protein
- 126 million children underweight because of inadequate food intake and frequent disease
- over 2 billion people affected by a vitamin or mineral deficiency.

von Braun (2005) suggests that there was very little progress in reducing hunger during the 1990s and that what little progress there had been was very uneven. China markedly reduced its number of hungry people but rates in the rest of the developing world actually rose, e.g. by 20 per cent in sub-Saharan Africa since 1990. Likewise the number of underweight children rose in most parts of Africa in the period 2000–05 but decreased in the other developing regions. von Braun (2005) highlighted vitamin A deficiency, iron deficiency anaemia and zinc deficiency as increasing the probability of early death in women and children, impairing the intellectual development of children and generally reducing quality of life. He estimated that vitamin A deficiency adversely affects the immune system of 40 per cent of young children in the developing countries

and is responsible for an annual toll of a million child deaths. Perhaps half a million children go blind each year due to vitamin A deficiency and millions of children are stillborn, have a birth defect or are permanently mentally impaired by iodine deficiency.

Many severe problems remain despite massive increases in world food production since the 1970s. How was the massive growth in cereal production since 1970 achieved? Most of the increase has been the result of increased yields rather than increases in the land area under cultivation. In Asia, cereal yields have doubled and those in Latin America increased by about two-thirds. The three major factors responsible for this 'Green Revolution' are (IFPRI, 1996):

- increased use of modern high-yielding crop varieties
- increased irrigation of land
- increased use of fertilizers and pesticides. Use of fertilizers by farmers in developing countries quadrupled over this period.

In contrast with the other developing regions of the world, cereal production in Africa remained stagnant over the period 1970–95 largely for the reasons listed below.

- African farmers have lagged behind in the use of new crop varieties.
- Less arable land is irrigated in Africa; only 8 per cent of African farmland is irrigated compared with 37 per cent in Asia.
- African farmers make less use of agricultural chemicals; Asian farmers use seven times more fertilizer than African farmers.

Can the rate of increase in production seen in 1970–95 be maintained in future decades? According to von Braun (2005) world cereal production in 2004 was a record at well over 2 billion tons; an increase of 9 per cent on the 2003 production. So cereal production is still increasing according to the latest estimates although most of the increase is still occurring in the developed countries especially in the USA and European Union.

The increased production of food to feed the growing world population has had a number of adverse environmental consequences. This has increased concern about whether the increases in food production are sustainable in the longer term using current approaches. Discussion of these issues is beyond the scope of this book but some of the important issues are listed below (for further information and discussion see Food and Agriculture Organization (FAO) 1996; IFPRI, 1996; World Resources Institute (WRI), 1997).

- Destruction of forests to increase the availability of arable land which can increase soil erosion, affect global climate and deprive forest dwelling people of their source of food and way of life.
- Adverse ecological effects of excessive use of agricultural chemicals.
- Overuse of irrigation. This can lower the water table, lead to salinization of land and make it agriculturally unproductive.
- Depletion of the world's fish stocks.

Key points

- Food production is sufficient to satisfy the nutritional needs of the world population but this food is unevenly distributed.
- Affluent countries have almost three times the *per capita* grain consumption of developing countries. This extra grain is fed to animals to produce meat and milk.
- The rate of world population growth has fallen sharply since its peak in the 1960s and the Malthusian predictions of rapid population growth leading to worldwide famines and epidemics now look too pessimistic.
- The world population almost doubled over the period 1960–95 but *per capita* grain production and energy availability increased largely because of increasing grain yields.
- The number of chronically malnourished people fell during this period but malnutrition in children and adults, including vitamin and mineral deficiencies, remains a huge problem in much of the developing world.
- The massive increases in grain yields seen during the 'Green Revolution' have been largely achieved by increased use of modern high yielding varieties, greater irrigation of farmland and greater use of agricultural chemicals.
- Africa has been relatively slow to adopt these changes and the Green Revolution has largely bypassed Africa where grain production stagnated in the period 1970–95.
- Rates of malnutrition rose sharply in sub-Saharan Africa over this period.

- The increase in food availability has led to destruction of large areas of forest, salinization of land due to over-irrigation, overuse of agricultural chemicals and depletion of the world's fish stocks.

Effects of income on food selection in industrialized countries

Even in industrialized countries, the food choices of the wealthiest and the poorest may vary quite considerably. Data presented in the previous edition of this book showed that by the end of the millennium most households in Britain owned a deep freeze and a microwave oven but nearly a fifth of the poor unemployed did not own a freezer and about a third did not own a microwave oven. This has implications for the economic purchasing and preparation of food as discussed later in this section. In the UK Food and Expenditure Survey (Department for Environment, Food and Rural Affairs (DEFRA), 2006) there is a simple analysis of food expenditure according to household income; the participating households are divided up into fifths (quintiles) according to their household income and comparisons made between the food purchases of these quintiles and its nutrient content. This analysis shows a number of interesting general trends, and some of these are listed below.

- The amount of milk and cream purchased decreases progressively with increasing income, but cheese purchases rise with income.
- The amount of sugar and preserves decreases markedly with increasing income and the highest income quintile purchases less than half of the amount purchased by the lowest income quintile.
- Purchases of fats and oils decrease progressively with increasing income.
- Fruit purchases increase with increasing income.
- Potato and cereal purchases decline with increasing income.
- The amount spent on eating out increases sharply with rising income and the amount spent by the highest quintile is well over three times that spent by the lowest income group.
- Purchases of alcoholic drinks increase with increasing income especially that consumed outside of the home.

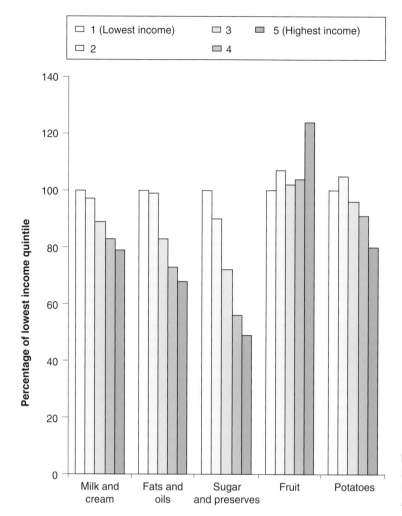

Figure 2.3 *Trends in amounts of household foods purchased according to income quintile. Data source: DEFRA (2006).*

Figure 2.3 illustrates some of these trends in household purchases across income quintiles.

Although this analysis is useful for highlighting such clear trends its usefulness is restricted in that the average size and composition of the households in the different quintiles varies markedly as does the average age of the household reference person (the HRP is the person whose occupation is used to classify the socioeconomic status of the family). For example the lowest quintile has an average of 1.2 adults and 0.3 children per household and the average age of the HRP is 59 years whereas in the highest quintile there are an average of 2.4 adults and 0.7 children and the average age of the HRP is only 45 years. An alternative mode of analysis used by DEFRA (2006) is to classify households according to the occupational category of the HRP. This classification also effectively splits families into income groups but in this case household composition and average age of the HRP is similar across the groupings. This analysis has been used to construct Tables 2.2 and 2.3.

Table 2.2 shows a comparison of the food-related spending of families in these different socioeconomic groupings based on the occupation of the HRP (DEFRA, 2006).

The average household income of the highest income group is more than five times that of the unemployed group shown in Table 2.2. Spending on household food and drink (excluding alcohol) is 60 per cent higher in the high-income group than the unemployed group and still 30 per cent higher than that of the group employed in routine occupations. Yet this household food spending represents over three times the proportion of household income in the unemployed group compared with

Table 2.2 Differences between the food and drink expenditure of rich and poor families in the UK*

	Group A	Group B	Group C
Total household income (£/week)	1299	460	231
Household food and drink (excluding alcohol, pence/per person/week)	2270	1741	1420
% Total household income	5	10.2	16.6
Eating out food and drink (excluding alcohol, pence/per person/week)	1243	575	511
All food and drink (excluding alcohol, pence/per person/week)	3513	2316	1931
% Total household income	7.8	13.6	22.6
All alcohol (pence/per person/week)	859	538	472
% Total household income	1.9	3.2	6.0
kcal obtained per penny (excluding alcohol)	1.5	2.5	2.6

*Data are from DEFRA (2006) and are based on the following classification using the occupation of the household reference person:
Group A: employed in a higher professional or managerial capacity by a large employer.
Group B: employed in routine work.
Group C: never employed or long-term unemployed.

the high-income group. These gaps widen still further if food and drink eaten outside the home and alcoholic drinks are included in the food spending. Despite spending much less on their food and drink, the poorer groups obtain almost as many calories per person per day and so they must inevitable obtain more calories for every penny they spend (see Table 2.2). The poorer groups are, of necessity, more economically efficient (judged on calories alone) in their food spending. This increased efficiency could be achieved in many ways such as:

- less purchasing of unnecessary items such as bottled water or alcohol
- buying cheaper brands
- shopping in the cheapest shops
- reducing waste
- buying lower quality (or lower prestige) items that provide more calories per penny, e.g. cheaper types of meat and fish and cheaper meat and fish products
- taking more advantage of special offers and promotions or simply taking more advantage of seasonal fluctuations in prices of many foods
- doing more food preparation at home rather than buying relatively more expensive prepared foods or eating out
- adopting a totally different, cheaper eating pattern with much larger quantities of starchy foods, inexpensive vegetables and legumes but less animal foods. This dietary pattern could be

described as more 'primitive' but could also be more in line with current nutritional guidelines.

Table 2.3 compares some of the purchasing practices of our three selected economic groups. Some of the trends in Table 2.3 are discussed briefly below.

- Compared with the highest income group, total meat purchases were slightly higher in the poorer employed group and markedly lower in the unemployed group. However, in the higher income group a larger proportion of the total meat purchased was fresh carcass meat. The poorer groups got considerably more meat for each penny they spent than the richer group, implying that they bought cheaper cuts and bulkier, lower quality meat products.
- As with meat, the poorer groups got more fish for each penny than the richer group again implying higher use of cheaper varieties of fish and fish products.
- The poorer groups bought more sugar and preserves and more fats and oils than the richest group.
- The poorer groups bought much less fruit and less vegetables (excluding potatoes) than the richer group. The unemployed bought only around half as much fruit as the richest group. People in Britain and the USA are being encouraged to eat more of these foods; at least five portions each day have been suggested. However, despite all of their nutritional merits (see Chapter 4), these

Table 2.3 Comparison of the food purchases and its nutrient content in different income groups in the UK*

	Group A	Group B	Group C
Meat and meat products (g/per person/week)	*1018*	*1091*	*903*
% Carcass meat	*21.7*	*20.3*	*19.4*
Spending (pence/per person/week)	*539*	*459*	*341*
Grams of meat/penny	*1.89*	*2.38*	*2.65*
Fish (g/per person/week)	*151*	*132*	*107*
Spending (pence/per person/week)	*110*	*68*	*52*
Grams of fish/penny	*1.37*	*1.94*	*2.06*
Fats and oils (g/per person/week)	*142*	*183*	*205*
Sugars and preserves (g/per person/week)	*86*	*144*	*135*
Vegetables (g/per person/week) (excluding potatoes)	*1127*	*966*	*774*
Fruit (g/per person/week)	*1400*	*844*	*723*
Vitamins and minerals (all %RNI)			
Calcium	*124*	*124*	*108*
Iron	*103*	*98*	*79*
Zinc	*101*	*100*	*86*
Vitamin A	*122*	*114*	*90*
Riboflavin	*152*	*148*	*125*
Folate	*141*	*130*	*107*
Vitamin C	*192*	*142*	*127*

RNI, recommended nutrient intake.
*Data are from DEFRA (2006) and are based on the following classification using the occupation of the household reference person:
Group A: employed in a higher professional or managerial capacity by a large employer.
Group B: employed in routine work.
Group C: never employed or long-term unemployed.

foods are relatively inefficient providers of energy because of their low energy density (see Chapter 6). Fresh fruit and vegetables (excluding potatoes) accounted for only 3.5 per cent of household food energy (excluding alcohol) but over 12 per cent of expenditure whereas fats, sugars and preserves provided over 12 per cent of household food energy but only accounted for about 2.5 per cent of the expenditure.

- The estimated vitamin and mineral intakes (calculated from food purchases) was generally lower in the lowest income group, i.e. those without employment. Some of these differences were large, e.g. compare the intakes of the highest income and unemployed groups for iron, zinc, vitamin A, folate and vitamin C as shown in Table 2.3.

In an analysis from the National Food Survey (Ministry of Agriculture, Fisheries and Food (MAFF), 1997) in the previous edition of this book, it was also found that poorer groups bought less of products that could be considered as non-essentials from a nutritional standpoint, e.g. they bought less than a quarter as much mineral water. There were also several examples of the poorer groups being less likely to make the healthier choice within a category such as:

- less of the bread bought by the poorer groups was whole grain and much more of it was standard white bread
- less of the milk bought by the poorer groups was low fat and much more of it was whole milk
- less of the soft drinks bought by the poorer group were low-calorie versions.

The most recent DEFRA (2006) household expenditure survey measures what people buy rather than what they eat. A number of assumptions about wastage and family distribution are made to estimate nutrient intakes (see Chapter 3 for details). The

National Diet and Nutrition Survey (NDNS) programme is a rolling programme of surveys that
record reported food consumption using weighed
inventories of different age groups of the British
population (this programme is described more fully
in Chapter 3). The latest NDNS survey of British
adults under 65 years (Hoare *et al.*, 2004) compared the intakes of men and women in households
who were and were not in receipt of state benefits.
Some of the differences found between these two
groups are listed below and in general they tend to
confirm the trends already discussed using the analysis from DEFRA (2006) in Table 2.3. Comparing
adults in household not in receipt of state benefits
with those in benefit receiving households, in those
receiving benefits:

- energy intakes were lower
- intakes of dietary fibre were lower
- added sugars made up a higher proportion of
  dietary energy in women
- average intakes of vitamins and minerals were
  generally lower and so were average blood levels
  of micronutrients.

A significantly higher proportion of women had
intakes of vitamin A and riboflavin that were
below the lower recommended nutritional intakes
(LRNI) (the point at which intakes are classified as
inadequate – see Chapter 3) and many more had
intakes of iron that were below the LRNI.

Key points

- Poorer families are less likely to own a freezer
  and less likely to own a microwave oven.
- Poorer families eat out much less often than
  richer ones and spend much less when they do
  eat out.
- Richer families spend more on household food
  than poorer ones but this represents a much
  smaller proportion of their total income.
- Poorer families are much more economically
  efficient in their food purchasing and obtain
  more calories per penny, e.g. they tend to buy
  cheaper types of meat and fish and meat and
  fish products.
- Poorer families buy more cereals, potatoes,
  sugar and fats than richer families but fewer
  fruit and fresh vegetables.

- Poorer households consume fewer non-essential
  items such as mineral water and alcoholic drinks.
- Poorer families are less likely to buy the
  'healthier' option within a category, e.g. bread
  made with less refined flour, low-fat milk and
  low-calorie soft drinks.
- Recorded energy intakes are lower in adults
  receiving welfare payments.
- Intakes of most vitamins and minerals were
  lower in the lowest socioeconomic groups as
  were average blood levels of micronutrients.
- Intakes of dietary fibre were lower in the lowest
  socioeconomic groups.
- More women in benefit-receiving households
  had intakes of vitamin A, riboflavin and iron
  that were below the lower reference nutrient
  intake (LRNI).

The minimum cost of a healthy diet

Welfare payments in the UK have traditionally been
calculated on the basis that enough money should
be provided to allow purchase of the essentials of
life but not enough to allow purchase of luxuries.
The same underlying philosophy governs the welfare systems of most industrialized countries. These
welfare payments should be enough to prevent
claimants from starving or being deprived of basic
shelter and clothing but not make their situation so
comfortable as to discourage them from seeking
employment or to encourage others to voluntarily
live off of the state. A more cynical Marxist interpretation of this principle would be that enough
money is provided to prevent social unrest but not
enough to reduce the competition for jobs and thus
risk increasing the cost of labour. Pressures on public expenditure may encourage governments to
economize by reducing the purchasing power of
those who are dependent on welfare payments.

Calculation of minimum subsistence levels of
income will be difficult ones. There are a host of
factors that will produce wide variations in the
quality of life that different families can achieve
with the same level of income. At the physiological
level, people vary in their energy and nutrient
requirements. Regional and individual variations in
housing, transport and fuel costs may make it difficult to produce a single welfare figure for a nation.
Differences in cultural and personal preferences

will affect the size of the required food budget. A minimally adequate income may make it difficult to live at maximum economic efficiency. For a variety of reasons such as those listed below it is often true that 'the poor pay more'.

- The poorest may be forced to buy in small expensive quantities; they can only afford to buy enough to meet immediate needs.
- They may be unable to stock up when a seasonal food is cheap or when special offers are made, e.g. because they do not own a freezer or simply lack capital.
- They may not have the transportation or personal mobility to allow them to shop at the most economic places.

Table 2.4 shows the potential magnitude of some of the differing costs of buying in small and large quantities. Webb and Copeman (1996) surveyed the differences in unit costs of the same brands of common grocery items in a large London supermarket. The general trend was for decreasing unit cost

with increasing pack size, penalizing those who need to buy in minimum quantities to satisfy immediate needs. There was often a sharp decrease in unit cost often between the smallest pack and the next smallest size to the disadvantage of those living alone or buying enough for one. Special offers tended to be concentrated in the largest packs and many special offers were in the form of discounts for multiple purchases. One would generally expect all household costs (e.g. replacement of capital items, rental charges and fuel costs) to rise on a *per capita* basis as the size of the household decreases, so increasing pressure on the food budget of poor, small households.

Those people who are forced to shop in smaller, more accessible shops may also have to pay much more. In a survey conducted in the Reading and Oxford areas of England in 1991, the cost of a basket of 21 food items was about a quarter higher in small independent grocery stores than in the supermarkets owned by the large multiple chains (Henson, 1992). The unit cost of milk bought in half gallons

Table 2.4 Differences in costs of small and large packs of a variety of grocery items obtained from a large London supermarket in early 1995. All comparisons are between same brands and prices are pence per unit (variable) and so are directly comparable within items[*]

Item	Small size	Unit price (pence)	Large size	Unit price (pence)	% Price difference
Cucumber	Half	70	Whole	49	43
Mushrooms	113 g	155	453 g	115[†]	35
Peas (can)	142 g	8.3	300 g	5.4	54
Margarine	250 g	14.8	1 kg	11.9	24
Corned Beef	198 g	36.4	340 g	28	30
Rice	500 g	11.8	4 kg	9.3	27
Baked beans	150 g	14	420 g	7.4	89
Chicken	Quarter chicken	99	Whole chicken	68[†]	46
Eggs	6	98	12	89	10
Cooking oil	500 mL	74	1 L	59	25
Weetabix	12	68	48	46	48
Tea bags	40	40.8	160	33.8	21
Milk	473 mL (1 pt)	28	2.8 L (6 pt)	22.2	26
Instant coffee	50 g	212	300 g	179	18
Washing-up liquid	500 mL	126	1 L	99[†]	26
Sugar	500 g	90	1 kg	62	45
Burgers (frozen)	4	43.7	20	36	15
White bread	400 g	6	800 g	4.4	36
Flour	500 g	48	1.5 kg	27.4	75

[*]From Webb and Copeman (1996).
[†]Denotes special offer.

(2.3 L) from large supermarkets in the UK is only half of that from the traditional doorstep delivery services. Major supermarkets are offering 'economy' white bread at less than a quarter of the cost in many small independent grocers.

Other demands on the household budget may greatly restrain food expenditure for some individuals or families. When financial resources are restricted, especially if there is a sudden decline in income (e.g. through loss of employment, retirement or long-term illness), then expenditure on food may be sacrificed to maintain spending upon other essentials such as housing, loan repayments, clothing or fuel. Food expenditure may be sacrificed to allow purchase or retention of some prestigious item or activity that helps maintain self-esteem, e.g. Christmas presents for children, a car, a cable/satellite television subscription, a computer, internet access, tobacco or going to the pub. Considerable savings can often be made in the food budget without obvious acute hardship, e.g. by switching to cheaper brands or varieties, by reducing wastage and by using cheaper alternatives such as margarine for butter or lower quality meat and fish products for fresh meat and fish.

Dobson *et al.* (1994) published a survey of the food buying and dietary habits of low-income families living in the English Midlands. Almost all of these families were in receipt of welfare payments (income supplement) and half of them had mothers as lone parents. Money and the cost of foods were seen as the most important factors in deciding what food could be bought. Other factors, such as taste, cultural acceptability and healthy eating, could only be considered in the light of what was economically available. These parents often saw incorporating advice about healthy eating as impractical or only partly practical in their economic circumstances. These families all reported great difficulties in managing on their incomes. Unexpected demands for money could derail their spending plans and at these times the food budget was often reduced to cope with these unexpected demands. These families needed to adopt various strategies to cope with their restricted food budgets.

- They needed to shop around for 'best buys' and this made shopping a time-consuming activity that they ceased to enjoy.
- Parents often reported going without food themselves to minimize the impact on their children.

- The need to avoid waste of food and money meant that children's preferences were given high priority. They did not have the means to provide foods that reflected the individual tastes of family members; parents often ate what their children would eat irrespective of their own likes and dislikes. They all had to eat the same food at the same time.

The burden of coping with the money available was largely borne by the mothers who did most of the shopping and food preparation. They tried to maintain a culturally usual 'mainstream' diet. This meant that they had to eat cheaper versions of mainstream meals. Parents went to great lengths to make sure that their children were seen to be eating the same things as their peers even if it meant making sacrifices themselves. They resisted radical changes to their diets.

To subsist on a minimum income is easier for those with some degree of budget management skill. Unfortunately those with the least of these skills may often be those most likely to be required to exercise them; poor educational attainment and poor socioeconomic status are strongly correlated. Strictly theoretical calculations of minimum subsistence levels cannot allow for food choices that appear irrational or even irresponsible using strictly biological criteria. People whose self-esteem has been dented by unemployment, disability or social deprivation may buy foods to boost their spirits and self-esteem rather than out of strict scientific necessity. In *The Road to Wigan Pier* George Orwell gives an example of an adequate but dull and low-prestige diet that in 1937 could be obtained for 20 pence (40 cents). He also gives an example of the real expenditure of an unemployed miner's family at the time. This real family spent only 4 pence each week on green vegetables and sweetened condensed milk, nothing at all on fruit, but 9 pence on sugar (representing 4 kg of sugar), 5 pence on tea and 3 pence on jam. Clearly white bread spread with margarine and jam and washed down with sweet tea was an important part of this family's daily diet. Orwell describes this mixture as being almost devoid of nutritional value and it certainly was low in several vitamins and minerals.

> When you are unemployed, which is to say when you are underfed, harassed, bored and miserable, you don't want to eat dull wholesome food. You

want something a little bit tasty ... Unemployment is an endless misery that has got to be constantly palliated, and especially with tea, the Englishman's opium. A cup of tea or even an aspirin is much better as a temporary stimulant than a crust of brown bread.

George Orwell (1937) The road to Wigan pier.
London: Victor Gollantz Limited.

Readers who would like a more scientific and detailed review of trends in the British diet between 1841 and 1994 should see Charlton and Quaife (1997). Orwell goes on to describe the poor people of a British industrial city as being small of stature and having universally bad or missing teeth – he suggests that it was rare to see a working class person with good natural teeth. He suggests that the death rate and infant mortality rate of the poorest area of any city were always at least double that in the wealthy areas, in some cases much more than double. He was writing about mid-twentieth century peacetime conditions in one of the wealthiest industrialized countries of the world. These few pages of Orwell's book underline how far social conditions and nutrition of most poorer people in Britain have improved over the past 70 years despite the disparity between the health and nutrition of rich and poor that still remains.

One practical consequence of the sort of effect described in the above quotation will be to make it even more difficult to persuade the less affluent to make dietary changes that they perceive as reducing either the palatability or prestige of their diet. It is important to their self-esteem that they and especially their children are seen to be eating like their peers (Dobson *et al.*, 1994). Diet-related disease is more prevalent in the poorer groups but they also seem to be more resistant to nutritional and other health education advice. The decline in prevalence of breastfeeding with social class (Hamlyn *et al.*, 2002) is a very clear example of this. This increases the onus on those seeking to effect dietary change among all social groups to suggest changes that are simple, economically feasible, easy to permanently incorporate in usual culinary practices and are not overly restrictive of highly palatable and high-prestige foods. Change must not require the consumption of a diet that, although wholesome by current nutritional criteria, is perceived as dull and unpalatable, uses low-prestige ingredients or is simply different from the mainstream.

Changes must also be within any group's economic means if they are really expected to be implemented. Groom (1993) and Leather (1992) review a number of attempts to devise 'healthy' diets that comply with UK dietary guidelines and are also within the economic means of poorer families. In 1991 in the UK, MAFF produced a 'low-cost, healthy diet' that could be purchased for £10 (US$20) per person per week at 1991 prices. However, it was suggested by Leather (1992) that this diet would be so different from the mainstream British diet as to be totally unrealistic. It would require, e.g.:

- almost total exclusion of meat and most dairy products from the diet
- a very large increase in bread consumption and most of this bread would have to be eaten dry without butter or margarine
- large increases in consumption of tinned fruit and frozen vegetables.

It is easy to produce lists of ingredients that meet any set compositional criteria within a very small budget but it is much more expensive to purchase a collection of ingredients that can also be combined into meals that make up a culturally acceptable diet. Dobson and colleagues' survey (1994) discussed earlier found that maintaining a mainstream diet was very important to low-income families. The Family Budget Unit at York University estimated the cost of a 'modest but adequate' diet which would not only be adequate and comply with current nutrition education guidelines but also be broadly in line with the usual diet of the UK population. Using these criteria their minimum cost for feeding an adult couple was about 70 per cent more than the minimum cost diet produced by MAFF in 1991(see Leather, 1992). This modest but adequate diet cost slightly less than average *per capita* food expenditure but significantly more than that spent by low-income families. To stay as close as possible to current eating patterns but to choose 'healthier' alternatives such as leaner meat, wholemeal bread and fruit leads to a substantial increase in food costs which may be beyond the practical means of many low-income families.

Families living in 'temporary' bed and breakfast type accommodation may face yet another extra financial burden. They may have little or no cooking facilities and thus be forced to rely on eating out, which is expensive, or rely largely upon cold foods that require no further cooking. Relying largely on cold foods also has its disadvantages; the diet is less varied and palatable, quite different from the diet of the culture. The minimum cost of eating a healthy diet is likely to be higher (perhaps around 15 per cent higher according to Leather, 1992).

Key points

- Welfare payments aim to provide enough money for the essentials of life but not enough to discourage people from working.
- Many factors will affect how much money any given family needs to provide a modest lifestyle, which makes setting the level of welfare payments a difficult and flawed process.
- Poverty may reduce the practical purchasing power of those on low incomes, e.g.:
  - if they cannot reach the cheapest shops
  - lack the storage facilities or capital to buy special offers
  - have to buy in small quantities to meet immediate needs.
- For low-income British families, financial considerations are the most important factors governing food choice. For these families, incorporating advice on healthy eating is seen as impractical.
- Poor families maximized economic efficiency by shopping around and avoiding waste. To avoid waste, children's preferences were given high priority.
- Poor families tried to maintain a mainstream diet and parents made personal sacrifices to prevent their children being stigmatized by eating differently from other children.
- Poor families resisted radical changes to their diets.
- During times of financial pressure, the food budget may be pared to allow spending on other essential items or bills.
- People struggling with difficult economic circumstances do not always make selections that are scientifically logical. They may buy foods that are palatable or help to maintain their self-esteem rather than those that are cheap and nutritious.
- It is possible to produce very low-cost lists of ingredients that meet particular nutritional criteria but these may involve eating a diet that is very different from the mainstream.
- The minimum cost of a healthy diet increases markedly if the ingredients must combine to make a culturally acceptable mainstream diet.
- Lack of cooking facilities will reduce the food choices of poorer people and raise the cost of a healthy diet.

CULTURAL AVAILABILITY

Beef is physically and economically available to devout Hindus in the UK but religious conviction makes it culturally unavailable. Under normal circumstances, people only eat things that are culturally recognized as foods. People choose things that in their culture are considered appropriate for the particular meal or occasion and that are suitable for the lifecycle group to be fed. This has been discussed earlier in the section dealing with consumer classification of food. The cultural acceptability of a food may change as it becomes physically more available and more familiar. The indigenous population may initially view unfamiliar immigrant foods with suspicion and even distaste but with time they may become more familiar and acceptable. Chinese foods and curry are now almost as much a part of British culture as fish and chips. Similarly, immigrants tend to gradually adopt some of the foods and dietary practices of the indigenous population. Exposure to alien foods through foreign travel may have a similar effect.

Dietary taboos

The word taboo is derived from the Polynesian name for a system of religious prohibitions against the use of sacred things. It has come to mean any sacred prohibition and, with common usage, the religious connotation is no longer obligatory. One could define a dietary taboo as any avoidance that is maintained solely because failure to do so would generate disapproval, ostracism or punishment within one's own cultural group or because it would compromise one's own ethical standards. A food taboo should be distinguished from a food avoidance that is based on sound empirical evidence of harm.

Many taboos are aimed at avoidance of flesh and these are often rigorously adhered to. It is said that the initial spark that ignited the Indian Mutiny against British rule in 1857 was the introduction of cartridges supposedly greased with animal fat. Hindu troops were unwilling to bite the ends off of these cartridges or, indeed, even to handle them. On 6 May 1857, 85 of 90 members of the third native cavalry in Meerut refused direct orders to handle cartridges which, according to a contemporary account, they mistakenly believed to be contaminated with animal fat. They were subsequently sentenced to terms of imprisonment of between 6 and 10 years. These men would undoubtedly have been aware of the likely consequences of their disobeying a direct military order, which underlines the potential strength of such taboos.

The taboos of other cultures tend to be viewed as illogical restraints often imposed upon individuals by authoritarian religious leaders. This model leads to the belief that taboos should be discouraged. This is almost certainly a misreading of the situation in most cases. Most taboos need little external compulsion to ensure adherence; people feel secure when maintaining cultural standards that have been ingrained since childhood. There are nonetheless a few examples of essentially religious taboos being incorporated into the secular law and of severe penalties being imposed upon transgressors. In many Indian states, the cow is legally protected and there are severe penalties for alcohol consumption in some Muslim countries.

Most people of western European origin would not consider dietary taboos to have any significant influence on their food selection but no society is completely free of dietary prohibitions. It is not too long ago that Roman Catholics were required to abstain from meat on Fridays and some Christians still avoid meat on Good Friday. In the UK, cannibalism is clearly prohibited but, equally, the consumption of animals such as cats, dogs and horses would result in widespread hostility and probably ostracism by other members of society. Most British people would not recognize these as taboos because they do not classify these creatures as potential food despite their being highly regarded as foods in some other countries. In France, for example, horsemeat is eaten, sometimes even meat from British horses!

In the UK, vegetarianism would seem to be an obvious candidate for an example of a dietary taboo that may have negative nutritional implications. Certainly many omnivores would like to think so, as the vegetarian's rejection of flesh is often perceived as a threat to highly desired and high-prestige foods. There are some problems associated with a strictly vegetarian (**vegan**) diet (see Chapter 17). However, a well-constructed vegetarian diet can be healthy and in the current climate of nutrition opinion may even be regarded as healthier than the typical omnivorous diet. Vegetarianism must be socially inconvenient where most of the population is omnivorous and where caterers may make only nominal provision for vegetarians. These inconveniences may, however, be more than compensated for by a comradeship, akin to religious fellowship, seemingly shared by many vegetarians and by enhancement of self-actualization.

Perhaps, taboo also played some part in the dramatic decline in breastfeeding that occurred in Britain in the decades following World War II or at least in thwarting current efforts to encourage breastfeeding. The inconvenience of breastfeeding and its 'prestige' can only have been worsened by a very strong taboo against breastfeeding amongst strangers; sometimes even amongst friends and relatives. The lack of provision of a suitable environment for feeding babies in most public places increases this problem. The arrival of a modern, scientifically developed and socially acceptable alternative provided women with an ideal opportunity to free themselves of the need to continue with this 'inconvenient and embarrassing process'. A survey conducted by the Royal College of Midwives in 1993 found that more than a third of the 700 restaurants surveyed either would not permit breastfeeding at the table or would ask women to stop if another customer complained. In a second survey, half of men disagreed with women breastfeeding 'in any place they chose'. They gave reasons for their objections like 'it's unnecessary' 'it's a form of exhibitionism' 'it's disgusting behaviour' (both of these surveys are briefly summarized in Laurent, 1993). Hamlyn *et al.* (2002) reported that a quarter of women said that one reason they chose not to breastfeed was because they did not like the idea or found it embarrassing (even higher numbers in previous versions of these quinquennial surveys). Clearly breastfeeding is seen by many men (and many women too) as a distasteful or embarrassing task that needs to be performed furtively. In Britain, images of bare female breasts are ubiquitous in popular newspapers, television, films and even on some beaches and yet the sight of a woman breastfeeding her baby apparently still has the potential to shock and embarrass a high proportion of British adults.

Many of the best-known taboos are permanent but some are only temporary. Some of the temporary ones may apply only during certain phases of the lifecycle or during illness. Some taboos may be restricted to certain groups of people. The familiar permanent religious taboos generally cause few nutritional problems. The temporary ones will also not usually give rise to adverse nutritional consequences unless they are imposed at times of rapid growth or other physiological stress. An extreme example quoted by Fieldhouse (1998) are the varied food avoidances among the women of the southern Indian state of Tamil Nadu. During lactation, for example, women should avoid meat, eggs, rice, dhal, chillies, cow milk, sardines, fruits, potato, yam, cashew nuts and onions. These avoidances would compound with previous restrictions during pregnancy and this could have serious nutritional consequences. There is a widespread belief among various peoples that sick children should not be fed or should only be offered very restricted diets, thus potentially precipitating **protein energy malnutrition**. There is also a widespread belief that many adult foods, especially meat and fish, are unsuitable for young children. This leaves only the starchy staple foods with their problems of low energy and nutrient density as the major permitted food at this time of high physiological demand for energy and nutrients.

If most dietary taboos are not usually associated with any major adverse nutritional consequences, then why should nutritionists and nutrition educators study them? They provide an insight into a culture and some understanding is necessary if the general philosophy of giving advice that is culturally compatible is to be maintained. If advice is given that involves breaking an important dietary taboo then all of the advice may be ignored and, perhaps, the future credibility of the adviser destroyed. Maybe, even worse, if certain individuals are persuaded to conform to this advice then this may provoke friction and divisions within a community or family.

If a taboo is nutritionally only marginally detrimental, neutral or perhaps even beneficial in its impact then, no matter how bizarre or irrational it may seem, the cultural choice of the client should be respected. Some of the practices of the adviser may seem equally bizarre to the client. If a taboo is manifestly harmful then the aim of the adviser should be to eliminate the harmful impact with the minimum disruption to the cultural life of the client.

The conclusion that a taboo is harmful should be based on a wide analysis of its impact. Fieldhouse (1998) used the example of the Hindu sacred cow to make this point. There are nearly 200 million cows in India and yet their slaughter for food is generally forbidden even in times of famine – illogical? harmful? He points out that cows provide milk and their dead carcasses provide leather and are used as food by the lower castes. Cows provide the oxen traditionally vital for Indian agriculture; cow dung is also a major source of fuel and fertilizer in rural India. Yet they scavenge much of their food which is basically inedible to humans. The conclusion that this taboo is harmful is now less secure and the value of the taboo in preventing destruction of these valuable and well-adapted animals in adverse conditions is, at least, arguable.

Taboos are often derived from some religious commandment, be it in the religious book of the group, the oral mythology or the edict of some historical religious leader or teacher. Many theories as to their origins exist such as in the list below; each can give plausible explanations of some taboos and often these different theories can be used to give equally plausible explanations of the same taboo.

- *Aesthetic.* Particular animals are rejected because of the perceived unpleasant lifestyle of the animal, e.g. some people consider the flesh of the mackerel as low-prestige or inferior fish because they regard the mackerel as a scavenger. All meat may be rejected because of the perceived cruelty involved in rearing and slaughter.
- *Health and sanitation.* The belief that there is, or was, some inherent logic underlying the exclusion of particular foods on health grounds. In effect, it is suggested that taboos originate from avoiding foods that are harmful. For example, the Jewish prohibitions against shellfish consumption may have been prompted by the risk of poisoning by the toxin produced by the plankton species *Gonyaulax tamarensis* that the shellfish may have consumed (see Chapter 18).
- *Ecology.* There is said to be some underlying environmental logic behind a particular prohibition. The exclusion of meat and fish at particular times to conserve stocks is an obvious example. The avoidance of meat by some present-day

vegetarians to prevent inefficient use of grain and thus to increase world food availability would be another.

- *Religious distinction.* Taboos serve to demonstrate the separateness of a religious group from non-believers and the self-restraint required to obey them may serve as a symbol of piety and obedience to the religious leaders.

The avoidance of pork by Jews is a well-known taboo and each of the above theories can be used to explain its origins (see below).

- *Aesthetic.* The pig is widely viewed as a dirty and scavenging animal even by people who value its flesh. Jewish dietary law states that only animals that have cloven hooves and that chew the cud are clean and therefore edible. The pig is considered unclean and therefore inedible.
- *Health and sanitation.* Pork in a source of a parasitic worm that causes the disease, trichinosis. Perhaps this is the origin of the Jewish taboo against pork which is shared by other Middle Eastern peoples? Opponents of this theory argue that this is merely a later attempt at scientific rationalization. The risk of trichinosis has also been used as an argument against horsemeat consumption in France.
- *Ecology.* It is suggested that supernatural prohibitions against the consumption of pork arose because the desert conditions of the Middle East were unsuitable for efficient pig rearing. Proponents of this theory argue that taboos rarely involve abundant species that can be eaten with no threat to total food supplies.
- *Religious distinction.* It is suggested that the pork taboo was originally part of a relatively lax and general prohibition against 'imperfect' animals, including flightless birds and shellfish. Its symbolic importance was heightened when Syrian invaders forced Jews to eat pork as a visible sign of submission and thus once Jews regained their independence, strict pork avoidance came to symbolize their Judaism and their opposition to pagan rule.

Key points

- People will normally only eat things that they recognize as food and things that they see as culturally acceptable and appropriate.

- Many religions have taboos against the consumption of particular foods but a religious context is not always present.
- People will often go to great lengths to avoid breaking a taboo and there is little need for external compulsion to ensure compliance.
- Some examples of taboos in western Europeans might be: vegetarianism, the avoidance of horsemeat in Britain, and perhaps even the avoidance of breastfeeding in public could be classed as a taboo.
- In general, the permanent religious taboos seem to have few adverse nutritional consequences but multiple taboos imposed at times of physiological stress, e.g. childhood, pregnancy or illness, may have greater potential to do harm.
- Dietary advisers need to be aware of taboos and avoid giving advice that would require breaking a taboo.
- There are several theories about the origins of taboos:
  - an animal or fish becomes taboo because of its unpleasant or 'dirty' lifestyle
  - they originate because the avoidance confers some biological or ecological benefit, e.g. avoidance of a foodborne disease or ecological damage
  - they are a mechanism for binding a religious group together and distancing them from non-believers.

Effects of migration on eating habits

Migrant groups are frequently used by epidemiologists when they try to distinguish between the environmental and genetic influences upon the disease patterns of populations (see Chapter 3). Migrants may also have nutrition-related problems that may be much rarer both in their native homeland and amongst the indigenous population of their new homeland. For example, migrants to the UK from the Indian subcontinent have suffered from mini epidemics of **rickets**, a condition that had been largely eliminated in the white population. These Britons of south Asian origin also have much higher rates of **type 2 diabetes** than the rest of the population and largely as a consequence of this have much higher mortality from coronary heart disease (see Chapter 16). It is, therefore, useful to try to establish and understand trends and patterns to the changes in dietary habits that inevitably occur after migration to answer questions such as:

- What factors influence the speed of change?
- Why is the health record of migrant groups often worse than that of the indigenous population?
- Are there any measures that might facilitate the healthful assimilation of migrant groups into their new environment?

Why should change occur at all? Culture, including food habits, is a learned phenomenon rather than something that is innate or biologically determined. Culture is transmitted between generations by the process of socialization. There is an inherent tendency of cultures to change over time. Although conflicts will inevitably arise between traditional influences and influences from the new culture, this process of change is almost inevitably greatly hastened by migration and exposure to the different cultural practices of the indigenous population. **Acculturation** is the term used to describe this acceleration of cultural change that occurs when different cultures interact. Both indigenous and migrant cultures are likely to be changed by their interaction but migrants may feel the need to adopt aspects of the indigenous culture to facilitate their acceptance and assimilation into their new country. They will usually be in a minority and be dependent on the goodwill of the indigenous population; they may therefore feel great pressure to conform to be accepted and to succeed in their new homeland.

Paradoxically, every culture also has a built in resistance to change. Culture is mostly internalized; routine activities done unthinkingly in a particular way because that is the way they have always been done. After migration, however, there is repeated exposure to different culture practices and familiarity may eventually lead to acceptance of initially strange and alien practices as normal. Dietary practices of the indigenous culture that are inconsistent with the values and beliefs of the migrants' culture may be the slowest to be adopted and also those most likely to cause social divisions within migrant communities or families. For example, migrants may be most reluctant to absorb dietary practices that would involve breaking of the food rules of their religion. The older, more conservative, migrants will probably be most resistant to such changes and may also be hostile to changes in the behaviour of younger, less ethnocentric members of their community or family. Dietary practices of migrants that are inconsistent with the values of the indigenous culture may also be a source of considerable friction between migrants and their fellow citizens. For example, Muslim and Jewish rules concerning the slaughter of animals have in the past provoked hostility in Britain from people concerned about animal welfare.

Bavly (1966) analysed changes over three generations in the diets of immigrants to Israel. She considered that several factors had a major accelerating effect on the speed at which change occurred:

- marriage between different ethnic groups
- the homemaker working outside the home
- children receiving nutrition education at school
- children having school meals
- nutrition education via the media for immigrants of European origin.

Although this work was done some time ago, these specific influences given by Bavly may be generalized to factors that increase interaction with the indigenous population and increase familiarity with, and understanding of, indigenous dietary practices. Conversely, any factors that tend to isolate the migrant from the indigenous population and culture may be expected to slow down acculturation, such as those listed below.

- Inability to read or speak the new language restricts interaction at the personal level and restricts access to the media.
- Cultural beliefs that discourage the homemaker from independent socializing outside the family.
- Religious beliefs and dietary rules that are at odds with the dietary practices of the indigenous majority.
- Living within a fairly self-contained immigrant area with shops that are run by fellow migrants and where familiar foods and even native language media are available.
- Many of these isolating influences would apply to many new immigrants from the Indian subcontinent to Britain.

Migration is often prompted by the attraction of improved economic opportunities and this encourages much migration from developing to industrialized countries. Thus large-scale migration is often accompanied by a complete change of social structure from a rural agrarian to a Western industrial-type of society. In the rural agrarian community, society is likely to be based on extended and close-knit family groupings with a constant flow of food between families and individuals. In Western industrialized societies, this informal family and community support may no longer be available because they are organized into relatively isolated family groups, food is normally shared only with the immediate family and this sharing may help to define the family. These changes in social organization may mean that in times of hardship, the missing informal neighbourhood and family support will have to be replaced by formal charitable or state welfare support. The impact of such changes may be ameliorated where movement is into an established ethnic community.

Migrants from a rural food-orientated economy may suddenly be confronted with a cash-dominated economy. Family incomes of new immigrants are likely to be relatively low (inappropriate skills, language problems, discrimination, etc.). This combination of low income and lack of experience in cash budgeting may make them unable to cope adequately, even though the income may be technically adequate. An educational induction programme might reduce the impact of this potential problem. Food selection for migrants may be complicated by the unavailability of recognizable traditional foods; even where they are available they may be relatively expensive because of their specialist nature. Food selection by immigrants may be particularly influenced by advertising pressures that encourage the excessive consumption of foods that are high in palatability and prestige but of relatively low nutritional value. Social and cultural pressures may discourage migrant women from breastfeeding their infants.

Migration from a rural agrarian society in a developing country to a Western industrial society will probably be associated with overall trends that are similar to the worldwide changes that accompany increasing affluence. The traditional starchy and predominantly vegetarian diet is likely to diversify, become more omnivorous, and sugars and fats will progressively replace some of the starch. The diseases associated with nutritional inadequacy will decline but the chronic diseases of industrialization will almost certainly become increasingly prevalent.

Wenham and Wolff (1970) surveyed the changes in the dietary habits of Japanese immigrants to Hawaii and their descendants. Japanese migrants began arriving in Hawaii at the end of the nineteenth century to become plantation workers. The typical Japanese diet at this time was a high-carbohydrate, predominantly rice and plant food diet. The major animal foods would have been fish and other seafood. Initially these migrants maintained their traditional diet; many regarded their stay in Hawaii as temporary and ate frugally in order to save for their return to Japan. After the annexation of Hawaii by the USA in 1898, these Japanese migrants started working outside of the plantations and businesses specializing in the importation of traditional Japanese foods sprang up. Initially this resulted in increased consumption of imported and high status Japanese foods. As these Japanese foods became cheaper, their status diminished and came to be regarded as old-fashioned by many younger Japanese who preferred to eat American foods. Note that a recent rapid influx of migrants into Britain from new European Union countries in eastern Europe has rapidly led to the opening of many shops specializing in the sale of eastern European foods in areas where large numbers of these migrants have settled.

Wenham and Wolff describe how among the Japanese migrants to Hawaii, the traditional Japanese social structure with its strong family tradition, worship of ancestors and subordination of personal desires to the welfare of the family was replaced by a more fragmented and personal-freedom orientated society. The traditional Buddhist restrictions on the consumption of meat became weaker as meat was plentiful in Hawaii. Public education seems to have been a catalyst for change amongst the second generation as the schools encouraged them to change their food and other habits. There also seems little doubt that World War II accelerated the 'Americanization' of Japanese in Hawaii. Wenham and Wolff describe a Japanese wedding in Hawaii before the war as being typically Japanese in character with no wedding cake, but by 1945 the food at such a wedding was likely to be much more cosmopolitan but with a Western wedding cake as the highlight. The authors concluded that in 1970, the Japanese in Hawaii could be classified into three groups:

- a traditional group of mainly older people who maintained a very Japanese cuisine
- a group that, despite being relatively acculturated, still consumed Japanese foods on some occasions

- an 'Americanized' group who rejected their Japanese heritage and the foods associated with it.

There may now exist yet a further category of Japanese-Americans who are moving back to traditional foods for health reasons and to reaffirm their ethnic identity (i.e. for reasons of self-actualization).

Williams and Qureshi (1988) suggested a similar 'four generation' concept that could be a useful way of explaining some of the variations in food choices within any particular ethnic minority group in the UK.

- *First generation A.* Made up of migrants who arrived as dependant relatives of migrant workers. They are usually retired and prefer to eat their native foods.
- *First generation B.* Migrants who arrived as workers. They are usually aged 21–65 years and they accept both native and British foods.
- *Second generation.* Young people aged 7–21 years who have been to school in Britain and in many cases are born here. They prefer the new diet and may strongly resist attempts to force them to consume their native diet, which is alien to them.
- *Third generation.* Children who are born in Britain, who feel British but who have become interested in tracing their ethnic roots. They accept both British and native foods.

Key points

- The disease patterns of migrants provide information upon the relative importance of genetic and environmental factors in the aetiology of diseases.
- Migrants often have poorer health than other members of the new community.
- Migrants tend to gradually adopt elements of the diet and lifestyle of their new country – they tend to acculturate.
- The indigenous population may also adopt some elements of the migrant culture and diet.
- Changes will be slowest where the dietary practices of the indigenous population are in conflict with the values and beliefs of the migrants, e.g. where they would involve breaking a religious taboo.

- The adoption of change by some migrants may be a source of conflict with their parents and elders.
- Anything that increases interaction between the migrants and the indigenous population and familiarizes the migrants with the indigenous diet will tend to speed up the rate of change, e.g. women working outside the home and children taking school meals.
- Anything that prevents interaction will slow down the rate of acculturation, e.g. language barriers, restrictions on women working and socializing outside the home or living within a fairly self-contained immigrant community.
- Migrants to an industrialized country from a rural area with an agricultural food-based economy may find it difficult to cope with the new cash-based economy, particularly as their incomes are likely to be relatively low.
- Several stages in the acculturation process have been recognized and these are summarized below.
  - People who have recently migrated may initially try to stick closely to their familiar diet and people who migrate later in life may remain in this category for the rest of their lives.
  - Younger adult migrants who enter employment will become familiar with the new diet and tend to eat both the new and traditional foods.
  - Children of migrants who attend school in the new country may become so acculturated that they prefer the new diet and resist eating their traditional foods, perhaps to increase their sense of belonging and acceptance by their peers.
  - Descendants of migrants born or brought up in the new country may seek out their ethnic roots and eat foods associated with these roots to reaffirm their ethnic and cultural identity.

'GATEKEEPER' LIMITATIONS ON AVAILABILITY

The housewife has traditionally been regarded as the family **gatekeeper** regulating the availability of food to her family. If most food is eaten within formal family meals and if food purchasing and meal construction is largely the province of the housewife then she has the potential to impose limitations on the availability of foods to the other family members. The personal beliefs and preferences of the gatekeeper may greatly affect their choices and thus the diet of the whole family. A vegetarian gatekeeper may effectively impose vegetarianism on other family members or conversely a non-vegetarian gatekeeper might refuse to provide a vegetarian alternative to a family member who would wish to be vegetarian. Convenience of preparation may affect the choices of the gatekeeper. Appreciation or criticisms by other family members will feedback and also be an important influence on her future choices. A number of social changes in industrialized countries might be expected to have undermined the traditional gatekeeper role of wives and mothers:

- more food tends to be eaten outside the home or is purchased by the individual consuming it
- ready made versions of dishes that have traditionally been home made shifts control over composition from the housewife to the food manufacturer
- other family members are more likely to participate in the shopping and food preparation
- within the home, there is more snacking or 'grazing' on self-selected foods available in the larder or refrigerator and less formal family meals.

Despite a diminution in this gatekeeper role of the mother, even within a traditional two-parent family, it may still be quite considerable. Certainly much food advertising is still directed towards the gatekeeper housewife. Advertisers emphasize factors such as the convenience of foods to a busy housewife and provide images of wives and mothers who have served the promoted food receiving acclaim from an appreciative and therefore loving family. Nicolaas (1995) conducted a survey of a representative sample of 2000 British adults on their attitudes to cooking and their cooking behaviour. This survey showed a marked divergence between attitudes and actual behaviour and suggested that the traditional gatekeeper role of the oldest adult female was still largely intact in British families. Almost all the participants thought that it was important that both sexes had basic cooking skills and to teach their children how to cook. Almost all agreed with the proposition that boys should be taught how to cook. When questioned about their actual behaviour, however:

- 80 per cent of women but only 22 per cent of men claimed to prepare every meal in their household
- 3 per cent of women and 18 per cent of men admitted to never preparing a meal.

Most of the women who never prepared a meal were in the 16–24 year age group and the frequency in this age group was similar to that of young men. The complete dataset strongly suggests that the majority of young people in this age group who live with their parents rely on their mothers to cook for them. In older age groups there is an even greater difference between male and female responses than those summarized above for the total sample. When adult men and women live together as partners it is usually the female who does most of the cooking.

Catering managers may exert a considerable gatekeeper influence over those living in institutions such as hospitals, prisons, retirement homes, boarding schools and to a lesser extent those taking lunches at school or work place. Older people living at home may have inexpensive weekday main meals delivered to them by a 'meals on wheels' service. The Caroline Walker Trust (CWT, 1995) has suggested nutritional standards and sample menu plans for 'meals on wheels' and meals provided in residential homes for the elderly.

If someone is subject to the gatekeeper influences of someone from a different cultural background then they may effectively be subject to a double dose of limitation due to cultural availability. The gatekeeper may only offer foods that are culturally available to them and only some of these may be culturally available to the consumer. Unless caterers make special provision for cultural/ethnic minorities then this may severely restrict the real choices of such people, e.g. hospital patients from minority groups.

Even those people seemingly immune to the influence of gatekeepers, such as the affluent person living alone, may still use staff dining facilities in the workplace. They may have limited time available for food preparation or low incentive to cook just for themselves. They may thus rely heavily on commercially pre-prepared meals or restaurants.

Key points

- Wives and mothers have traditionally been the gatekeepers in western European families but anyone who caters for someone else is acting as a gatekeeper.

- Despite major social changes, the gatekeeper role of women is largely intact in British families and women are still largely responsible for selecting and preparing the family meals.

- Gatekeepers can have almost total control over what some people eat and thus their scope for making dietary changes may be dependent on the goodwill and co-operation of their gatekeeper.

- The range of food that is truly available may be considerably narrowed if a person is reliant on a gatekeeper from a different cultural background, e.g. someone from an ethnic minority relying on a white gatekeeper.

- Almost everyone is subject to some gatekeeper influences.

3

Methods of nutritional surveillance and research

INTRODUCTION AND AIMS OF THE CHAPTER

The methods used to study nutrition range from the high precision measurements of the analytical chemist through to the inevitably much less precise methods of the social scientist and behavioural psychologist. All approaches can be equally valid and rigorous, and the complete range of approaches is necessary to study all of the various aspects of nutrition.

The aims of this chapter are:

- to make readers aware of the range of methods that are available for nutritional surveillance and research, how they are performed, their strengths and limitations, their general theoretical basis and the circumstances in which different methods are more or less appropriate. This is a first step towards successful use of these methods
- to give readers a sufficient insight into the methods of nutritional surveillance and research to enable them to read the literature critically. An understanding of the relative strengths and the limitations of the methods used is essential for any critical evaluation of the conclusions drawn from reported data. Some perception of the errors inherent in methods of measurement is necessary for realistic appraisal of the results that they produce.

NUTRITIONAL ASSESSMENT AND SURVEILLANCE

Strategies for nutritional assessment

There are two ways of approaching the assessment of dietary and nutritional status.

1 One can try to determine whether the nutrient intake (or nutrient supply) is adequate to meet the expected needs of the individual or group under investigation. Three key tools are need to make this assessment:
   - a method of measuring the amounts of foods being eaten (or perhaps the available food supply)
   - a way of translating the amounts of foods being consumed into quantities of energy and essential nutrients, i.e. tables of food composition
   - some yardstick of adequacy that can be used to determine whether the measured intakes of energy and essential nutrients are sufficient for that individual or group. These standards of dietary adequacy are called **dietary reference values (DRVs)** in the UK. The term(s) **recommended dietary/daily allowances (RDAs)** have been widely used elsewhere, including the USA.
2 One can make observations and measurements on the individuals concerned to determine whether they have been receiving adequate

amounts of energy and essential nutrients. The three types of indicator that can be used to make this assessment are:

- *clinical signs.* One can look for clinical signs or the symptoms of a nutrient deficiency
- *anthropometry.* Anthropometric measurements such as body weight and height can be compared with appropriate standards or used to monitor changes within the individual or group over time
- *biochemical assessment.* Biochemical measurements, usually on blood or urine samples, can indicate either the general nutritional status of the donor or the status with regard to any specific nutrient.

Key point

- Dietary and nutritional status can be determined either by assessing the adequacy of the nutrient intakes of the subjects or by monitoring clinical, anthropometric or biochemical indicators of nutritional status.

Measurement of food intake

Measures of food intake have a variety of purposes:

- to assess the adequacy of the diets of populations, groups or individuals and to identify any problem nutrients
- to relate dietary factors in populations or individuals to disease incidence or **risk factors** such as plasma cholesterol concentration
- to compare the diets of different countries, regions, socioeconomic groups and different age and ethnic groups
- To monitor changes in the diets of populations, groups or individuals over time and thus, for example, to monitor the effectiveness of nutrition education programmes.

Population or group methods

Food balance sheets
These are used to estimate the average *per capita* food and nutrient consumption of nations (see Figure 3.1 for summary). Food balance sheets usually yield no information about distribution within the population. They will not show, for example, regional differences in nutrient intakes, socioeconomic influences on

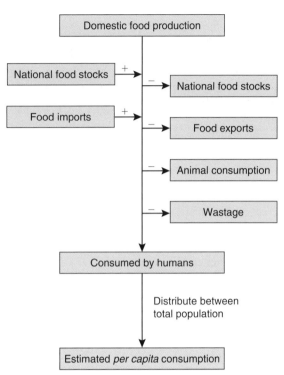

Figure 3.1 *Schematic diagram to illustrate how food balance sheets can be used to estimate* per capita *food consumption in a country.*

nutrient intakes or age and sex differences in nutrient intakes. Domestic food production is first estimated. Governments and international agencies (e.g. the Food and Agriculture Organization of the United Nations, (FAO)) routinely make estimates of total crop yields and total agricultural production of countries. Allowance is made for any change in food stocks within the country during the period. Any food imports are added to the total and any exports are subtracted from it. This estimate of food available for human consumption must then be corrected for wastage and any food not consumed by humans, e.g. animal fodder and pet foods (see Figure 3.1). Such methods allow crude estimates of population adequacy and crude comparisons of actual intakes with nutrition education guidelines to be made. They also allow international comparisons, e.g. comparison of the average *per capita* energy intake of different populations, or relating average *per capita* sugar consumption to rates of dental caries in different populations.

Home-produced food and small-scale production sites will be a potentially large source of error in these estimates. Wastage will be difficult to estimate accurately and will probably depend on the affluence of the population – the rich are likely to waste more than the poor. In the European Union (EU), construction of national food balance sheets has been complicated by the introduction of the single market and the consequent reduction in checks on movements of food between member states.

The average intakes of residents of an institution can similarly be estimated from the amount of food entering the institution over a period of time.

Household budget surveys

The **National Food Survey** of the UK is an example of a national household survey that was undertaken annually for about 60 years (e.g. Ministry of Agriculture, Fisheries and Food (MAFF), 1997). This survey ended in 2001 when it was replaced by the **Expenditure and Food Survey**, which is an amalgamation of the National Food Survey and another national survey that had been running since 1957, the Family Expenditure Survey. Data from the Expenditure and Food Survey relating to food and drink are now published under the title Family Food (e.g. Department for Environment, Food and Rural Affairs (DEFRA) 2004). These three surveys provide an important historical record of changes in the British diet over more than half a century; MAFF (1991) reviews the changes recorded in the first 50 years of the National Food Survey.

In the National Food Survey, one member of a nationally representative survey of 7000–8000 households was asked to record in a diary all food entering the household for human consumption during 1 week; both the amounts of food and the expenditure on food were recorded. Records were collected at different times throughout the year and home-grown food was included in the log. Until 1992 no information was collected about alcoholic drinks, soft drinks (soda) or confectionery (candies), as these are often purchased by individual family members. From 1992 onwards such purchases made for home consumption were recorded and the nutritional analyses presented both including (total household food and drink) and excluding these products (household food excluding soft drinks, alcohol and confectionery); this allowed comparisons to still be made with results from earlier years. For most of its existence no detailed information was collected in the National Food Survey on meals eaten outside the home, merely the number of such meals consumed

by each family member was recorded. In the latter years of the survey some information on meals eaten outside the home was recorded and reported separately from household food and drink.

The Family Expenditure Survey which also ended in 2001, used a similar sized representative sample to that of the National Food Survey. In this survey, every household member aged over 16 years was issued with a diary to record all expenditure including food expenditure, but amounts of food were not recorded. The recording period was 14 days and once again the sampling was spread throughout the year.

The Expenditure and Food Survey uses similar representative samples of UK households to those used in the two surveys it replaced. The recording period in this survey is 14 days and all household members aged 7 years or over complete a diary. Each person's expenditure on all items including food and drink is recorded and where possible amounts of food purchased are also recorded; where this is not possible (e.g. food eaten out) amounts are estimated using standard portion sizes. It is intended that free food such as free school meals and meals provided by employers will eventually be included in this survey. However, this was not done in the first 2 years. Information is also recorded concerning the composition of the household, the ages and sexes of the family members and their ethnic origin, the family's income and socioeconomic status and the region of the country in which it lives.

When data from the old National Food Survey and Family Expenditure Survey were compared, substantial differences in estimates of food expenditure between the two surveys were found (Paterakis and Nelson, 2003). The data from the new Expenditure and Food Survey was considered by DEFRA (2003) to be more comparable with the old Family Expenditure Survey than the National Food Survey. Complex adjustments have been applied to the results of this new survey to make them comparable with those obtained from the National Food Survey and so allow historical comparisons and trends followed; details of this adjustment procedure can be found in DEFRA (2003).

The Expenditure and Food Survey and its antecedents can be used for many purposes such as those listed below. Many other countries also conduct household budget surveys that can be used for some or all of these functions depending on exactly how they have been conducted.

- The UK household budget surveys can be used to monitor changes in UK food purchasing practices over time. They can thus, for example, be used to monitor the effects of health promotion campaigns, price changes, the effects of 'food scares' (like the bovine spongiform encephalopathy (BSE) crisis in Britain) and to correlate changes in diet with changes in measures of health and disease. In Chapter 4, the Expenditure and Food Survey and its antecedents will be used to quantify some of the major changes in the British diet over recent decades, such as the massive switch from animal-derived cooking and spreading fats to those made from vegetables oils. Changes in the scope and execution of these surveys over time have to be borne in mind and allowed for when making historical comparisons.
- These surveys provide information about regional differences in dietary habits within the UK. These data may explain some of the regional differences in the health and disease patterns within the UK.
- They provide information on differences in food purchasing practices of different ethnic groups within the UK.
- They provide information on seasonal patterns of food purchasing.
- They provide information about differences in the diets of different socioeconomic groups. One can compare the diets of rich and poor, the diets of young and old, the diets of the employed, unemployed and retired. One can compare diets of households with 'reference adults' in different occupational categories.
- The Expenditure and Food Survey gives us information about how food purchasing and eating habits differ according to family structure. One can compare the diets of single adult or two adult families with those that have varying numbers of children.
- It is possible to make crude estimations of the supply of energy and essential nutrients in UK diets and thus the probable levels of dietary adequacy and highlight nutrients whose intakes may be less than satisfactory. One can also make crude estimations of the degree to which current diets comply with current dietary guidelines. One can monitor how intakes of nutrients are changing with respect to both standards of adequacy and dietary guidelines for the prevention of chronic disease.

There are several errors and uncertainties when household budget surveys such as the UK. Expenditure and Food Survey are used to quantify what people eat. Some examples are given below.

- These surveys do not measure what people eat; they measure what they buy. Differences in wastage rates and preparation practices will not show up in the Expenditure and Food Survey. For example, if a family buys 500 g of meat but trims the fat off before they eat it, this will give the same record as another family that buys this meat and eats all of the fat. Similar temporal changes in food preparation practices may also occur, but not show up in these surveys.
- Families may change their purchasing behaviour during the survey period, e.g. they may buy more food than usual and this tendency may be proportionately greater in lower-income groups.
- The survey may not be truly representative of the whole population. Some groups are excluded from the survey such as the single homeless and those low-income families housed 'temporarily' in bed and breakfast type accommodation. Some poorer groups may be deterred from participating in the survey because of embarrassment about the diet they can afford (see Leather, 1992). According to DEFRA (2004) only 60% of those families selected for the Expenditure and Food Survey responded, which was a lower response rate than in past surveys.
- No attempt is made to record distribution of the purchased food between family members although assumptions about wastage, distribution and losses of nutrients during cooking and preparation are made to estimate individual intakes of food and nutrients. These surveys can only estimate average consumption per person. One consequence of this is that, for example, the average *per capita* expenditure on food decreases with increasing family size, partly because children tend to eat less than adults (it may also be more economic to buy in bulk).
- When the recording is done by a single family member, as with the old National Food Survey, then snacks, drinks and sweets brought by other family members, which they consume outside the home, go unrecorded in the household log; this should be less likely with the Expenditure and Food Survey where all family members aged 7 years and above keep an expenditure diary.

- Paterakis and Nelson (2003) noted marked differences in the food expenditure data provided by the old National Food Survey and Family Expenditure Survey. They noted that there were also substantial differences in time trends between the two surveys, which could lead to different conclusions regarding changes in consumption patterns. This means that the absolute values recorded by any household budget survey will certainly be affected by differences in methodology, making comparisons between surveys problematical, e.g. comparing results from different countries within the EU. Even within countries, conclusions about temporal changes in food purchasing, one of the major strengths of these surveys, may also vary according to the precise methodology.

Individual methods

Individual methods of assessing food intake may either involve prospective recording of food as it is eaten or may assess intake retrospectively by the use of interviews or questionnaires. These methods, almost inevitably, rely to a large extent on the honesty of the subjects.

Retrospective methods

Twenty-four hour recall is frequently used to retrospectively assess the food and nutrient intakes of subjects. An interviewer asks subjects to recount the types and amounts of all food and drink consumed during the previous day. This recalled list is then translated into estimates of energy and nutrient intakes by the use of food tables. The method has often been used in large-scale epidemiological surveys where large numbers of subjects need to be dealt with quickly and cheaply, and where precision in assessing the intake of any individual is deemed not to be essential. The method requires relatively little commitment from the subject and thus co-operation rates tend to be good. As the assessment is retrospective, subjects do not alter their intakes in response to monitoring. Some of the limitations and sources of error in this method are given below.

- *Memory errors.* Subjects can forget some of the items that have been consumed. This method tends to significantly underestimate total calorie intake and seems to particularly underestimate, for example, alcohol intake. This method, even when used

with probing to try to improve memory, probably under-records energy and most nutrients by at least 20 per cent. This makes any assessment of the prevalence of dietary inadequacy using this method highly suspect.

- *Quantification errors.* It is difficult to quantify portions in retrospect. It may be particularly difficult for the very young and the very old to conceptualize amounts. Several lists of standard portion sizes have been published. For example, Mills and Patel (1994) have produced a list of weights of individual items (such as chocolate bars) and average UK portion sizes for many foods. The Food Standards Agency in the UK is currently sponsoring research to produce up-to-date information on average food portion weights for adults aged 16–64 years, older adults and different age groups of children. These portion sizes are based on those recorded in the rolling programme of **National Dietary and Nutrition Surveys** (discussed at the end of this section). Food models or photographs are sometimes used to aid this quantification process; subjects are shown photographs of different sized portions and asked to indicate which is closest to the one they ate and a weight for this portion is given. Nelson *et al.* (1997) have published a photographic atlas of food portion sizes.
- *Intra-individual variation.* Intake may not be representative of the subject's usual intake. The day chosen for the record may not be typical of the subject's usual daily intake. Weekend and weekday intakes may be very different in some subjects. Illness or stress may affect the appetite of a subject. Some social occasion or event may exaggerate the subject's usual intake. Even where subjects are of regular habits and no particular factors have distorted that day's intake, the intake of many nutrients tends to fluctuate quite markedly from day to day and thus one day's intake cannot be taken to represent the subject's habitual intake.
- *Interviewer bias.* Any interview-based survey is liable to bias. The interviewer may encourage subjects to remember particular dietary items more than others and thus may obtain a distorted picture of the real diet. If the interviewer indicates approval or disapproval of certain foods or drinks this may also encourage distorted recall. It requires skill and training to take a proper diet history.

It might seem logical to extend the recall period to get a more representative picture of a subject's usual dietary pattern but, of course, memory errors can be expected to increase exponentially as the recall period is extended. It is possible to use a succession of 24-hour recalls to get a more representative picture of an individual's habitual intake. A more representative picture of dietary pattern may be obtained by taking detailed **dietary histories** or, as is more frequently done, by using **food frequency questionnaires**. The investigators may be interested in the intakes of particular nutrients and thus the frequency of consumption of the types of foods that contain these nutrients may give a useful indication of the usual intake of that nutrient. For example, assessing the frequency, types and amounts of fruit and vegetables consumed would be a useful guide to vitamin C or β-carotene intakes. Food frequency questionnaires are not suitable for assessing actual intakes of nutrients but are useful for categorizing individuals into low, medium and high intakes for any selected nutrient.

Prospective methods

The **weighed inventory** requires that the subjects weigh and record all items of food and drink consumed over a predetermined period (a week is often used). The operator must then translate this food inventory into nutrient intakes with food tables. Household measures (e.g. cup, spoon, slice) can be recorded in a **food diary** rather than subjects being required to weigh everything. This clearly involves some loss of accuracy in determining the size of portions of many food items. However, as a whole, these prospective methods have the advantage of being direct, accurate, current and of variable length, allowing more representative assessments of average intakes to be made. Some disadvantages of these methods are:

- subjects may still forget to record some items that they consume, especially snacks
- they are labour intensive for both subject and operator, and considerable motivation and skill on the part of the subject is required for accurate and complete recording. Participation rates may therefore be low and this may make the population sampled unrepresentative of that being surveyed
- this type of recording usually requires that subjects are numerate and literate. To obtain records

from subjects who do not have these skills, a variety of methods have been tried, e.g. subjects can photograph their food and drink, or subjects have been given balances that have a tape recorder incorporated so that the subject's oral description of the weighed food can be recorded

- prospective methods may be invalidated if subjects modify their behaviour in response to monitoring, e.g. in an attempt to impress the operator, to simplify the recording process, or, simply because their awareness of their food and drink intake has been heightened by the recording process. There is evidence that subjects involved in clinical trials may conform to the recommended diet more closely on recording days.

All of the methods of recording food intake described so far require that the estimated amounts of food eaten be translated into amounts of energy and nutrients by the use of some food composition database, i.e. paper food tables or a computerized version of the database. With **duplicate sample analysis**, a duplicate sample of all food eaten is prepared and may be subject to direct chemical analysis. This method does not therefore have to depend on the use of a food composition database. Use of food tables may, for example, overestimate the intake of labile vitamins such as vitamin C in people relying on hospital or other institutional food that has been kept hot for extended periods. For example, Jones *et al.* (1988) found very low vitamin C intakes among a group of long-stay hospital patients when assessed by analysis of representative samples of the food eaten. These intakes were much lower than would have been obtained using conventional food tables. They indicated that prolonged warm holding of food was an important factor in this low intake and suggested it might also apply to other heat-labile nutrients. This method is obviously labour intensive, expensive and requires good analytical facilities. It is most appropriately used in a metabolic research setting.

Box 3.1 summarizes the relative advantages and disadvantages of retrospective and prospective methods of dietary assessment.

Even though the weighed inventory method of assessing food and nutrient intake is very labour intensive, it has been used in Britain to periodically assess the diets and nutritional status of large representative, samples of various age groups of the UK

Box 3.1   Relative merits of retrospective and prospective methods of measuring food intake

Problems with all methods

- *Honesty.* Most methods rely on the honesty of subjects. Records that are clearly invalid may need to be identified and excluded, e.g. recorded energy intakes that are below 1.2 × the basal metabolic rate in non-dieting subjects
- *Under-recording.* For one reason or another most methods tend to under-record energy intakes and there is considerable evidence that this under-recording is more pronounced in obese people
- *Intra-individual variation.* It is assumed that the intake of nutrients during the monitored period is representative of habitual intakes. It will require several days of monitoring to get a reasonable assessment of habitual intakes for most nutrients. For some nutrients (e.g. vitamin A) for which intra-individual variation is particularly great, it may require longer
- *Population sampling bias.* When sampling populations one assumes that the sampled group is representative of the total test population. The more commitment and skill a method requires the less likely this is to be true. Some groups may be difficult to access, e.g. homeless people, disabled people. When sampling some groups, e.g. young children or the very elderly, one may need a proxy to carry out the recording
- *Food table errors.* All methods except duplicate sample analysis rely on the use of food tables. This may be a particular problem in determining intakes of residents in hospitals and care institutions where prolonged warm holding may destroy much of the heat-labile vitamin content

- *Coding errors.* When subject records are analysed, some entries may be ambiguous and misclassified

Retrospective methods

Advantages

- Tend to be quick and cheap
- Require little commitment from subjects so tend to get high participation rates
- Honest subjects cannot change their habits in response to monitoring because the food has already been eaten

Disadvantages

- Very prone to memory errors
- Retrospective quantification can be difficult
- Interviewer may influence the subject

Prospective methods

Advantage

- Greater accuracy because less prone to memory and quantification errors

Disadvantages

- Require commitment and competent record keeping by subjects and this can reduce participation rates
- Subjects may deliberately or unwittingly modify their eating in response to monitoring, e.g. to simplify recording, to deceive/impress the recorder or simply because of heightened awareness

population. Since 1986 there has been a rolling programme of **National Dietary and Nutritional Surveys** (the NDNS programme). These surveys aim to provide comprehensive information of the dietary habits and nutritional status of Britons in all age groups and to monitor changes in these over time. The programme began in 1986/7 with the collection of data for the first NDNS survey of British adults aged 16–64 years (Gregory *et al.*, 1990), and it has been followed up by a series of other reports on other age groups:

- the NDNS survey of children aged 1.5–4.5 years (Gregory *et al.*, 1995)

- the NDNS survey of people aged over 65 years (Finch *et al.*, 1998)
- the NDNS survey of young people aged 4–18 years (Gregory *et al.*, 2000).

The most recent survey in this programme is the new NDNS survey of adults aged 19–64 years, published in five volumes with the fifth being a summary volume (Hoare *et al.*, 2004). The first survey of Gregory *et al.* (1990) was jointly commissioned by the then **Ministry of Agriculture Fisheries and Food** and the Department of Health. The **Food Standards Agency** has now taken over responsibility for the NDNS programme and all five volumes of the latest survey can be accessed free on the internet (www.food.gov.uk/science/dietarysurveys/ndnsdocuments). These surveys have other elements that are relevant to diet, health and nutritional status as well as the results of the weighed inventory. For example, the latest survey of adults (summarized by Hoare *et al.*, 2004) consists of the following elements:

- a dietary interview which determines information on the eating and drinking habits and socio-demographic information such as age, marital status, social class
- a 7-day weighed inventory of all food and drink consumed
- results of a 24-hour urine analysis
- physical measurements such as height, weight (for calculation of **body mass index (BMI)**), waist and hip circumference and blood pressure
- a 7-day activity diary
- results of a blood test for biochemical indicators of nutritional status and plasma cholesterol levels.

Key points

- Measurements of food intake can be used to assess dietary adequacy, to monitor the degree of compliance with nutritional guidelines, to make comparisons between groups or populations and to relate dietary variables to disease risk.
- The food intakes of populations can be determined by the use of food balance sheets, by representative surveys of household food purchases (such as the UK Expenditure and Food Survey) or even by assessing the individual diets of representative population samples.
- Individual methods of assessing food intake can be retrospective or prospective. One can either ask subjects to provide information about what they have already eaten (e.g. 24-hour recall or a food frequency questionnaire) or ask subjects to record what they consumed over a period, e.g. 7-day weighed inventory.
- Choice of method of measuring food intake will depend on the time and resources available and also on the purpose of the measurement.
- The advantages and disadvantages of the various methods are listed in Box 3.1.

- The rolling NDNS programme in the UK uses a weighed inventory together with blood and urine analysis and physical measurements to periodically assess the dietary practices and nutritional status of the different age groups of Britons.

Tables of food composition

Food tables are an essential tool of both nutritional surveillance and research. Printed food tables contain lists of thousands of foods and the amounts of each nutrient in a standard amount (100 g) of each food are given. They are based on standard databases such as that maintained by the **US Department of Agriculture (USDA)** or that maintained in Britain by the Royal Society of Chemistry on behalf of the DEFRA. To translate food intakes into nutrient intakes with such printed tables is very tedious and time-consuming. The content of each nutrient in the consumed portion of each food has to be calculated from the tables and eventually the total consumption of each nutrient determined.

Nowadays, the information in the printed tables is available electronically. The investigator merely keys in the foods and portion sizes and computer software automatically translates these into nutrient intakes. The program not only accept weights of foods but will translate household measures or descriptive portions into estimated weights of food or use a database of standard portion sizes that have been incorporated into the software. These programs will also calculate the nutrient intakes as proportions of the standard reference values appropriate for a subject whose size, age, sex, activity level and reproductive status has also been entered. Both forms of these tables are the result of thousands of hours of meticulous analytical work. To give the nutrient contents of 1000 foods requires more than 30 000 individual determinations and many more if individual amino acids and fatty acids are included. A detailed discussion of these analytical methods is beyond the scope of this book. A few of these methods are discussed in other sections of the book, e.g. determination of the energy content of foods is outlined in Chapter 6 and the protein content of foods in Chapter 10.

The analytical methods used to determine the nutrient content of foods are often extremely precise with a very low level of measurement error.

However, several sources of error are inherent in the use of food tables and these may produce errors and uncertainties that are orders of magnitude greater than the errors in the analytical methods. Food tables can only give an indication of the typical or average composition of a food and that may in some cases be very different from the actual composition of the sample of food that has been eaten. Some of these errors are given below.

Food tables – problems and errors

Limited range of foods covered by tables

The major databases mentioned above each contain several thousand different food items, including many menu items from the major restaurant chains. Despite this, there will inevitably be foods eaten that are not specifically listed in the printed tables or computer software that uses them. In such circumstances the operator either has to find other sources of information (such as nutritional information on the food label) or has to judge what food is the nearest equivalent in the food tables. For example, British tables do not specifically list goat meat, which is frequently used as an ingredient in curry, so one would use the composition of generic curried meat. Continued innovation on the part of food manufacturers and increased availability of foods from different parts of the world means that this will be an ongoing problem. In fairness, it is now quite difficult to find gaps in the British database and the range of foods listed has increased substantially over the past couple of decades. It includes many foods traditionally eaten by Britain's long-established minority ethnic communities, although the recent influx of migrants from eastern Europe will not yet have been fully catered for in the existing database.

Recipe variations

Many dishes are extensive mixtures of foods and it often not practical in diet records or histories to obtain the precise mixture of ingredients used in the preparation of a particular dish. Even though the food tables may list this dish, the recipe used for the analysis in the tables may be quite different from that consumed. Thus, for example, bolognese sauce is something that will be listed in the tables but will vary markedly in its composition from cook to cook. The range and proportions of the main ingredients used, leanness of the meat, the amount of thickening agent (e.g. flour) and salt, and the proportion of water may all vary considerably. When estimating the nutrients in something like a slice of pie, the proportions of crust and filling used by the analyst may be different from those that were actually eaten.

Brand variation

Different brands of the same commercially prepared foods will also vary and the composition of any single brand may vary significantly from batch to batch. There are several brands of 'baked beans canned in tomato sauce'; food tables can only give an average or typical composition.

Nutrient supplementation

Some foods may be supplemented with nutrients; this could be a source of considerable error if the supplementation in the analysed and eaten food is different, e.g. if only some brands of a food are supplemented or if American food tables are used to analyse British bread.

Biological variation

Just as different brands and recipes of prepared foods vary in their composition so different varieties of natural foods will vary in their composition. There may even be marked variation, particularly seasonal variation, within the same variety. Rump (buttock) steak from different cattle may have markedly different proportions of fat and lean. The vitamin C content of apples varies greatly between different varieties. The vitamin D content of milk varies between summer and winter. Once again food tables can only indicate an average or a typical composition.

Method and duration of storage

The nutrient content of foods changes during storage. Milk left in strong sunlight loses much of its riboflavin (vitamin B_2). The vitamin C content of main crop potatoes after 8–9 months of storage will be only about a quarter of that when they were freshly dug and stale vegetables generally may have lost much of their original vitamin C. Foods on which mould has grown may acquire dietetically significant amounts of vitamin B_{12}. Warm holding of food before it is eaten may lead to destruction of most of the heat-labile vitamins.

Vitamin precursors and variants

Some vitamins may have several different chemical forms or may be present in the form of a precursor. When the vitamin activity of foods is assessed then the activity contributed by the different chemical forms must be estimated and added together. Vitamin A activity in food is due to vitamin A itself (retinol), the plant-derived pigment β-carotene and other plant pigments that have vitamin A activity, such as cryptoxanthin and α-carotene (see Chapter 12). The niacin (vitamin B_3) derived from food may either come directly from vitamin in the food or indirectly by conversion of the amino acid tryptophan to niacin.

Bioavailability of vitamins and minerals

Food tables can give a precise estimate of the amount of a chemical in a food, but they give no indication of its bioavailability, e.g. how much of it is absorbed in the gut. Iron from meat is much better absorbed than that from vegetable sources and iron absorption is increased by vitamin C and alcohol but decreased by fibre and tannin. The calcium in milk is much better absorbed than that in most other foods. There may also be doubt about the biological activity of some forms of a vitamin in foods, e.g. some of the conjugated forms of folic acid.

Use of table and cooking salt

Salt is often added to food during cooking and at the table. A weighed inventory and standard food tables are therefore regarded as an unreliable means of estimating an individual's total salt intake.

Calcium from bone

Pieces of bone in meat and fish may greatly increase the calcium content. With canned fish, the bones are softened and made more readily edible and cutting meat with a saw produces powdered bone that sticks to the meat and is eaten.

Contamination from utensils and cooking vessels

Contact of foods with processing machines or with cooking utensils may significantly affect the content of metallic elements. Cooking or brewing in iron pots may enhance the iron content of foods very considerably, e.g. beer brewed in iron vessels has been a cause of frequent toxic iron overload among the Bantu people of South Africa.

Minerals from cooking water

Cooking food in hard tap water may significantly increase the content of calcium and other minerals. Variation in the content of drinking water may greatly affect the intake of some minerals, e.g. fluoride.

Minerals from adhered soil

Contamination of food with small amounts of soil may affect its mineral content.

Key points

- Food tables contain lists of the nutrient contents of thousands of foods either in paper form or electronically.
- They can be used to convert amounts of food into amounts of energy and nutrients.
- They can only give a typical or average composition and are prone to many limitations and sources of error, such as:
  - some foods may be missing from the database
  - biological variations in the composition of plants and animals and brand, and recipe variations in the composition of prepared foods
  - variation in the method and duration of food storage will affect its composition
  - they take no account of variations in the bioavailability of nutrients
  - the mineral content of foods may be affected by the addition of salt, the presence of adhered bone, mineral content of the cooking water, or leeching of minerals into food from utensils and storage vessels.

Dietary standards and nutrient requirements

Origins of dietary standards

Almost 60 years ago the National Research Council (NRC) in the USA established a committee to produce a comprehensive set of dietary standards. These standards were intended to be a yardstick against which diets or food supplies could be assessed to determine their likely adequacy. The first printed version of these standards appeared in 1943 and they were called **recommended dietary allowances (RDAs)**. These were the first official and comprehensive set of dietary standards. Many other governments and international agencies now regularly publish their own dietary standards and the American RDAs have been revised and republished regularly since 1943. The first edition of these American RDAs (NRC, 1943) covered just six pages and dealt with only 10 nutrients; the current British version of these standards (Committee on the Medical Aspects of Food (COMA), 1991) covers more than 200 pages and deals with more than 30 nutrients.

The first British RDAs were published by the British Medical Association in 1950. In 1969 the first truly official set of UK standards was published by the then Department of Health and Social Security (see Webb, 1994).

Definitions and explanations

For the purposes of setting dietary standards, the population is divided up into subgroups: children are divided up into bands according to their age and sex; and adults are subdivided according to their age and sex with separate standards for pregnant and lactating women. Then standards are set for energy and each nutrient for each of these population subgroups (Table 3.1). These standards are intended for use with healthy people and they make no allowance for the effects of illness and injury on nutrient needs.

The RDA in the USA is the suggested average daily intake of that nutrient that is sufficient to meet the needs of nearly all healthy people in that age and sex grouping. It represents the best estimate of the requirement of those people in the population with a particularly high need for that nutrient. The RDA does not represent the minimum requirement when it is used to assess the diets of individuals. Rather, it should be thought of as lying within a 'zone of safety'; the further intake is below the RDA then the greater is the risk of deficiency and the further above the RDA then the greater is the risk of toxic effects.

Until 1991, the British standards were also termed RDAs, and this term is still to be found on British food labels where it refers to the RDA set by the EU. However, in the current version of the British standards (COMA, 1991), the general term **dietary reference values (DRVs)** is used to cover a range of differently defined values. The word 'recommended' has been specifically avoided as it was felt to wrongly imply that the RDA represented the minimum desirable intake for health and thus that intakes below the RDA represented inadequacy. Instead of a single RDA three reference values are offered for protein, vitamins and minerals in these new British standards. The highest of these three values is called the **reference nutrient intake (RNI)**. It is essentially equivalent to the old RDA as it also represents the estimated requirement of those people with the highest need for the nutrient. In practice it is still the value that is used in most circumstances. The other two DRVs offered for these nutrients are the **estimated average requirement (EAR)** which is self-explanatory and the **lower reference nutrient intake (LRNI)**. The LRNI is the best estimate of the requirement of those individuals with a low need for the nutrient. The requirement of almost everyone should lie within the range covered by the LRNI and the RNI.

COMA (1991) assumed that the variation in nutrient requirements of individuals follows a **normal distribution** (Figure 3.2). Approximately half of the population should require more and half less than the EAR. The **standard deviation** is a precisely defined statistical measure of the variation of individual values around the mean or average in a normal distribution. The RNI is set at a notional two standard deviations above the mean and the LRNI a notional two standard deviations below the mean (Figure 3.2). The characteristics of a normal distribution mean that the requirements of all but 5 per cent of the population should lie within the range covered by two

Table 3.1 A plan of the layout of tables of dietary standards (e.g. recommended dietary allowance (RDA) or reference nutrient intake (RNI))

Age group (examples)	Nutrient 1	Nutrient 2	Nutrient 3	Nutrient 4, etc.
0–3 months				
7–10 years				
11–14 years (female)				
19–50 years (male)				
50+ years (female)				
Pregnant				
Lactating				

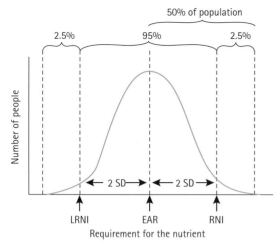

Figure 3.2 *Normal distribution of individual nutrient needs within a population with the theoretical positions of the UK dietary reference values. RNI, reference nutrient intake; LRNI, lower RNI; EAR, estimated average requirement; SD, standard deviation. From Webb (1994).*

standard deviations on either side of the mean. Thus the RNI and LRNI should theoretically satisfy the needs of 97.5 per cent and 2.5 per cent of the population, respectively. The RNI should represent an amount sufficient, or more than sufficient, to satisfy the needs of practically all healthy people (essentially the same definition as the American RDA). The panel considered that the RNI would be sufficient for everyone despite the theoretical risk that 2.5 per cent of the population are not provided for. There is considerable lack of precision in most of the estimations used to set dietary standards and so they tend to be set generously.

COMA (1991) suggested that this system of standards allows for more meaningful interpretation of measured or predicted intakes that fall below the RNI (i.e. the old RDA). At the extremes, if an individual's habitual intake is below the LRNI then the diet is almost certainly not able to maintain adequacy as it has been defined for that nutrient. If intake is above the RNI then it is safe to assume that the individual is receiving an adequate supply. In between these two extremes the chances of adequacy fall, to a statistically predictable extent, as the intake approaches the LRNI, e.g. an individual consuming the EAR has a 50 per cent chance of adequacy. Note that the iron requirements of women are an example where requirements for a nutrient are known not to be normally distributed; high iron

losses in menstrual blood in some women skew or distort the distribution. Note that when interpreting the results of nutrition surveys (e.g. in Chapter 12 and 15) those individuals with intakes below the LRNI are classified as having inadequate intakes and this definition is used to estimate the prevalence of dietary inadequacy for vitamins and minerals. While the LRNI is theoretically sufficient for 2.5 per cent of the population it is unlikely that all of those with the lowest intakes will have the lowest needs.

The RDAs for energy have traditionally been set at the best estimate of *average* requirement, rather than at the upper extremity of estimated requirement. Whereas for most nutrients, a modest surplus over requirement is not considered likely to be detrimental, this is not so with excessive energy intake that may lead to obesity. Consistent with this traditional practice, the latest UK standards give only an EAR for energy. Any individual's energy requirement will depend on many factors, particularly their size and activity level, and appetite should ensure that adequate intakes of energy are consumed by healthy non-dieting subjects. The EAR for energy is set for a person of average weight and with a specified (low) level of physical activity. The COMA panel considered that, for eight nutrients, it did not have sufficient information to estimate the rather precisely defined set of values discussed above. In these cases, therefore, the panel merely suggested a **safe intake** 'a level or range of intakes at which there is little risk of either deficiency or toxic effects'.

The 1991 UK standards also, for the first time, set reference values for the various fat and carbohydrate fractions, including dietary fibre. These values are clearly directed towards reducing the risk of chronic disease. At the time, this broke new ground for these standards because their traditional function has been solely to set standards of nutritional adequacy. COMA (1991) attempted to integrate the functions of standards of adequacy and that of nutritional guidelines aimed at reducing the risk of chronic disease. The reference values for fat and carbohydrate fractions are discussed in Chapter 4.

The formal and precise statistical definitions used by COMA (1991) should not be allowed to obscure the major role that judgement has in the setting of these values. The criterion that any dietary standards committee uses to define adequacy is almost inevitably a matter of judgement and opinion. There may also be considerable errors and uncertainties in estimating the average amount required to satisfy this criterion and in estimating the standard deviation of requirement. Thus any particular reference value is the consensus view of one panel of experts based on the information available and the prevailing social, political and economic climate. Views of individual panel members may differ so it is also likely to be the result of compromises between the views. There may also be genuine differences of opinion between different panels of experts. Some non-scientific considerations may also influence different committees to differing extents. Thus, the dairy industry might lobby for the calcium standard to be high, fruit growers lobby for a high vitamin C standard and meat and fish suppliers may be keen to keep the protein standard high. Where fruit is cheap and plentiful a committee may be generous with vitamin C allowances because the cost of erring on the high side is perceived as minimal. However, where fruit is, for much of the year, an expensive imported luxury a panel may be more conservative in its vitamin C standard.

In the USA, the last (ninth) single volume of RDAs was published in 1989 (NRC, 1989a). Since 1994, American and Canadian scientists have collaborated in updating and expanding the concept of the RDA and have issued a series of publications (e.g. Institute of Medicine (IOM), 2000) that have set a series of values in addition to the RDAs and given a detailed account of the evidence and rationale for the values for each nutrient. The term **dietary reference intakes (DRIs)** has been used to collectively cover this expanded set of dietary standards as briefly defined below.

- The RDA as defined previously.
- The EAR as used in Britain since 1991 and the term estimated energy requirement (EER) is the equivalent value used for energy.
- Adequate intake (AI) is the value used when an accurate RDA cannot be set; it is essentially the same as the 'safe intake' used in the British standards.
- The tolerable upper intake level (UL) is the highest average daily intake that is likely to pose no adverse risk to health to almost all individuals within the general population. This value was seen as a necessary addition because of the increased use of fortified foods and nutrient supplements.

- The acceptable macronutrient distribution range (AMDR) is the range of intakes of energy yielding nutrients such as carbohydrates and fats that are associated with reduced risk of chronic disease while still providing adequate intakes of essential nutrients. These values are the American equivalent of the DRVs for the energy yielding nutrients set by COMA (1991) and in both cases they are set as percentages of energy intake.

Significant variations have occurred in these dietary standards over the years and there are still quite marked variations in the dietary standards used in different countries. Historical differences can be partly explained by the differences in scientific information available to different panels but current international differences are largely due to variations in the way the same information has been interpreted by different panels of experts. There are several quite marked differences between the American RDA and the British RNI even though they are essentially equivalent in their definition. In general, American RDAs are higher than UK RNIs; Table 3.2 gives many examples of standards in Britain and the USA for adults under 50 years. For example, Table 3.2 shows that the American RDA for vitamins C is more than double the British RNI. In Chapter 10, the huge historical variations in protein standards for children are reviewed and discussed. In Chapter 15, the differences in the current UK and US standards for pregnant women are highlighted and discussed. Table 3.3 shows the RDA used for food labelling purposes with the EU and thus found on many British food labels.

Uses of dietary standards

A set of dietary standards allows nutritionists to predict the nutritional requirements of groups of people or of nations. Governments and food aid agencies can use them to identify the needs of populations, to decide whether available supplies are adequate for the population to be fed, and to identify nutrients whose supply is deficient or only marginally adequate. They thus provide the means to make informed food policy decisions, for example about:

- the amount and type of food aid required by a population or group
- the priorities for agricultural production and food imports

Table 3.2 Comparison of the reference nutrient intake (RNI), lower reference nutrient intake (LRNI) and American recommended dietary allowance (RDA) for selected micronutrients for adults aged 19–50 years

Nutrient	Male			Female		
	RNI	LRNI	RDA	RNI	LRNI	RDA
Vitamin A (μgRE/day)	700	300	900	600	250	700
Thiamin (mg/day)	1.0	0.6	1.2	0.8	0.45	1.1
Riboflavin (mg/day)	1.3	0.8	1.3	1.1	0.8	1.1
Niacin (mgNE/day)	17	11	16	13	9	14
Vitamin B_6 (mg/day)	1.4	1.0	1.3	1.2	0.9	1.3
Folate* (μg/day)	200	100	400	200	100	400
Vitamin B_{12} (μg/day)	1.5	1.0	2.4	1.5	1.0	2.4
Vitamin C (mg/day)	40	10	90	40	10	75
Vitamin D[†] (μg/day)	–	–	5	–	–	5
Vitamin E (mg/day)	Above 4[‡]	15	–	Above 3[‡]	15	–
Calcium (mg/day)	700	400	1000	700	400	1000
Chromium (μg/day)	Above 25[‡]	35	–	Above 25[‡]	25	–
Iron (mg/day)	8.7	4.7	8	14.8	8	18
Iodine (μg/day)	140	70	150	140	70	150
Magnesium (mg/day)	300	190	400	270	150	310
Potassium (mg/day)	3500	2000	4700	3500	2000	4700
Selenium (μg/day)	75	40	55	60	40	55
Zinc (mg/day)	9.5	5.5	11	7	4	8

*It is now recommended that women of child-bearing age take 400 μg/day supplement of folate.

[†] In Britain it is assumed that most adults can make sufficient vitamin when their skin is exposed to summer sunlight; the US value is for ages 25–50 years.

[‡] Safe intake, used where the panel felt that they did not have enough information to set formal RNI and LRNI.

Table 3.3 The recommended daily allowances (RDAs) used for food labelling in the European Union

Nutrient	'Labelling' RDA
Vitamin A (μgRE)	800
Thiamin (mg)	1.4
Riboflavin (mg)	1.6
Niacin (mg NE)	18
Vitamin B_6 (mg)	2
Folate (μg)	200
Vitamin B_{12} (μg)	1
Biotin (μg)	150
Pantothenic acid (mg)	6
Vitamin C (mg)	60
Vitamin D (μg)	5
Vitamin E (mg)	10
Calcium (mg)	800
Iodine (μg)	150
Iron (mg)	14
Magnesium (mg)	300
Phosphorus (mg)	800
Zinc (mg)	15

- which foods might be beneficially subsidized or, if foods need to be rationed, the size of rations that are needed
- whether to fortify foods with added vitamins or minerals.

Similarly, they are used by institutional caterers (e.g. in prisons or schools), and those catering for the armed forces to assess the food requirements of their client population and also to check proposed menus for their nutritional adequacy. Those devising therapeutic or reducing diets can check any proposed diets for adequacy using these standards.

These standards also provide the means to assess nutritional adequacy after an intake survey. They can be used as a yardstick for assessing the adequacy of groups or individuals. In the UK, the LRNI is regarded as the cut-off point below which an individual intake is classified as inadequate and the RNI would indicate that intake is certainly adequate. In the USA, the RDA is set such that if the average intake of a group is above the RDA then this should ensure that practically all members of the group are obtaining an adequate amount for their needs and in the UK the RNI is regarded as a similar ideal minimum for the group average. When individuals are being assessed, it must be borne in mind that intakes below the RDA (and RNI in the UK) do not necessarily represent inadequacy. When assessing the nutritional adequacy of individuals, remember that there are substantial fluctuations in the intakes of some nutrients from day to day. The habitual intake of the individual over a period of some days should ideally be the one that is compared with the standard.

Most consumers will be exposed to these standards when they are used on food labels to give a meaningful indication of nutrient content. Absolute numerical amounts of nutrients will be meaningless to most consumers but when expressed as a percentage of the RDA they become more meaningful. COMA (1991) suggested that the EAR was the most appropriate reference value to use for food labelling in Britain. As Britain is a member of the EU, the RDAs seen on British food labels are actually set by the European Directive on food labelling, and these differ slightly from the recommendations in the UK DRV (see Table 3.3 for a list of the labelling RDAs). In America, the reference daily intake (RDI) is used to indicate essential nutrient content on food labels. It is set at the higher of the two adult RDA values and referred to on the label as simply the 'daily value'.

Inaccurate standards

Setting dietary standards too low will negate their purpose. A yardstick of adequacy that does not meet the criterion of adequacy is of no use and is probably worse than no standard at all because it will tend to induce a false sense of security and complacency. A serious underestimation of the standards for a nutrient could result in a nutrient deficiency being falsely ruled out as the cause of some pathology. Perhaps more probably, it could result in a suboptimally nourished group being reassured as to their dietary adequacy. Such arguments about the obvious hazards of setting standards too low means that there will be a strong temptation to err on the side of generosity when setting them. This may be especially true in affluent countries where the need to avoid waste of resources is less acute. Potentially adverse consequences of setting standards too high include the following.

- Some nutrients (e.g. iron and some fat-soluble vitamins) are toxic in excess. An unrealistically high standard might encourage sensitive individuals to consume hazardous amounts.
- High standards may encourage the production or supply of unnecessary excesses, which will result in wasteful use of resources.
- High standard values may create the illusion of widespread deficiency and result in unnecessary and wasteful measures to combat an illusory problem.
- Unreasonably high 'target' values for particular nutrients may lead to distortion of the diet with deleterious effects on the intake of other nutrients.
- If an unreasonably high standard results in the classification of large numbers of people as deficient but there are no other manifestations of deficiency then this may discredit the standards and may, in the longer term, undermine the credibility of nutrition education in general.

Some of the consequences of earlier exaggeration of human protein requirements are discussed in Chapter 10, and this may serve as a case study to illustrate most of these points.

Defining requirement

The first problem that has to be confronted when devising a set of dietary standards is to decide the criteria that will be used to define adequacy. Ideally the determined intake should maximize growth, health and longevity, but these are not a readily measurable set of parameters. Overt deficiency of a nutrient will often produce a well-defined deficiency syndrome so that the minimum requirement will be an intake that prevents clinical signs of deficiency. Optimal intakes are assumed to be some way above this minimum requirement. Subclinical indications of impairment or depletion of nutrient stores may occur long before overt clinical signs of deficiency. COMA (1991) decided that the EAR should allow for 'a degree of storage of the nutrient to allow for periods of low intake or high demand without detriment to health'. This is actually a rather loose (vague) definition and the committee had to translate this into a quantitative and measurable criterion case by case.

The problem of defining an adequate intake is well illustrated by the example of vitamin C. It is generally agreed that in adults, about 10 mg per day of this vitamin is sufficient to prevent the deficiency disease, **scurvy**. Below 30 mg/day negligible levels of the vitamin are detectable in plasma, at intakes of between 30 mg and 70 mg/day plasma vitamin levels rise steeply, and they start to plateau at intakes of between 70 mg and 100 mg/day. COMA (1991) chose an adult RNI of 40 mg/day because at this intake most individuals would have measurable amounts of vitamin C in their plasma that is available for transfer to sites of depletion. Essentially the same data have resulted in American RDA of 90 mg/day for men and 75 mg/day for women. Some people advocate daily intakes of gram quantities of this vitamin to maximize resistance to infection. COMA (1991) listed numerous suggested benefits of very high vitamin C intakes and yet none of these influenced its DRVs. The underlying criterion in setting the DRVs is dietary adequacy even though the additional requirement for adequate stores represents a large safety margin over that required for minimal adequacy, i.e. prevention of scurvy.

The following sections cover the various methods that have been used to assess nutrient requirements and to set dietary standards for these nutrients. Examples of the use of each approach are also explained. Many readers may find it sufficient to select a small number of nutrients to use as illustrative case studies of how standards are set. Note that the method used to set the EAR for energy is explained in Chapter 6.

Deprivation studies

The most obvious and direct way of assessing the minimum requirement for a nutrient is to use an experimental diet that lacks the nutrient and see how much of it needs to be added to this diet to prevent or cure the signs of deficiency. Experiments in Sheffield, England, during World War II demonstrated that volunteers started to develop signs of the deficiency disease **scurvy** after a couple of months on a vitamin C-free diet. Intakes of around 10 mg/day were shown to prevent the development of scurvy and to cure the clinical signs (see COMA, 1991). Thus 10 mg/day is the minimum requirement for vitamin C and COMA chose this as the LRNI for vitamin C. Deprivation studies of this type may require the consumption of very restricted diets for long periods before clinical signs of deficiency develop in previously well-nourished adults. For example, it takes up to 2 years of depletion before such adults develop even limited signs of vitamin A deficiency. This is because

the liver contains large amounts of stored vitamin A. Volunteers need to consume a very restricted and unpalatable diet for a long time, and this may also have some adverse consequences on their long-term health. It would be ethically unacceptable to deliberately subject vulnerable groups to this type of deprivation, e.g. children and pregnant or lactating women. This means that the extra requirements of these groups usually have to be inferred from less direct methods.

As an alternative to controlled experiments it is possible to use epidemiological data relating average intakes of a nutrient to the presence or absence of clinical signs of deficiency in populations. For example, it has been observed that the deficiency disease **beriberi** occurs when average population intake of thiamin falls below 0.2 mg/1000 kcal (0.2 mg/4.2 MJ) but when average intake is above this level beriberi does not occur (Passmore and Eastwood, 1986).

Radioactive tracer studies

If a known amount of radioactively labelled vitamin, or other nutrient, is administered to a volunteer then, assuming that this labelled vitamin disperses evenly in the body pool of that vitamin, the dilution of the radioactivity can be used to estimate the total size of that body pool. A sample of plasma is taken and the amount of vitamin and the amount of radioactivity in the sample measured. The **specific activity** of vitamin in the plasma sample (i.e. the radioactivity per unit weight of vitamin) can be used to calculate the total pool size, provided that the amount of radioactivity administered is known (see below), e.g.:

- administer 1 million units of radioactivity
- specific activity in sample is measured as 1000 units of radioactivity per mg of vitamin
- so radioactivity has been diluted in 1000 mg of vitamin, i.e. in a 1000 mg body pool of the vitamin.

If after administration of a radioactive vitamin load, the body losses of radioactivity are monitored this will allow the rate of vitamin loss or depletion to be determined.

Using this approach, Baker *et al.* (1971) found that the average body pool of vitamin C in a group of healthy, well-nourished American men was around 1500 mg. On a vitamin C-free diet, this pool depleted at a rate of around 3 per cent/day. This 3 per cent depletion rate is termed the **fractional catabolic rate** and was found to be independent of the pool size, i.e. 3 per cent of whatever is in the body is lost no matter how much or how little is present in the body. When the body pool fell below 300 mg, symptoms of scurvy started to appear. Baker *et al.* estimated that to maintain the body pool above 300 mg and thus to prevent scurvy their subjects needed to consume 9 mg/day (i.e. 3 per cent of 300 mg). This agrees very well with the reported approximately 10 mg/day to prevent scurvy in the much earlier depletion study in Sheffield.

Balance studies

These methods rely on the assumption that in healthy, well-nourished adults of stable body weight the body pool size of some nutrients remains constant. Healthy adults are, for example, in approximate daily balance for nitrogen (i.e. protein), calcium and sodium. Over a wide range of intakes and suitable measurement period, the intake is approximately equal to the output. Any variations in intake are compensated for by changes in the rate of absorption from the gut, changes in the rate of excretion, or changes in the rate of metabolism. If say calcium intake is progressively reduced then initially losses of calcium in urine and faeces will also decline and balance will be maintained. Eventually, however, a point will be reached when balance can no longer be maintained and output starts to exceed input. It seems reasonable to propose that the minimum intake at which balance can be maintained represents the subject's minimum requirement for calcium. Such short-term experiments do not exclude the very real possibility that long-term adaptation to chronically low calcium intakes will occur.

COMA (1991) assumed that the average daily loss of calcium via urine and skin in British adults was 160 mg/day. To replace this daily loss it estimated that an intake of 525 mg/day would be required assuming that around 30 per cent of dietary calcium is absorbed. COMA chose this as the adult EAR for calcium, adding or subtracting 30 per cent to allow for individual variation. It therefore came up with 700 mg/day and 400 mg/day as the RNI and LRNI, respectively.

Factorial methods

Factorial calculations are essentially predictions of the requirements of particular groups or individuals taking into account a number of measured variables (or factors) and making a number of apparently logical assumptions. For example, during growth or pregnancy certain nutrients will be retained and accumulate in the growing body or pregnant woman. On the basis of knowledge of the rate at which these nutrients accumulate during pregnancy or growth one can then make predictions of the amount required. For example:

> Estimated requirements for pregnancy = amount to achieve balance (from value for non-pregnant women) + (daily accumulation rate of nutrient during pregnancy × factor to allow for assumed efficiency of absorption and assimilation)

COMA (1991) predicted the increase in EAR for energy of women during lactation using the following factorial calculation.

> Increase in EAR for energy during lactation = average energy content of daily milk production × 100/80 (assuming 80% conversion of dietary energy to milk energy) − an allowance for the contribution from the extra maternal fat stores laid down during pregnancy

It should always be borne in mind that, no matter how logical they may seem, such values are theoretical predictions and they may not represent actual physiological need. Physiological adaptations may occur which will reduce the predicted requirement, e.g. the efficiency of calcium and iron absorption from the gut increases during pregnancy (see Chapter 15).

Measurement of blood or tissue levels

COMA (1991) defined some reference values according to the intake required to maintain a particular circulating level or tissue level of the nutrient. As we have already seen, the LRNI for vitamin C is set at the intake that prevents scurvy (10 mg/day in adults). The RNI is set at a level that maintains a measurable amount of vitamin C in plasma in most adults (40 mg/day); the EAR (25 mg/day) is set half way between the LRNI and the RNI. The reference values for vitamin A in the UK are based upon the intake that is estimated as necessary to maintain a liver concentration of 20 μg vitamin A per gram of liver. To estimate the intake of vitamin A required to maintain this target liver concentration, the panel had to perform quite an elaborate factorial calculation (summarized in Figure 3.3).

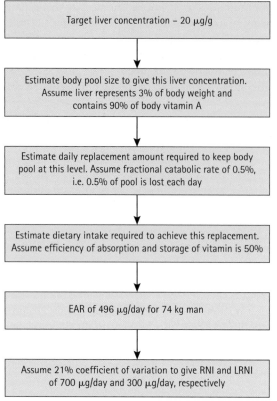

Figure 3.3 *Scheme to illustrate the calculations and assumptions required to estimate the vitamin A intake required to maintain a designated liver concentration and thus to set the dietary reference values for vitamin A. After COMA (1991). RNI, reference nutrient intake; LRNI, lower RNI; EAR, estimated average requirement.*

First the panel had to predict the size of the body pool required to achieve this liver concentration. To do this assumptions had to made about what proportion of the body is liver and also about how the total body pool of vitamin A partitions between the liver and other tissues. The fractional catabolic rate of vitamin A has been measured at 0.5 per cent of the body pool lost per day and so an amount equivalent to 0.5 per cent of this estimated pool would have to be replaced each day. Finally assumptions had to be made about the efficiency with which ingested vitamin A is stored in the liver to convert this replacement requirement into an intake requirement.

Biochemical markers

COMA (1991) used the intake required to 'maintain a given degree of enzyme saturation' as another

criterion for determining reference values. An example of this is the use of the erythrocyte glutathione reductase activation test to assess and define nutritional status for riboflavin (vitamin B_2). Glutathione reductase is an enzyme present in red blood cells whose activity is dependent on the presence of a cofactor (FAD) derived from riboflavin. The enzyme cannot function in the absence of the cofactor. In riboflavin deficiency the activity of this enzyme is low because of reduced availability of the cofactor. In red blood cells taken from well-nourished subjects, the activity of this enzyme will be higher because it is not limited by the availability of the cofactor. To perform the activation test, the activity of glutathione reductase is measured in two samples of red cells from the subject – one has had excess FAD added the other has not had FAD added. The ratio of these two activities is called the **erythrocyte glutathione reductase activation coefficient (EGRAC)**. It is a measure of the extent to which enzyme activity has been limited by riboflavin availability in the non-supplemented sample and thus is a measure of the subject's riboflavin status. The RNI is set at the intake that maintains the EGRAC at 1.3 or less in almost all people. Similar enzyme activation tests are used to assess status for thiamin (vitamin B_1) and vitamin B_6.

- Activation of the enzyme transketolase in red cells is used to determine thiamin status – a thiamin-derived cofactor is necessary for transketolase to function.
- Activation of the enzyme glutamic oxaloacetic transaminase in erythrocytes can be used to assess vitamin B_6 status.

Biological markers

Blood haemoglobin concentration has been widely used in the past as a measure of nutritional status for iron. It is now regarded as an insensitive and unreliable indicator of iron status for reasons such as:

- haemoglobin concentration changes in response to a number of physiological factors such as training, altitude and pregnancy
- iron stores may be depleted without any change in blood haemoglobin concentration (see under 'biochemical assessment' later in this chapter for further discussion of iron status assessment).

Vitamin K status is frequently assessed by functional tests of prothrombin levels in blood. Prothrombin is one of several clotting factors whose synthesis in the liver depends on vitamin K as an essential cofactor. Thus in vitamin K deficiency, prothrombin levels fall and blood clotting is impaired. To measure the **prothrombin time** excess calcium and tissue thromboplastin are added to fresh plasma that has been previously depleted of calcium to prevent clotting. The time taken for the plasma to clot under these conditions depends on the amount of prothrombin present and thus the vitamin K status of the donor. Anticoagulant drugs, such as warfarin, work by blocking the effect of vitamin K. Prothrombin time is thus a useful way of monitoring vitamin K status and thus of regulating drug dosage during anticoagulant treatment.

Animal experiments

Animal experiments are of limited value in quantifying the nutrient needs of human beings. They may even encourage widely erroneous estimates to be made. It is extremely difficult to allow for species differences in nutrient requirements and to scale between species as different in size as rats and people. The following examples illustrate some of the difficulties of predicting human nutrient needs from those of laboratory animals.

Most rapidly growing young animals need a relatively high proportion of their dietary energy as protein but human babies grow more slowly and thus are likely to need proportionally less than most other young mammals. Rat milk has around 25 per cent of its energy as protein compared with only about 6 per cent in human milk. Predicting the protein needs of human children from those of young rats is likely to exaggerate the needs of children.

Pauling (1972) used the measured rate of vitamin C synthesis in the rat (which does not require dietary vitamin C) to support his highly controversial view that gram quantities of the vitamin are required for optimal human health. He scaled up the rat's rate of production on a simple weight-to-weight basis and estimated that rats of human size would make 2–4 g/day of the vitamin. He suggested that this gave an indication of human requirements. This procedure seems extremely dubious on several grounds, e.g. the decision to scale up the rat's rate of vitamin C synthesis on a simple weight-to-weight basis. Vitamin needs may be more related to metabolic needs than simple body weight, and if one scales according to relative metabolic rate then one

might predict that the human size rat would only make around a quarter of the amount predicted by body weight scaling.

The expected nutritional burdens of pregnancy and lactation are also relatively much greater in small laboratory animals than in women. Laboratory animals have relatively larger litters, short gestations and more rapidly growing infants than human beings. Extrapolating from laboratory animals is thus likely to exaggerate any extra nutritional requirements of pregnant and lactating women (see Chapter 15).

Despite these reservations about the use of animal experiments to quantify human nutrient needs, they have had a vital role in the identification of the essential nutrients and their physiological and biochemical functions. Several of those awarded Nobel prizes for work on vitamins used animals in their work. The need for essential fatty acids was, for example, demonstrated in the rat 40 years before unequivocal confirmation in an adult human being. Animal experiments may also be very useful in providing in-depth information on the pathological changes that accompany prolonged deficiency and in determining whether prolonged marginal adequacy is likely to have any long-term detrimental effects.

Key points

- Dietary standards are yardsticks of nutritional adequacy; they are called dietary reference intakes (DRIs) in the USA and dietary reference values (DRVs) in the UK.
- Reference values are set for each nutrient for each of the various age and sex groups within the population.
- The recommended dietary allowance (RDA) in the USA and the reference nutrient intake (RNI) in the UK represent an estimate of the requirements of those healthy in the age group with the highest need.
- The RNI is set at a notional two standard deviations above the estimated average requirement (EAR).
- The lower reference nutrient intake (LRNI) is set at two standard deviations below the EAR.
- The LRNI is the estimated requirement of those with the lowest need for the nutrient and thus is assumed to be insufficient to meet most people's needs.

- The standards for energy are set at the estimated average requirement.
- The setting of dietary standards depends on the judgement of panels of experts, and so they vary from country to country and over time.
- Reference values are dependent on the definition of adequacy used.
- COMA (1991) defined the EAR as an amount that would prevent deficiency and allow some degree of storage.
- These standards can be used to:
  - assess whether food supplies or nutrient intakes are adequate
  - estimate the needs of groups or populations
  - check whether menus or prescribed diets are adequate.
- Use of RDAs on food labels makes nutrient contents more meaningful to consumers.
- On labels in the USA, the higher of the two adult RDAs is present as the 'daily value' whereas in the UK, the RDA set by the EU is used.
- Standards that are set too low are obviously of no use but setting values too high may also produce other more subtle problems.
- Many different methods can be used to define and determine what is an adequate intake of a particular nutrient, such as:
  - direct measurement of the amount needed to cure or prevent deficiency
  - use of radioactively labelled nutrient to measure body pool size and fractional catabolic rate or rate of excretion
  - estimation of the amount necessary to maintain balance between input and losses of the nutrient
  - factorial estimates of the amount of nutrient required, e.g. to produce milk in lactation to support growth or growth of the products of conception in pregnancy
  - estimates of the amount necessary to achieve a particular blood or tissue level, a specified level of enzyme activity or some biological marker.
- Animal studies have been invaluable in identifying essential nutrients and the effects of deficiency but are of little value in quantifying human nutrient requirements.

Clinical signs for the assessment of nutritional status

Nutrient deficiencies ultimately lead to clinically recognizable deficiency diseases. Identification of the clinical signs of these deficiency diseases (see Box 3.2) usually requires little or no specialized equipment, is cheap, simple and quick, thus enabling assessment surveys to be conducted rapidly and cheaply even in the most inaccessible places. Even non-medical personnel can be trained to conduct clinical surveys of nutritional

> **Box 3.2   Some clinical signs that may indicate a nutritional deficiency** (one possible dietary cause is given in parenthesis)
>
> - Loose, hanging clothes or a wasted appearance (energy/protein deficit and weight loss)
> - Loss of hair pigment and easy 'pluckability' (energy/protein deficit in children? – kwashiorkor)
> - White foamy spots on the cornea (Bitot's spots – vitamin A)
> - Dry and infected cornea (vitamin A)
> - Oedema (thiamin, B_1– beriberi)
> - Several types of dermatitis (in skin exposed to sunlight, niacin – pellagra)
> - Enlargement of the liver (energy/protein deficit – kwashiorkor)
> - Loss of peripheral sensation (thiamin)
> - Spongy, bleeding gums (vitamin C – scurvy)
> - Angular stomatitis – spongy lesions at the corners of the mouth (riboflavin)
> - Pale conjunctiva (iron deficiency anaemia)
> - Red inflamed tongue (riboflavin)
> - Spontaneous bruising (vitamin C)
> - Tiny subdermal haemorrhages or petechiae (vitamin C)
> - Swelling of the thyroid gland in the neck or goitre (iodine)
> - Bowed legs (vitamin D – rickets)
> - Mental confusion (water – dehydration)
> - Confusion or dementia (niacin)
>
> Note that several of these symptoms can be indicative of more than one nutritional deficiency or they may indicate other non-nutritional conditions. They can be profitably used to construct screening checklists to identify individuals in need of further investigation or to assess the level of nutrient deficiency in a population.

status by recording the presence or absence of various clinical signs from checklists of clinical signs that are likely to be associated with nutrient deficiencies.

The potential problem of population sampling bias as mentioned in Box 3.1 is one that can affect any type of dietary or nutritional survey. Those conducting the survey must take steps to actively ensure that the subjects are representative of the whole population under investigation. Those most badly affected by deficiency diseases may well be those least accessible to the survey team – the weak, the frail, the elderly, pregnant and lactating women, and babies are the least likely to be out and about. Sampling people in the street or those people who are mobile enough to attend a centre may well overestimate the nutritional status of the population. This may be particularly important when clinical signs are used because these are often present only in those most severely affected by dietary deprivation.

The clinical signs of deficiency usually become recognizable after severe and prolonged deficiency and thus they are relatively insensitive indicators of nutritional status. It is generally assumed that suboptimal intakes of nutrients producing subclinical impairment of physiological functioning occur long before overt symptoms of deficiency become clinically apparent. That is, long before any deficiency disease becomes clinically apparent. In surveys in affluent countries, few cases of clinical deficiency would be found in most sectors of the population. Surveys that use clinical signs would therefore tend to provide only limited information about the nutrient status of the population, e.g. that there are no deficiencies severe enough or long-standing enough to induce overt clinical deficiency. Clinical signs are therefore not useful as early indicators of nutritional problems that can warn of the need to implement preventative measures. They may be much more useful in providing a quick guide to the extent of nutritional deficiency in less affluent countries, during famine and even in high-risk groups in affluent countries, e.g. the homeless, alcoholics, under-privileged children and frail, elderly people.

Clinical signs tend to be qualitative and subjective. Any attempt to grade or quantify clinical signs is likely to depend on subjective judgements on the part of the operator. For example, grading the severity of **goitre** (swelling of the thyroid gland due to iodine deficiency) depends on the judgement of the assessor about the degree of thyroid enlargement; different clinicians may produce considerably different grades for the same population. Also, clinical signs are not very specific indicators of nutrient deficiencies. Some symptoms are common to several deficiency diseases and also to non-nutritional causes. Some form of dermatitis is, for example, common to several deficiency diseases and may also be induced by a variety of non-nutritional causes. Oedema may be a symptom of beriberi, protein-energy malnutrition, heart failure, kidney disease, etc.

Anthropometric assessment in adults

Box 3.3 lists of some anthropometric measures that may be used to assess nutritional status.

| **Box 3.3** | **Anthropometric measures used for nutritional assessment** |

3 months' unintentional weight loss

- Up to 5 per cent: mild depletion
- 5–10 per cent: moderate depletion
- Over 10 per cent: severe depletion

Useful for screening new admissions to hospital or residential care homes

Body mass index

BMI = weight (kg)/height (m)^2

- Under 18.5 kg/m^2 – underweight*
- 18.5–25 kg/m^2 – ideal

- 25–30 kg/m^2 – overweight
- 30+ kg/m^2 – obese
- 40+ kg/m^2 – severely obese

BMI is standard way of classifying people on the basis of their height and weight

Demiquet index

Weight (kg)/demi-span (m)^2
Alternative to BMI in people who cannot stand erect, e.g. the elderly. Demi-span or knee height can be used in regression equations to predict height and then BMI can be estimated

Measures of mid-upper arm circumference

- Mid-arm circumference (MAC)

Useful as a simple indicator of nutritional status when compared with standards or as an indicator of weight change when measured sequentially. Can be used in those confined to bed

- Mid-arm muscle circumference (MAMC) = MAC − ($\pi \times$ triceps skinfold)

Indicator of lean body mass or to monitor changes in it

- Arm muscle area = $(MAMC)^2/4\pi$

Skinfold calipers

Skinfold thickness can be measured at several sites to indicate the amount of fat stored subcutaneously in these sites and then translated into an estimate of per cent body fat with a calibration chart or table. A more direct assessment of body fat than weight, particularly useful for athletes who have unusually high amounts of muscle for their weight

Bioelectrical impedance

On passing a weak alternating current between two points on the body, the impedance (resistance) depends on the relative amounts of fat and lean in the body. Not strictly an anthropometric method but included here for convenience. Gives a rapid and direct estimate of body fat using an internal calibration with little technical skill required

Body density

Fat is less dense than lean tissue. If one assumes that fat has a density of 0.9 kg/L and lean tissue 1.10 kg/L, it is possible to estimate the per cent of body fat from the body density. Not suitable for routine use. Traditionally the method used for calibration of other methods of measuring fatness, e.g. skinfold measurements and bioelectrical impedance. Volume is usually measured by underwater weighing, but this is technically difficult and requires specialist facilities

*Until recently 20 kg/m² was used as the lower limit for normal. This has now been lowered to 18.5 kg/m², but some of the sources cited later in this book have continued to use 20 kg/m² as the cut-off point for normal.

Uses of anthropometric assessment

Anthropometry is the scientific study of the measurement of the human body. Anthropometric assessment means making nutritional assessment by means of physical measurements of body weight and dimensions. Body composition may be estimated from anthropometric measurements, and this can have a variety of uses.

- It allows assessment of nutritional status. Anthropometric measurements can be used to detect under-nutrition or obesity in adults and children and to indicate whether the growth of children has been satisfactory.
- It allows useful comparisons of metabolic rates of individuals or groups. Adipose tissue has a low metabolic rate and so expressing metabolic rate per unit of lean body mass is more meaningful than simply expressing it per unit total weight.
- Certain drug dosages may be calculated per unit of lean body weight.

Changes in body weight may be due to gain or loss of water, lean tissue and/or fat. Longitudinal measurements of body composition may help to decide the composition of any weight change. Most of the measures currently available for assessing body composition are relatively insensitive and thus could only be reliably used for this purpose if the weight change were substantial.

Height and weight

Body weight alone will be a useful indicator of nutritional status in adults only if it is measured repeatedly over a period of time. It can then, for example, be used to monitor changes in the nutritional status of patients in hospital or those living in residential homes for the elderly. Unintentional weight loss can be an indicator of disease or deteriorating nutritional status as a result of adverse socioeconomic status. Many hospital admission forms have a question about weight change in the previous 3 months (see Box 3.3) designed to help identify patients who are nutritionally 'at risk'.

An individual's 'ideal' weight will obviously depend on how tall they are – one expects tall people to weigh more than short ones. In the past, weight-for-height tables were the most common way of assessing people's weight status. These tables give the desirable weight ranges for men and women of any particular height and age. Three desirable ranges are usually given for each height for both sexes, depending on frame size, i.e. whether the person is of light, medium or heavy build. Obesity was then defined as more than 20 per cent over the person's ideal weight range and underweight defined as more than 10 per cent below their ideal weight range. The tables produced by the Metropolitan Life Insurance Company have been widely used for this purpose. Note that the original purpose of these tables was for commercial use in assessing actuarial risk in people taking out life insurance policies. They were produced by recording the heights and weights of large numbers of life insurance applicants and then relating initial weight to risk of dying (and thus claiming on the policy) in the succeeding years. These ideal ranges were those associated with the lowest death rates. People above or below these ranges (i.e. underweight or overweight) had higher death rates. These tables are relatively cumbersome and inconvenient to use especially as they require some assessment of frame size. Objective measures of frame size such as wrist circumference and elbow breadth are not difficult to measure in a clinic or laboratory, but they add to the inconvenience of weight-for-height tables particularly for studies with large groups or populations.

Body mass index

In recent years, the **BMI** has become the standard way of classifying adults using their heights and weights. This measure has been shown empirically to be the best simple and quantitative anthropometric indicator of body composition and thus of nutritional status.

$$BMI = \frac{Body\ weight\ (kg)}{Height\ (m)^2}$$

Note that BMI can be calculated from heights and weights in imperial units using the following approximation:

$$BMI = \frac{Weight\ (pounds)}{Height\ (inches)^2} \times 705$$

The normal range for the BMI has for some years been set at $20–25\,kg/m^2$, and any value significantly below this range is taken to indicate underweight and values above this range to indicate varying degrees of overweight or obesity (see Box 3.3). This classification is still used in the NDNS survey of British Adults (Hoare *et al.*, 2004) and in some other sources of population data (e.g. the NDNS survey of older adults of Finch *et al.*, 1998) and so will be used in this book unless specifically stated otherwise. In recent years, however, there has been some reconsideration of where the lower level of normality should lie. Many people with BMI slightly below 20 are perfectly well and healthy and have good appetites and apparently healthy diets. The range of normality has thus been extended from $18.5\,kg/m^2$ to $25\,kg/m^2$ rather than the traditional $20–25\,kg/m^2$. Below is a system for classifying varying degrees of underweight using BMI (after Heymsfield and Baumgarter, 2006).

- $<16\,kg/m^2$ – grade III protein-energy malnutrition
- $16–17\,kg/m^2$ – grade II protein energy malnutrition
- $17–18.5\,kg/m^2$ – underweight
- $18.5–25\,kg/m^2$ – normal.

When the BMI is being used to classify people as underweight or too fat, then it is being implicitly assumed that variations in weight for a given height are primarily due to variations in adiposity, i.e. that heavy means fat and that light means lean. This assumption generally holds reasonably well but there are some circumstances where it clearly does not hold. Some examples are given below.

- *Body builders.* People with very well-developed musculature like body builders will be heavy but have very low fat content. In this case their BMI may falsely indicate obesity. In the past, some very muscular American footballers were rejected for military service because they were heavy and so mistakenly classified as obese.
- *The elderly.* As people become elderly, so the mass of muscle and bone in the body tends to fall and is replaced by fat. A group of elderly people will have a higher average body fat content than a group of young adults of the same height and weight. In elderly women, in particular, loss of lean tissue and bone mass may mean that BMI remains within the normal range even though more direct measures of fatness may indicate excess adiposity.

- *Oedema and dehydration.* Changes in body fluid content can produce major changes in body weight without any change in body fat content. Excess accumulation of tissue fluid, oedema, can lead to a substantial increase in body weight and may obscure the person's malnourished state. Oedema is a common symptom of malnutrition and of many other conditions such as heart failure, kidney disease, liver disease and pregnancy. Oedema may be a major hindrance to the anthropometric assessment of nutritional status in hospital patients and malnourished children in developing countries if body weight plays any part in that assessment.

Alternatives to height

Accurate measurement of height requires that the person be able to stand erect. In people who cannot stand erect, another measure of skeletal size is needed. **Demi-span** is one such measure; it is the distance from the web of the fingers (between the middle and ring fingers) and the sternal notch when the subject's arm is held horizontally to the side (with support if necessary). Some disabled people and many very elderly people are unable to stand upright for height to be accurately measured. The 1992 COMA report on the nutrition of elderly people recommended that demi-span measurements should be included in all nutritional surveys of older people. White *et al.* (1993) derived the following equations for estimating height (cm) from demi-span (cm) measurements in people aged over 55 years:

$$\text{Height for men} = (1.2 \times \text{demi-span}) + 71$$

$$\text{Height for women} = (1.2 \times \text{demi-span}) + 67$$

This enables BMI to be estimated from measurements of weight and demi-span. The Royal College of Nursing (RCN), UK, has published a set of nutritional standards for elderly people (RCN, 1993) which included a ready reckoner for estimating BMI from body weight and demi-span. Webb and Copeman (1996) have also compiled a list of anthropometric norms for elderly people. Demi-span measurements can be also be used to derive indices with body weight, which are analogous to the BMI, the **mindex** and **demiquet** indices.

$$\text{Mindex} = \frac{\text{Weight (kg)}}{\text{Demi-span (m)}}$$

$$\text{Demiquet index} = \frac{\text{Weight (kg)}}{\text{Demi-span (m)}^2}$$

White *et al.* (1993) found that both mindex and demiquet correlated very highly with BMI but concluded that mindex was probably a better index of obesity than demiquet. **Knee height** is another way of estimating skeletal size that is used less often than demi-span. It is measured in a seated position and is the height from the floor to the knee joint space. The following equations can be used to estimate height (cm) from knee height (cm):

$$\text{Male height} = 64.19 + (\text{knee height} \times 2.03) - (0.04 \times \text{age})$$

$$\text{Female height} = 84.88 + (\text{knee height} \times 1.83) - (0.24 \times \text{age})$$

Skinfold calipers

The traditional method for more direct estimation of fatness in people is measurement of skinfold thickness using skinfold calipers. Spring-loaded calipers are used which exert a constant pressure on a fold of skin and the thickness of the skinfold is indicated on a meter. The thickness of the skinfold will largely depend on the amount of fat stored subcutaneously in the region of the skinfold. Skinfold thicknesses are measured at several sites and the assumption is made that the amount of fat stored subcutaneously at these sites (as measured by the skinfold thickness) will be representative of the total amount of body fat. Using the method of Durnin and Womersley (1974), skinfold thickness in millimetres is determined at four sites: over the triceps muscle; over the biceps; in the subscapular region; and, in the supra iliac region. The total of these four skinfolds is then translated into an estimate of percentage body fat using a calibration table or formula. Figure 3.4 shows the relationship between the sum of these four skinfolds and percentage body fat (estimated by body density) in 17–29-year-old men and women. Table 3.4 shows a table that can be used to estimate percentage fatness from these four skinfolds.

The single triceps skinfold thickness is sometimes used in nutritional surveys. It has the obvious advantage, in such circumstances, that it can be measured quickly and without the need for people to undress. Some problems associated with use of skinfold calipers are:

- it is a relatively time-consuming method

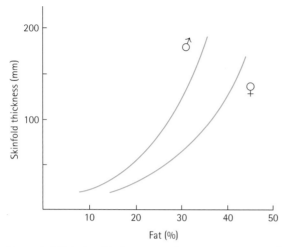

Figure 3.4 *Relationship between caliper measurements of skinfold thickness at four sites and body fat content estimated from body density in young adults. Data from Durnin and Womersley (1974).*

- people need to undress to have their skinfolds measured
- it requires a great deal of skill and care to obtain accurate and reliable skinfold measurements
- the process of translating skinfold measurements into estimates of fatness relies upon calibration tables derived from body density measurements, and so any errors in the use of density are also inherent in this method
- there is considerable inter-individual variation in the distribution of body fat as well as pronounced inter-racial differences. Standards need to be appropriate for the racial group being assessed.

Bioelectrical impedance

Bioelectrical impedance as a method of measuring body composition is now being used in many health centres and fitness clubs. I have included it in the anthropometry section for convenience. The devices that use this principle are becoming much cheaper and their operation is fairly simple. These devices give an almost instant estimate of the amount of fat and lean in the body and so their use is likely to grow

Table 3.4 Converting the sum of four skinfolds into estimates of percentage body fat. Data of Durnin and Womersley (1974) who used density measured by underwater weighing to estimate fatness in a sample of Scottish people

Skinfolds (mm)	Males (age in years)				Females (age in years)			
	17–29	30–39	40–49	50+	16–29	30–39	40–49	50+
20	8.1	12.2	12.2	12.6	14.1	17.0	19.8	21.4
30	12.9	16.2	17.7	18.6	19.5	21.8	24.5	26.6
40	16.4	19.2	21.4	22.9	23.4	25.5	28.2	30.3
50	19.0	21.5	24.6	26.5	26.5	28.2	31.0	33.4
60	21.2	23.5	27.1	29.2	29.1	30.6	33.2	35.7
70	23.1	25.1	29.3	31.6	31.2	32.5	35.0	37.7
80	24.8	26.6	31.2	33.8	33.1	34.3	36.7	39.6
90	26.2	27.8	33.0	35.8	34.8	35.8	38.3	41.2
100	27.6	29.0	34.4	37.4	36.4	37.2	39.7	42.6
110	28.8	30.1	35.8	39.0	37.8	38.6	41.0	43.9
120	30.0	31.1	37.0	40.4	39.0	39.6	42.0	45.1
130	31.0	31.9	38.2	41.8	40.2	40.6	43.0	46.2
140	32.0	32.7	39.2	43.0	41.3	41.6	44.0	47.2
150	32.9	33.5	40.2	44.1	42.3	42.6	45.0	48.2
160	33.7	34.3	41.2	45.1	43.3	43.6	45.8	49.2
170	34.5		42.0	46.1	44.1	44.4	46.6	50.0
180	35.3					45.2	47.4	50.8
190	35.9					45.9	48.2	51.6
200						46.5	48.8	52.4
210							49.4	53.0

at least in the short term. Bioelectrical impedance is based on the much poorer conductance of fatty tissue compared with lean tissue. Electrodes are placed on one of the subject's hands and feet, a current is generated by the machine's battery in one limb, passes through the body and is picked up by the electrode on the other limb. The machine uses the resistance to the current or the 'impedance' (because it is alternating current) to estimate lean body mass and body fat. If the subject's age, sex, height and weight are keyed in, the machine gives a rapid prediction of the amount and percentage of fat in the body. Simple, inexpensive machines that use this principle are now widely sold for home use.

Estimation of fatness from body density

The calibration of the skinfold method of determining fatness (Table 3.4) has been obtained by using body density as a reference method. The density of fat (0.9 kg/L) is less than that of lean tissue (1.1 kg/L), and so measurement of whole body density enables one to estimate the proportion of fat in the body.

$$\text{Density} = \frac{\text{Mass}}{\text{Volume}}$$

Mass may be determined by simple weighing. Volume is measured by comparing the weight of the body in air and its weight when fully immersed in water. The difference between these two values is the weight of water displaced by the body (Archimedes' principle). Knowing the density of water (1 kg/L), the volume of water displaced, i.e. the volume of the body, can be calculated. The principle is very simple but the technical procedures required to obtain accurate and valid values are quite elaborate, e.g.:

- subjects wear a weighted belt to ensure that they are fully immersed and correction has to be made for this
- corrections will need to be made for the residual air in the lungs during the immersion, which will greatly distort density measurements.

This method requires sentient and co-operative subjects. It is not suitable for routine use or for use with young children. It has traditionally been used as the reference method against which other methods are calibrated and validated, e.g. skinfold calipers and bioelectrical impedance.

Body water content as a predictor of body fat content

Measurement of body water content should allow good estimates of body fatness to be made. The body can be seen as consisting of two compartments, lean tissue with a constant proportion of water (around 73 per cent) and water-free fat. A measure of body water allows one to estimate proportions of lean and fat in the body. In order to estimate body water content in a living person or animal, one needs some chemical substance that is non-toxic, will readily and evenly disperse in all of the body water and is readily measurable. Water that is labelled with the deuterium isotope of hydrogen (heavy water) or the radioactive isotope of hydrogen (tritiated water) seems to fulfil these criteria.

After allowing time for dispersal, the concentration of the chemical in a sample of body fluid is measured. Knowing the amount of the substance introduced into the body one can estimate the amount of diluting fluid (i.e. the body water). The principle is illustrated by the hypothetical example below.

1 Administer 100 units of chemical.
2 Allow time for dispersal in body water.
3 Measure concentration in body water sample, let us say 2 units per litre.
4 Volume of body water estimated at 50 L, i.e. 50 kg of water.
5 Estimate lean body mass assuming this 50 kg of water represents, let us say 73 per cent of lean tissue, i.e. 50 × 100/73.
6 Total weight – lean weight = weight of body fat.

This method should yield reliable and valid measures of body water and thus good estimates of body fat.

Mid-arm circumference measures

In immobile adults who cannot be weighed (e.g. unconscious hospital patients) **mid-arm muscle circumference** of the upper arm can be a useful anthropometric indicator of nutritional status. A single measurement needs standards for interpretation but longitudinal changes in this measure are a reasonably sensitive indicator of changes in body weight. Mid-arm circumference has been widely used as a simple and rapid means of assessing nutritional status in children. A piece of previously calibrated and colour-coded tape can be used. If the circumference lies in the green region then this can be taken to indicate normality, in the yellow region mild malnutrition and a circumference in the red region indicates frank malnutrition.

Mid-arm muscle circumference has been widely used as a simple measure of lean body mass. The circumference of the mid-arm is measured with a tape and the triceps skinfold measured with calipers. Then:

$$\text{MAMC} = \text{MAC} - (\pi \times \text{triceps skinfold})$$

Changes in MAMC are taken to indicate changes in lean body mass and once again may be a useful longitudinal measure of nutritional status in hospital patients.

Anthropometric assessment in children

Anthropometric measurements are cumulative indicators of the nutritional status and general health of children. Low values for height or length provides evidence of the chronic effects of malnutrition – weight for height is a more acute measure and indicates current nutritional status. These simple measures require little equipment or professional training and so even non-specialists can easily and cheaply produce reliable results. Interpretation of these results requires that they be compared with standards. The need for reliable standards is a recurrent problem when interpreting anthropometric measurements. If standards of height and weight for children are derived from children in affluent countries then poor children in developing countries may not correspond well with such standards. These differences between rich and poor are largely a reflection of chronic adaptation to undernutrition by the poor, which may make interpretation of results and deciding on appropriate responses difficult. An anthropometric survey of children in rural Bangladesh is likely to show that their average heights and weights are some way below those of typical American children of the same age but they may be typical of children living in rural Bangladesh and thus they are not specifically 'at risk'. This point is well illustrated by considering some of the changes that have occurred in the anthropometric characteristics of affluent populations during the twentieth century.

- Britons are on average several inches taller than they were at the start of the twentieth century and are maturing earlier. Britons in the higher socioeconomic groups have always been taller than those in the lower groups but this gap narrowed considerably during the twentieth century.

- Sexual maturation occurs earlier now than at the start of the twentieth century, e.g. girls are starting menstruate 2–3 years earlier than before and boys reach their adult stature at 19 years rather than in their mid-twenties.

- The normal or average values of height and weight of British children have also changed significantly during the course of the twentieth century. Note that large cross-sectional measurements of height in British adults have found a decrease in average height with increasing age. Part of this is a real tendency for people to decrease in height as they grow old but most of it is due to the tendency for younger generations to be taller than their parents and grandparents (e.g. White *et al.*, 1993).

Body size not only depends on environmental factors, like diet, but is also genetically determined. Some races of people may be genetically smaller than others and this is another factor that makes the use of non-local standards problematical. Within races there is a natural biological variation in the genetic component of height. This will obviously create difficulties in assessing the nutritional status of an individual child from a single set of anthropometric measurements. Are short children short because they are genetically small or because they are chronically malnourished? Growth curves are more useful ways of monitoring the nutritional status of individual children. Provided children remain on their predicted growth curve then whether the absolute values are low or high is in most cases unimportant. If a child on a high growth curve dips significantly below that curve it may indicate a nutrition or health problem even though he or she may be close to average for their age. Children who remain on a low growth curve will be assessed as growing satisfactorily even though they may be below average size for their age.

Centiles are frequently used to interpret anthropometric measures in children. If the growth curves of a population are plotted, growth curves that are typical of each per cent (or centile) of the population can be produced, i.e. the largest 1 per cent through to the smallest 1 per cent. If, for example, point measurements on a group indicate an average height for age that is substantially below the 50th centile, this suggests impaired growth in the sample group. A point measurement on an individual showing a value at the extremes of the range, e.g. below the 5th centile, indicates a probability that growth has been unsatisfactory. Figure 3.5 shows the World Health Organization (WHO) standards of height for age in girls up to 5 years of age; the 3rd, 10th, 50th, 90th and 97th centiles are given. If a girl has a height for age below the 3rd centile then there is a less than 3 per cent probability that she has been growing satisfactorily.

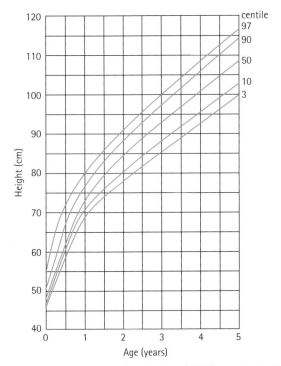

Figure 3.5 *World Health Organization (WHO) standards of height (length) for age, in girls aged up to 5 years. The 97th, 90th, 50th, 10th, and 3rd centiles are shown. After Passmore and Eastwood (1986).*

BMI in children

Although BMI is the single most widely used anthropometric measure in adults, its use in children has been hindered by a lack of universally agreed standards and 'cut-off' points like those that exist for adults. If such standards could be established then, as in adults, BMI could be used in children to assess and classify them, to monitor changes in levels of adiposity over time and also to make regional or international comparisons. The main difficulty is that BMI changes markedly with age. The following examples of median BMI at different ages illustrate this (Cole et al., 2000):

- birth – 13 kg/m^2
- 1 year – 17 kg/m^2
- 6 years – 15.5 kg/m^2
- 20 years – 21 kg/m^2.

Two main systems of standards have been used in Britain. Firstly values have been compared with a 1990 reference sample of British children (Cole et al., 1990). This large representative sample was used to construct centile curves of BMI with age from birth until adulthood. Values that fall above the 95th centile are taken to indicate obesity and those above the 85th centile classified as overweight. A similar set of reference data for American children has also been used in the USA. Such a system is useful for monitoring changes over time in a given population but it is rather arbitrary in its classification and of limited value for making international comparisons. Cole et al. (2000) devised a set of international standards based on the adult 'cut-off' points for obesity (BMI >30 kg/m^2) and overweight (BMI <25 kg/m^2). They used a sample of almost 100 000 children from six countries and plotted the centile curve of BMI against age for these children and used the centile curves that at 18 years went through the adult 'cut-off' for obesity and overweight. Selected values from this set of 'cut-off' points are shown in Table 3.5; in the original source (Cole et al., 2000), which can be accessed free online (www.bmj.com/cgi/content/full/320/7244/1240), a more extensive list is given at half-yearly intervals from 2 years of age onwards.

Table 3.5 Selected values for the estimated equivalent of an adult body mass index (BMI; kg/m^2) of 25 (overweight) and a BMI of 30 (obese) at various ages*

Age (years)	BMI (kg/m^2)			
	Indicating overweight		Indicating obese	
	Boys	Girls	Boys	Girls
2	18.41	18.02	20.09	19.81
4	17.55	17.28	19.29	19.15
6	17.55	17.34	19.78	19.65
8	18.44	18.35	21.60	21.57
10	19.84	19.85	24.00	24.11
12	21.22	21.68	26.02	26.67
14	22.62	23.34	27.63	28.57
16	23.90	24.37	28.88	29.43
18	25	25	30	30

*Data taken from Cole et al. (2000), based on a sample of almost 100 000 children from six countries.

Key points

- Weight for height is a measure of acute nutritional status in children but oedema may distort weight measurements.
- Height for age (or weight for age) is a cumulative or chronic measure of past status.
- Failure to grow and gain weight may be directly due to nutritional inadequacy or a secondary consequence of ill health.
- Genetic variation in size hinders the interpretation of height and/or weight measurements in children.
- Centiles (hundredths) are one way of allowing for genetic differences in size.
- If an individual value is below the appropriate 5th centile then this means that there is only a 5 per cent chance that that child has been growing satisfactorily.
- The average for a well-nourished population of children should be close to the 50th centile.
- If serial measurements are made, children should approximately follow their centile line.
- The body mass index (BMI) changes with age in children and so its use has been hindered by a lack of accepted standards.
- In one classification system for BMI in children, values are compared with an historical representative national dataset and values above the 85th centile for age classified as overweight and those above the 95th centile classified as obese.
- A less arbitrary and more internationally useful system determines from the centile lines for a large international sample of children the lines that correspond to a BMI of 25 kg/m^2 or 30 kg/m^2 at age 18 years.
- These centile lines allow values for each age that correspond to these adult values to be calculated and tabulated (examples shown in Table 3.5).

Estimating fatness in animals

The fat content of dead animals can be measured directly by extracting the fat with a suitable solvent (e.g. chloroform). Animal experimenters thus have

the option of using this precise analytical method at the end of their experiment. This analytical method also provides an absolute standard against which other methods of estimating fatness can be calibrated and validated. In humans, of course, any method of estimating fatness can only be validated and calibrated against another estimate.

Experimental animals can be used to show that there is an almost perfect negative correlation between the percentage of body water and the percentage of body fat (see Figure 3.6). This validates the use of body water measurements to predict body fatness. In the mice used to derive Figure 3.6, when body water was expressed as a percentage of the fat-free weight, all values were within the range of 74–76 per cent. This validates the earlier assumption that the body is made up of lean tissue with a constant proportion of water plus water-free fat. Other methods, similar to those described for people, are also available to estimate the fatness of animals: weight/length indices; density; and, in animals that store fat subcutaneously, like pigs, skinfold thickness. Rodents do not store much of their fat subcutaneously but dissection and weighing of one fat storage organ may be used to predict total fat content in dead animals (Webb and Jakobson, 1980).

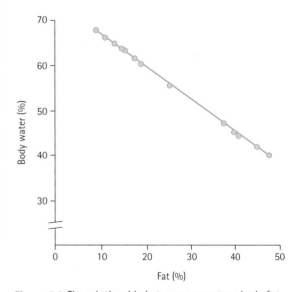

Figure 3.6 *The relationship between percentage body fat and percentage body water in mice. To illustrate the value of body water measurements in predicting body fat content. Data from Webb and Jakobson (1980). After Webb (1992a).*

Key points

- Body composition of animals can be measured accurately and directly by chemical analysis of the carcass.
- Carcass analysis can be used to calibrate and validate other less direct methods of estimating body composition. In humans, any method of estimating body composition can only be calibrated and validated by comparison with other estimates.
- Chemical analysis of animal carcasses shows that percentage body water is highly negatively correlated with percentage fat and that the water content of the fat-free mass is constant.

Biochemical assessment of nutritional status

Biochemical measures of nutrient status yield objective and quantitative measures and are the most sensitive indicators of nutritional status. They can usually be measured with great precision as is common with such analytical procedures. Several of these biochemical measures of nutrient status were discussed in the section dealing with the methods used to assess nutrient requirements, such as:

- measures of blood and tissue levels of nutrients or metabolites
- measures of nutrient excretion rates
- enzyme activation tests
- functional biochemical tests such as prothrombin time.

Table 3.6 gives a short list of some commonly used biochemical tests of nutritional status and the values that indicate normality and/or deficiency.

Biochemical measurements need laboratory facilities and they are relatively expensive and time consuming to perform. Interpretation of the values obtained will depend on the limits of normality that have been set and this will often be a matter of judgement. For example, blood haemoglobin concentration can be measured with considerable precision but deciding on the level that should be taken to

Table 3.6 Examples of biochemical tests of nutritional status*

Nutrient	Test	Deficiency	Adequacy
Protein/energy	Serum albumin		35–45 g/L
Protein/energy	Serum transferrin		2.5–3.0 g/L
Vitamin C	Plasma vitamin C	$<11\,\mu mol/L$	
Thiamin (B_1)	erythrocyte transketolase activation coefficient (ETKAC)	>1.25	
Riboflavin (B_2)	Erythrocyte glutathione reductase activation coefficient (EGRAC)	>1.3	
Vitamin B_6	Erythrocyte aspartate transaminase activation coefficient (EAATAC)	>2.00	
Niacin	Urinary N' methyl nicotinamide excretion (mg nicotinamide/g creatinine)	<0.5	>1.6
Folic acid	Serum folate (acute status)	$<6.3\,nmol/L$	$>7\,nmol/L$
	Red cell folate (long-term status)	$<337\,nmol/L$	$>422\,nmol/L$
Vitamin B_{12}	Serum B_{12}		$>118\,pmol/L$
Vitamin A	Plasma retinol used for long-term status (clinical tests are often used)	$<0.35\,\mu mol/L$	$>0.7\,\mu mol/L$
Vitamin D	Plasma 25-OH cholecalciferol (D_3)		$>25\,nmol/L$
Vitamin E	Total tocopherol in serum	$<11.6\,\mu mol/L$	
	Plasma tocopherol to cholesterol ratio	$<2.25\,\mu mol/mmol$	
Iron	Blood haemoglobin (men)	$<13\,g/dL\;(<130\,g/L)$	
	Blood haemoglobin (women)	$<12\,g/dL\;(<120\,g/L)$	
	Serum ferritin (men)	$<20\,\mu g/L$	
	Serum ferritin (women)	$<15\,\mu g/L$	
Zinc	Serum zinc	$<10\,\mu mol/L$	$>18\,\mu mol/L$

*Critical values for micronutrients in adults are largely taken from Ruston et al. (2004).

indicate anaemia will be a matter of judgement. Thus translating surveys of haemoglobin measurements into assessments of the prevalence of anaemia will depend very much on the limits of normality that are used. A figure of 12 g of haemoglobin per 100 mL of blood (120 g/L) at sea level was traditionally taken as the level below which there is a progressively increasing risk of anaemia; this is still used as the critical value for women (130 g/L for men). If this value is taken as the lower limit of normality then the prevalence of iron deficiency anaemia in menstruating women is high even in industrialized countries (10–20 per cent). However, clinical symptoms of anaemia may only become apparent with haemoglobin levels well below 120 g/L. Conversely, substantial depletion of iron stores (as measured by serum ferritin concentration) and some symptoms of iron deficiency may occur without any decrease in blood haemoglobin concentration. Assessment of iron status and prevalence of deficiency is discussed further in Chapter 14.

Perhaps the most striking recent illustration of the difficulties in setting realistic and useful thresholds for adequacy with biochemical methods of assessment is that of riboflavin. Riboflavin status is assessed biochemically by measuring EGRAC as described earlier in the chapter. An EGRAC of greater than 1.3 is taken to indicate riboflavin inadequacy. In the latest NDNS survey of British adults aged 19–64 years (Hoare et al., 2004) around two-thirds of adults were classified as riboflavin deficient using this criterion, rising to around 80 per cent in those under 25 years (details in Chapter 12). The average intake of riboflavin recorded in this survey was around 1.5 times the RNI. It is difficult to reconcile these two values. The biochemical classification at face value suggests that the RNI is set too low and that riboflavin inadequacy is a major problem in Britain and perhaps that food fortification with this vitamin needs to be considered. It seems more probable, as suggested by Hoare et al. (2004) that the biochemical assay is very sensitive and considerably overstates the real prevalence of riboflavin deficiency, and that consideration should be given to adjusting the biochemical criterion for riboflavin deficiency. Note that Finch et al. (1998) also found high prevalence of riboflavin deficiency in their NDNS survey of older adults using this same criterion (see Chapter 15).

Measurements made on urine samples have the obvious advantage of requiring no invasive procedures and of giving relatively large samples and thus avoiding the need for special micro-analytical techniques. They can be useful if excretion rate of an intact nutrient or readily identifiable derivative can be related to nutritional status. Rates of urine flow, and thus the concentration of solutes in urine samples, are very variable and greatly influenced by, e.g.:

- recent fluid consumption
- physical activity
- consumption of substances that have diuretic or antidiuretic activity (e.g. caffeine or nicotine).

Twenty-four-hour samples may give more meaningful results but their collection will be impractical in many survey situations. Even where they are feasible, checks will be required to ensure that the samples are complete in non-captive subjects. As an example, it is generally agreed that the best method of assessing salt intake on any particular day is to measure the sodium excreted in the urine in a 24-h period (see Chapter 14). To ensure that the 24-hour urine sample is complete, subjects may be asked to take doses of a marker substance (para-amino benzoic acid) with their meals. Only where there is practically complete recovery of the marker in the urine sample will the sample be accepted as complete. Note that the sodium excreted in a single 24-hour sample may not be a reliable indication of *habitual* salt intake (see Chapter 14). Urinary levels of the B vitamins have traditionally been used as measures of nutritional status for these vitamins. The values are often expressed as amount of nutrient (or nutrient derivative) per gram of creatinine in the urine sample as seen for niacin in Table 3.6. It is assumed that the excretion of creatinine is approximately constant and thus this gives a more meaningful value than the amount of nutrient per unit volume of urine because the latter depends on the rate of urine flow.

Blood samples give much greater scope for assessing nutrient status. Plasma, serum or blood cell concentrations of nutrients are extensively used as specific measures of nutritional status. Enzyme activation tests using red blood cell enzymes (as discussed earlier in the chapter) are also used. Plasma albumin concentration drops in severe protein energy malnutrition, and it has been widely used as a general biochemical indicator of nutritional status. Many medical conditions also result in a reduced plasma albumin concentration, e.g. liver and kidney disease, some cancers and infection. Albumin has a relatively long half-life in plasma, and it is now regarded as too insensitive and non-specific to be a good biochemical indicator of nutritional status.

Other plasma proteins with a shorter half-life in plasma may give a more sensitive indicator of protein energy status, e.g. **transferrin** (the protein that transports iron in plasma) and **retinol-binding protein** (the protein that transports vitamin A or **retinol**).

Blood tests require facilities and personnel capable of taking and safely handling, transporting and storing blood samples. Analysis of blood samples often requires special micro-analytical techniques because of the limited volumes that can be taken for analysis.

Key points

- Clinical signs, anthropometric measurements and biochemical analyses of body fluid samples can all be used to assess nutritional status. Examples of these methods are given in Boxes 3.2 and 3.3, and Table 3.6.
- With any nutritional assessment of groups or populations, steps must be taken to ensure that the sampled group is representative of the whole population under investigation.
- Clinical signs can be incorporated into checklists that can be used for screening and assessment by non-specialists and without the need for specialist equipment. They have the following merits and disadvantages:
  - they are quick, simple, and cheap to record
  - they are insensitive indicators of malnutrition and do not give early warning of an impending nutritional problem
  - some signs are common to several nutrient deficiencies and to non-nutritional problems and so they are not specific
  - they are qualitative and subjective because they depend upon the opinion of the assessor and often yield just a yes/no response or a descriptive grading of severity.
- Merits and disadvantages of anthropometric methods of assessment are:
  - they are quantitative and objective
  - many are quick and simple to perform, require only simple equipment and do not require specialist personnel
  - accurate assessment of fatness with skinfold calipers does require care and technical expertise
  - they often need reliable standards to interpret their results. Some are more useful if measured sequentially to monitor changes in nutritional status

- previous obesity can reduce their sensitivity in detecting deteriorating nutritional status
- oedema can substantially distort body weight and undermine any method that relies on accurate body weight measurement.
- Merits and disadvantages of biochemical methods are:
  - they are quantitative and objective
  - they are the most sensitive methods of nutritional assessment
  - in many cases, they are highly specific indicators of the status for a particular nutrient
  - they are time consuming, expensive and they need specialist laboratory facilities and personnel
  - standards of normality may be difficult to set in some cases
  - if concentration of a nutrient or metabolite in urine is measured then either some mechanism has to be found to correct for the wide variation in rates of urine flow or a complete 24-hour sample should be collected
  - blood analyses require an invasive collection procedure and often require a micro-analytical technique because of the small volumes available for the analysis.

Measurement of energy expenditure and metabolic rate

Metabolic rate is the rate at which energy is expended by the body. Energy expenditure may be rather crudely and indirectly assessed from measurements of energy intake. As energy can neither be created nor destroyed, energy expenditure over any given period must be equal to the intake plus or minus any change in body energy stores.

$$\text{Energy expenditure} = \text{energy intake} \pm \text{change in body energy}$$

When expenditure is measured in this way, the errors in measuring intake and changes in body energy will compound. The methods of measuring changes in body energy are insensitive, making this method unreliable for measurement of expenditure over short periods. Tens of thousands of calories may be added to or lost from body energy without their being quantifiable by the simple routine methods of measuring body composition. This error is minimized if the time period is long, but this means that subjects will be required to monitor their intakes for extended periods.

All of the energy expended by the body is ultimately lost as heat. It is theoretically possible to measure this directly in a whole body calorimeter. This is a chamber surrounded by a water jacket in which the heat released by the subject in the chamber is measured by a rise in temperature in the surrounding water. It is more usual to predict energy expenditure from measures of oxygen consumption and/or carbon dioxide evolution. Foodstuffs are metabolically oxidized to carbon dioxide, water and, in the case of protein, nitrogenous waste products such as urea. This oxidation process consumes atmospheric oxygen and produces carbon dioxide. The chemical equations for the oxidation of the various foodstuffs can be used to predict the **energy equivalent of oxygen**, which is the amount of energy released when a litre of oxygen is used to metabolically oxidize food. For example, the equation for the oxidation of glucose is:

$$C_6H_{12}O_6 \quad + \quad 6O_2 \quad = \quad 6CO_2 \quad + \quad 6H_2O$$

| $180\,g$ | $6 \times 22.4\,L$ | $6 \times 22.4\,L$ | $6 \times 18\,g$ |
| Glucose | Oxygen | Carbon dioxide | Water |

Oxidation of $180\,g$ of glucose yields about 665 kcal (2800 kJ).

Thus 1 L of oxygen yields approximately 4.95 kcal (20.8 kJ) when it is being used to metabolize glucose, i.e. 665 divided by (6×22.4). Similar calculations can be performed using the other substrates. They yield energy equivalents for oxygen that are not very different from that for glucose. If a mixture of substrates is being oxidized, a figure of 4.86 kcal (20.4 kJ) per litre of oxygen can be used as the approximate energy equivalent of oxygen. If more precise estimation is required, the ratio of carbon dioxide evolution to oxygen consumption, the **respiratory quotient (RQ)**, gives an indication of the balance of substrates being metabolized. The RQ is 1.0 if carbohydrate is being oxidized but only 0.71 if fat is being oxidized. Tables are available listing the energy equivalent of oxygen at various RQs.

The simplest way of measuring oxygen consumption (and carbon dioxide evolution) is to use a Douglas bag. This is a large plastic bag fitted with a two-way valve so that the subject who breathes through a mouthpiece attached to the valve sucks in air from the atmosphere and then blows it out into the bag. All of the expired air can be collected over a period of time, and the volume and composition of this expired air can be measured. Knowing the composition of the inspired atmospheric air means that the subject's oxygen consumption and carbon dioxide evolution can be calculated. Note that the collection period is limited to a few minutes even if the capacity of the bag is large (100 L).

The static spirometer is essentially a metal bell that is filled with oxygen and is suspended with its open end under water. The subject breathes through a tube connected to the oxygen-containing chamber of the bell. The bell rises and falls as the volume of gas inside the bell changes; thus it will fall and rise with each inspiration and expiration. If the system contains a carbon dioxide absorber then the bell will gradually sink as the subject uses up the oxygen in the bell. This change in volume of oxygen inside the bell can be recorded on a calibrated chart and thus the rate of oxygen consumption can be determined. This is a standard undergraduate practical exercise. It is limited to a few minutes of measurement of resting oxygen consumption or short periods of consumption with static exercise, e.g. on an exercise bicycle.

Portable respirometers have been developed that can be strapped onto the back and thus used and worn while performing everyday domestic, leisure or employment tasks. These respirometers, such as the Max Planck respirometer, monitor the volume of gas expired by the wearer and divert a small proportion of the expired gas to a collection bag for later analysis. They are once again only suitable for relatively short-term recording, but they can be used to quantify the energy costs of a variety of tasks. If subjects keep a detailed record of their 5 minute by 5 minute activities over a day (**activity diary**), total energy expenditure can be roughly estimated using the measured energy costs of the various activities.

Many research units have respiration chambers that allow relatively long-term measurement of energy expenditure of subjects performing any routine tasks that may be done within the chamber. The respiration chamber is essentially a small room with controlled and measured flow of air through it. Oxygen consumption and carbon dioxide production by the subject can be measured by the difference in the composition of air as it enters and leaves the chamber. These pieces of equipment are, in practice, complex and expensive, and thus restricted to a relatively few well-funded research units. They can be used to monitor long-term energy expenditure of subjects who can live in the chamber for several days and perform everyday tasks that simulate normal daily activity.

Over the past few years, the **doubly labelled water method** has been widely used to determine the long-term energy expenditure of free-living subjects going about their normal daily activities. Subjects are given a dose of doubly labelled water ($^2H_2^{18}O$), i.e. water containing the heavy isotopes of hydrogen (^2H) and oxygen (^{18}O). The subjects lose the labelled oxygen more rapidly than the labelled hydrogen because the hydrogen is lost only as water whereas the oxygen is lost as both water and carbon dioxide. This is due to the action of the enzyme carbonic anhydrase that promotes the exchange of oxygen between water and carbon dioxide. The difference between the rate of loss of labelled hydrogen and labelled oxygen is a measure of the rate of carbon dioxide evolution, and it can be used to estimate long-term rate of carbon dioxide evolution and thus long-term energy expenditure. Comparisons of total energy expenditure measurements by respiration chamber and by doubly labelled-water method suggest that this method gives an accurate measure of energy expenditure. Using this method, investigators at last have an acceptably accurate means of estimating the long-term energy expenditure of free-living people.

Comparisons of metabolic rates between individuals

Basal metabolic rate (BMR) is the minimum rate of energy expenditure in a conscious, resting animal or person. It is the metabolic rate measured in a rested, fasted individual who has been lying in a room at thermoneutral temperature for half an hour. Absolute BMR obviously tends to increase with increasing body size. Large animals have higher absolute BMRs than small ones. Fully grown adults have larger BMRs than small children. However, relative BMR (i.e. per unit body mass) declines with increasing body size. Small animals have larger relative metabolic rates than large ones. Small children have higher relative metabolic rates than adults. This equation approximately predicts the BMR of mammals of different sizes both within and between species:

$$\text{Basal metabolic rate} = \text{Constant (k)} \times \text{Weight}^{3/4}$$
$$\text{\small (kcal/day)} \qquad \text{\small (70)} \qquad \text{\small (kg)}$$

For more information on BMR and its prediction from body weight see Chapter 6. Human metabolic rates have traditionally been expressed per unit of body surface area, e.g. kcal(kJ)/hour/m². Even in human adults, if BMR is expressed per unit of body weight, large variations between individuals are found, particularly between fat and thin individuals. Adipose tissue has a much lower metabolic rate than lean tissue and so increasing adipose tissue mass has relatively much less effect in increasing whole body metabolic rate than increasing lean tissue mass. Increasing adipose tissue mass also has relatively little effect in increasing body surface area. Thus expressing BMR per unit surface area tends to reduce the individual variation and has been a useful way of comparing BMR in different individuals. Nomograms are available that allow surface area to be predicted from measurements of height and weight.

Nowadays, it is considered that the best way of comparing and expressing BMR of people is to express it per unit weight of lean tissue, e.g. kcal(kJ)/hour/kg lean tissue. When expressed in this way, the BMRs of men and women are not different whereas when expressed per unit surface area those of women are about 10 per cent less than those of men. This is an artefact due to the much higher body fat content of women.

Key points

- Metabolic rate is the rate of energy expenditure of the body and basal metabolic rate (BMR) is the minimum metabolic rate measured in a conscious person who is rested, warm and fasted.
- Metabolic rate can be measured directly by measuring heat output but it is usually calculated from the rates of oxygen consumption and/or carbon dioxide production.
- Conventional methods of measuring metabolic rate by oxygen consumption only allow it to be monitored for a few minutes at a time. Even in a respiration chamber, subjects are restricted to the activities that can be carried out in a small room.
- The doubly labelled water method allows long-term energy expenditure to be measured in free-living subjects.
- Absolute BMR increases with body size but relative BMR (i.e. per unit body weight)

decreases with size. Small animals or people have smaller absolute but larger relative BMRs than larger animals.

- BMR (in kcal/day) can be roughly predicted by multiplying the body weight (in kg) raised to the power 0.75 by a constant (70).
- Metabolic rates of people have traditionally been expressed per unit of body surface area and if this method is used, men have higher relative BMRs than women.
- It is better to express relative metabolic rate per unit of lean tissue mass; the sex differences in relative BMR then disappear because it is an artefact caused by the higher body fat content of females.

METHODS USED TO ESTABLISH LINKS BETWEEN DIET AND DISEASE

Strategic approaches – observational versus experimental

Two main strategies can be used for investigating possible links between dietary or other lifestyle variables and diseases or disease risk factors such as high blood pressure or high plasma cholesterol concentration.

- *The observational approach.* Observational, epidemiological methods are used to relate differences in the diets or lifestyle characteristics of populations or individuals to their risk of developing a disease or their measured level of a disease risk factor. Descriptive epidemiological methods rely on looking at the occurrence and distribution of diseases in groups or populations whereas with analytical epidemiological methods data are collected from individuals with the aim of testing an hypothesis. Analytical studies may include a control group.
- *The experimental approach.* In this approach, investigators attempt to produce a controlled change in the diets or other behaviour of individuals or populations to determine the effect that this has on the disease/mortality risk or the measured level of a risk factor such as blood pressure or plasma cholesterol.

Box 3.4 classifies the methods available for investigating possible links between diet and disease under three headings – descriptive epidemiology, analytical epidemiology and experimental methods. In the following sections, the principles and problems of these methods are discussed with examples chosen to illustrate the methodology and its problems. Often well-known classic studies and older studies have been chosen for illustrative purposes. Several of these classic papers highly influenced the later direction that research took and the scientific opinion of their time. Some studies have been chosen because they illustrate some of the pitfalls of their methodology.

Box 3.4	Research methods used to investigate possible links between diet and disease

Observational methods

Descriptive epidemiology

- *Cross-cultural comparisons.* Correlation is made between the level of a dietary factor and the frequency of a disease in different populations. These may be comparisons between nations or between special groups within a nation (e.g. between Seventh Day Adventists and the rest of the population in the USA)
- *Time trends.* Changes in the dietary habits of populations are correlated with changes in disease frequency

- *Migration studies.* The changes in dietary habits that follow migration are correlated with changes in disease frequency in the migrant population
- *'Experiments of nature'.* These are studies of people with some genetic mutation or other accident of nature that increases (or decreases) their exposure to some suggested disease risk factor. Does the increased exposure to the risk factor result in increased rate of disease?

Analytical epidemiology

- *Cohort studies.* The dietary characteristics of a large sample of individuals are measured. The samples are selected and the measurements made to test a hypothesis. The deaths and the causes of mortality and/or morbidity of individuals within the sample are then monitored over the succeeding years. Disease risk is correlated with the level of exposure to possible dietary risk factors

- *Case–control studies*. Established cases of the disease are identified and matched to a sample of non-sufferers, the controls. The past diet (or other exposure) of the cases and controls are then compared to see if this provides evidence of greater exposure to the suggested risk factor in the case group (or greater exposure to a possible protective factor in the control group)

Experimental methods

- *Animal experiments*. Dietary changes are tested in short- or long-term controlled experiments with laboratory animals to see if they result in the postulated change in risk factor or disease frequency
- *Short-term human experiments*. Dietary changes are tested in short-term controlled experiments to

see if they result in the postulated change in risk factor measurement

- *Clinical trials*. A dietary change that is expected to lead to improved prognosis in patients is tested under controlled conditions to see if it yields the expected benefits. Ideally the treatment is compared with the effects of a **placebo** (dummy) treatment and neither the investigators nor the patient knows who has received the real and placebo treatments until after the study is completed (double-blind trial)
- *Intervention trial*. A population-level trial. An attempt is made to change the exposure of a test population to the postulated dietary factor, e.g. by encouragement or possible by a nutrient fortification programme. The change in disease frequency is compared with that in a control population that has not received the intervention
- *Systematic reviews and meta-analyses*. All trials of a particular intervention that meet set quality criteria are identified. These are then weighted according to sample size and their data used in a combined statistical analysis. This allows several smaller studies to be combined together to produce a single study of much greater statistical power

Key points

- Observational (epidemiological) and experimental approaches are used to investigate links between diet and disease.
- Epidemiological methods can be subdivided into observational epidemiology and analytical epidemiology.
- In the experimental approach, there are experimental and control groups and the investigators impose some 'intervention(s)' on the experimental group, which is designed to test an hypothesis.
- Box 3.4 summarizes the principles of the various methods.

Some general characteristics and problems of epidemiological methods

Association does prove cause and effect

Epidemiological methods produce evidence of an association between two variables. In this context, evidence of an association between some measured

dietary variable and a disease or risk factor such as high blood pressure. Such epidemiological association does not necessarily mean that there is a 'cause and effect' relationship between the dietary factor and the disease. The association may be coincidental and dependent on a relationship between both tested variables and a third unconsidered or **confounding variable** (or many confounding variables). It is even possible that in some cases that there may be an 'effect and cause' relationship, i.e. the disease results in a change in the dietary variable. This important distinction has already been discussed in Chapter 1 and several examples are described there. The problem of confounding variables pervades all types of epidemiological investigation and epidemiologists use various means and statistical devices to correct for variables they suspect to be confounding but this is an imperfect process and the quality of this correction is likely to vary considerably from study to study.

If, as claimed by McCormick and Skrabanek (1988) there really are 250 risk markers for coronary heart disease then the task of identifying any one of them as independent of all of the others is a formidable one. An apparent protective effect of moderate doses of alcohol against coronary heart disease has been reported many times (see Chapter 4) but how many authors will have considered or corrected for level of physical activity as a potential confounding variable? One large English survey reported a strong positive association between alcohol consumption and level of physical activity (White *et al.*, 1993). Barker *et al.* (1998) list six characteristics which make it more likely that a demonstrated association is causal.

- *Strength of the association.* The stronger the association the less the likelihood that it is due to some unforeseen confounding factor.
- *It is graded or dose dependent.* There is usually a graded effect of true causes rather than a threshold effect.
- *Independence of the association.* The relationship remains significant even after correction for potentially confounding variables.
- *Consistency of the finding.* If the association is found in a variety of studies using different investigative approaches this makes it more likely that it is due to cause and effect.
- *Reversibility.* If reduced exposure to the suspected cause leads to reduced incidence of the disease this increases the likelihood of it being a true cause.
- *Plausibility.* The association is more likely to be 'cause and effect' if there is a believable mechanism to explain the causality of the association, which can be supported by laboratory studies. A plausible mechanism unsupported by corroborating laboratory studies probably adds little weight to the argument. It is quite possible to devise plausible mechanisms for most observations, often equally plausible mechanisms for opposing findings. The most plausible and intellectually satisfying mechanism may not be the one that ultimately proves to be correct.

Sources and quality of data

Information about the diets of individuals and populations is derived from the methods discussed earlier in this chapter. Food balance sheets or household expenditure surveys (such as the UK Food and Expenditure Survey) are often the basis for international dietary comparisons. Methods that correlate dietary factors with disease risk in individuals clearly require individual methods of dietary assessment. Dietary surveys of large representative samples can be properly used for international comparisons, e.g.

the rolling programme of NDNS surveys in the UK. Small, unrepresentative survey results that are extrapolated and taken to represent whole populations can be major sources of error. The many sources of error and uncertainty in estimating dietary intakes have been discussed earlier in the chapter. Acceptably accurate and representative measures of habitual dietary intake are clearly a prerequisite for detecting associations between diet and disease risk.

Information about mortality from specific diseases is usually obtained through some analysis of information recorded on death certificates. Efforts have been made to standardize death certificates internationally and to standardize the nomenclature and diagnostic criteria for the various causes of death. The WHO publishes the *International classification of diseases, injuries and causes of death* (ICD), which is regularly revised. Death certificates in the UK list both the underlying (main) cause and contributory causes of death. There will, however, still be differences between individual doctors and this variation is likely to be even greater between those in different regions or nations. There may be straightforward errors of diagnosis, different diagnostic criteria or terminology may be used at different times or in different centres, even the accuracy of the age recording on death certificates may vary. When autopsies have been used to confirm the accuracy of previously recorded causes of death, they show that errors in diagnosing the causes of death in individual patients may be common. Both false positives (i.e. people falsely diagnosed as dying of the disease) and false negatives (i.e. people dying of the disease but not recognized as such) tend to occur. If individuals are the unit of comparison then these two errors compound but they do tend to cancel out if population mortality is calculated. Even though the number of individual errors of diagnosis may be quite large, provided false negatives and false positives occur at similar rates then the accuracy of the estimate of population mortality may be little affected. Systematic over- or under-recording of deaths from any cause will seriously distort population comparisons, e.g. any attempt to play down the prevalence of a disease to protect the tourist industry or for other commercial or political reasons.

Accurate and representative measures of morbidity in populations are probably more difficult to obtain than mortality data. Investigators almost certainly have to rely on less rigorous and uniform methods of collecting data than death certificates. Some sources of information about disease frequency in populations are:

- notification or registration of particular diseases. Any variations in the efficiency of these collection procedures in different areas will distort the estimates of disease frequency
- analysis of reasons for hospital admission or general practitioner consultation. Multiple recordings of the same individuals is one source of error here
- social security data on reasons for absences from work
- extrapolation from relatively small scale and possibly unrepresentative survey samples.

Incidence and **prevalence** are terms used to indicate disease frequency. Incidence is the number of new cases of the disease occurring within a specified time period. Prevalence is the number of cases of the disease existing at any particular point in time. Prevalence depends both on the incidence and the duration of the disease. A chronic disease will have a much greater prevalence than an acute one of similar incidence. As an example, the incidence of **cystic fibrosis** in the UK remained fairly constant for many years at about 300–400 per year but the prevalence has increased because the survival time of people with the disease has increased. The chronic diseases of industrialization, almost by definition therefore, have high prevalence. Not only do they cause reduced quality of life for large numbers of people but they also exert a considerable drain on health and social care budgets.

If an asymptomatic risk factor, such as plasma cholesterol level or blood pressure, is being related to diet then investigators will have to rely on data obtained from their own or published surveys. If these surveys are used to make international comparisons then they may have been conducted in the various countries by different investigators using different protocols. Since the early 1990s annual health surveys of representative samples of English adults have included anthropometric measurements and measurements of major risk factors as a result of the 1990 *Health of the Nation* white paper (and similar Welsh and Scottish surveys). The rolling programme of NDNS surveys also includes anthropometric measurements and measurements of some key diet-related risk factors such as blood pressure and blood lipoprotein concentrations.

Age standardization

Whenever comparisons of the death (or disease) rates between different populations or groups are made, some allowance has to be made for any differences in their age structures. The simplest measure of mortality is the **crude death rate** for the specified cause:

$$\frac{\text{Number of deaths (by cause) in one year}}{\text{Number of people in the population}} \times 1000$$

This measure is often of limited value because mortality from many causes is so highly age-dependent and because of the widely varying age structures of some populations. Higher birth rates and shorter life expectancies mean, for example, that populations in developing countries tend to have a lower average age than in the Western industrialized countries. A more useful measure for international or regional comparisons is the age-specific death rate, e.g.:

$$\frac{\begin{array}{c}\text{Annual number of deaths (by cause)}\\ \text{in men aged 45–54 years}\end{array}}{\begin{array}{c}\text{Number of men in this age}\\ \text{group in the population}\end{array}} \times 1000$$

To make more complete comparisons the **standard mortality ratio (SMR)** is a useful and widely used measure. To calculate the SMR, it is necessary to use as a standard or reference population, a population in which all of the various age-specific mortality rates for the cause under investigation have been established. Then for each age band of the test population, one must calculate how many deaths would be expected or predicted given:

- the number of persons of that age in the test population
- assuming the same age-specific death rate as in the reference population.

For example:

Number of men aged 45–49 years in the test population $\times$ death rate from the cause for men aged 45–49 years in the reference population = number of predicted deaths in 45–49-year-old men in the test population

This calculation is made for each relevant age group in the population, and the total number of predicted deaths in the test population is calculated.

The total number of actual deaths in the test population is then expressed as a percentage or ratio of the predicted number of deaths from that cause in that test population:

$$SMR = \frac{\text{Actual number of deaths in test population}}{\text{Predicted number of deaths}} (\times 100)$$

The SMR can be used for international comparisons, to make regional comparisons within any given country or to make comparisons between other groups. When used for regional comparisons within a country, the whole national population can be used as a reference population. For example, comparisons of the SMRs for gastric cancer in different regions of Britain in the early 1980s showed that the SMR was over 115 in Wales but less than 85 in parts of East Anglia. People in Wales have more than a 1.15 times greater risk of dying of this disease than the national population whereas those in East Anglia has less than 0.85 times the risk of the whole population. Regional differences in diet, lifestyle and environment in Britain can be compared to see if any are associated with this variation in gastric cancer mortality. This might provide important clues about the aetiology of gastric cancer.

Key points

- Epidemiological methods provide evidence of association between dietary variables and disease risk.
- Epidemiological association between two variables does not necessarily mean that they are causally related.
- Association may arise because both of the tested variables are linked to other confounding variables.
- An association is more likely to be causal if it is strong, consistent between studies, dose-dependent, independent of likely confounding variables, reversible, and can be explained by a plausible mechanism that can be supported by experiment.
- Information about causes of death is usually obtained directly or indirectly from death certificates.

- There is an international classification system for causes of death (the ICD) and a standardization of the format of death certificates.
- Errors do occur in the diagnosis of cause of death – false negatives and false positives. These tend to compound when individuals are the unit of study but tend to cancel out when population mortality rates are calculated.
- Accurate information on frequency of non-fatal diseases or disease risk factors is likely to be more problematical than calculation of mortality rates.
- Information on non-fatal disease frequency is obtained from the following sources:
  - disease notifications or registers
  - analysis of reasons for hospital admission, physician consultations or absences from work
  - from surveys.
- Incidence is the number of new cases of a disease that occur within a specified time period.
- Prevalence is the number of cases of a disease that exist at any point in time. It is a product of the incidence and duration of the disease.
- Comparisons of crude death rates between groups or populations may be of little value if they are not age (and sex) standardized because the age and sex structures of different populations may be very different.
- Age-specific death rate is the rate of death from a disease within a specified age and sex group.
- Standard mortality ratio is the ratio of predicted deaths to actual deaths in test populations.
- The predicted number of deaths is calculated as those that would occur in a population of this age structure if the age-specific death rates were the same as those in a reference population.

Cross-cultural comparisons

An early indication that diet may be implicated in the aetiology of a disease often comes from cross-cultural associations between a population measure of the dietary variable and population mortality or morbidity rates from the disease. Some examples are given below.

- A positive association between the average saturated fat intakes of populations and their mortality rates from coronary heart disease points towards high saturated fat intakes as a causal factor in coronary heart disease.

- A positive association between *per capita* sugar consumption in different countries and the average number of decayed, missing and filled teeth in young people implicates sugar in the aetiology of dental caries.
- A positive association between *per capita* salt consumption and blood pressure in various adult populations implicates high salt intake in the aetiology of hypertension.
- A negative association between *per capita* fibre consumption and bowel cancer mortality in various populations has been used to implicate the fibre depletion of Western diets in the aetiology of bowel cancer.

There are large variations between nations in mortality and morbidity rates from the diet-related diseases of industrialization. It is, therefore, common to see cross-population associations between a dietary variable and one of these diseases used to implicate diet as a major cause of the disease as in the four above examples. It is, of course, premature to then assume a cause and effect relationship between that dietary factor and the disease. As populations become more affluent numerous changes in diet, lifestyle and environmental conditions tend to occur simultaneously, opening up the likelihood that there will be many confounding variables. For example, all of the following changes may accompany increasing affluence and industrialization:

- increased fat and saturated fat consumption
- lower consumption of starches and fibre
- increased use of simple sugars, salt and perhaps alcohol and tobacco
- increased consumption of animal protein
- reduced incidence of nutritional deficiencies
- reduced physical activity
- increased proportions of overweight and obese people
- improved medical care
- many other changes in diet, lifestyle and environment.

Accompanying these trends for change in diet and lifestyle are general trends in patterns of mortality and morbidity. Life expectancy increases, mortality from infectious diseases and other acute causes declines, but there is increased prevalence of and mortality from the various chronic diseases of industrialization. Cross-cultural studies tend to focus on individual associations between one of these lifestyle or dietary changes and one of these chronic diseases. Thus the association between saturated fat intake and coronary heart disease mortality is used to support the proposition that high intake of saturated fat causes heart disease, and the negative association between fibre intake and bowel cancer used to support the proposition that low intakes of fibre cause bowel cancer. As high-fat diets tend to be low in fibre and vice versa, it would certainly be possible to produce equally convincing correlations between fibre intake and coronary heart disease (negatively correlated) and between saturated fat intake and bowel cancer.

The classic paper of Gleibermann (1973) on the relationship between the average salt intake and blood pressure of adult populations illustrates several of these problems of cross-cultural studies. From the literature, she gleaned estimates of the salt intakes and blood pressures of middle-aged people in 27 populations from various parts of the world. The data for the male populations have been used to construct a simple scatter diagram (Figure 3.7). The correlation coefficient and line of best fit have also been calculated. There is a highly significant, positive and apparently linear relationship between the average salt intake and the mean blood pressure of these populations, consistent with the hypothesis that high salt intake is causally linked to the development of hypertension.

The two variables in Figure 3.7 were measured by numerous investigators. The methods, conditions of measurement and quality of measurement are therefore not consistent across the groups. As has already been noted earlier in the chapter, salt intake is a particularly problematical measurement. The methods used to determine salt intakes in these 27 populations varied and in some cases were unspecified, ranging from the high precision 24-hour sodium excretion method to 'educated guesses' made by Gleibermann herself. Recorded blood pressure may be very much influenced by the method used and the care taken by the measurer to standardize the conditions, e.g. blood pressure may be affected by how long the subjects are allowed to relax before measurement and it may be raised if measured in anxious subjects.

Although the correlation shown in Figure 3.7 was highly significant, there is a considerable scatter of points around the line of best fit. The correlation coefficient (r) was 0.61, suggesting that only about 37 per cent (r^2) of the variation in population blood pressures is accounted for by variation in their salt intake. It is possible that this association is due to some confounding variable or variables, e.g. the populations with the lowest blood pressures and lowest salt intakes would also tend to be active, have low levels of obesity, have relatively low alcohol intakes, have high potassium intakes. All of these factors are thought to favour lower blood pressure. More recent investigators have suggested that the inclusion of different races may have increased the scatter with Gleibermann's data because black populations may be genetically more sensitive to the hypertensive effects of salt (e.g. Law *et al.*, 1991a).

The range of salt intakes shown in Figure 3.7 was huge, from around 1 g/day to well over 25 g/day. The average salt intakes in the UK and USA are some way below the middle of this range. If one takes the linear relationship at face value, it could be predicted that specified falls in any population's average salt intake would be associated with specified falls in average blood pressure. One could then go on to make predictions about the expected benefits for that population (reductions in the prevalence of hypertension and hypertension-related diseases). It would be hard to show conclusively that this association was linear over the whole range. This is what is being assumed when predicting that small or moderate reductions in salt intakes of the populations around the centre of the range will have predictable effects on average blood pressure.

Numerous studies in Western industrialized countries have measured blood pressure and salt intakes in large samples of individuals living in particular towns or regions. In many of these studies no association was found between individual salt intake and individual blood pressure. One explanation for this disparity is that the gold standard method for measuring salt intake (24-hour sodium excretion) is probably a poor measure of an individual's habitual salt intake. This fact alone would make it improbable that one would find a correlation between individual salt intake measured in this way and blood pressure even if habitual salt intake is a major determinant of individual blood pressure (see Chapter 14 for further discussion).

Such disparity between cross-cultural and within population studies is common in epidemiological studies and also tends to be found, for example, when dietary saturated fat intake and plasma cholesterol are correlated. Taking these results at face value, one might conclude that whereas average salt intake is an important determinant of average population blood pressure, individual differences in salt intake are not a major factor in producing the differences in blood pressure within a single population. This may initially seem like a contradiction because, of course, the influence of salt on population blood pressure would have to be a summation of its effects on the blood pressure of individuals. However, numerous other factors may also affect an individual's blood pressure, such as:

- individual genetic variation
- levels of activity and obesity
- alcohol consumption
- genetic variation in susceptibility to the hypertensive effects of salt.

These other influences on blood pressure may mask any effect of salt on individual blood pressure. Some people may have high blood pressure because they are overweight, inactive and consume large amounts of alcohol yet their salt consumption may be low. Other people may have low blood pressure despite high salt intake because they are fit, abstemious and

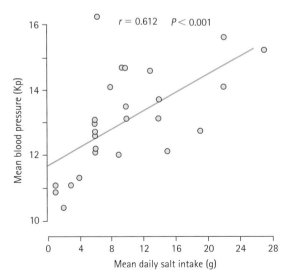

Figure 3.7 *Simple scatter diagram showing the relationship between estimated salt intake and mean blood pressure in 27 male populations. Data of Gleibermann (1973).*

relatively salt insensitive. Large numbers of such people would, of course, make it difficult to find a significant association between salt intake and blood pressure, especially as most people within any given population will be concentrated around the mean value and the total range of salt intakes may be relatively narrow. This problem is discussed further in the section dealing with short-term human experiments later in this chapter.

Anomalous populations

Cross-cultural studies may highlight anomalous populations that deviate significantly from the general trend. These anomalous populations may provide useful information that can lead to modification of existing theories or to additional areas of investigation. Observations that Greenland Eskimos had low rates of heart disease despite a diet high in fats of animal origin were important in focusing attention on the potential dietary and therapeutic benefits of fish oils (Dyerberg and Bang, 1979, see Chapter 11 for further discussion). Mckeigue *et al.* (1985) found that the south Asian population living in one area of London had much higher rates of coronary heart disease than the white population living in the same area. This was despite their apparently lower exposure to many of the traditional risk markers for coronary heart disease, e.g. they had lower serum cholesterol levels, smoked less, drank less alcohol, consumed less saturated fat and cholesterol, and many were lactovegetarian (see Chapter 17 for further discussion).

Special groups

There are 'special groups' within populations that because of their religion or occupation behave differently from most of the people around them. Such groups are often intensively studied because there should be less confounding variables between these groups and the rest of their own population than are seen in other cross-cultural studies. For example, Seventh Day Adventists in the USA are a religious group who abstain from alcohol and tobacco and around half of them are ovolactovegetarian. They have lower rates of coronary heart disease and many types of cancer (including bowel cancer) than the American population as a whole (e.g. Fraser, 1988).

Despite the use of such groups because of better matching than in most cross-cultural studies, there may still be numerous differences in the diet and lifestyle of these groups compared with say, the average American. Picking out one dietary or other lifestyle difference between such groups and the rest of the population may still produce false assumptions about cause and effect. A religion may 'impose' numerous lifestyle and dietary constraints on its adherents; religious groups may be socially, intellectually or even genetically unrepresentative of the population as a whole; and of course their religious faith may provide emotional comfort that lessens the impact of stresses on mental and physical health. One report even suggests that being religious itself protects against the development of bowel cancer (Kune *et al.*, 1993).

Key points

- Cross-cultural comparisons aiming to identify associations between diet and disease risk are particularly prone to confounding effects.

- Increasing affluence and industrialization bring multiple changes in diet composition and lifestyle as well as major changes in life expectancy and disease frequencies.

- Several associations between diet and disease risk factors that are consistently found in between-population studies are not apparent in samples of individuals from within the same population, e.g. the association between daily salt intake and blood pressure. Some of the possible reasons for this dichotomy are:
  - measures of the average nutrient intakes of populations may be much more valid than measures of the habitual intakes of individuals
  - within populations there is likely to a much narrower range of nutrient intakes and risk factor levels
  - many factors other than the dietary variable may influence an individual's risk factor level and so obscure the relationship.

- In cross-cultural studies, anomalous populations who deviate markedly from the general trend may open up new areas of investigation or generate new hypotheses.

- Special groups within populations whose diet and behaviour differ markedly from the bulk of the population are of special interest. There are likely to be fewer confounding variables than with other cross-cultural comparisons.

Time trends

Populations' diets and lifestyles tend to change with the passage of time, these changes may be particularly rapid and pronounced if there has been rapid economic development and industrialization. Epidemiologists may look for associations between the changes in a population's diet and its mortality and morbidity rates for particular diseases. Seasonal changes may also be important if an acute event is being studied.

In America and western Europe, salt consumption declined during the twentieth century as salting was largely replaced as a means of preserving food by refrigeration and other preservation methods. This decline in salt consumption in these countries was associated with reduced mortality for stroke and gastric cancer (note that high blood pressure is a risk factor for stroke). These observations were used to support the proposition that salt is an aetiological influence for both of these diseases (Joossens and Geboers, 1981). Figure 3.8 shows a very strong correlation between average death rates from stroke and gastric cancer in 12 industrialized countries between 1955 and 1972. This is consistent with the hypothesis that a change in exposure to a common causal influence was responsible for the decline in mortality from both diseases, i.e. reduced intake of dietary salt. The apparent, relative acceleration in the rate of stroke mortality after 1972 is attributed to the population impact of antihypertensive drugs, which would be expected to reduce mortality from stroke but not gastric cancer. MacGregor and de Wardener (1998) give several more examples of associations between falling salt consumption and falling blood pressure, but the decline in salt intake in these studies was partly induced by active publicity campaigns rather than being wholly spontaneous and so cannot be classified as descriptive epidemiological studies.

In Chapter 8, Figure 8.4 (p. 189) shows a marked increase in the prevalence of obesity in England over the past 25 years. Later in the same chapter (Figure 8.13, p. 208) shows that the average *per capita* calorie intake has declined markedly in recent decades, i.e. we are eating less but getting fatter. These paradoxical time trends are used to support the hypothesis that declining physical activity is a major underlying cause of the rising levels of overweight and obesity.

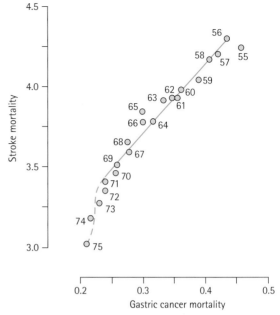

Figure 3.8 *Time trends in mortality from gastric cancer and stroke over 20 years. Each point represents average death rates from these diseases in 12 industrialized countries for that year, e.g. 55 represents rates in 1955. Source: Webb (1992a). Simplified from Joossens and Geboers (1981).*

The Japanese are frequently used by those investigating links between diet and disease as an example of a nation that, though affluent and industrialized, has a diet very different from the typical American and western European diets. The Japanese diet has much less meat and dairy produce but much more vegetable matter and seafood. Since World War II, however, the Japanese diet has undergone considerable 'Westernization'. For example, since 1950 total fat intake has trebled; the ratio of animal to vegetable fat has doubled; and American-style fast-food outlets have mushroomed. Mortality patterns of the Japanese have also changed over this time scale. Two-thirds of deaths in Japan are now due to cardiovascular diseases, cancer and diabetes whereas in 1950 only one-third were due to these causes. Deaths from cancer have increased two and a half times since 1950 as have deaths from heart disease, e.g. in Chapter 9 it is noted that in 1960 age standardized rates of bowel cancer in Japan used to be about a third of UK levels but are now very similar to UK rates.

These changes in Japanese mortality patterns are consistent with current views on the causal influences of diet on particular chronic diseases. Note, however, that Japanese boys are now more than 20 per cent taller than they were in 1950 and total life expectancy of the Japanese has also shown very big increases over the same time scale making them now one of the most long-lived population in the world. Fujita (1992) reviewed these changes in the Japanese diet since World War II and concluded that 'they have greatly improved the nutritional status of the Japanese people'. He further suggested that the rise in crude mortality rates from the diseases of industrialization is 'mainly due to increases in the actual numbers of elderly people, rather than to westernising effects in dietary habits'. Of course, this does not mean that the current Japanese diet is optimal, and it certainly does not mean that further 'westernization' of the Japanese diet will lead to further benefits but the example does illustrate the potential hazards of focusing too narrowly on individual causes of mortality or morbidity.

Key points

- Temporal changes in disease frequency can be associated with corresponding changes in diet in genetically stable populations.
- These changes may take place rapidly if there is rapid industrialization in a country.
- Many of the problems of cross-cultural studies also apply to analysis of time trends.
- Increases in the proportion of deaths due to chronic diseases are inevitable when the life expectancy of a population rises.

Migration studies

One possible explanation of the differences between the morbidity and mortality patterns of different nations is that they are due to genetic differences between the populations. Studies on migrants are a useful way of distinguishing between environmental and genetic influences on disease frequency. People who migrate are immediately exposed to the new environmental conditions and they also tend to **acculturate**, i.e. they progressively adopt aspects of the dietary and lifestyle habits of the indigenous population. However, unless widespread inter-marriage occurs, migrants retain the genetic characteristics of

their country of origin. Migrant populations generally also tend to progressively acquire the morbidity and mortality characteristics of their new homeland (Barker *et al.*, 1998). These trends indicate that although there are undoubtedly variations in genetic susceptibility to different diseases both within and between populations, environmental factors have a predominant influence on disease rates in populations. The differences in the mortality and morbidity patterns in different nations are predominantly due to differences in environment, lifestyle and diet rather than to the genetic differences between populations. In some instances where the change in risk exposure occurs at the time of migration then the time lag between migration and change in disease frequency may suggest the length of the latent period between the initiating event and the appearance of symptoms.

In Chapter 18, it is suggested that when women from areas such as China and Japan, where consumption of soya products is high and rates of breast cancer comparatively low, migrate to countries where soya consumption is low rates of breast cancer remain low in the migrants themselves but rise in subsequent generations. This observation has been used to support the hypothesis that exposure to the **phytoestrogens** in soya products in early life or even in the womb has a lifelong effect in reducing the risk of breast cancer.

Mortality rate for stroke has for a long time been much higher in Japan than in the USA whereas mortality from coronary heart disease has been much higher in the USA than in Japan. In Japanese migrants to the USA and their descendants, mortality rates for these diseases moved over time towards those typical of other Americans. This indicates that these differences in mortality rates in the two countries are due to diet or other lifestyle factors and thus that they are potentially alterable by intervention.

Key points

- Migration is accompanied by immediate changes in the environment and usually more gradual changes in diet as migrants acculturate to their new surroundings.
- Unless there is extensive inter-marriage, migrant populations remain genetically similar to those in their country of origin.

- Migration is usually accompanied by a gradual shift in disease frequencies away from that in the country of origin towards that typical of the new country.
- Migration studies suggest that many of the differences in disease frequencies seen between populations are due to environmental and lifestyle factors rather than to genetic differences between races.

Cohort studies

In a **cohort study**, a sample of people, or cohort, is selected from either within the same population or, less commonly, from several populations. Details of the individual diets, lifestyle and other characteristics of all members of the cohort are then recorded and their subsequent health and mortality monitored for a period of years or even decades. The sample is selected and the data are collected with the aim of testing an hypothesis about the cause of a disease. The investigators then look for associations between the measured characteristics and the subsequent risks of mortality or morbidity. They look for dietary, lifestyle or other characteristics that are predictive of increased risk of a particular disease. To use a simple non-health example, a university could record the entry qualifications of its new students and see if these predict the eventual level of achievement of students at the end of their course. Is there a significant association between level of entry qualification and final level of attainment?

Cohort studies usually require large sample groups and long follow-ups to get enough cases of a disease for meaningful statistical analysis, e.g. a sample of 100 000 middle-aged northern Europeans would be required to get 150 cases of colon cancer within a 5-year follow-up period. Cohort studies therefore inevitably require major commitments of time, effort and money and are generally not suitable to study uncommon diseases. Many famous cohort studies have been conducted using tens or even hundreds of thousands of subjects and some of these are still ongoing after several decades. Such studies are not limited to investigating any one diet–disease relationship, but can be used to provide data on dozens of such relationships. For example, data from the American Nurses' Health Study has been used to investigate several relationships between environmental factors and diseases, e.g.:

- obesity and coronary heart disease (Manson *et al.*, 1990)
- vitamin E and coronary heart disease (Stampfer *et al.*, 1993)
- meat, fat, fibre and colon or breast cancer (Willett *et al.*, 1990)
- *trans*-fatty acids and coronary heart disease (Willett *et al.*, 1993).

Many problems of such studies are common to other areas of epidemiology, such as:

- the accuracy of the endpoint diagnosis
- the reliability, range and validity of the original measurements (note that several long running, sophisticated cohort studies have made repeat measurements on surviving members of the cohort at regular intervals)
- the problem of confounding variables.

Large and well-conducted cohort studies are considered to be the most powerful and robust of the epidemiological methods. Many large and sometimes ongoing cohort studies have been major influences on our current views about the ways in which diet and lifestyle influence health and disease risk. Some examples of the better known of these large cohort studies are briefly described below. Internet addresses are provided, where further details of these studies can be found.

- The European Prospective Investigation into Cancer and Nutrition (EPIC) is at the time of writing the largest study of diet and lifestyle ever undertaken and it is made up of a cohort of over half a million people from 23 centres in 10 European countries. The study was started in 1992 and between 1993 and 1999 it recruited a sample of 520 000 European adults aged over 20 years. Detailed information was collected about diet and lifestyle using a questionnaire and anthropometric measurements and blood samples were collected at the time of recruitment. The aim of this study is to investigate the relationship between diet and other lifestyle factors and the incidence of chronic diseases, particularly cancer. Some of the results from this study are discussed in Chapter 9 in the section dealing with dietary influences upon bowel cancer risk. See www.iarc.fr/epic/Sup-default.html for further details.

- The Framingham study was started in 1948 when a cohort of just over 5000 men and women resident in the town of Framingham in Massachusetts in the USA were recruited. Detailed physical examinations and lifestyle questionnaires were completed on each of these subjects with the aim of identifying common factors and characteristics that related to cardiovascular disease risk. Detailed medical histories and physical examinations were carried out at 2-yearly intervals. In 1971 a second, similar-sized cohort was recruited from the adult children of the original cohort along with their spouses. See www.nhlbi.nih.gov/about/framingham for further details.
- The Nurses' Health Study was started in 1976 when about 120 000 married American nurses were recruited and asked to fill in health-related questionnaires. The primary motivation with this first cohort of participants (aged 30–55 years in 1976) was to assess the long-term consequences of oral contraceptive use. The participants were sent follow-up questionnaires at 2-yearly intervals and in 1980 food frequency and diet questionnaires were first included. In 1989, a second slightly younger cohort was recruited with the aim of looking not just at the effects of oral contraceptive use but also at diet and lifestyle as risk factors for subsequent disease. See www.channing.harvard.edu/nhs/index.html for further details.

As a practical example of a cohort study, Morris *et al.* (1980) asked 18 000 middle-aged British civil servants to complete a questionnaire on a Monday morning detailing, among other things, a 5-minute by 5-minute record of how they spent the previous Friday and Saturday. They found that over the next 8 years, those who had reported engaging in vigorous leisure time activity, had only half the incidence of coronary heart disease of those who reported no such vigorous activity (even allowing for differences in smoking of the two groups). This finding is consistent with the hypothesis that exercise reduces the risk of coronary heart disease. It does not prove that the differences in heart disease rates were caused by differences in exercise levels. They are several other possible explanations such as:

- perhaps those best equipped for vigorous physical activity and thus more inclined to participate are also less prone to coronary heart disease

- perhaps a reluctance to participate in vigorous leisure time activity is an early indication of existing but undiagnosed coronary heart disease
- perhaps participation in leisure time activity is a marker for those who are most health conscious and who eat healthier diets and generally lead healthier lifestyles.

When cohort studies are used to assess the relationships between exposure to an environmental factor and disease, the term **relative risk** is widely used:

$$\text{Relative risk} = \frac{\text{Incidence in exposed group}}{\text{Incidence in unexposed group}}$$

In the example of Morris *et al.* (1980) the relative risk of coronary heart disease (CHD) in the inactive smokers could be compared with that of the active non-smokers:

$$\text{Relative risk} = \frac{\text{CHD incidence in inactive smokers}}{\text{CHD incidence in active non-smokers}}$$

In many dietary studies, the population is divided up into fifths or **quintiles** according to their level of consumption of a particular nutrient, i.e. the fifth with the lowest consumption (or exposure) through to the fifth with the highest consumption. The relative risk in each quintile can then be expressed in relation to that of the lowest quintile, e.g.:

$$\text{Relative risk} = \frac{\text{Incidence of disease in any other quintile}}{\text{Incidence in lowest quintile}}$$

Figure 3.9 shows the relative risk of developing colon cancer in differing quintiles of a cohort of almost 90 000 American nurses (i.e. using data from the Nurses' Health Study) divided according to their consumption of animal fat (Willett *et al.*, 1990). The results indicated that increased animal fat consumption was associated with a progressive increase in risk of colon cancer; the effect was statistically significant.

Positive results from an apparently rigorous cohort study are usually given particular weight when conclusions are made about relationships between lifestyle factors and disease.

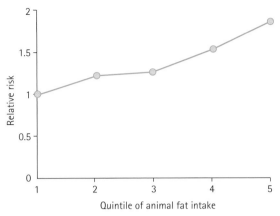

Figure 3.9 *Relative risk of colon cancer according to quintile of animal fat intake. A cohort of almost 90 000 American nurses was followed for 6 years, and there were 150 recorded cases. Simplified from Willett* et al. *(1990).*

Key points

- Cohort studies are expensive and time-consuming because they require large samples of subjects to be followed for long periods of time.
- Cohort studies are usually impractical for investigating the causes of uncommon diseases but can be used to investigate the causes of several diseases simultaneously.
- Deaths in the first few years of the study may represent those with existing disease at the start of the study and may need to be excluded from the analysis.
- Relative risk is the ratio of the incidence of disease in the exposed group to that in the unexposed group.
- Relative risk can be calculated in quintiles of the population divided according to their level of exposure to the independent variable (e.g. the dietary factor). The incidence in each quintile is expressed as a ratio of that in the lowest quintile of exposure.

Case–control studies

In **case–control studies,** investigators try to identify differences in the diet, lifestyle or other characteristics of matched groups of disease sufferers and controls. Often such studies are retrospective. A group of those suffering from or dying of a particular

disease is matched with a group that can act as control. The investigators then retrospectively identify differences in the past diets, behaviours or occupations of the two groups that might account for the presence of the disease in the case group. Returning here to the example of predicting final degree results from entry qualifications: a case–control study could be used to identify the characteristics of students who have attained first class degrees. One could take a group of students attaining first class degrees (cases) and match them with some obtaining lower grades (controls) and see if the entry or other characteristics of the two groups are different.

Matching of cases and controls is clearly a critical factor in such investigations. Sample sizes are usually small which means that testing and correction for the effects of confounding variables cannot be undertaken in the final analysis of the results. Ideally one would match only for confounding variables, i.e. those that are independently linked to both the suspected cause and the disease under investigation. Matching for factors that are linked to the cause but not independently to the disease will actually tend to obscure any relationship between the suspected cause and the disease. Barker *et al.* (1998) use the example of a suspected link between taking oral contraceptive and deep vein thrombosis. Religious belief may be linked to use of contraceptive but is unlikely to be causally linked to the disease. They make the point that 'perfect matching of influences which determine exposure to the suspected cause will result in the frequency of exposure in cases and controls becoming identical'.

In addition to the problem of control selection, it may be extremely difficult to obtain reliable information about past behaviour, especially past dietary practices. Present behaviour may be an unreliable guide to past behaviour because the disease or awareness of it may modify current behaviour; differences between controls and cases may be as a result of the disease rather than its cause. Some diseases, such as cancer, are probably initiated many years before overt clinical symptoms appear. This may make it desirable to compare the behaviours of the two groups many years previously. If one tries to assess things such as past smoking habits or the position in which a baby was laid down to sleep then one could expect reasonably accurate responses. Trying to assess habitual salt intake 5 years ago will present a much greater challenge.

Case–control studies helped to highlight the apparently causal link between prone (front) sleeping and risk of cot death. More than 20 case–control studies were published over a 20-year period from the early 1970s. Each of these found that babies who had died from cot death were more likely to have slept on their fronts than those who did not die (see Department of Health (DH), 1993; Webb, 1995).

Cramer *et al.* (1989) tried to test the hypothesis that high dietary galactose consumption (from lactose or milk sugar) was implicated in the aetiology of ovarian cancer. Approximately equal numbers of sufferers and non-sufferers from the disease were asked to fill in a food frequency questionnaire, focusing on the dietary patterns in the previous 5 years but asking the 'cases' to ignore changes in food preferences since their diagnosis of cancer. Lactose consumption was not significantly different in the cases and controls, nor were there any significant differences when several other specific dairy foods were considered separately. However, eating yoghurt at least once a month was associated with significantly increased relative risk of ovarian cancer. The implication was that yoghurt consumption is causally linked to the development of ovarian cancer but there are many other explanations for these results such as those given below.

- Yoghurt is a food with a 'healthy image' and ovarian cancer is sometimes called the silent cancer because the disease has often progressed to an advanced stage before its clinical recognition. Perhaps minor subclinical effects of the disease persuaded the cases to include more healthy foods in their diets prior to the onset of clinically overt symptoms.
- The more associations one tests, the more likely it is that one of them will be statistically significant simply by chance. Lactose consumption *per se* was not associated with risk of ovarian cancer and so these authors then looked for a link with several individual dairy foods.
- The sufferers also differed from the controls in several other respects. The cases were more likely to be Jewish, college educated, never been married, never had children and never to have used oral contraceptives. It is not unreasonable to suggest that women with such characteristics might also be more likely to eat yoghurt. The differences

in yoghurt consumption may be due to some other characteristic of women who develop ovarian cancer, rather than yoghurt consumption being directly, causally linked to the development of ovarian cancer.

Case–control studies may be prospective. Clinical records or stored samples may be used to yield information that is more reliable or at least less subject to bias than asking questions about past behaviour, e.g. levels of carotenoids in stored blood samples can be used as an objective marker for fruit and vegetable consumption around the time of the blood collection. On occasion, such information may be recorded or stored with the specific intention of referring back to it when cases have become apparent. Wald *et al.* (1980) investigated the possibility of a link between vitamin A status and risk of cancer. Serum samples were collected from 16 000 men over a 3 year period and frozen; 86 men from this large sample subsequently developed cancer. They were matched for age, smoking habits and time at which the samples were collected with 172 men who did not develop cancer. The serum retinol (vitamin A) concentrations were then measured in the stored samples from both groups of men. Serum retinol concentrations were found to be lower in the cases than in the controls, consistent with the hypothesis that poor dietary vitamin A status increases cancer risk. There are several reasons (see below) why these results and those of other similar studies need to be interpreted cautiously.

- The time between sample collection and clinical diagnosis was short (i.e. 1–4 years). It is quite likely that an existing undiagnosed cancerous condition may have resulted in reduced serum retinol concentration. The difference in serum retinol concentrations of cases and controls may be a product of early cancer rather than its cause.
- Serum retinol concentration is an insensitive measure of dietary status for vitamin A in individuals. Serum retinol concentrations only start to fall when liver stores are seriously depleted. Other factors, like infection, may influence plasma retinol concentrations.

In cohort studies, relative risk can be calculated directly, but in case–control studies an indirect measure of relative risk, the **odds ratio**, has to be used. This is defined as the odds of exposure to the suspected cause among the cases divided by the odds of exposure amongst the controls.

$$\text{Odds ratio} = \frac{\text{Odds of case exposure}}{\text{Odds of control exposure}}$$

In most case–control studies this is calculated using the equation:

$$\text{Odds ratio} = \frac{\begin{array}{c}\text{No. of exposed cases} \times \\ \text{no. of unexposed controls}\end{array}}{\begin{array}{c}\text{No. of unexposed cases} \times \\ \text{no. of exposed controls}\end{array}}$$

If the experiment has been designed using matched pairs of cases and controls then:

$$\text{Odds ratio} = \frac{\begin{array}{c}\text{No. of pairs with case exposed} \\ \text{but control unexposed}\end{array}}{\begin{array}{c}\text{No. of pairs with case unexposed} \\ \text{but control exposed}\end{array}}$$

As with relative risk in cohort studies, the odds ratio can be calculated at each of several different levels of exposure, e.g. with quintiles of exposure (see Figure 3.9).

Case–control studies of some type account for many of the putative links between diet or lifestyle and disease that fleetingly attract the attention of the health correspondents of the media. They can be conducted cheaply and quickly and so are available even to those with very limited research facilities. This type of study is clearly an important tool for the epidemiologist seeking to identify causes of many diseases. Many of these studies relating to diet have major methodological difficulties and are open to several interpretations. Often these studies do no more than point to the possibility of a causative link that is worthy of further investigation.

Key points

- In case–control studies, the matching of cases to controls is of paramount importance. Ideally they need to be matched only for likely confounding variables that are independently linked to both the suspected cause and the outcome measure.
- Ideally one should compare diets of cases and controls at the time of disease initiation.

- It may be difficult to obtain reliable measures of past diet. Current diets of disease sufferers may be a product of the disease rather than a cause.
- Stored blood or other samples may be used to give more objective measures of past nutritional status.
- Odds ratio is the measure of relative risk used in case–control studies. In most studies it is the product of the number of exposed cases and unexposed controls divided by the product of the unexposed cases and the exposed controls.

Cross-sectional studies

By using a risk marker or a symptom as the measure of outcome it is possible to get 'immediate' results using a survey of a cross-section of the population. If one assessed the diet and nutritional status of a large sample of people and then measured a disease risk marker or symptom, one could look for correlations between consumption of a particular substance and the measured outcome, e.g. the relationship between measured saturated fat intake and blood cholesterol concentration or between habitual salt intake and blood pressure. The ongoing programme of NDNS surveys provides an opportunity for such cross-sectional analysis. In the first survey of adults, Gregory *et al.* (1990) found no significant correlation between dietary saturated fat intake and serum low-density lipoprotein (LDL) cholesterol concentration in men (see Chapter 11).

'Experiments' of nature

Observations on victims of some congenital or acquired disorder may provide useful evidence about the relationships between diet and disease. For example, the observation that people with familial hypercholesteraemia (an inherited tendency to very high plasma cholesterol concentration) are prone to premature coronary heart disease supports the belief that plasma cholesterol levels and coronary heart disease risk are positively associated. The Nobel prize winning work of Brown and Goldstein (1984) indicates that the high plasma cholesterol in these people is a primary consequence of their genetic defect and this supports the proposition that the association is causal.

Animal experiments

This topic has previously been the subject of two critical reviews by the author (see Webb, 1990, 1992b). Animal experiments allow researchers to perform high precision, well-controlled and, if necessary, long-term experiments to directly test hypotheses. Technical, ethical or financial constraints would often make it difficult or impossible to undertake such experiments using human subjects. The **reliability** of well-designed and competently executed animal experiments should be high. The researcher can thus have confidence that a statistically significant difference between, say, an experimental group and a control group is due to the treatment. It should be repeatable if the experimental circumstances are replicated. Epidemiologists, on the other hand, have to rely on finding statistical associations between naturalistic observations of diseases or disease markers and potential causes. These are not truly experiments because the investigator does not impose any constraint or intervention on the subjects to test a hypothesis. These observational human studies cannot be properly controlled. Confounding variables may lead to a false assumption that two associated variables are causally linked and, conversely, other influences on the dependent variable (the disease) may obscure a causative association.

Animal experiments are thus likely to be much more reliable than human epidemiology and even many human experiments. The problem with animal experiments is their questionable **validity**. It may be difficult to decide to what extent hypotheses generated or supported solely by the results of animal experiments may be applied to people. Strictly speaking, animal experiments can only be used to generate hypotheses about humans. The hypothesis should then be tested by direct experiment with humans or if that is not possible then the extent to which human observations are consistent with the animal-generated hypothesis can be assessed. In practice, however, results from animal experiments may be extrapolated to people with little experimental confirmation in people and sometimes with little consideration of biological factors which may make such projections unsafe. It is a measure of the robustness of animal experimentation that often, despite such lack of rigour, essentially correct conclusions about humans are drawn from these experiments.

Animal experiments have had a key role in progressing our knowledge of human biology. They have also, therefore, made an important contribution to producing the practical medical, surgical and nutritional benefits that have resulted from the application of that knowledge. Only about 20 per cent of the Nobel prize winners in physiology and medicine have used human subjects for their research, and only about 10 per cent have not made use of some non-human species (Webb, 1992b). These Nobel prizes represent a yardstick to assess the contribution of animal experiments because they acknowledge landmark achievements in advancing physiological and medical knowledge. Almost all prize winners have made use of non-human species in their research. There is also clear evidence that animal experiments have sometimes misled those doing research in human biology and medicine. Two examples are given below.

- Dietary cholesterol was once widely regarded as the dominant influence on plasma cholesterol concentration. Frantz and Moore (1969) in a review of 'the sterol hypothesis of atherogenesis' concluded that although saturated fat was an important influence on plasma cholesterol its effect was probably to potentiate the effects of dietary cholesterol. Dietary cholesterol is now considered to be a relatively minor influence on plasma cholesterol concentration for most people. According to Frantz and Moore, experiments with herbivorous laboratory rabbits were the major evidence directly supporting their view of dietary cholesterol as the dominant influence on blood cholesterol concentration.
- In Chapter 10 it is argued that experiments with laboratory rats were an important factor in exaggerating the protein requirements of children and thus in falsely indicating a huge deficit in world protein supplies.

Animal experiments are an important research tool in the study of human nutrition and they have made major contributions to advancing understanding of all aspects of human biology. Animal experiments also have a considerable potential to mislead the human nutritionist, especially if results generated in experiments with small laboratory animals are extrapolated to people with little consideration of the factors that might invalidate such projections and with little attempt to corroborate the animal-generated hypothesis with studies in people.

Several problems that may make it difficult to extrapolate the results of nutrition experiments with laboratory animals to people are given below.

Species differences in nutrient requirements

There may be both qualitative and quantitative differences in the nutritional requirements of different species. Most mammals, unlike primates and guinea-pigs, make their own vitamin C and therefore do not require a dietary supply. All mammals require an exogenous source of protein but the requirements of children and other young primates are low compared with other mammals because of their slow growth rate. The milk of most mammals has 20–25 per cent of the energy as protein whereas in humans and chimpanzees this figure is only about 6 per cent (see Chapter 10).

Species differences in feeding pattern and diet character

Animals may be exposed to a type of diet or a mode of feeding that is totally different from their natural one. Their response in such an experiment may not be a good guide to the response of people, especially if the experimental diet or feeding pattern is much more akin to the natural one in humans. For example, rabbits are herbivores and would not normally encounter cholesterol in their diets because cholesterol is found exclusively in foods of animal origin. Rabbits may be metabolically ill equipped to handle large dietary loads of cholesterol. They certainly seem to be much more sensitive to the atherogenic effects of cholesterol than many other laboratory species. Omnivorous and carnivorous species should be better adapted to handling dietary loads of cholesterol and thus less susceptible to its atherogenic effects. With the benefit of hindsight, the assumption that the rabbit's response to dietary cholesterol would predict the human response seems unsafe. This partly explains why dietary cholesterol was regarded as a much greater influence on plasma cholesterol and atherogenesis than it is now.

Some animals spend long periods of time nibbling or grazing whereas other species consume large amounts of food rapidly in short duration and in relatively infrequent meals. The idea that nibbling regimens might be useful in the treatment of human obesity were largely based on experiments that monitored the effect of meal feeding upon naturally nibbling species such as rats and mice.

Controlled experimental conditions versus real life

Animal experiments are usually performed under highly controlled conditions. Experimental and control groups are matched and treated identically except for imposed differences in the experimental variables. Strictly speaking one should assume that the test treatment only produces the results obtained under the specified conditions of the experiment. In practice, one tends to assume that essentially similar effects would result from the treatment even if some of the background conditions were changed (e.g. in free-living, genetically diverse, wild animals of the same species). Changes in background conditions might sometimes substantially alter the response of even the experimental species to the experimental treatment, i.e. controlled experiments with laboratory animals might sometimes not even predict the response of free-living wild animals of the same species, let alone the response of human beings.

Take as an example the key role that animal experiments play in the toxicological testing of food additives (see Chapter 18 for further discussion of this topic). Such tests often involve exposing experimental animals to huge doses of single additives over their whole lifespan under laboratory conditions. If additives show no adverse effects under these test conditions it is assumed that they are generally nontoxic to that species in those doses. Under different conditions, however, the additive might have harmful effects. There might be interactions between the additive and some other factor. The additive might, for example, become harmful:

- in the presence of other additives, drugs or chemicals
- when there is a particular nutrient inadequacy or the diet is low in antioxidants
- when there is exposure to cigarette smoke or alcohol
- if animals with differing genotypes are exposed.

There is, for example, a well-known interaction between certain older antidepressant drugs (monoamine oxidase (MAO) inhibitors) and certain foods containing tyramine (e.g. cheese). The tyramine causes a dangerous rise in blood pressure in people taking these drugs.

Differences in species' sizes

One of the major advantages of using laboratory animals for experiments is their small size, which greatly reduces research costs. More than 90 per cent of all animals used for experiments in the UK are rodents or rabbits (Webb, 1992b). This small size also leaves experimenters with the difficulty of how to allow for differences in size when projecting results from animal experiments to humans. It is usual to scale dosages and requirements according to body weight but this is more because of convention and convenience than because there is convincing evidence of its validity. Earlier in the chapter, fourfold differences were obtained when projecting the rat's rate of vitamin C synthesis to human size depending upon whether relative body weight or relative metabolic rate was used as the basis for the scaling.

Let us try to model in a mouse experiment the sugar consumption of two human populations, one consuming about 40 kg/person/year and one consuming about half this amount. These amounts represent somewhere near 20 per cent and 10 per cent of total energy intake respectively for the human populations. If one scales this human consumption according to relative body weight to set the experimental consumption in the mice then sugar would only represent around 2.5 per cent and 1.3 per cent of total calories in the two groups of mice. As discussed earlier in this chapter, the relative metabolic rate (i.e. energy expenditure per unit weight) declines with increasing body size in mammals. Small animals such as rats and mice have much more rapid metabolic rates than larger species such as man. This accounts for the large differences produced when the scaling is by relative body weight or relative metabolic rate in the two examples above.

Rodents are widely used in studies on energy balance that are directed towards increasing understanding of human energy balance regulation (see Chapter 7). The size difference in relative metabolic rate is just one of several factors that greatly complicate the human nutritionist's interpretation of energy balance studies conducted with small mammals. It is sometimes difficult to project even qualitatively the results from energy balance studies on rodents to humans. Two examples are given below.

- The relative energy costs of locomotion (i.e. energy required to move a specific mass a specific distance) declines with increasing body size. There is also the added complication that, in humans, bipedal locomotion seems to double the energy cost of walking compared with that of a similarly sized quadruped. This makes it difficult to assess the impact of activity level on overall human energy expenditure from small animal studies.

- Small animals rely upon heat generation as their principal physiological response to cold whereas large animals and people rely much more upon heat conservation to maintain body temperature in the cold. When mice are used then the situation may be still further complicated because mice have been shown to become torpid when fasted, i.e. they allow substantial and prolonged falls in body temperature in order to conserve energy (e.g. Webb et al., 1982). Most investigators, in the past, have assumed that mice are always homeothermic. Such factors would clearly make it difficult to predict the effects of environmental temperature on human energy needs from experiments with mice. They may also complicate more fundamental decisions about the relative importance of variations in energy intake or expenditure to overall energy balance and thus to the development of obesity. In Chapter 7 it is argued that experiments with rodents were largely responsible for encouraging the belief that much human obesity might be triggered by a reduced metabolic or thermogenic (heat-generating) response to overfeeding, i.e. that some thermogenic defect was an important cause of human obesity.

Key points

- Use of laboratory animals for experiments extends the range of experiments that are ethically and technically feasible.
- Well-designed animal experiments should yield reliable and repeatable results.
- The results from experiments with laboratory animals may not validly predict the responses of free-living people.
- Animal experiments have made a major contribution to understanding of human biology and to the practical benefits that have resulted from the application of that knowledge.
- Animal experiments also have the potential to mislead human biologists, particularly if the results are simply extrapolated to humans.

- There are species differences in the quantitative requirements for nutrients and even some differences in the range of nutrients that are essential to different mammals.

- Different species have different types of diet and different patterns of feeding. The response of a species to a foreign diet or feeding pattern may be a poor guide to the response of a species for which it is normal.

- The effects of a dietary alteration under a set of controlled conditions may not predict what would happen under a different set of background conditions and thus that of free-living animals or people.

- It is very difficult to scale doses or nutrient requirements between species of vastly different sizes. Scaling according to body weight may be misleading.

- It can also be difficult to scale the energy costs of exercise and homeothermy between large and small species. This is a particular problem if small animals such as mice are used as models for humans in energy balance studies.

Human experimental studies – an overview

Human experimental studies have been divided up into three categories for ease of discussion, i.e. short-term experiments, clinical trials and intervention trials, but these divisions are rather arbitrary. The overall design strategy is similar in the three types of study, the differences are to do with the scale and duration of the study, the nature of the experimental constraints and outcome measurements and whether or not the subject is expected to gain therapeutic benefit from the experimental treatment. The issues listed below are discussed at various points within the next three sections but they apply to most human experiments and in many cases to animal experiments as well.

- *Subject selection.* If the control and test groups are not matched at the start of an experiment for factors that can affect the outcome (e.g. age or initial disease severity) then this can bias the outcome. If healthy subjects are used in a trial of a preventive change then this is called a primary intervention trial but in a secondary trial the

intervention is tested in those with previous disease history.

- *Measures of outcome.* Outcomes may be long term and holistic, e.g. effect on disease prevalence or mortality or even total mortality. More often they are more acute and/or reductionist, e.g. changes in symptom severity, risk factor level (e.g. plasma cholesterol concentration) or some objective measure of disease progression such as narrowing of the joint space in arthritis.

- *The placebo effect.* A placebo is a dummy treatment that should be indistinguishable from the real treatment; its purpose is to allow researchers to differentiate between the physiological benefits of treatment and psychological benefits due to the subject's expectation of benefit. The more subjective the measure of outcome, the more important it is to account for any psychological effects of an intervention. For example, in trials of therapies for depression it is common for the placebo to result in benefits for more than 25 per cent of subjects and in studies on the treatment of menopausal hot flushes placebos may produce benefits in up to 50 per cent of subjects.

- *Operator bias.* The person conducting an experiment may influence the outcome – if the outcome is subjective their judgement may be affected if they know which subject is being treated or they may inadvertently affect the response of the subject. In a double-blind trial neither subject nor researcher know whether they are receiving the real or placebo treatment until after the data collection has been completed.

- *Treatment compliance.* In an animal experiment or with human subjects in a controlled environment (e.g. hospital ward) one can ensure that each subject complies with the experimental protocol. In free-living human subjects one cannot ensure compliance (e.g. that they take a vitamin pill) or with a dietary change (e.g. a calorie-controlled or low-fat diet) or even reliably assess the degree of compliance in different subjects.

Short-term human experiments

Most of the hypotheses relating diet to the risk of chronic disease suggest that prolonged exposure to the dietary risk factor eventually leads to increased risk of developing clinical disease. Clearly such hypotheses are not directly testable in acute experiments. However, these diet–disease hypotheses often involve hypothetical chains of apparently reversible steps between exposure to the initial dietary risk factor and the onset of clinical disease. The **diet–heart hypothesis**, for example, envisages changes in plasma cholesterol resulting from high intake of dietary saturated fats leading to lipid deposition in artery walls, atherosclerosis and ultimately increased risk of coronary heart disease (see Chapter 11 for details). It may be possible to test individual steps in such an hypothesis in short-term experiments without exposing the experimental subjects to any significant long-term risks.

Keys *et al.* (1959) began a classical series of studies that have had a tremendous influence on thinking about the relationship between diet and heart disease. They were able to show that changing the ratio of polyunsaturated to saturated fats in the diet had predictable acute effects on plasma cholesterol concentration. When subjects switched from diets high in saturated fat and low in polyunsaturated fat to low-saturated, high-polyunsaturated-fat diets (i.e. from low to high **P:S ratio**) their plasma cholesterol concentration fell (see Figure 3.10). All of the subjects showed some decline in plasma cholesterol even

though the degree of responsiveness varied. The total fat content of the two diets was matched. Two particular problems with this type of experiment are:

- the results of such short-term experiments may not necessarily predict the long-term response. The subjects may adapt to any change in the longer term
- support for one element of any hypothesis does not confirm the whole hypothesis. In the example above, even if high-polyunsaturated, low-saturated-fat diets reduce plasma cholesterol, it does not necessarily follow that this will lead to improved health and longevity or even necessarily to a reduced risk of coronary heart disease. All that one has shown is a short-term decline in an asymptomatic risk marker.

Further consideration of the data in Figure 3.10 may help to explain the apparent contradiction between the results of between population and within population studies of the relationship between saturated fat intake and plasma cholesterol concentration. Saturated fat intake appears to be a major determinant of average population plasma cholesterol even though, within populations, there seems to be no significant association between serum cholesterol concentration and saturated fat intake. In this experiment, the dietary change in P:S ratio had a cholesterol-lowering effect in the individuals and the appropriate statistical test (a paired 't' test) would show that this effect was highly statistically significant. This dietary change seems to have shifted the whole distribution of individual serum cholesterol concentrations downwards. If the sample was large enough, one would expect this would significantly reduce average plasma cholesterol of the sample population. Yet, the range of cholesterol concentrations of subjects consuming a matched diet, say diet A, is huge and the average reduction in cholesterol resulting from the dietary change to diet B is relatively small in comparison. The difference between the two means is less than a third of the difference between the highest and lowest values on diet A. This is despite the fact that the magnitude of this experimental dietary change was enormous; it is probably towards the extreme ends of the range of practical feasibility with regard to P:S ratio on a high-fat diet. Although the ratio of polyunsaturated to saturated fat clearly affects individual plasma cholesterol levels, and therefore average population levels, it is not the

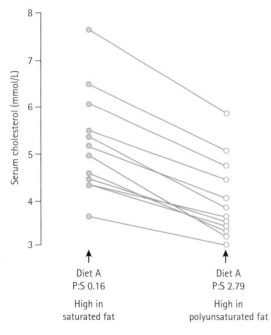

Figure 3.10 *Effects of different types of fat on serum cholesterol in 12 men. Total fat in the two diets was matched. Data of Keys* et al. *(1959). Source Webb (1992a). After NACNE (1983).*

primary factor determining where any individual lies within the population range of plasma cholesterol concentrations.

Key points

- A dietary factor may contribute to the cause of a disease by initiating a reversible chain of events that eventually results in clinical disease.
- It may be possible to test elements of this chain of events in short-term, human experiments without exposing the subjects to significant risk.
- In the diet heart hypothesis, high saturated fat intake is postulated to raise plasma cholesterol concentration, which ultimately can lead to increased risk of coronary heart disease, this element of the hypothesis can be tested experimentally.
- The experimental confirmation of one step in the hypothetical chain does not prove the whole hypothesis.
- Short-term responses to dietary change may not always be the same as long-term responses.

Clinical trials

Clinical trials are usually used to test the effectiveness of a treatment on the course or severity of a disease or symptom. The aim of such trials is to isolate and quantify the effect of the treatment under test. It is, therefore, necessary to eliminate, minimize or allow for other influences on the disease progression or severity such as those listed below.

- There may be variation in disease progression or severity that is unrelated to the intervention. This requires that there be a matched control group or control period.
- There may be considerable variation in the initial disease severity and this could be a source of bias if the control and experimental groups are not initially well matched. If the sample is large enough then simply allocating subjects randomly to control and experimental groups will make it likely that groups will be initially well matched. In some studies, particularly small-scale studies, there may need to be more formal matching for disease severity.

- A placebo effect of treatment may occur, i.e. a psychologically based improvement that results from the patient's expectation that treatment will yield benefits. If the outcome measure involves any subjective grading of symptom severity this placebo effect is likely to be particularly important. Ideally the control subjects would be given a placebo treatment which they cannot distinguish from the real treatment.
- There may be unconscious bias on the part of the operator who measures outcomes and who administers the real and placebo treatments. Ideally the experimenter should also be unaware of which patients are receiving real and placebo treatments until after the data collection has been completed. This is particularly important if the outcome measure involves any subjective judgement to be made by the experimenter. If the operator knows which are the real and dummy treatments it may affect the way they instruct or interact with the subject and thus partly undermine the effects of the placebo control.

In clinical trials of dietary interventions, particular problems may make it impossible to achieve the design aims listed above, e.g.:

- a dietary intervention aimed at varying intake of a particular nutrient will usually involve consequential changes in the intakes of other nutrients
- if the intervention is a special diet, then it may be difficult or impossible to allow for the placebo effect and to eliminate operator bias. This will be easier if the dietary change can be accomplished by the use of a supplement in tablet form
- if the intervention is a special diet there are likely to be variations in the degree of compliance and it may be difficult or impossible to objectively assess the level of compliance.

One ideal model of a clinical trial is the double-blind, random-crossover trial. Patients are given indistinguishable real or placebo treatments during two consecutive trial periods and some measure of treatment success made at the end of both treatment periods. Patients would be randomly assigned to receive either real or placebo treatment first. Neither patient nor experimenter knows whether real or placebo treatment is being given at any particular time. It may even be possible to ensure uniform compliance by administering treatment (e.g. a tablet) in the presence of the experimenter. An example to illustrate this type of experimental design follows.

MacGregor *et al.* (1982) prescribed patients with mild to moderate hypertension a diet designed to be low in sodium. All subjects were required to remain on this experimental diet throughout the 10 weeks of the experiment. After a 2-week adjustment period, the subjects then received either slow-release sodium tablets or placebos during two consecutive monthly periods. The sodium tablets raised salt intake and negated the effects of the low-salt diet. The real and placebo tablets were identical and were administered using the double blind, random-crossover model (see Figure 3.11 for a summary of the experimental protocol). Blood pressure was found to be significantly lower at the end of the placebo period compared with the

salt-supplementation period. This supports the hypothesis that moderate salt restriction can have at least some short-term effect of lowering blood pressure in this category of patient.

In Chapter 15, a large double-blind clinical trial is described which was set up to test whether folic acid supplements given to high-risk pregnant women reduced the risk of babies being born with **neural tube defects**. The subjects were almost 2000 women, from 7 countries and 33 centres, who were at high risk of having babies with neural tube defects (because of a previously affected pregnancy). They were randomly assigned to receive one of four treatments starting when they planned to become pregnant again:

- folic acid supplements
- other vitamin supplements
- both of these
- neither of these, just a placebo.

There were many less affected babies in the two folic acid supplemented groups compare with the two groups not receiving folic acid supplements (MRC, 1991). It has since been demonstrated that folic acid supplements are also effective in preventing first occurrence of neural tube defects in random samples of women (see Chapter 15).

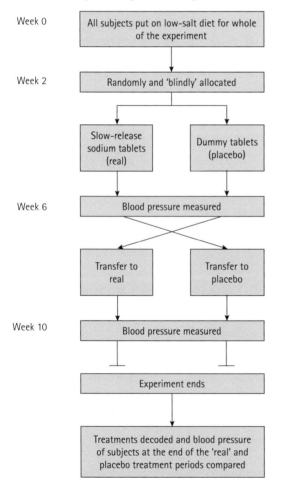

Figure 3.11 *A plan of the experimental protocol of MacGregor* et al. *(1982) to illustrate a double-blind, randomized, crossover trial.*

Key points

- Clinical trials aim to isolate and quantify the effects of a treatment on the course or severity of a disease.
- With large samples it may be sufficient to randomly allocate subjects to control and test groups but in small studies there often needs to be more direct matching of subjects for initial severity.
- The use of a placebo (dummy) treatment in the control group can allow for any psychological effects of treatment.
- In the double-blind design, neither patient nor researchers know who has been allocated to the treatment and control groups until the end of the study.
- Clinical trials of dietary interventions have particular difficulties, such as:
  - it may be difficult to produce isolated changes in diet

> – it may be difficult to design a placebo treatment that is not easily recognizable by either subjects or researchers
> – there may be variation in compliance with the prescribed diet that may be difficult to quantify.

Intervention trials

These are essentially long-term, population-level experiments. The design aim is to make the intended variable or variables the only difference between matched control and experimental groups. The scale and duration of most intervention trials and perhaps also the nature of the intervention itself may make it impossible to impose the level of rigour in design that can be accomplished with small-scale, short-term experiments or clinical trials. Some of the problems that may be encountered when designing intervention trials are given below.

- *Selection of subjects.* In some intervention trials, a 'high-risk' group may be used as subjects. Even if an intervention is convincingly shown to benefit such subjects then this does not necessarily mean that the intervention will yield net benefit to the population as a whole.
- *Ethics of withholding treatment or information from the control group.* When such high-risk subjects are used, then there may be an ethical dilemma about how to treat the control group. If they are made aware of their high-risk status, the control group may significantly alter their behaviour during the course of the experiment.
- *Multiple intervention.* Most of the chronic diseases of industrialization are assumed to have a multifactorial aetiology. Multiple risk factor interventions may be used to maximize the likely benefits of intervention. In some cases, the experimental aspects of the trial may be given low priority because the primary purpose is to promote health within a population rather than to test the efficacy of the intervention. Using such multiple interventions may make it impossible to quantify the contribution of any particular intervention to the overall benefits (or harm) demonstrated for the experimental group. Factorial design of experiments can aid in this respect but may not be practical in many trials. Note that the previously discussed clinical trial of folic acid supplementation in pregnant women is an example of a factorial design. With such a design it is possible to statistically test the effects of several interventions and also to test for any possible interaction between interventions.

- *Measure of outcome.* An intervention trial may be designed to test the effect of the intervention upon a particular disease risk marker or upon morbidity or mortality from a particular disease. Even if the intervention produces the expected beneficial effect in such cases, the ultimate holistic test of the benefit of the intervention is whether such narrow benefits result in a reduction in total morbidity or mortality. Statistically significant reductions in these holistic measures may require impossibly large subject groups and long periods of study.

Passmore and Eastwood (1986) summarized studies on the effects of water fluoridation upon the dental health of UK children. These come closer to an 'ideal' design than most intervention trials. In 1956, three experimental areas of the UK started to fluoridate their water supply and three neighbouring areas were used as controls. Prevalence of caries in the teeth of the children in the control and experimental areas was similar prior to fluoridation but by 1961 the experimental areas had shown a considerable relative improvement. One of the experimental areas later discontinued fluoridation and within 5 years, caries prevalence had gone back up to the level in the control areas. This trial provided very convincing evidence of the benefit of fluoridation to the dental health of children. The controversy that has prevented widespread fluoridation of water supplies in the UK revolves around its long-term safety rather than its efficacy in preventing dental caries. Absolute, long-term safety is, of course, much more difficult to demonstrate convincingly.

In the Multiple Risk Factor Intervention Trial (MRFIT) (1982), a third of a million American men were screened to identify 13 000 who were classified as at 'high-risk' of coronary heart disease. These high-risk men were then randomly assigned to experimental and control groups. The experimental group received intensive dietary counselling aimed at both normalization of plasma cholesterol concentration and body weight, and they received aggressive treatment for hypertension and intensive counselling to help them reduce their use of tobacco. The control group received no counselling but they, and their general practitioners, were advised of their high-risk status and the results of annual physical examinations sent to them. This group was called 'usual care'. The intervention was apparently successful in modifying behaviour and in producing measurable reductions in the objective risk markers (e.g. plasma cholesterol concentration). However, the study failed to show any beneficial effects of intervention, i.e. there was no difference in either total mortality or even coronary heart disease mortality between the two groups after 7 years of follow-up. This failure has been partly explained by the behaviour of the control group, who also seemed to modify their behaviour once they became aware of their high-risk status. It has also been suggested that harmful effects of the antihypertensive treatment may have cancelled out and obscured the beneficial effects of other aspects of the intervention.

Both of these trials could be described as primary intervention trials – they aimed to prevent the onset of disease in asymptomatic subjects. Rarely have such trials produced significant reductions in total mortality when dietary interventions have been used. Other trials are described as secondary intervention trials because they use subjects who have already experienced a disease event (e.g. have already had a myocardial infarction). These subjects are an extreme example of a high-risk group and one would need to be particularly cautious about assuming that any benefit demonstrated in such a group would have net beneficial effects on the population as a whole. Burr *et al.* (1991) tested the effects of three dietary interventions upon total 2-year mortality in 2000 men who had recovered from a myocardial infarction. The three dietary interventions were advice to:

- increase cereal fibre consumption
- reduce total fat intake
- eat oily fish or take fish oil capsules twice weekly.

The subjects were randomly allocated to receive or not to receive advice on each of these three interventions and the allocations were made independently of allocations for the other two interventions. Thus there were eight possible combinations of interventions or non-interventions, including a group who received no intervention at all. The fish oil intervention almost uniquely, for a dietary intervention, did produce a significant reduction in total all-cause mortality. One suggestion why this trial alone has produced a statistically significant fall in total mortality is because there appeared to be almost no tendency for non-fish advised men to increase their fish consumption. At the time, the potential therapeutic effects of fish oils were not widely known in the UK. In many other intervention trials, control subjects have also tended to modify their behaviour in the direction of that counselled for the intervention group.

Key points

- Intervention trials are long-term, population-level experiments.
- The scale and duration of these studies and the nature of the interventions may pose considerable problems in designing these studies.
- If high-risk subjects are used then it cannot be assumed that any net benefit demonstrated in the study will translate to a net benefit for the general population.
- It may pose ethical problems if high-risk control subjects are denied the intervention that is expected to be beneficial.
- It will undermine the study if control subjects alter their behaviour in the direction of that suggested for the experimental groups.
- If multiple interventions are used then it may be difficult to decide which intervention has produced any study benefits.
- A reduction in mortality for a particular disease or disease risk factor does not necessarily mean that the intervention has produced a net benefit.
- Significant reductions in total mortality may require impossibly large groups and long periods of study. Primary dietary interventions have rarely produced significant reductions in total mortality.
- A secondary intervention trial uses subjects who have already experienced a disease event.

Systematic reviews and meta-analyses

The costs and difficulties of conducting a controlled trial increase with the size and duration of the study. For this reason many clinical trials have used relatively small numbers of subjects. This means that even well-designed and executed studies may not have the statistical power to provide a definitive judgement of the value of the intervention. This means that even though the scientific literature may contain many individual studies of a particular intervention it may still be difficult to make a clear judgement of its effectiveness. Such studies vary in size and quality and in the details of their design, so simply counting how many studies are for, against or inconclusive is not a helpful or valid procedure.

A systematic review aims to identify, using preset and objective search methodology, as many as possible of the studies that have addressed a particular topic. One or more electronic databases of published papers will be used to identify all papers that use the key search words. Other preset and systematic search methods may be used to find additional studies, e.g. the reference lists of papers from the primary search and perhaps some method for trying to get data from studies that have not been formally published.

In the meta-analysis of studies identified from a systematic review, all studies that meet predetermined quality and eligibility criteria are statistically pooled. In this way several small studies of limited statistical power can be combined as if they were a single study of much greater statistical power. Individual component studies in the meta-analysis are weighted according to the sample size used. In theory, a well-conducted systematic review and meta-analysis should give a much better indication of the true answer to a question than a simple for and against count or a qualitative and subjective interpretation by the reviewer.

When studies are combined in a meta-analysis, it is assumed that they are all essentially homogeneous and that any differences between them in terms of outcome are due to chance. This is often not the case, e.g. differences in outcome may be due to 'real' differences in the nature of the subjects, i.e. a treatment may have different effects in different categories of subject. Some of the other pitfalls of this approach are as follows (after Naylor, 1997).

- *Publication bias.* There is much evidence that studies with positive outcomes are more likely to be published than those with negative or inconclusive outcomes (Easterbrook *et al.*, 1992). This issue was discussed in Chapter 1 where it was also noted that citation rates for papers with positive outcomes can be much higher than for those that report negative outcomes (Ravnskov, 1992). If

studies are funded by organizations or companies that have a commercial interest in the outcome of a trial, this might lead to lack of publication of trials with negative outcomes and perhaps selective publication or highlighting of positive findings. This is seen as a major problem in the area of dietary supplements because of the high level of involvement of manufacturing companies in the funding of trials. It is now common to see authors of scientific papers and clinical trials acknowledge sources of funding and any 'conflicting interests'.

- *Multiple publishing.* Some trials may be published more than once and so if these are all included in a meta-analysis then this can bias its outcome. Naylor quotes the example of a single study being the source for seven different publications. These different publications of the same trial had different authorship, which make it more difficult to identify that they all related to the same study.
- *Selection bias.* Unless the selection of papers for inclusion in the meta-analysis is done strictly using pre-set objective criteria then this may be a source of bias.

Several examples of meta-analysis will be found in later chapters of this book, e.g. in Chapter 12 there is discussion of a meta-analysis by Vivekanathan *et al.* (2003). These authors used for their analysis, seven large randomized trials of the effects of vitamin E supplements on long-term mortality and morbidity from cardiovascular disease and eight trials of β-carotene supplements. This analysis found no suggestion of any benefits for vitamin E supplements and evidence that β-carotene supplements caused a small but significant increase in both all-cause and cardiovascular mortality. The authors concluded that their analysis provided no support for routine supplementation with vitamin E and that supplements of β-carotene were contraindicated.

Key points

- A systematic review aims to identify all trials of a particular hypothesis using predetermined and systematic searching of the literature.
- In a meta-analysis, studies that meet set quality criteria are combined into a single study of much greater statistical power.

- Studies with positive outcomes are more likely to be published than those with negative outcomes; this publication bias can bias the results of meta-analysis as can multiple publication of the same dataset in the literature.

In vitro studies

In vitro studies are, literally translated, studies that have been done in glass in contrast with studies using whole animals or people which are termed *in vivo* or in life. These include:

- simple analytical studies measuring the level of a substance presumed to be 'protective' in a food, e.g. measuring levels of antioxidants in berries
- experiments with isolated cells including tumour cells, e.g. what effect does a food extract have on growth of tumour cells?
- experiments using micro-organisms, e.g. the mutagenic potential of a substance with bacteria may be a guide to its likely carcinogenicity
- effect of a food extract or component on a receptor or enzyme system, e.g. phytoestrogens in soya beans bind to and weakly stimulate mammalian oestrogen receptors.

The dietary supplement glucosamine is widely used to prevent or alleviate the symptoms of arthritis. There is evidence that it can stimulate the production of cartilage in cultured chondrocytes and this has been used as support for the view that it may help in joint repair and maintenance even though the concentrations required are high in relation to those found *in vivo* after glucosamine supplementation (Bassleer *et al.*, 1998).

The results of such experiments must be interpreted conservatively until there is collaboration from more holistic studies. Extravagant media claims are often made about specific foods or supplements on the basis of such studies:

- a substance with high levels of potential antioxidants may be claimed as being able to prevent cancer
- a substance that reduces the growth of isolated tumour cells may be claimed to have value in treating cancer
- a food substance able to kill bacteria in culture may be claimed to have potential anti-infective properties when eaten.

Key points

- *In vitro* studies are those not done with whole animals or people – literally done in glass.
- They include:
  - analysing for the presence of a particular chemical constituent
  - measuring effects on micro-organisms or isolated cells
  - measuring the effects on an enzyme's activity or the ability to bind with a receptor.

4

Dietary guidelines and recommendations

THE RANGE OF 'EXPERT REPORTS' AND THEIR CONSISTENCY

Over the past 30 years dozens of expert reports have been published in the industrialized countries that have produced sets of dietary guidelines or recommended changes in national diets. These guidelines and recommendations have been aimed at reducing morbidity and mortality from the diseases of industrialization and so ultimately at promoting health and longevity. Prior to this, most published dietary recommendations and guidelines were geared towards assuring adequate intakes of the essential nutrients and preventing the consequences of deficiency. The first fairly comprehensive standards of adequacy were published as early as 1943 in the USA (National Research Council (NRC), 1943). Truswell (1999) reviewed dietary guidelines around the world at the end of the millennium.

Some of these sets of dietary guidelines have focused on one aspect of diet and health. For example, in the UK, Committee on the Medical Aspects of Food (COMA, 1994a) focused on 'nutritional aspects of cardiovascular disease' whereas COMA (1998) was concerned with 'nutritional aspects of

the development of cancer'. Other reports have attempted to synthesize current ideas on the relationship between diet and individual diseases and produced more general and comprehensive guidelines aimed at 'reducing chronic disease risk' and promoting health, e.g. NRC (1989b) in the USA and COMA (1991) in the UK.

These many reports from around the world inevitably vary somewhat in the way the recommendations are framed, the scope of their recommendations, the precise quantitative targets and the priority attached to the various recommendations. Nevertheless, in general qualitative terms, there is a striking level of agreement and consistency between almost all of these reports; examples of fundamental disagreement are rare. This certainly adds a cumulative weight to these recommendations and guidelines. Most of these reports directly or indirectly recommend the changes listed below or at least make recommendations that are consistent with them.

- Maintain **body mass index (BMI)** within the ideal range (i.e. avoid excessive weight gain) either by restricting energy intake and/or increasing energy expenditure (exercise).

- Eat a variety of foods with ample amounts of starchy, fibre-rich foods and plenty of fruits and vegetables.
- Reduce the proportion of fat and especially saturated fat in the diet and perhaps reduce or not increase cholesterol intake.
- Reduce salt consumption.
- Reduce or not increase the consumption of added sugars (i.e. those not naturally present in fruit, vegetables and milk).
- Limit the consumption of alcohol.

In the UK, the report of the National Advisory Committee on Nutrition Education (NACNE, 1983) had a great influence on nutrition education. This committee, for the first time in the UK, attempted to offer a comprehensive set of quantitative dietary targets for the UK population. Its publication generated considerable debate and controversy in the UK and this debate helped focus attention on the relationships between diet and chronic degenerative disease. NACNE suggested that its full recommendations could be implemented within 15 years (by 1998) and that a third of the recommended changes could be achieved within 5 years (by around 1988). In retrospect, several of the NACNE targets now look unrealistic to achieve within a 15-year time scale, e.g. their aim of reducing total fat intake by almost a quarter and almost halving intakes of saturated fat and added sugars. NACNE's short-term target for total dietary fat (i.e. to reduce total fat to no more than about 35 per cent of food energy by 1988) appeared in the Department of Health (DH) report *The health of the nation* as a target for the year 2005! (DH, 1992). The latest National Dietary and Nutrition Survey of British adults (Hoare *et al.*, 2004) indicates that at last this short-term goal may have been achieved. The COMA reports *Dietary reference values, Nutritional aspects of cardiovascular disease, Nutritional aspects of the development of cancer* (COMA, 1991, 1994a, 1998 respectively) are still currently regarded as the authoritative sources of UK dietary recommendations and guidelines. In this chapter, I will use a synthesis of the recommendations in these three reports as the current UK position.

In the USA, *Dietary goals for the United States*, published in 1977, was the first report to focus specifically on reducing the risk of chronic degenerative disease. It also aroused considerable critical comment and discussion at the time the time of publication. According to Truswell (1999), one collection of commentaries on this report contains almost 900 pages. Some of the criticisms of this report seem very familiar and many of them are still commonly made about all reports of this type. Some examples of these criticisms are (after Truswell, 1999):

- technical – some of the recommendations are wrong, too extreme or that some important issues are not adequately covered. In this particular report, there were criticisms that the target for salt was too ambitious and that there were no targets for obesity
- the report is premature and based on inadequate scientific evidence
- the recommendations might not be appropriate for the whole population. In particular, the guidelines might be more appropriate for overweight middle-aged men than for active, rapidly growing children and perhaps even for women
- the report is unnecessary because health and life expectancy are already improving
- the recommended changes might have serious negative impact on important industries such as the sugar industry and the dairy industry
- a general resentment that governments and their experts are trying to tell people what to eat.

The NRC report of 1989 offered a comprehensive set of dietary recommendations and goals (NRC, 1989b) and although several sets of guidelines have been offered since then, these still represent a very concise set of targets that would still be regarded as consistent with current more complex and lengthy advice. *Dietary guidelines for Americans* is published every 5 years and the latest edition was jointly published in 2005 by the Departments of Health, and Human Services and Agriculture (DHHS/USDA, 2005). These new guidelines offer tailored recommendations to different lifecycle groups in the US population. The general recommendations are consistent with the international consensus summary offered at the start of this chapter. These new American guidelines place heavy emphasis on control of body weight through reduced calorie intake and especially by encouraging increases in physical activity. They offer detailed recommendations on activity targets for different lifecycle groups; this issue is discussed in Chapter 17. Some of the other recommendations in these new guidelines also address issues that are dealt with in other chapters in this book:

* recommendations on food safety measures (Chapter 18)
* iron and folic acid intakes in pregnancy (Chapter 15)
* vitamin B_{12} and vitamin D in the elderly (Chapter 15).

The **World Health Organization** (WHO, 1990) also published a set of nutritional goals in the form of suggested minimum–maximum ranges for selected nutrients. The minimum suggested intake of the nutrient should be sufficient to prevent deficiency whereas the maximum should be consistent with the aim of reducing the risk of chronic degenerative disease. These goals were intended to have worldwide application and are summarized below.

* Total fat should make up between 15 per cent and 30 per cent of energy intake and countries consuming high amounts of fat should ultimately work towards the lower end of this range.
* Saturated fatty acids should not exceed 10 per cent of total energy with no lower limit.
* Polyunsaturated fatty acids should make up between 3 per cent and 7 per cent of energy intake.
* Cholesterol intake should be below 300 mg/day with no lower limit.
* Carbohydrate should provide 55–75 per cent of dietary energy and complex carbohydrate (starch) 50–75 per cent.
* Dietary fibre intake should be 27–40 g/day (which corresponds to approximately 20–25 g of **non-starch polysaccharide**).
* Added sugars should contribute no more than 10 per cent of dietary energy with no lower limit.
* Protein from mixed sources should provide 10–15 per cent of dietary energy.
* Salt intake should be less than 6 g/day with no lower limit specified (although some small amount of salt intake is essential).

Key points

* In recent decades the focus of nutrition education has been on preventing chronic disease rather than simply ensuring dietary adequacy.

* Many sets of recommendations and guidelines have been produced in the past 30 years, and there is a remarkable consistency about the general qualitative changes that they recommend for industrialized countries.
* Consumers should eat more starch, fibre and fruits and vegetables but less fat, saturated fat, added sugar and salt. Excessive alcohol consumption should be avoided.
* Criticisms of these reports, particularly the earlier ones have been on the following grounds:
  - a recommendation is wrong or impractical
  - a recommendation is premature and there is insufficient evidence to justify it
  - a recommendation may be inappropriate for some sectors of the population
  - implementing the recommendation(s) will have adverse economic consequences
  - governments should not try to control what people eat.
* The World Health Organization has published a set of nutritional goals that are intended to have worldwide application.

VARIATIONS IN THE PRESENTATION OF GUIDELINES AND RECOMMENDATIONS

Some reports on diet and health frame their advice in the form of simple qualitative or semiquantitative recommendations that are easy to understand by the general public, e.g. 'eat five portions of fruits and vegetables each day', 'reduce consumption of fatty foods especially those rich in saturated fat'. Other more technical reports aimed at scientists and health professionals usually frame their recommendations in a more quantitative way, like the WHO goals listed earlier. It is expected that health professionals and health promoters will interpret these quantitative ideals and translate them into practical dietary recommendations for their clients.

Some quantitative recommendations such as those for salt and fibre are given simply as grams per day. However, for the energy-yielding nutrients (fats, carbohydrates and proteins) these recommendations are often framed as a percentage of the dietary energy as seen in some of the WHO recommendations listed earlier. This method of presentation allows the amount of the nutrient to be expressed in a single number that does not have to be adjusted as energy intake varies or qualified by a statement of the energy intake at which it applies. It effectively represents the concentration of the nutrient in the diet. Further discussion of this procedure and the calculations can be found in Chapter 6. A recommendation that carbohydrates should be 50 per cent of total energy means that carbohydrates should provide 50 per cent of the total energy consumed. Sometimes recommendations are expressed as a percentage of the food energy rather than total energy to eliminate the distorting effects of alcohol. Recommendations to Britons to reduce fat to 33 per cent of their total average energy intake is approximately equivalent to 35 per cent of their average food energy excluding alcohol. Alcohol usually has a diluting effect on the proportion of energy derived from fat (and carbohydrate and protein).

In the UK dietary recommendations have usually been framed as targets for average population consumption, e.g.:

- to reduce the average percentage of food energy from fat from about 40 per cent in 1990 to no more than 35 per cent by 2005 (DH, 1992)
- back in 1989 the US NRC (1989b) gave its recommendations in the form of individual minimum or maximum intakes
- fat should make up no more than 30 per cent of an individual's energy intake.

If a percentage of energy target is set as an individual maximum (or minimum) it would require a much greater change than if the same target were set as an ideal population average. This is illustrated in Figure 4.1 by reference to the apparently common 30 per cent target for proportion of total energy from fat in the old NRC (1989b) guidelines and those of the NACNE committee set back in 1983. If individuals are all to meet this 30 per cent target then the average population intake must be some way below 30 per cent because of individual variation in fat intakes. Current dietary reference values (DRVs) for macronutrients in the USA (summarized in National Academy of Sciences (NAS), 2004) are presented in a much more detailed format with specific amounts (g/day) offered for each age group for carbohydrate, dietary fibre, total fat and ω-6 and ω-3 polyunsaturated fatty acids just as they are for vitamins and minerals. Some recommendations may be targeted at specific groups

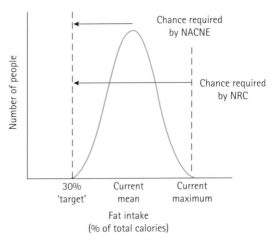

Figure 4.1 *Theoretical changes in the current 'normal' distribution of population intakes required to meet the recommended fat intakes of NACNE (1983) and NRC (1989b). NACNE recommended a new population average of 30% of energy from fat whereas NRC recommended 30% as an individual target.*

(e.g. guidelines for pregnant women) or they may exclude particular groups (e.g. children under 5 years). In this chapter, I will generally only consider recommendations that are intended for all healthy people over 5 years of age. Recommendations for specific groups are dealt with in Chapter 15.

Key points

- Some reports frame their recommendations in simple qualitative terms that can be interpreted by the general public.

- Others reports offer quantitative targets that health professionals and health promoters need to translate into practical terms for their clients.

- Quantitative fat, carbohydrate and protein targets are sometimes expressed as a percentage of total energy or food energy (excluding alcohol).

- This method of expression means that the numerical recommendation does not need to be qualified by the energy intake at which it applies and effectively represents the concentration of fat, carbohydrate or protein in the diet.

- In the UK, targets are usually expressed as population averages whereas in the past US targets were given as individual maxima and minima.

- Current American dietary standards give numerical values in grams per day for each life stage group for carbohydrates, dietary fibre, total fat and ω-6 and ω-3 polyunsaturated fatty acids.

'FOOD' RECOMMENDATIONS

Consumers in the UK, America and elsewhere are encouraged to eat a variety of foods each day. Different foods have different profiles of essential nutrients and different profiles of potentially toxic substances in them. Eating a variety of foods makes it more likely that adequate amounts of all the essential nutrients will be consumed and less likely that any toxins in food will be consumed in hazardous amounts. Consumers in most countries are encouraged to eat foods from different categories or food groups to ensure the adequacy of their diets (see later). Japanese consumers are advised to eat at least 30 foods each day!

In both the UK and the USA, consumers are being advised to increase their consumption of fruits and vegetables. More specifically, there is an active campaign in the UK that urges consumers to eat a minimum of five portions of fruit and vegetable each day with only one of this five being fruit juice. Diets low in fruits and vegetables have been associated in numerous epidemiological studies with increased rates of cancer and cardiovascular disease. Some of the possible reasons why fruits and vegetables might exert a protective effect against these diseases are given below.

- They are major sources of dietary fibre including the soluble components of dietary fibre.
- They are low in energy and so they make the diet bulky, which may help in weight control.
- They increase the proportion of dietary energy that is derived from carbohydrate and so reduce the proportion from fat and also alter the balance of dietary proteins, increasing the proportion of total protein that is of vegetable origin.
- They are the major sources of vitamin C and other antioxidants, e.g. β-carotene and the other carotenoids and non-nutrient antioxidants. These antioxidants inhibit the oxidative damage to cells caused by free radicals that may be important in the aetiology of both cancer and cardiovascular disease (see Chapter 12 for further critical discussion).

- They are important sources of potassium, and high potassium intake may help in the prevention of high blood pressure.

Some nutritionists might be sceptical about the putative health benefits of any one of these compositional changes but almost all would support the recommendation to increase consumption of fruits and vegetables. The cumulative evidence supporting this food change is overwhelming although there is a real possibility that other non-nutritional differences may contribute to the association between high fruit and vegetable intake and reduced risk of chronic disease, i.e. that people consuming more fruit and vegetables may be more health conscious or more affluent and thus have other lifestyle characteristics favourable to long-term health. For example, those who eat more fruit and vegetables may be:

- more physically active and leaner
- less likely to smoke or consume excessive amounts of alcohol.

It is recommended in both the UK and the USA that starchy foods such as cereals and potatoes should be more prominent in the diet. This would increase the amount of dietary fibre and the proportion of dietary energy coming from starch. This would almost inevitably lead to a reduction in the proportion being derived from fat and/or sugar because there is not much variation in protein intake. Britons and Americans are also encouraged to increase their consumption of oily fish (e.g. mackerel, herring, salmon, trout and sardines). These oily fish are the only rich sources of the long chain **n-3** (ω-3) polyunsaturated fatty acids. These fatty acids may have several effects regarded as beneficial for many people, such as:

- anti-inflammatory effects
- anti-aggregating effects on blood platelets, which reduces the tendency of blood to clot and increases bleeding time
- beneficial effects on blood lipoprotein profiles.

There is a more detailed discussion of the actions of fish oils in Chapter 11. Concentrated fish oil supplements are not advised for the general population although they may be useful for some individuals and some preparations have medicinal licences in the UK for the treatment of high concentrations of blood triacylglycerol and for use in people with existing cardiac disease.

Key points

- People should eat a variety of foods selected from each of the major food groups.

- Dietary variety helps to ensure adequacy and reduces the risk of toxins being consumed in hazardous amounts.

- Five daily portions of fruit and vegetables are recommended in the UK.

- Fruits and vegetables are good sources of dietary fibre, potassium and antioxidants. High fruit and vegetable diets tend to be bulky and low in fat which may aid weight control.

- High fruit and vegetable intake may be a marker for people who are generally more health conscious and have other healthy lifestyle characteristics.

- Starchy cereals and potatoes should be more prominent in UK and US diets.

- Increased consumption of oily fish is recommended.

ENERGY AND BODY WEIGHT

Most dietary guidelines emphasize the importance of maintaining an ideal body weight (BMI in the range 18.5–25 kg/m^2) by matching energy intake to expenditure. Details of current activity levels and targets for increasing activity are given in Chapter 17. Well over half of British and American adults are either overweight or obese and these figure have been rising alarmingly during the past three decades. Obesity and being overweight are associated with reduced life expectancy, increased illness and disability as well as having social and psychological consequences that further reduce the quality of life. In particular, obesity is associated with increased risk of **type 2 diabetes**, hypertension, cardiovascular diseases and several types of cancer (see Chapter 8 for details on the prevalence and consequences of obesity).

In both the UK and the USA, increased physical activity is recognized as a key factor in the maintenance of an ideal body weight. Both the US and UK populations have become increasingly sedentary in recent decades. There is clear evidence in Britain that as a consequence of our increasingly sedentary lifestyle, average energy intakes have fallen substantially in the past few decades (Prentice and Jebb, 1995). Over the same period, the average BMI has increased and the numbers of overweight and obese adults have also increased sharply. A national survey of activity and physical fitness of British adults found very high levels of inactivity and low levels of aerobic fitness among the majority of the adult population (Allied Dunbar, 1992, see Chapter 17 for further details). In Chapter 8, it is argued that inactivity is a major cause of the epidemic of obesity that is sweeping through most industrialized and many developing countries. Increased activity should ultimately lead to a reduction in average BMI and some moderation in the numbers of obese and overweight people in these countries. Concentrating on reducing energy intake still further does not seem to be the solution to this still increasing problem of obesity. Increased activity and fitness have many other health benefits (see Chapter 17).

Key points

- The body mass index should be kept within the ideal 18.5–25 kg/m^2 range.

- Increased activity is important in control of body weight and inactivity is an important cause of obesity.

- Dietary guidelines around the world generally recommend increased levels of physical activity to prevent excessive weight gain.

- Britons eat much less now than 50 years ago but are now much fatter.

- Increased activity and fitness have numerous other health benefits.

RECOMMENDATIONS FOR FATS, CARBOHYDRATES, PROTEIN AND SALT

UK targets

- The contribution of fat to total energy should be reduced. In the UK the aim is to get fat down to a population average of 35 per cent of food energy (33 per cent of total energy).

- The contribution of saturated fatty acids should be reduced to an average 11 per cent of food energy (10 per cent of total energy).
- Polyunsaturated n-6 (ω-6) fatty acid intake should not increase any further. COMA (1991) suggested a population average of 6 per cent of total energy from these fatty acids with no individual's intake exceeding 10 per cent.
- Cholesterol intakes in the UK should not increase. Cholesterol is generally regarded, at least in the UK, as a relatively minor influence on plasma cholesterol. If saturated fat intake is reduced then this may well also cause a drop in cholesterol intake as some foods are important contributors of both cholesterol and saturated fat to the diet.
- COMA (1994a) recommended increasing intake of long chain n-3 (ω−3) polyunsaturated fatty acids from an average of 0.1 g/day to 0.2 g/day. This is effectively a recommendation to eat twice as much oily fish.
- COMA (1991) recommended that carbohydrates should provide an average 50 per cent of food energy (47 per cent of total energy).
- Added sugars or **non-milk extrinsic sugars** should make up less than 11 per cent of food energy (10 per cent of total energy intake). The term non-milk extrinsic sugars covers all of the sugars that are not present in milk or within the cell walls of fruits and vegetables – it is almost synonymous with added sugars except that it would include the sugar in extracted fruit juices. **Intrinsic sugars** are those that are found naturally in fruits and vegetables; Britons are encouraged to eat more of these along with the complex carbohydrates.
- If Britons are to obtain 50 per cent of their food energy from carbohydrate and only 11 per cent from added sugars, it follows that 39 per cent should come from starches and intrinsic sugars combined.
- COMA (1991) recommended a 50 per cent increase in the intakes of dietary fibre or non-starch polysaccharide, i.e. to aim for a daily intake of about 18 g of non-starch polysaccharide (equivalent to around 25 g of dietary fibre).
- Current protein intakes should be maintained. Both COMA (1991) and NRC (1989a) specifically counselled against taking in more than double the reference nutrient intake (RNI) (recommended dietary allowance (RDA)) of protein.

- An upper limit of 6 g/day for salt intake has been suggested. This amounts to a reduction of more than a third for Britons.

In Table 4.1 these varied recommendations and targets have been synthesized into a British diet of 'ideal' composition. As noted earlier there are detailed guidelines given for each life stage group for Americans, but some more general recommendations are as follows.

- Less than 10 per cent of calories should come from saturated fat.
- Total fat intake should represent between 20 and 35 of calories with most coming from polyunsaturated and monounsaturated fatty acids.
- Cholesterol intake should be less than 300 mg/day.
- Adequate intakes of dietary fibre are set at 14 g per 1000 kcal of the energy requirement.
- A maximum intake for sodium is suggested which translates to approximately 6 g/day of salt.
- Adults are recommended to consume 4.7 g/day of potassium.

Table 4.1 The composition of a diet that would meet current UK guidelines

Nutrient	'Ideal' intake
Total fat	33% of total energy
Saturated fatty acids	10% of total energy
n-6 (ω-6) Polyunsaturated fatty acids	7% of total energy
n-3 (ω-3) Polyunsaturated fatty acids	At least 0.2% of total energy
Total carbohydrate	47% of total energy
Added sugars	10% of total energy
Alcohol	5% of total energy
Protein	15% of total energy
Non-starch polysaccharide	>18 g/day
Salt	<6 g/day

These recommendations are generally consistent with American guidelines.

Rationale

Overall, the changes discussed in the previous section would be expected to make the diet more bulky and to reduce the amount of energy derived from each gram of food. Reducing the content of fat and sugar and replacing it with foods rich in starch, fibre and also probably with a higher water content would reduce the **energy density** of the diet (amount of energy per gram of food). This bulky and less energy dense diet should aid weight control and lessen the risks of excessive weight gain and obesity. Such a diet would also have more nutrients per unit of energy (higher nutrient density) because fats and sugars (and alcohol) add a lot of energy but few nutrients. The changes in fat consumption would be expected to lead to the following benefits:

• better weight control (fat is palatable, a concentrated source of energy, less satiating than carbohydrate and very efficiently converted to body storage fat)
• reduced plasma (low-density lipoprotein (LDL)) cholesterol concentrations and a corresponding reduction in atherosclerosis and risk of cardiovascular diseases. High intakes of saturated fat raise plasma cholesterol concentrations and replacing saturated fat with unsaturated fat reduces plasma cholesterol concentrations. A raised plasma cholesterol concentration is causally linked to increased risk of coronary heart disease. These changes may also reduce the tendency of blood to clot and form thromboses.
• reduced risk of some cancers such as bowel cancer which are associated with a high-fat, low-carbohydrate diet.

A reduced consumption of added sugars should lead to improved dental health. Both dental decay (caries) and gum disease are strongly linked to high sugar consumption especially frequent consumption of sugary snacks and drinks between main meals. The priority should therefore be to concentrate on reducing this between-meal sugar and reducing the frequency of consumption of sugary drinks and snacks. Increased intakes of complex carbohydrate are an inevitable requirement if fat and sugar intakes are to be reduced. Non-starch polysaccharide should additionally lead to improved bowel function, less constipation and reduced incidence of minor bowel conditions like haemorrhoids (piles) and diverticulosis. High-fibre diets are also associated with reduced risk of bowel cancer and some forms of fibre may have a plasma cholesterol lowering effect.

A reduction in salt intake is expected to lead to a reduction in average population blood pressure and a reduced rate of rise of blood pressure with age. This should lead to reduced incidence of hypertension and ultimately to reduced incidence of strokes, coronary heart disease and renal failure. High salt intake may also be a factor in the aetiology of stomach cancer and so a reduction in salt intake should further decrease the prevalence of this form of cancer. High intakes of potassium may also have beneficial effects on blood pressure.

Key points

• Dietary targets for average of population in UK are:
  – fat – no more than 35 per cent of food energy
  – saturated fat – no more than 11 per cent of food energy
  – intakes should not increase
  – long chain n-3 (ω-3) polyunsaturated fatty acid intake doubled
  – no increase in n-6 (ω-6) polyunsaturated fatty acids with individual maximum of 10 per cent of energy
  – carbohydrates should make up at least 50 per cent of food energy
  – added sugars should be less than 11 per cent of food energy
  – non-starch polysaccharide intakes should be over 18 g/day
  – salt intake should be cut to 6 g/day.

• Similar recommendations have been made in the USA.

• These changes should:
  – produce a diet that is less energy dense but more nutrient dense
  – improve body weight control
  – reduce plasma cholesterol concentrations and so reduce the risk of cardiovascular diseases
  – reduce the risk of bowel and some other cancers
  – improve dental health
  – reduce constipation and other bowel disorders like haemorrhoids and diverticulosis
  – reduce average blood pressure and the prevalence of hypertension and so lead to reduced incidence of strokes, renal failure and coronary heart disease.

ALCOHOL

There is a practically unanimous belief that excessive alcohol intake is damaging to health, and that alcohol should therefore be used only in moderation or not at all. What constitutes an acceptable and healthy alcohol intake is a rather more contentious issue. There is persuasive evidence that small amounts of alcohol may have some beneficial effects on health but excessive alcohol consumption has severe health and social consequences. High alcohol consumption leads to an increased risk of liver disease, strokes, fatal accidents, birth defects, hypertension, and several forms of cancer. COMA (1998) suggested an annual social cost of excessive alcohol consumption in Britain of £2.5 billion at 1998 prices.

Many studies have reported higher mortality in those who abstain from alcohol completely than in those consuming moderate amounts of alcohol. High alcohol intakes are on the other hand associated with sharply increasing mortality, the so-called J curve (or U curve) of mortality. It has been argued that this J curve of mortality is merely an artefact due to the inclusion of reformed alcoholics in the abstaining group. However, many reports support the idea of a protective association between moderate alcohol consumption and, in particular, coronary heart disease, and that this remains even after correcting for this effect (e.g. Rimm *et al.*, 1991).

A 10–12-year cohort study conducted in Denmark (Gronbaek *et al.*, 1994) confirmed the J-shaped relationship between total mortality and alcohol consumption, with lowest relative mortality risk in those consuming 1–6 units of alcohol per week. Only with weekly alcohol consumption in excess of 42 units per week was total mortality significantly higher than in those consuming low amounts of alcohol. Age did not change the relationship between mortality risk and alcohol consumption and the apparent benefits of small amounts of alcohol applied to all adults. Some other studies in the USA (e.g. Klatsky *et al.*, 1992) have reported that the relative risk of dying as a result of alcohol consumption is higher in younger people than older people because of the alcohol-related increase in deaths from violence and traffic accidents in younger adults. Gronbaek *et al.* (1994) suggest that this difference in findings between the American and Danish studies may be because accidents and violence are less prominent as causes of death among young Danes than among young Americans.

With alcohol, the priority is to moderate the intakes of high consumers rather than to aim for a more universal reduction. Despite a substantial body of evidence that alcohol in moderation may have some beneficial effects, expert committees have generally shied away from recommending people to drink alcohol. Many people find it difficult to gauge and regulate their intake of alcohol; this explains the general reluctance of expert committees to recommend that people should consume alcohol. Back in 1983, NACNE recommended a reduction in alcohol consumption from an average 6 per cent of total energy to 4 per cent of total energy. It suggested that this should be achieved by curtailing the consumption of high consumers rather than shifting the whole distribution of intakes as with their other recommendations. Current US guidelines recommend that if people do drink alcohol then they should limit their consumption to no more than about 2 units of alcohol in any one day for men and just 1 unit for women. They further suggest that alcoholic beverages should not be consumed at all by those who cannot control their alcohol intake, women who are or might become pregnant, lactating women and adolescents.

A unit of alcohol is defined as 8 g of pure alcohol, which is equivalent to half a pint of ordinary beer (about 250 mL), a small glass of wine (75 mL) or a single measure of spirits. In Britain, the recommended maximum intake of alcohol was for some time 21 units per week for men and 14 units for women. In 1995 the Department of Health rather controversially raised these safe drinking limits to 28 units per week for men and 21 units for women. This alcohol should be spread fairly evenly throughout the week and high consumption on particular days (binge drinking) should be avoided. Given this need to avoid binge drinking the recommended maximum alcohol intakes are now usually presented as daily maxima of 4 units for men and 3 units for women. This Department of Health report (DH, 1995) also contained some positive encouragement for older people who do not drink to consider taking 1–2 units per day. It is generally recommended on both sides of the Atlantic that pregnant women should avoid alcohol. Alcohol impairs judgement and co-ordination and slows down reflexes so should be avoided when driving or participating in any other activity where such impairments could be hazardous, e.g. operating machinery.

Table 4.2 shows the distribution of reported alcohol intakes in British men and women. This table shows that 60 per cent of men and 43 per cent of women in this survey reported that they exceeded the recommended maximum number of daily units on at least one day in the sampled week. The proportions exceeding these daily maxima were substantially higher in the youngest age group. Half of young men and a third of young women consumed more than double the recommended levels on at least one day in the sample week.

Table 4.2 Distribution of alcohol in British men and women based on maximum number of units consumed during a 7-day dietary record of British adults aged 19–64 years*

	All (% recording)	19–24 years (% recording)
Men		
Nothing in 7 days	20	20
Up to 4 units[†]	20	14
4–8 units	21	15
8+ units	39	50
Mean no. daily units	7.8	9.4
Women in 7 days		
Nothing	33	29
Up to 3 units[†]	23	14
3–6 units	21	23
6+ units	22	34
Mean daily units	3.6	5.3

*Data from Hoare et al. (2004).
[†] Note that UK recommendations are that men should consume a maximum of 4 units in any one day and women a maximum of 3 units, i.e. 60 per cent of men (43 per cent of women) and 65 per cent of the younger men (57 per cent of younger women) exceeded these maxima on at least one day.

Mechanisms by which alcohol may reduce risk of coronary heart disease

Low to moderate alcohol intake seems to be associated with reduced total mortality largely as a result of reduced mortality from coronary heart disease. Even though heavy drinkers have higher total mortality this is largely due to causes other than coronary heart disease. Listed below are several suggested mechanisms by which alcohol may protect against coronary heart disease (see COMA 1998 for primary sources).

- Alcohol intake is associated with increased levels of **high-density lipoproteins (HDL)** in plasma. This is the cholesterol-containing lipoprotein fraction in plasma that removes excess cholesterol to the liver and affords protection against atherosclerosis and coronary heart disease (see Chapter 11 for further details on HDL).
- Some alcoholic drinks (especially red wine) may contain substances that act as antioxidants and help to prevent the free radical damage that is implicated in the aetiology of atherosclerosis. Polyphenols in red wine (particularly a substance called *trans*-resveratrol) have been the subject of much study. On the basis of *in vitro* studies with vascular endothelium and short-term studies in animals these are claimed to be cardioprotective. One widely publicized study found that wines from two particular regions had the highest concentrations of these polyphenols. It was widely implied on the basis of this limited evidence that these wines were the healthiest, and this was a factor in the longevity of the people living in these particular wine-producing regions (see Corder *et al.*, 2006).
- Alcohol may reduce the tendency of blood to clot and for thromboses to form. Alcohol consumption is associated with reduced plasma fibrinogen levels and reduced activity of platelets (fibrinogen is a key protein in blood clotting and platelet activation is also a key step in blood coagulation).

Key points

- Alcohol should be consumed in moderation or not at all. Alcohol should be avoided during pregnancy and when driving.

- High alcohol consumption has serious health and social consequences and is associated with steeply increasing mortality. Low alcohol consumption is associated with lower mortality than complete abstention and seems to afford some protection against coronary heart disease.

- The relationship between alcohol consumption and mortality risk is a J-shaped curve.

- Alcohol consumption raises the high-density lipoprotein cholesterol concentration in blood and reduces the tendency of blood to clot.

- Some alcoholic drinks contain antioxidants that may afford protection against damage by free radicals.

- Recommendations for alcohol in the UK are a maximum of 3 units per day for women and for 4 units per day for men.

- American men are advised to drink up to 2 drinks per day and women only 1 per day.

- A unit of alcohol is a small glass of wine, a half-pint of ordinary beer or a standard measure of spirits (approximately 8 g of pure alcohol).

Table 4.3 The macronutrient composition of the typical adult British diet. Values are percentage of food energy unless otherwise stated

	Nutrient as percentage of food energy		
	Men	Women	Target (DRV)
Fat	35.8	34.9	35
Saturated fat	13.4	13.2	11
Protein	16.2	16.1	n/a
Total carbohydrate	47.7	48.5	50
Non-milk extrinsic sugars	13.6	11.9	11
Salt (g/day)[†]	11.0	8.1	<6
NSP (g/day)[‡]	15.2	12.6	18+

DRV, dietary reference value; NSP, non-starch polysaccharide.
*Data from Hoare et al. (2004).
[†]85 per cent of men and 69 per cent of women did not meet the target for salt.
[‡]72 per cent of men and 87 per cent of women did not meet the target for NSP.

HOW DO CURRENT UK DIETS COMPARE WITH 'IDEAL' INTAKES?

Table 4.3 summarizes the macronutrient composition of the British adult diet as determined by the latest National Diet and Nutrition Survey (NDNS) (Hoare *et al.*, 2004). These values represent substantial improvements on those recorded in the 1990 NDNS survey (Gregory *et al.*, 1990). The percentage of food energy from fat in this survey was less than half a per cent higher than the dietary reference value (DRV, 35 per cent) when the average of the two sexes is used; this is compared with 38 per cent in the 1990 NDNS. Although the values for saturated fat are still somewhat higher than the DRV they are nonetheless an improvement on the 16 per cent recorded in 1990. There has been a reduction in the energy derived from non-milk extrinsic sugars towards the target DRV and a substantial increase in the proportion of energy that comes from all carbohydrates. The average salt intakes shown in Table 4.3 are still around 60 per cent higher than the DRV and three-quarters of the adult population exceeded the recommended maximum. Although there has been some small increase in average recorded intakes of non-starch polysaccharide in this latest NDNS survey compared with the 1990 survey, about 80 per cent of adults still do not consume the recommended 18+ g/day.

Key points

- According to the latest NDNS adult survey, the average British diet when compared with current UK guidelines:
  - was close to the target of 35 per cent of dietary energy as fat
  - was just 2.3 per cent over the target of 11 per cent of food energy as saturated fat
  - was about 2 per cent below the target of 50 per cent of food energy from carbohydrate
  - was about 2 per cent over the target of 11 per cent of food energy as non-milk extrinsic sugars
  - was 60 per cent higher than the target of no more than 6 g salt/day
  - had 4 g/day too little non-starch polysaccharide (NSP) and 80 per cent of people did not consume the recommended 18+ g NSP/day.

- These values (see Table 4.3) represent significant movements towards the target values since the 1990 NDNS survey report with the exception of those for salt.

OTHER NUTRIENTS

The importance of obtaining intakes of all the essential nutrients in line with current dietary standards is generally acknowledged, i.e. of ensuring that the diet contains adequate amounts of energy and all of the essential nutrients.

Calcium and iron

Milk and milk products are the most important sources of calcium in British and American diets. Meat is a major source of dietary iron in its most readily absorbed form as haem. There has been concern that calcium and iron intakes might fall along with any fall in saturated fat consumption. Iron and calcium intakes can be maintained despite cuts in fat and saturated fat if low-fat dairy products, fish, lean meat and poultry are substituted for fatty meats, full-fat dairy products and other fried and fatty foods. Back in 1983, NACNE recognized the importance of milk in maintaining adequate calcium intakes. It suggested that the wider availability of lower-fat milk would allow calcium intakes to be maintained despite the recommended cuts in saturated fat intake. Low-fat milk has indeed become more available in the UK and semi-skimmed milk now accounts for most of the milk drunk in Britain. The issue of calcium and its importance in bone health is discussed at length in Chapter 14.

Fluoride

NAS (2004) recommended optimal intakes of fluoride, especially in children whose teeth are developing. COMA (1991) endorsed the more widespread fluoridation of public water supplies up to a level of 1 ppm and set a safe intake of fluoride for infants of 0.05 mg/kg body weight/day. The effects of fluoride on dental health are discussed in Chapter 9.

Potassium

Increased consumption of fruits and vegetables leads to an increase in potassium intakes. COMA (1994) specifically recommended an increase in average potassium intake to about 3.5 g/day in adults (4.7 g/day in the USA). There is evidence that high potassium intake protects against the hypertensive effects of salt. Hoare et al. (2004) found that average potassium intakes were below the 3.5 g/day

RNI for both men and women with an average of only 2.8 g/day in women; 20 per cent of women recorded intakes that were below the lower RNI (LRNI) of only 2 g/day.

Key points

- It is important that adequate amounts of all essential nutrients are consumed.

- Calcium and iron intakes can be maintained despite reductions in saturated fat if lean meat, poultry and low-fat milk replace fatty meats, full fat dairy products and other fatty foods.

- In both Britain and the USA minimum intakes of fluoride are recommended, especially in young children, to protect against dental decay.

- High potassium intakes may help to prevent high blood pressure. Increased fruit and vegetable consumption leads to increased potassium intakes and British adults have been recommended to increase potassium intake to 3.5 g/day (4.7 g/day in the USA).

- 20 per cent of British women recorded potassium intakes of less than 2 g/day.

WILLINGNESS TO CHANGE

It is sometimes argued that health promotion and nutrition education in particular are doomed to be ineffective because consumers are unwilling to make changes to their diets on health grounds. For example, in a short article that was largely critical of health promotion, Watts (1998) suggests that 'no one has yet fathomed out how to persuade anyone to live more healthily'. To support his argument, he uses the failure of several major intervention trials to demonstrate significant benefits for the intervention group. However, health advice and health promotion can produce major shifts in national behaviour. In the 1970s and early 1980s many parents in Britain and elsewhere were persuaded to use a front sleeping position for their babies rather than the traditional back sleeping position. In the early 1990s many were then persuaded to revert to the traditional back position to reduce the risk of cot death (see Chapter 1 and Webb, 1995). Smoking is much less prevalent now than it was when the links between smoking and lung cancer were first established and publicized. In several sectors of British society, smoking has gone from being accepted as the accepted social norm to a minority and anti-social activity.

There is also ample evidence that Britons and Americans made huge changes to their diets in the last quarter of the twentieth century. These changes were largely driven by the desire to control body weight and the publicity about the links between diet and health. Table 4.4 shows a comparison of fat purchases for home consumption in the UK in 1975 and 1996 with some indication of changes since 1996. Some other health-driven changes to British diets are given below.

Table 4.4 Fats purchased for home consumption in the UK in 1975 and 1996*

	1975	1996
'Yellow fats'		
(as % of yellow fat sales)		
Butter	*68*	*25*
Soft margarine	*14*	*21+*
Other margarine	*18*	*<3*
Low fat spreads	*–*	*51†*
Cooking fats		
(as % of cooking fat sales)		
Vegetable oils	*22*	*77†*
Other fats (mainly lard)	*78*	*23*
Fats as percentage of food energy§		
Total fat	*41.3*	*39.7*
Saturated fatty acids	*20.3*	*15.4*
Polyunsaturated fatty acids	*4.6*	*7.2*
P:S ratio	*0.19*	*0.46*

*Data source: National Food Survey.
† In 2004–05 low and reduced fat spreads accounted for 60 per cent of the spreading fat market.
‡ Vegetable oils in 2004–05 had a market share of 81 per cent of cooking fat sales.
§ More recent data on dietary fats as a percentage of food energy can be seen in Table 4.3.

- Low-fat milks only became readily available in the early 1980s in Britain and so before this almost all of the fresh liquid milk sold was whole-fat milk. Between 1986 and 2005 low-fat milk increased from 19 per cent of liquid milk sales to around 70 per cent.

- In 1986 about 7 per cent of the soft drinks purchased for home consumption were low-calorie versions and by 2005 this had risen to 30 per cent.
- In the late 1960s sales of sugar amounted to about 0.5 kg per person per week but by 2005 this had fallen to 35 g/week. (Note that total added sugar consumption has not dropped by anything like this amount because it has to some extent been offset by greater consumption of sugar in manufactured products.)
- In 1976, sales of wholemeal bread made up a negligible proportion of total bread sales. Improvements in the texture of wholemeal bread coupled with health messages about dietary fibre have caused sales to rise so that in 2005 just under a quarter of loaves of bread sold were wholemeal loaves.

Many of the changes in recent decades are the result of simple replacement of a traditional product with another of similar or better utilitarian value so they have been easy to understand and implement. Butter and hard margarine have been replaced by soft margarine and low-fat spreads in most British homes (Table 4.4). Semi-skimmed (1.7 per cent) and skimmed milk have largely replaced whole milk. Even though the new 'healthier product' is often considered slightly less palatable than the traditional product, people have been prepared in large numbers to make this relatively small sacrifice for their health or to try to lose weight. Table 4.4 shows that there have been dramatic changes in the types of cooking and spreading fats used in British homes but until recently there were only relatively small changes in the overall prominence of fat in British diets. Health promoters and nutrition educators should consider this when framing their dietary advice or devising their campaigns. People need to be offered simple, realistic and relatively painless ways of achieving or moving towards the desired nutritional goals.

Key points

- Despite assertions to the contrary, consumers have made substantial dietary changes as a result of health information and heath promotion.
- Since 1975 the following changes to the British diet have occurred:
  - a massive switch from the use of butter and hard margarine to soft margarine and low-fat spreads

- – a huge switch from the use of animal-derived cooking fats such as lard to use of vegetable oils for cooking
- – replacement of whole milk with low-fat milks, which now account for 70 per cent of liquid milk sales
- – large increases in the sales of low-calorie soft drinks and wholemeal bread.

● Many of these dietary changes made in Britain involve the simple replacement of a traditional product by an alternative that although possibly less palatable has similar utilitarian characteristics and is perceived as healthier.

● Past experience thus suggests that if consumers are offered simple, realistic and relatively painless ways of improving their diets then many will make such changes.

SOME BARRIERS TO DIETARY CHANGE

Figure 1.4 (p. 25) summarized the pathway by which a health promotion message is transmitted to the public and successfully results in improvements in health. At each step on this pathway potential barriers are there that may prevent effective change being made. Many factors may discourage consumers from changing their diets in the direction suggested in this chapter – a number of potential barriers to change.

Palatability

Fat and sugar are major contributors to the palatability of Western diets. Starch and fibre are bland and so high-fibre, high-starch diets are often perceived as deficient in taste, smell and having an unappealing texture. As populations become more affluent their natural inclination is to replace much of the starchy food that makes up the bulk of peasant diets and replace it with foods that are much higher in fat and sugar.

Sugar–fat seesaw

It may prove particularly difficult to reduce simultaneously the contribution of both fats and sugars to the diet. This would inevitably involve a substantial increase in starch consumption. In free-living affluent population there tends to be an inverse relationship between sugar and fat consumption. People who get a low proportion of their energy from fat tend to get a high proportion from sugar and *vice versa*, this is the so-called '**sugar–fat seesaw**'. Survey data quoted by McColl (1988) suggested that people who consumed less than 35 per cent of their calories as fat, derived, on average, more than 25 per cent of their calories from sugars. Back in 1990 Gregory *et al.* found that whereas 13 per cent of their representative sample of British adults met the target of no more than 33 per cent of total energy from fat only 1 per cent met both this fat target and that for added sugars. Those men and women who met the fat targets and sugar targets had higher alcohol intakes than those who did not, i.e. alcohol tended to dilute the fat and sugar and so help some individuals to meet sugar or fat targets. This sugar–fat seesaw might, in practice, increase the difficulty for individuals of meeting both fat and sugar targets.

Availability of healthy alternatives

We saw in the previous section that many of the most striking changes in the British diet in the past 30 years have resulted from the substitution of a traditional food by one perceived as more healthy. If people are to continue to make these substitutions then the healthy alternatives must be readily available, affordable and acceptable in terms of their palatability. The massive switch from whole- to low-fat milk coincided with the much greater availability of low-fat milks, especially semi-skimmed milk, in the early 1980s. The increase in sales of wholemeal bread was partly the result of improved texture of these products. Low-fat spreads were unavailable 25 years ago but now account for 60 per cent of the 'yellow fat' market in Britain. It may be argued that public demand will be sufficient to ensure increasing availability of these 'healthier' alternatives. However, to demonstrate demand, the public must be given reasonable access to a product. Will a perceived future demand always be sufficient incentive for manufacturers and retailers to provide health options, particularly for a product likely to yield no increase in or perhaps even lower profit margins? The range of these low-fat, low-sugar and low-salt products is increasing all the time but some of them may be relatively expensive or perceived as poor value for money by low-income families trying to satisfy their appetites with strictly limited funds, e.g.:

- extra lean mincemeat (hamburger) is more expensive than the standard version
- low-fat milk costs the same as whole milk but provides fewer calories, i.e. the healthier version provides far fewer calories per penny (this applies to most low fat and sugar products)
- fruits and vegetables are an expensive source of energy, especially the more exotic and appealing varieties
- the cheapest white bread in British supermarkets costs much less than a wholemeal loaf.

Skills and knowledge

It is easier for people to reduce their fat intake or increase their fibre intake if they have a reasonable idea of the relative amounts of these in different foods. Have people got the skills and knowledge to prepare meals that are both appetizing and more in tune with current guidelines? Are food, nutrition and food preparation given sufficient weighting in our schools?

Traditional nutritional beliefs

Some consumers may be reluctant to increase their consumption of starchy foods because they still perceive then as fattening. A reduction in consumption of meat and cheese may be hindered by their perception as valuable sources of first class protein.

Key points

- Several factors may act as barriers or hindrances to the implementation of current nutritional guidelines.
- Sugar and fat add palatability to the diet whereas starch and fibre are bland – this may discourage the replacement of some fat and sugar by starchy foods.
- In affluent diets there is often a sugar–fat seesaw, which makes it more difficult to simultaneously reduce the proportions of energy derived from both fat and sugar.
- Substitution of traditional foods by 'healthier' alternatives requires that the healthier options are readily available, affordable and palatable.

- Many of the 'healthier' options are more expensive than the traditional product particularly when costed as calories per penny. This may hinder dietary improvement in low-income groups.
- People may lack the knowledge and skills to implement the guidelines.
- Some outdated beliefs may discourage beneficial dietary change, e.g. 'starchy foods are fattening' 'high intakes of meat and cheese are necessary to meet protein needs'. They may simply provide those reluctant to change with an excuse for not changing.

AIDS TO FOOD SELECTION

Selecting food solely according to biological criteria requires considerable knowledge of nutrition and food composition. It takes some skill to routinely translate current views on optimal intakes into meals and diets. Dieticians and nutrition educators need ways of translating complex technical guidelines about diet composition into simple, practical advice that is easy to understand, remember and implement. When adequacy was the nutritional priority then **food groups** were a simple and effective means of helping people to select food on a constituent basis. Foods were grouped together according to the nutrients that they provided – consumers could then be advised that if they consumed specified minimum numbers of portions from each of the groups then nutritional adequacy would probably be assured.

The most widely used of these food group systems was the **four food group plan**. Foods were divided up into four basic food groups and a specified minimum number of servings from each group were recommended. Several generations of American schoolchildren and college students were taught the basic four food group plan since its development in 1955. Thus this classification system will still be familiar to many American adults although it would be much less familiar to most Britons. The four food groups and an outline of their essential nutrient profiles are listed below.

- *The milk group* (milk, cheese, yoghurt and other milk products) – these provide good amounts of energy, good quality protein, vitamin A, calcium and riboflavin.

- *The meat group* (meat, fish, eggs and also meat substitutes such as pulses and nuts) – these provide protein, vitamin A, B vitamins and iron.
- *The fruit and vegetable group* (fruits and those vegetables not classified as meat substitutes) – these provide carotene, vitamin C, folate, riboflavin, potassium and fibre.
- *The bread and cereals group* (bread, rice, pasta, breakfast cereals and products made from flour). Whole-grain cereals are good sources of B vitamins, some minerals and fibre. White flour still provides reasonable amounts of fibre and it is often fortified with vitamins and minerals (in the UK, with iron, calcium and some B vitamins).

People were advised to eat a minimum of two portions each day from the meat and milk groups and a minimum of four portions from the other two groups each day. As the foods in these four groups have differing profiles of essential nutrients, provided consumers ate enough to satisfy their appetite and ate these minimum numbers of portions, nutritional adequacy was practically assured. Many foods are not covered by any of these categories, e.g. butter, oil and other fats, sugar, alcoholic drinks, etc. This is because they are largely sources of energy and provide few nutrients so no minimum portions were recommended. They were to be used sparingly because of their low nutrient density.

Such food group schemes were originally designed to ensure nutritional adequacy rather than to guide consumers towards a diet that helps to prevent chronic disease. Many foods in the milk and meat groups are now seen as rich sources of dietary fat and cholesterol as well as nutrients, e.g. whole milk, cheese, fatty meat. Many foods in the cereals group are seen as low in fat and sugar and high in fibre and starch in addition to being sources of some nutrients. Many foods in the fruit and vegetables group are very low in energy density and practically fat free in their natural unprocessed state. To comply with the compositional guidelines discussed in this chapter, consumers need to be encouraged to:

- increase their consumption of cereals, vegetables and fruit
- moderate their consumption of meats and dairy foods
- minimize their consumption of fatty and sugary foods that do not fit into any of the four groups
- choose foods within the food groups that are low in fat and added sugars but high in fibre.

For some time, nutrition educators tried to adapt this four food group guide to modern nutritional priorities, e.g. highlighting the low-fat/low-sugar options within each group. However, a food guide that merely suggested minimum quantities from the food groups was unsuited to modern dietary guidelines with their emphasis on moderating intakes of some foods and food groups and increasing the prominence of other food groups in the diet.

In 1992, the US Department of Agriculture (USDA, 1992) published a new guide to food selection intended to update and replace the basic four plan – the **food guide pyramid** (see Figure 4.2). This food pyramid is a development of the food groups and was designed to reflect the dual aims of selecting a diet that is not only adequate but also meets nutritional guidelines aimed at reducing the risk of chronic disease. At the base of the food pyramid are the starchy grain foods that should contribute more servings than any other single group to the ideal diet – 6–11 servings depending upon total energy intake (in the range of 1600–2800 kcal or 6.7–11.8 MJ). On the next tier of the pyramid are the fruit and vegetable groups – a total of 5–9 servings from these groups depending upon energy intake. At the third level on the pyramid are the foods of animal origin (including the vegetarian alternatives to meat and milk such as pulses, nuts, soya milk and modern meat substitutes). There should be 2–3 servings from each group on this tier, i.e. from the meat and milk groups. At the top of the pyramid are the fats, oils and sweets – foods such as salad dressings, cream, butter, margarine, soft drinks, sweets (candies), sweet desserts and alcoholic drinks. These foods provide few nutrients but are high in energy, sugars and fats and thus should be used sparingly in the ideal diet, especially for those seeking to lose weight. In Figure 4.2, a triangle symbol is distributed lightly within the cereal, fruit and milk groups to show that some foods from these categories may contain added sugars, e.g. sweetened breakfast cereals, fruit canned in syrup, some flavoured yoghurts, milk shake and ice cream. Also in Figure 4.2, a circle symbol is distributed lightly throughout the cereal and vegetable groups to show that these may contain added fats and more densely in the meat and milk groups to show that many of the foods in these groups contain substantial amounts of naturally occurring fat. The top layer of the pyramid contains a high density of both triangles and circles to emphasize its role as a major contributor of fats and added sugar to the

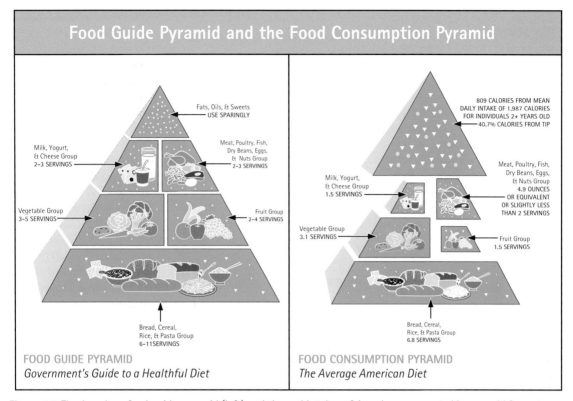

Figure 4.2 *The American food guide pyramid (left) and the real intakes of Americans presented in pyramid format (right). Source: US Department of Agriculture/US Department of Health and Social Services; Pyramid servings intakes by US children and adults 1994–1996, 1998, Community Nutrition Research Group, Beltville Human Nutrition Research Center, Agricultural Research Service, US Department of Agriculture, 2000. Food consumption pyramid reproduced by permission of Cattlemen's Beef Board and National Cattlemen's Beef Association.*

diet. The food pyramid thus indicates a general dietary structure that should ensure adequacy and yet at the same time make it more likely that other nutrition education guidelines aimed at reducing chronic disease will also be met. Highlighting the likely sources of fat and added sugars in the diet with the circle and triangle symbols should aid consumers in making choices that reduce intakes of fat and added sugars.

Figure 4.2 also shows alongside the standard food guide pyramid, an estimate of what the average American really eats, laid out in the form of a pyramid. This 'real' pyramid is much more top heavy than the ideal one with foods from the fats and sugars group providing 41 per cent of the calories. The milk and meat group provide around 3.5 servings compared with the 4–6 suggested and fruits and vegetables 3.6 servings (including a large contribution from potatoes) compared with the suggested 5–9 servings. The bread and cereals group provide

6.8 servings which is just within the 6–11 servings suggested. This shows just how large are the dietary changes required by the US food guide pyramid.

Following the launch of the food guide pyramid in the USA, a British version of this pyramid appeared in 1993. This was an unofficial attempt to provide Britons with some form of nationally accepted food guide for the first time. It was produced jointly by the Flour Advisory Bureau and the Dunn Nutrition Laboratory in Cambridge. 'The British Healthy Eating Pyramid' was in most of its essentials identical to the US version except that potatoes were included with the cereals at the base of the pyramid (rather than with the other vegetables). The fruits and vegetables were represented as a single group on the second tier of the pyramid with a recommended 5–9 daily servings. In early 1994, the Nutrition Task Force had identified the need for a national pictorial food guide as a priority for implementing the dietary and nutritional targets set out in *The health of the nation* (DH, 1992). Research on the best form that this food guide should take was undertaken on behalf of the Health Education Authority. A variety of different formats were tested with both the general public and with health professionals. This research showed that such pictorial guides could improve people's understanding of nutritional concepts. A plate shape was found to be more effective at conveying those nutritional concepts than an American-type pyramid. The tilted plate model proved most appealing to members of the public (Hunt *et al.*, 1995). As a result of these findings, The Health Education Authority in Britain published the first official national food guide in mid-1994. It used the image of a tilted plate with five food groups occupying different sized segment of this plate (Figure 4.3, now published on the eatwell website).

Two large segments occupy about 30 per cent of the plate each:

- starchy foods, the bread, cereals and potatoes group
- the fruit and vegetables group.

Two medium-sized segments occupy about 15 per cent of the plate each:

- meat, fish, eggs and pulses
- milk and milk products like cheese and yoghurt.

The smallest sector of the plate represents less than 10 per cent of the area and contains:

- fatty and sugary foods.

The general dietary structure indicated in the tilted plate model is essentially the same as that suggested by the American pyramid. The diet should contain large amounts of starchy foods and fruit and vegetables, more moderate amounts of foods from the meat and milk groups and strictly limited amounts of fatty and sugary foods. In the form that is used for general display, e.g. in supermarkets and for general guidance to the public, it contains no recommended numbers of portions. It is felt that the wide variation in individual energy intakes and thus the wide variation in numbers of recommended portions would make this information difficult for the general lay person to interpret. The 'eatwell' tilted plate on general release (Figure 4.3) does contain additional advice for selection within each food group:

- choose low-fat options from the meat and milk groups where possible
- eat a variety of fruits and vegetables
- eat all types of starchy foods and choose high-fibre varieties where possible.

There is a version of this tilted plate model that does contain recommended numbers of portions of foods. It is intended for use by health professionals

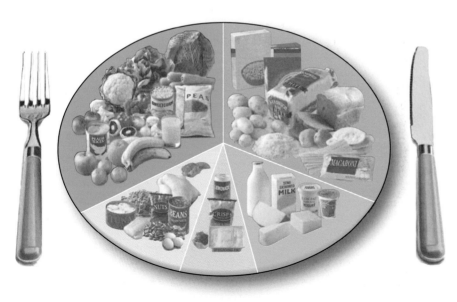

Figure 4.3 *The eatwell plate model used as the national food guide in the UK. Crown copyright. www.eatwell. gov.uk/ healthydiet/eatwellplate reproduced by kind permission of Her Majesty's Stationery Office.*

in one-to-one counselling with their clients where they can interpret this quantitative information in a way that is appropriate to the individual. These portion guides are similar to those suggested on the American pyramid guide:

- 5–9 measures of fruits and vegetables
- 5–14 measures of bread cereals and potatoes
- 2–3 measures of meat, fish and alternatives
- 2–3 measures of milk and dairy foods
- 0–4 measures of fatty and sugary foods.

Key points

- Nutrition educators have used a variety of guidance tools to translate technical nutritional guidelines into practical and comprehensible dietary advice.

- Food groups helped to guide consumers towards a nutritionally adequate diet. Foods were grouped into four or more categories with differing nutrient profiles and consumers were advised to eat a minimum number of portions from each category daily.

- The milk, meat, cereals and fruit and vegetables were the four groups of the basic four group plan. Sugary and fatty foods were in a separate category outside the main food groups.

- New food guides became necessary when 'preventing chronic disease' became a major nutritional priority and when guidelines often stressed reducing or moderating intakes of certain dietary components.

- The USA now has a food guide pyramid. Foods are arranged on the pyramid in order to indicate their ideal prominence in the diet. The large base section of the pyramid is occupied by the bread and cereals group, on the next level are the fruit and vegetable groups, then the meat and dairy groups. The small section at the top of the pyramid is occupied by fatty and sugary foods, emphasizing the need to restrict intake of these.

- In Britain a tilted plate model is used. Two large sectors of the plate are occupied by starchy foods (cereals and potatoes) and the fruit and vegetable group, two moderate-sized sectors by the meat and alternatives group and the milk group. The last small section of the plate is occupied by fatty and sugary foods.

- In the American pyramid, the density of circular and triangular symbols indicates the likely sources of fat and added sugar, respectively.

- In the UK, text messages on the plate urge consumers to choose low-fat and high-fibre options from within the appropriate groups.

- The American pyramid has suggested ranges for ideal numbers of daily portions from each of the food groups. Only the version of the British guide intended for use by health professionals has these portion guidelines.

CONCLUDING REMARKS

Although many nutritionists would argue about specific diet/disease issues, few would disagree with the proposition that significant health benefits would be likely to accrue if Americans and Britons were leaner, more active, consumed alcohol moderately, ate less fat, sugar and salt but more fruit, vegetables and cereals. The basic qualitative message transmitted by the American food guide pyramid and the British tilted plate enjoy consensus support of nutritionists and dieticians.

In this chapter, recommendations have only been considered in terms of their effects on the health of people eating them. Dietary changes will also inevitably have social, economic and environmental consequences. Some dietary changes that might be deemed nutritionally desirable may not be sustainable if everyone adopts them. If those in the wealthy industrialized countries make dietary changes that soak up more of the world's resources, then health promotion in wealthy countries may be at the expense of still greater deprivation in poorer ones. Some examples of these issues are given below.

- The world's oceans are already suffering depletion of fish stocks due to over-fishing. If people are encouraged to eat more fish, will this situation worsen still further? Is fish farming a realistic alternative to wild fish? Is it capable of producing fish on a huge scale without heavy inputs of energy and other negative ecological repercussions?
- If all Western consumers start eating five portions of fruits and vegetables each day, will many of them be transported into northern countries with all the resultant fuel costs? What effects will their

growth have upon groundwater resources in the producing country? Will they be grown as cash crops for export at the expense of the staple crops needed to feed the local population?

- If Western consumers reduce their consumption of meat and dairy foods and replace them with starchy cereals and roots, then this should have a positive impact upon sustainability. It takes 3–10 kg of grain to produce 1 kg of meat or poultry. However, what if these Western consumers are encouraged to waste many of the expensively produced calories in animal foods? If they only eat the leaner cuts of meat and discard much of the fat in animal carcasses, if skimmed milk and lean meat are seen as a healthy nutrient rich products but the market for butterfat, lard and beef fat shrinks still further? How many millions of starving children in the developing world could have been fed with the millions of tonnes of grain used to produce the beef burnt in Britain since 1988 in order to protect British consumers from bovine spongiform encephalopathy (BSE; 'mad cow disease', see Chapter 18 for details of BSE)?
- The dietary changes brought about by health promotion have already had a noticeable effect on the nature of farming and the countryside. In Britain, huge yellow swathes of land devoted to the growth of oilseed rape have become a feature of many parts of the British countryside. Can the hill land in the more mountainous parts of Britain be used productively for purposes other than grazing animals?
- Some of the recommended dietary changes seem to be encouraging a more artificial and less natural diet, e.g. use of low-fat spreads, low-calorie drinks and use of some meat substitutes.
- As an alternative to the American food guide pyramid, Walter Willett and his colleagues at the Harvard School of Public Health have suggested a pyramid based on the traditional Mediterranean diet in which most of the dietary fat would come from olive oil. Olive oil is a relatively expensive (and delicious) regional product; is it practical to recommend such a diet for mass consumption, e.g. in northern Europe and the colder regions of North America?

Detailed discussion of such issues is beyond the scope of a book such as this and beyond the capabilities of its author but they are issues that need to be considered by those advocating dietary change.

Key points

- Most nutritionists would agree with the broad thrust of current nutritional guidelines despite questioning particular elements of them.

- The environmental, economic and cultural impacts of recommended dietary changes need to be considered as well as simply their nutritional desirability for residents of the home country.

- Expert committees must ensure that any recommendations they make are sustainable if implemented on a mass scale by many populations.

5

Cellular energetics

INTRODUCTION AND AIMS OF THE CHAPTER

This brief and greatly simplified outline of the energy conversions within the cell is not intended to be an introduction to the study of biochemistry. Only the minimum of factual biochemistry to allow illustration of the broad principles and concepts has been included. The purpose is to give the reader with no biochemical background enough perception of the biochemical processes of the cell to help their understanding of nutrition. This short summary may also provide a useful overview for readers who have studied biochemistry. Certain nutritionally important observations should be clarified by this discussion, such as those listed below.

- Fatty acids cannot be converted to glucose but glucose can be converted to fat.
- The human brain cannot use fatty acids as substrates but during starvation it obtains more than half of its energy from the metabolism of **ketone bodies** that are derived from fatty acids.
- Many vitamins are essential as precursors of the coenzymes that are necessary to allow enzyme-mediated reactions to occur.
- Amino acids can serve as energy sources and can be used to generate glucose during fasting.
- Certain substances can 'uncouple' the link between oxidation (energy production) and phosphorylation **(adenosine triphosphate (ATP)** synthesis) and thus cause this energy to be released as heat. This is how **brown fat** in some animals generates heat for maintaining body temperature in the cold.

OVERVIEW OF METABOLISM

The catabolism (breakdown) of carbohydrates, fats and proteins within cells releases chemical energy. This energy is used to drive all of the energy requiring processes of the cell, e.g. synthetic processes, muscle contraction, transport of materials across cell membranes, nerve conduction. Adenosine triphosphate has a pivotal role as a short-term energy store within the cell. The chemical energy released during the catabolic metabolism of foodstuffs is stored as high-energy ATP and then the breakdown of ATP is used to drive the other energy-requiring processes. Each cell produces its own ATP; it is not transported between cells.

Although they will not discussed in the following outline, it should be borne in mind that every cellular reaction is catalysed (speeded up) by a specific **enzyme**. The reactions would not occur to any significant extent in the absence of the specific enzyme – it is the enzymes within the cell that determine what reactions can occur within the cell, and thus they determine the nature of the cell. Enzymes are proteins and the genetic code (contained in the DNA molecule) codes for the proteins of the cell. It is the proteins an organism produces that determines its characteristics. Genetic diseases are the result of an error in one of the proteins produced by that individual. Many enzymes require non-protein moieties known as **coenzymes** or cofactors in order to function. Several of these coenzymes are derivatives of vitamins and it is their roles as precursors of coenzymes that accounts for the essentiality of several vitamins. Cofactors that are bound strongly to the enzyme and become an integral part of the enzyme structure are termed **prosthetic groups**. Other substances that are sometimes taken as dietary supplements can also act as coenzymes: these are not classified as vitamins because endogenous synthesis is considered sufficient to meet our needs (see Chapter 12).

Nature and functioning of ATP

Adenosine triphosphate comprises a purine base (adenine), a pentose sugar (ribose) and three phosphate groups. The hydrolysis of ATP to adenosine diphosphate (ADP), by removal of one of the phosphate groups, is a highly **exergonic reaction**, i.e. a considerable amount of chemical energy is released during the reaction. This energy would be released as heat if the ATP hydrolysis were conducted in a test tube. Similarly, the hydrolysis of ADP to adenosine monophosphate (AMP) is also highly exergonic. Conversely, the conversions of AMP to ADP to ATP are highly **endergonic reactions**, they absorb large amounts of energy; if these reactions were conducted in a test tube then one would expect to need to provide heat energy to make the thermodynamics of the reactions favourable.

ATP: adenine — ribose — P — P — P

ADP: adenine — ribose — P — P

AMP: adenine — ribose — P

P = Phosphate group (PO_4)

Within the cell, highly exergonic reactions in the catabolism of foodstuffs are coupled to ATP synthesis. The combined reaction remains slightly exergonic but much of the chemical energy of the exergonic, catabolic reaction is stored as ATP rather than being released into the cellular fluids as heat. For example, take the hypothetical exergonic catabolic reaction:

A ——→ B + large output of heat energy

In the cell:

A ——→ B + a smaller output of heat energy

ADP   ATP

Other reactions within the cell are endergonic (energy consuming) and one would expect that if these reactions were being carried out in a test tube, heat would have to be provided to make them

thermodynamically favourable and allow them to occur. Within the cell, however, such an endergonic reaction can be coupled to ATP hydrolysis to make the combined reaction exergonic and thus thermodynamically favourable at body temperature. For example, take the hypothetical endergonic reaction:

X + heat energy ——→ Y

In the cell:

X ——→ Y + small net output of heat energy

ATP   ADP

Substrate level phosphorylation

In catabolic pathways, some highly exergonic steps are directly linked to ATP formation (substrate level phosphorylation) as illustrated by the theoretical A → B reaction above. For example, in the glycolysis pathway one reaction involves the conversion of diphosphoglyceric acid to monophosphoglyceric acid, and this reaction is directly coupled to ATP synthesis:

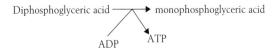

Diphosphoglyceric acid ——→ monophosphoglyceric acid

ADP   ATP

Oxidative phosphorylation

Much of the energy released in the catabolic pathways of metabolism occurs as a result of oxidation. Many oxidative steps involve the removal of hydrogen atoms from substrate molecules and their acceptance by hydrogen acceptor molecules such as **nicotinamide adenine dinucleotide (NAD)**. For example, take the hypothetical oxidative reaction:

XH_2 + NAD ——→ X + $NADH_2$

In this reaction, XH_2 has been oxidized to X and NAD has been reduced to $NADH_2$. As a real example, in the citric acid cycle (discussed below) malic acid is oxidized to oxaloacetic acid by the removal of hydrogen and this reaction is coupled to the reduction of NAD by hydrogen addition:

Malic acid ——→ oxaloacetic acid

NAD $NADH_2$

NAD is derived from the vitamin niacin. Niacin is essential because it is a precursor of NAD and the phosphorylated derivative NADP. Re-oxidation of these reduced hydrogen acceptors in the **mitochondria** of cells results in the production of large quantities of ATP (three molecules of ATP per molecule of $NADH_2$ re-oxidized):

$$NADH_2 + O_2 \longrightarrow NAD + H_2O$$
$$3\ ADP \qquad 3\ ATP$$

This mitochondrial process is called **oxidative phosphorylation**. In this process, there are a series of oxidation–reduction reactions, which culminate in the reduction of molecular oxygen to water. Reduced NAD ($NADH_2$) reduces the next compound on the **electron transport chain** and is itself re-oxidized, this reduced compound then reduces the next compound and so on to molecular oxygen. This sequence is called the electron transport chain because reduction can be defined either as the addition of electrons or the addition of hydrogen.

During this sequence of oxidation–reduction reactions, there is considerable release of chemical energy. Some of this energy is released as heat, which helps to keep the body warm but some of it is used to force hydrogen ions or protons (H^+) through the inner mitochondrial membrane. As the inner mitochondrial membrane is generally impermeable to protons this creates a considerable proton gradient across this membrane. There are pores in the inner mitochondrial membrane through which protons can pass back into the mitochondrion and this controlled flow of protons provides the energy that drives ATP synthesis in the mitochondrion. This is the chemiosmotic theory of oxidative phosphorylation, which explains how the oxidation of reduced cofactors (e.g. $NADH_2$) is linked to ATP synthesis.

If the inner mitochondrial membrane becomes more permeable to protons, it will compromise or 'uncouple' this link between oxidation and ATP synthesis. Uncouplers make the inner mitochondrial membrane more permeable to protons and so they cause oxidation to accelerate but the energy is released as heat rather than used to drive ATP synthesis. In a tissue known as **brown fat**, there is an uncoupling protein (UCP1), which when activated by sympathetic nerve stimulation allows protons to leak though the inner mitochondrial membrane, and this generates heat. This tissue is capable of producing large amounts of heat to warm the body and brown fat is prominent in small mammals, hibernating animals and human babies. There are other uncoupler proteins in other tissues (UCP2 and UCP3), and their significance is discussed in Chapter 7. Some drugs and poisons also uncouple oxidative phosphorylation, e.g. dinitrophenol. These substances increase body heat production and can cause rapid weight loss but those currently available are too toxic to be used therapeutically for this purpose.

Oxidative phosphorylation normally yields the vast bulk of the energy released in catabolic metabolism. Cells which do not have mitochondria (e.g. red blood cells) or which have insufficient oxygen supply (e.g. a muscle working beyond the capacity of the blood system to supply oxygen) have to rely upon the anaerobic metabolism of glucose to supply their energy needs. One molecule of glucose when metabolized anaerobically to lactic acid gives a net yield of only two molecules of ATP, whereas when it is metabolized aerobically to carbon dioxide and water it yields 38 ATP molecules.

METABOLISM OF GLUCOSE AND THE MONOSACCHARIDES

Dietary carbohydrates are digested to their component monosaccharides before being absorbed. Digestion of starch yields glucose and digestion of disaccharides yields glucose plus other monosaccharides, fructose from sucrose (cane or beet sugar) and galactose from lactose (milk sugar).

Glycolysis

Glycolysis is the initial pathway involved in the metabolism of carbohydrates and is summarized in Figure 5.1. The first three steps in this pathway involve activation of the glucose molecule by the addition of phosphate groups and a molecular rearrangement (**isomerization**) of glucose phosphate to fructose phosphate. There is consumption of two ATP molecules during these activating steps. The fructose diphosphate thus produced is much more reactive (unstable) than glucose and the six carbon (6C) molecule can be split by an enzyme into two, three carbon (3C) molecules. The other major dietary monosaccharides, fructose and galactose, also feed into the early stages of this glycolysis

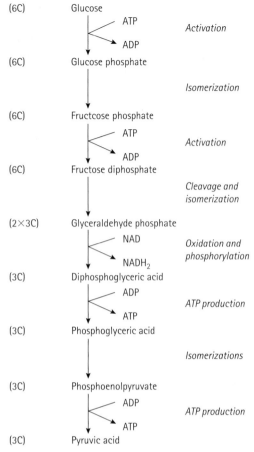

Figure 5.1 *The glycolytic sequence. C, carbon atom.*

pathway as does glucose phosphate derived from the breakdown of body glycogen stores.

During the steps that convert glyceraldehyde phosphate into pyruvic acid, there is production of two molecules of reduced NAD and four molecules of ATP from each starting molecule of glucose. Taking into account the two molecules of ATP used to generate fructose diphosphate, there is a net yield of two molecules of ATP at the substrate level for each molecule of glucose. Under aerobic conditions, the reduced NAD will be re-oxidized in the mitochondria using molecular oxygen and will yield a further six molecules of ATP in oxidative phosphorylation. Under anaerobic conditions, this reduced NAD must be re-oxidized by some other means, otherwise the very small quantities of oxidized NAD within the cell would be quickly exhausted and the whole process halted. In mammalian cells

this NAD is regenerated under anaerobic conditions by the reduction of pyruvic acid to lactic acid:

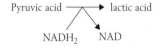

Lactic acid is the end product of anaerobic metabolism in mammalian cells and anaerobic energy production is only possible from carbohydrate substrate. Red blood cells do not have mitochondria and thus they metabolize glucose only as far as pyruvic acid and lactic acid. During heavy exercise, the oxygen supply to a muscle limits aerobic metabolism and so the muscles will generate some ATP anaerobically and produce lactic acid as a by-product. Accumulation of lactic acid is one factor responsible for the fatigue of exercising muscles. Note also that in thiamin deficiency (beriberi) there is effectively a partial block in the metabolism of carbohydrate beyond pyruvic acid because the conversion of pyruvic acid to acetyl coenzyme A requires a coenzyme, thiamin pyrophosphate, which is derived from thiamin. Lactic acid and pyruvic acid therefore also accumulate in people with beriberi because of this metabolic block.

The lactic acid produced by anaerobic metabolism is used for the re-synthesis of glucose in the liver (Cori cycle). This re-synthesis of glucose is effectively a reversal of glycolysis and thus it is possible to synthesize glucose from any intermediate of the glycolysis pathway, although the process does consume ATP.

Aerobic metabolism of pyruvic acid

Under aerobic conditions pyruvic acid will normally be converted to acetyl coenzyme A (effectively activated acetate):

$$\text{(3C) Pyruvic acid + coenzyme A} \xrightarrow[\;\;\;\;\text{NAD}\quad\text{NADH}_2\;\;\;\;]{\quad CO_2\quad} \text{(2C) acetyl coenzyme A}$$

Coenzyme A is a large moiety that is derived from the B vitamin, pantothenic acid – addition of the coenzyme A moiety increases the reactivity of acetate. It is released in the next reaction and recycled. This step cannot be reversed in mammalian cells and thus glucose cannot be synthesized from acetyl coenzyme A. The acetyl coenzyme A (2C) then enters a sequence known as the **Krebs cycle** or the **citric acid cycle** (Figure 5.2), and it combines with oxaloacetic acid (4C) to give citric acid (6C). The citric acid goes through a sequence of eight reactions, which ultimately result, once again, in the production of oxaloacetic acid, i.e. a cyclic process. During two of the reactions, a molecule of carbon dioxide is produced and in four of them a molecule of reduced coenzyme (e.g. $NADH_2$) is produced; in only one reaction is there direct substrate level ATP production. Each starting molecule of glucose yields two molecules of acetyl coenzyme A and thus each molecule of glucose metabolized under aerobic conditions results in two 'turns' of the citric acid cycle.

multiple units of acetyl coenzyme A, in a pathway known as the **β-oxidation pathway**. A 16-carbon fatty acid (e.g. palmitic acid) would thus yield eight, 2C units of acetyl coenzyme A (summarized in Figure 5.3). Note that as the conversion of acetyl coenzyme A back to pyruvic acid is not possible in mammalian cells, fatty acids cannot be used to generate glucose.

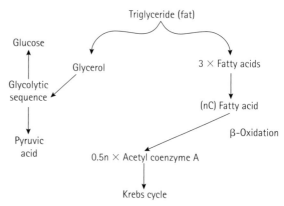

Figure 5.3 *Outline of fat metabolism. nC, number of carbon atoms.*

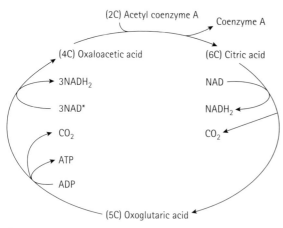

Figure 5.2 *Krebs cycle. C, carbon atom.*

After undergoing the reactions of glycolysis and the citric acid cycle, all of the six carbon atoms of the original glucose molecule will thus have been evolved as carbon dioxide. Re-oxidation of the reduced coenzyme (e.g. $NADH_2$) in the mitochondria results in the production of water. Thus overall, the glucose is metabolized to carbon dioxide and water.

METABOLISM OF FATTY ACIDS AND GLYCEROL

Dietary fat, or the fat stored in adipose tissue, is largely **triacylglycerol (triglyceride)** and it yields for metabolism, one molecule of glycerol and three fatty acid molecules. The 3-carbon (3C) glycerol is converted to glyceraldehyde phosphate and enters glycolysis – it can thus be used directly as a source of energy or it can be used to generate glucose (by reversal of glycolysis). Fatty acids are metabolized to

Brain cells do not have the enzymes necessary for β-oxidation, and therefore they cannot directly use fatty acids as an energy source. When carbohydrate is available (e.g. when carbohydrates are eaten regularly) brain cells use glucose as their substrate but they are not, as was previously thought, totally dependent on carbohydrate as a substrate. During fasting, they can use certain ketones or **ketone bodies** that are made from acetyl coenzyme A. This means that during starvation the brain can indirectly use fatty acids that have been converted to these ketones in the liver (discussed more fully under metabolic adaptation to starvation in Chapter 6).

Fatty acids are synthesized by a process that is essentially a reversal of β-oxidation, e.g. to synthesize 16C palmitic acid, 8 units of 2C acetate (as acetyl coenzyme A) are progressively assembled. Thus fatty acids can be synthesized from carbohydrates via acetyl coenzyme A. Breakdown of fatty acids to acetyl coenzyme A is an oxidative process (hence β-oxidation) thus the synthesis of fatty acids from acetyl coenzyme A is a reductive process. The reduced form of the phosphorylated derivative of

NAD, $NADPH_2$, is used as the source of reducing power in this pathway – $NADPH_2$ is generated in the **pentose phosphate pathway** (see later).

METABOLISM OF AMINO ACIDS

Surplus amino acids from protein can be used as an energy source. The nitrogen-containing amino group is removed to leave a moiety, the keto acid, which can be converted to pyruvic acid, acetyl coenzyme A or one of the intermediates of the citric acid cycle. The amino group can be converted to the waste product urea or it can be transferred to another keto acid and thus produce another amino acid; a process called **transamination**.

It is possible to make glucose from protein. If the amino acid (e.g. alanine) yields pyruvic acid, glucose synthesis merely involves the effective reversal of glycolysis. If the amino acid (e.g. glutamic acid) yields a citric acid cycle intermediate, this intermediate will be converted to oxaloacetic acid, which can then be converted to the phosphoenolpyruvate of glycolysis:

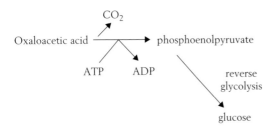

Note that acetyl coenzyme A (and thus fatty acids) cannot be used to synthesize glucose via this route because the two atoms of the acetate that enter the citric acid cycle have been lost as carbon dioxide by the time oxaloacetic acid has been regenerated. Utilization of existing citric acid cycle intermediates to synthesize glucose is theoretically possible but they would be so rapidly depleted that their contribution to glucose supply would be insignificant. Metabolic routes for the metabolism of the different foodstuffs are summarized in Figure 5.4.

During starvation or carbohydrate deprivation, the only routes available for the maintenance of carbohydrate supplies are by manufacture from amino acids or the glycerol component of fat. This process of generation of glucose from amino acids (**gluconeogenesis**) occurs in the liver but it is inefficient and energy expensive, and will of course lead to depletion of the protein in muscle and vital organs.

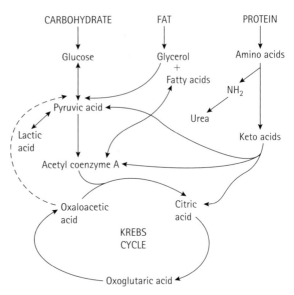

Figure 5.4 *Summary of metabolic routes for foodstuffs.*

Note, however, that the need for gluconeogenesis is limited during starvation or carbohydrate deprivation by the use of ketone bodies as an alternative to carbohydrate substrate.

THE PENTOSE PHOSPHATE PATHWAY

This pathway generates reducing power in the form of $NADPH_2$ (necessary, for example, in fatty acids biosynthesis) and also generates the pentose sugar, ribose phosphate, essential for nucleotide (e.g. ATP) biosynthesis and nucleic acid (RNA and DNA) synthesis. The first part of this pathway involves the conversion of glucose phosphate to ribose phosphate.

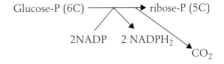

If the demand for $NADPH_2$ and ribose phosphate is balanced, these two will represent end products of the pathway. If, however, the demand for $NADPH_2$, say for active lipid synthesis, exceeds the demand for ribose phosphate, the excess ribose is converted, by a complex series of reactions, to 3-carbon glyceraldehyde phosphate and 6-carbon fructose phosphate. The overall reaction is:

$$3 \times \text{Ribose-P} (3 \times 5\text{C}) \longrightarrow \text{glyceraldehyde-P} (3\text{C}) + 2 \times \text{fructose-P} (2 \times 6\text{C})$$

The enzymes used in this series of reactions are called transketolase and transaldolase – transketolase requires thiamin pyrophosphate, derived from vitamin B_1, thiamin, as a coenzyme. The glyceraldehyde phosphate and fructose phosphate produced by these reactions can both enter glycolysis, either to be metabolized to pyruvic acid or used to regenerate glucose phosphate. If the demand for ribose phosphate exceeds that for $NADPH_2$, the reverse of the transketolase/transaldolase reaction can generate ribose phosphate from glyceraldehyde phosphate and fructose phosphate.

Wernicke–Korsakoff syndrome is a neuropsychiatric disorder caused by lack of dietary thiamin (see Chapter 13). In industrialized countries, it is usually associated with thiamin deficiency brought on by alcoholism. The symptoms of this syndrome are probably due to inadequate $NADPH_2$ synthesis leading to impaired synthesis of **myelin**, the fatty sheath that surrounds many neurones.

AN OVERVIEW OF MACRONUTRIENT HANDLING IN THE GUT

This chapter has been concerned with the final metabolic fate of the monomeric components of fats, carbohydrates and proteins, i.e. how monosaccharides, amino acids and fatty acids are metabolized in the cell. However, most of the energy in food is present as complex macromolecules which must first be broken down into these monomers before they can be absorbed and used within cells. The process of digestion of these macromolecules is briefly discussed in Chapters 9–11 (dealing with carbohydrates, fats and proteins), but digestion and absorption of all three is overviewed briefly here.

Carbohydrates

Most of the available carbohydrate in food is consumed as either starches or the disaccharides sucrose (beet or cane sugar, glucose–fructose) and lactose (milk sugar, glucose–galactose) with usually just small amounts of free glucose and fructose (Chapter 9, Figure 9.1, p. 226, gives a brief classification of the carbohydrates and Figure 9.2, p. 236, shows the structure of some carbohydrates and illustrates the nature of α 1–4 and α 1–6 links between glucose residues in starch). In the mouth, saliva contains the enzyme α-amylase which breaks

down α 1–4 links between glucose residues in starch. Under most circumstances the contribution of salivary α-amylase to overall starch digestion will be relatively small because food usually only spends a short time in the mouth and the enzyme is denatured by the acid environment of the stomach. However, food entering the stomach will buffer the stomach acid and raise stomach pH for a while and the enzyme within a bolus of food may be protected from the effects of stomach acid.

Pancreatic juice secreted into the duodenum also contains an α-amylase. The end products of starch digestion by α-amylase are mainly maltose (glucose–glucose), maltotriose (three glucose residues joined by α 1–4 links), and so-called α-limit dextrin, which is a small oligosaccharide produced from amylopectin with an α 1–6 link that cannot be broken down by α-amylase.

On the mucosal surface of the small intestine are a series of enzymes which complete the digestion of carbohydrates into their component monosaccharides.

- Maltase breaks α 1–4 links between maltose, maltotriose or slightly larger oligosaccharides with glucose residues joined solely by α 1–4 links to yield glucose.
- Lactase digests any lactose present to glucose and galactose.
- Sucrase breaks sucrose into glucose and fructose.
- Isomaltase breaks the α 1–6 links in the α-limit dextrin enabling it to be broken down into glucose. (Sucrase and isomaltase can also break α 1–4 links between glucose residues.)

Glucose and galactose are absorbed actively across the intestinal brush border. They bind to a transporter protein called SGLT1 which also binds to sodium ions on the mucosal surface of the gut cell. Inside the cell the concentration of sodium is kept low by an active sodium–potassium pump and this low sodium concentration causes release of both sodium and glucose (or galactose) from the transporter protein. The high sodium gradient requires energy to maintain it and this accelerates glucose/galactose transport and makes it 'active' transport. High sodium concentration increases glucose or galactose binding to SGLT1 but low sodium concentration inhibits glucose or galactose binding. Fructose binds to a GLUT-5 transporter protein at the brush border but this does not bind sodium and so fructose absorption is said to be sodium independent and not active; it is absorbed more slowly than the other monosaccharides. Fructose concentration within the mucosal cell is kept very low and so fructose absorption is essentially complete even though it is not active and fructose can only pass down a concentration gradient, i.e. it is absorbed by facilitated diffusion.

Protein

Amino acids are ingested as proteins which contain 20 different amino acids linked together in sometimes very long chains joined together by peptide bonds. Figure 10.1 (p. 248) illustrates the way in which amino acids are joined to make proteins and shows that at one end of every protein there is a free amino group (the N-terminal) and at the other end a free carboxyl group (the C-terminal). The different types of amino acids are described in the text.

In the acid environment of the stomach, the enzyme pepsin starts to cleave the peptide bonds between amino acids in proteins. It is a type of proteolytic enzyme called an endopeptidase because it breaks peptide bonds within the protein molecule. Exopeptidases break off the terminal amino acids from a peptide. Complete digestion of protein still occurs in conditions where there is an absence of pepsin and so it is not necessary for protein digestion. In the duodenum proteolytic enzymes from the pancreas convert 70 per cent of dietary protein into oligopeptides of up to six amino acids and the remaining 30 per cent has been broken down to free amino acids. These pancreatic proteases are:

- *trypsin* – breaks the links within proteins at lysine or arginine residues
- *chymotrypsin* – breaks links at aromatic or neutral amino acids
- *elastase* – breaks bonds at aliphatic amino acids
- *carboxypeptidases* – break off certain C-terminal amino acids from proteins and peptides.

On the surface of the brush border there are a series of 20 further peptidases which complete the breakdown of dietary protein into free amino acids plus dipeptides and tripeptides. There are several amino acid transporter proteins and some that transport the small peptides – these have different amino acid specificities and some are sodium dependent.

Any di- and tripeptides absorbed are digested by peptidases within the cytoplasm of the mucosal cells.

Fat

The digestion and absorption of fat has been discussed fairly fully in Chapter 11 and so will only be outlined here. Most dietary fat is in the form of triacylglycerol made up of a glycerol 'backbone' to which are attached three fatty acid residues (see Figure 11.1, p. 264). Fat is insoluble in water and so to allow water-soluble digestive enzymes to act on it, it must first be emulsified (dispersed as small particles within the fluid gut contents). Churning of fats in the stomach with phospholipids and the effect of bile within the duodenum emulsify the dietary fat so that the pancreatic enzyme lipase can act on it to convert dietary triacylglycerol into monoacylglycerol plus two free fatty acids. Some shorter-chain fatty acids pass directly into the mucosal cell but most of the products of fat digestion form microscopically small particles with bile salts and phospholipids called micelles. An emulsion formed when fats are emulsified is cloudy because the particles are large enough to scatter light but micelles are so small that they appear clear as if a true solution has been formed.

Fat digestion products (and fat-soluble vitamins) within the micelles are in equilibrium with tiny amounts of these products that are in true solution within the intestinal contents. These small amounts in true solution diffuse across into the mucosal cells and are immediately replaced by amounts from within the micelles. Once inside the mucosal cell the monoacylglycerol and fatty acids are re-esterified into triacylglycerol and thus the concentration gradient across the mucosal cell membrane is maintained and more fat digestion products can diffuse across; in this way fat absorption from the intestine is normally almost 100 per cent. The triacylglycerol produced within the mucosal cells is coated with protein to form particles called chylomicrons which then enter into the lymphatic vessels that supply the intestine and these drain into the venous system. In the tissues, lipase in the capillaries breaks down triacylglycerol within chylomicrons to fatty acids and monoacylglycerol and fatty acids which diffuse into the tissues and may once again be re-esterified into triacylglycerol for storage or transport.

PART TWO

ENERGY, ENERGY BALANCE AND OBESITY

6

Introduction to energy aspects of nutrition

SOURCES OF ENERGY

Although the range of nutrients required by living organisms varies enormously, all organisms require an external supply of energy. Plants 'trap' energy from sunlight and use it to make sugars in the process of photosynthesis. Photosynthesis is the ultimate source of all the energy in living systems and fossil fuels. In human diets, the food macronutrients, fat, carbohydrate and protein (plus alcohol) are the sources of energy.

UNITS OF ENERGY

The Standard International (SI) unit of energy is the **joule,** which is defined as the energy expended when a mass of 1 kg is moved through a distance of 1 m by a force of 1 N (newton). For nutritionists the **kilojoule (kJ,** a thousand joules) and the **megajoule (MJ,** a million joules) are more practical units. Traditionally, nutritionists have used a unit of heat, the **kilocalorie (kcal),** as their unit of energy. Although a kilocalorie is strictly 1000 calories, most people, when dealing with nutrition, tend to use the terms calorie and kilocalorie as if synonymous. A kcal is defined as the heat required to raise the temperature of a 1 L of water by 1 °C. In practice, the kilocalorie is still widely used both by nutritionists and by non-scientists. The kilocalorie is a

convenient unit because people with a limited knowledge of physics can understand its definition and because nutritionists may use heat output as their method of measuring both the energy yields of foods and the energy expenditure of animals and people.

To inter-convert kilocalories and kilojoules:

$$1 \, kcal = 4.2 \, kJ$$

Key points

- A joule is the energy expended when a mass of 1 kg is moved through a distance of 1 m by a force of 1N.
- A kilojoule (kJ) = 1000 J.
- A megajoule (MJ) = 1 000 000 joules (1000 kJ).
- A kilocalorie (kcal) is 1000 calories, but in nutrition the term calorie usually means kilocalorie.
- 1 kcal = 4.2 kJ.

HOW ARE ENERGY REQUIREMENTS ESTIMATED?

Table 6.1 shows some selected UK **estimated average requirements (EARs)** for energy. Remember

Table 6.1 Selected current UK estimated average requirements (EARs) for energy. Corresponding American recommended dietary allowances (RDAs) from the 1989 edition of dietary reference values are given for comparative purposes

Age (years)	UK EAR		American RDA*	
	kcal/day	MJ/day	kcal/day	MJ/day
1–3 boys	1230	5.15	1300	5.44
1–3 girls	1165	4.86	1300	5.44
7–10 boys	1970	8.24	2000	8.37
7–10 girls	1740	7.28	2000	8.37
15–18 men	2755	11.51	3000	12.56
15–18 women	2110	8.83	2200	9.21
19–50 men	2550	10.60	2900	12.14
19–50 women	1940	8.10	2200	9.21
75+ men	2100	8.77	2300	9.63
75+ women	1810	7.61	1900	7.96

*Note that since 2002 (NAS, 2004) the American standards for energy have allowed an estimated energy requirement for an individual adult to be determined that takes account of their exact age, height category, weight category and activity level. This is discussed more fully in the text.
Data sources: COMA (1991) and NRC (1989a).

that these UK dietary standards for energy represent the best estimate of average requirement whereas the most commonly used reference values for most nutrients, the **reference nutrient intake (RNI)** or **recommended dietary allowance (RDA)**, are the estimated needs of those with the highest requirement (see Chapter 3 for discussion and rationale).

The **basal metabolic rate (BMR)** is the minimum rate of energy expenditure in a conscious person or animal. It is determined by measuring the metabolic rate (see Chapter 3) of a subject who has been resting for some time in a warm room and after an overnight fast. It represents the energy required to keep the body's internal organs and systems functioning, e.g. for breathing, circulation of blood and brain function. In a sedentary person, BMR accounts for more than two-thirds of total energy expenditure and only in those who are extremely active will it make up less than half of total energy expenditure. If BMR is measured in large samples of individuals then, within specified age and sex bands, there is a linear relationship between BMR and body weight. This means that one can derive regression equations that allow the average BMR of a group of people

within an age band to be predicted from the average weight of the group. For example, in women aged 18–29 years the following regression equation allows prediction of average BMR from average weight:

$$BMR \text{ (kcal/day)} = 14.8 \times weight \text{ (kg)} + 487$$

So, if the average weight of women in this age band is 60 kg, then:

$$Average\ BMR = (14.8 \times 60) + 487$$
$$= 1375\ kcal/day$$

To estimate the average daily energy requirement of this group, one must multiply the BMR by a factor that reflects the level of physical activity of the group. This is called the **physical activity level (PAL)**. If this population is assumed to be sedentary in both their occupation and in their leisure time, a PAL value of 1.4 would be appropriate. So the average energy expenditure of the group (and thus their average requirement) would be estimated at:

$$BMR \times PAL = 1375 \times 1.4 = 1925\ kcal/day$$

This is essentially how the UK panel setting the dietary standards (Committee on the Medical Aspects of Food (COMA), 1991) arrived at the figure of 1940 kcal/day (8.1 MJ/day) for women aged 19–50 years in Table 6.1 (the slight difference in numbers occurs because of interpolation over the larger age band).

In principle, this is the method COMA (1991) used to set the EARs for energy for all adults and older children. The panel used regression equations such as the one above to predict BMR from the average weight of Britons in each age group. For most groups the BMR was multiplied by a PAL of 1.4 to reflect the generally sedentary nature of the British population. In adults aged over 60 years the panel used a PAL of 1.5. This higher PAL for elderly people seems surprising given the clear evidence that activity decreases in the elderly (the reasons for this anomaly are outlined in the next section). For younger children, estimates of energy requirements are largely based on survey measurements of average energy intakes.

Also shown simply for comparison in Table 6.1 are the past American RDAs for energy set in 1989 – the current American standards for energy set dietary reference intakes for individuals and these are discussed briefly later in this section. The American panel that set the 1989 energy RDA (National Research Council (NRC) 1989a) used similar regression equations to predict the average BMR (or the resting energy

Table 6.2 A guide to predicting the physical activity level (PAL) multiple of an individual or group*

Non-occupational activity	Occupational activity					
	Light		Moderate		Moderate/heavy	
	M	F	M	F	M	F
Non-active	1.4	1.4	1.6	1.5	1.7	1.5
Moderately active	1.5	1.5	1.7	1.6	1.8	1.6
Very active	1.6	1.6	1.8	1.7	1.9	1.7

*After COMA (1991).
M, male; F, female.
It takes about half an hour's brisk walking to raise the PAL by 0.1 on that day.

expenditure (REE)) of Americans in the various age bands and multiplied by an activity (PAL) factor. The large differences between the British and American values in Table 6.1 are mainly due to differences in the activity factor used by the two panels. Americans also tend to be a little heavier than Britons. The American panel used PAL multiples of between 1.55 and 1.7 in older children and adults up to 50 years compared with the UK panel's 1.4. Like the British panel, NRC used a PAL multiple of 1.5 for older people.

It must be borne in mind when using figures such as those in Table 6.1 that these are estimates of average requirements. They are not intended to be used as an accurate statement of the requirements of individuals. Many factors affect the energy expenditure and thus the energy requirements of an individual, e.g.:

- size – in general, the bigger the body the greater the energy expenditure
- body composition – lean tissue is metabolically more active and uses more energy than adipose tissue
- activity level (as discussed above)
- environmental conditions such as the ambient temperature
- physiological factors such as hormone levels
- rate of growth in children
- individual genetic variability.

It is possible to roughly estimate the energy requirements of an individual. One could use the regression equation appropriate for the person's age to estimate their BMR from their weight (a list of regression equations can be found in COMA, 1991). Alternatively, it can be assumed that in adults under 50 years, the BMR is 0.9 kcal/h for a woman

(1.0 kcal/h for a man). Such approximations assume average proportions of fat and lean in the body and so they become increasingly unreliable as one moves towards extremes of fatness or leanness. Using this rule of thumb, the estimated BMR of a 65 kg man would be:

$$65 \times 1.0 \times 24 = 1560 \, \text{kcal/day}$$

This estimated BMR must then be multiplied by an appropriate PAL. Table 6.2 was offered by COMA (1991) as a guide to deciding on the appropriate PAL multiple. It uses three categories each for both occupational and non-occupational activity levels. Only those who are extremely active (e.g. athletes in training) or extremely inactive (e.g. elderly housebound people) will fall outside this range.

The current American dietary reference intakes for energy do try to allow one to derive a more specific estimated energy requirement (EER) which reflects the height, weight, exact age and activity category of the individual. There is a standard table which gives the EER for a 30-year-old man and woman and there are 24 numerical values listed for each sex. There are three heights and two body weights for each height (corresponding to a BMI of either $18.5 \, \text{kg/m}^2$ or $25 \, \text{kg/m}^2$). For each of the six height and weight categories given for each sex there are four different activity levels to choose from (sedentary, low active, active and very active). Of course these 48 numerical values are only for men and women aged exactly 30 years and for each year less than 30 one must add on 10 kcal/day for men and 7 kcal/day for women; for each year above 30 years one must subtract these same amounts. This table can be accessed online (http://iom.edu/Object.File/Master/21/372/0.pdf).

Key points

- The average basal metabolic rate (BMR) of a group can be estimated from their average body weight using regression equations derived from measurement of BMR and body weight in a large sample of people.
- This BMR can be used to estimated average energy requirements by multiplying it by a factor that reflects the activity level of the group – the physical activity level (PAL).
- This PAL can vary from under 1.3 in elderly house-bound people to well over 2 in athletes during training.
- In the UK, the dietary standard for energy is the estimated average requirement (EAR) and up until 2002 in the USA it was the recommended dietary allowance (RDA).
- Both the EAR and the RDA are estimates of average requirements and any individual's requirements will depend on many factors such as their size, body composition, activity level, physiological state and environmental conditions.
- Current US energy standards allow an estimated energy requirement for an individual to be calculated which takes into account their exact age, height category, weight category and activity level category.

VARIATION IN AVERAGE ENERGY REQUIREMENTS: GENERAL TRENDS

Table 6.1 suggests quite large differences between the estimated average energy requirements of Britons and Americans, which largely reflect the different assumptions about activity levels and average body weights made by the panels who set these values. Other trends that are apparent on close inspection of this table are summarized below.

- The energy requirements of males are generally higher than those of females. This is largely because the average male is bigger than the average female. In older children and adults, females also have a higher proportion of adipose tissue, which is metabolically less active than lean tissue.
- The relative energy requirement (per unit body weight) of growing children is higher than that of adults – a 2-year-old child may be only around a fifth of the weight of an adult but requires more

than half of the adult energy intake. In the case of older teenagers, even the absolute energy requirement is higher than in adults. This relatively high energy requirement of growing children partly reflects the energy requirements for growth but, particularly in small children, it is also partly a manifestation of the general inverse relationship between the relative metabolic rate and body size (see Chapter 3). Younger children also tend to be more active than adults.

- The values given in Table 6.1 imply that there is a considerable reduction in energy needs in the elderly. This suggests that older people will need less energy and eat less food than younger adults. As requirements for most other nutrients are not thought to decline with age, then this increases the vulnerability of elderly people to nutrient inadequacies (see Chapter 15 for further discussion). The amount of metabolically active lean tissue declines in old age and the proportion of body fat increases. There is also no doubt that activity levels show an accelerating decline in middle age and old age. This decline in activity is reflected in the use of a reduced PAL multiple for elderly people in the American values. However, the British panel took the surprising decision to use a PAL multiple of 1.5 for older adults compared with only 1.4 in younger adults. This decision was made because in younger people, the panel was keen to discourage over-consumption of energy because of the prevalence of obesity. In elderly people, their priorities were to maintain sufficient energy intake to allow adequate intake of other nutrients and to prevent elderly people becoming underweight. The values in Table 6.1 almost certainly understate the real decline in energy intake that occurs in very elderly people. The real PAL of elderly housebound people may be 1.3 or even less.

Key points

- Children have higher relative metabolic rates than adults and thus require more energy per kilogram of body weight.
- Men have higher average energy requirements than women because they are bigger and have a higher lean to fat ratio in their bodies.

● Basal metabolic rate declines in the elderly due to reduced lean body mass and this compounds with declining activity levels to substantially reduce the average energy requirements in very elderly people.

ENERGY CONTENT OF FOODS

The oxidation of foodstuffs in metabolism is often likened to the oxidative processes of combustion or burning. This would suggest that the heat energy released during the burning of a food should be an indicator of its metabolic energy yield. In a **bomb calorimeter**, a small sample of food is placed in a sealed chamber, which is pressurized with oxygen to ensure complete oxidation (burning). The food is then ignited electrically and the heat energy released during combustion of the food sample is measured. In practice, the heat energy released during combustion will significantly overestimate the energy that is metabolically available from most foods. The predictive value of the energy of combustion is worsened if the food is high in indigestible material or high in protein.

Some components of a food may burn and release heat energy but not be digested and absorbed, so this fraction of the energy of combustion will be lost in the faeces, e.g. some components of **dietary fibre**, and indigestible proteins such as those in hair. In the bomb calorimeter there is complete oxidation of protein to water, carbon dioxide and oxides of nitrogen whereas in metabolic oxidation most of the nitrogen is excreted in the urine as urea. Urea will burn and release energy and so this means that some energy released from protein when it is burnt is lost in the urine when it is metabolized. The metabolic energy yield from protein is only about 70 per cent of the heat energy released during combustion; the other 30 per cent is lost in the urine. To determine the **metabolizable energy** using a bomb calorimeter, the heat energy released during combustion has to be corrected for this energy lost in the faeces and urine.

The usual way of determining the energy value of foods is to measure the available carbohydrate, fat, protein and alcohol content of the food and then to use standard conversion values for the metabolizable energy of each of these nutrients (Box 6.1).

In the main, these approximations hold irrespective of the type of fat, carbohydrate or protein; the carbohydrate figure is applied to both starches and sugars. Small variations in these conversion factors are of little significance given the many other sources of error in estimating dietary energy intake. **Nonstarch polysaccharide (NSP)** or dietary fibre has traditionally been assumed to contribute nothing to metabolizable energy but recent studies suggest that it may yield up to 8 kJ (2 kcal) per gram (via its fermentation by intestinal bacteria to volatile fatty acids and the subsequent absorption and metabolism of those acids).

Key points

● Food yields less energy when metabolized than when burnt because of losses in faeces (undigested material) and in urine (mainly urea).
● The energy yields of the macronutrients are listed in Box 6.1.
● The metabolizable energy of foods is determined by measuring the content of fat, carbohydrate and protein and using the energy equivalents of these nutrients.

SOURCES OF DIETARY ENERGY BY NUTRIENT

Dietary recommendations and survey reports often quote carbohydrate, fat, protein and even alcohol intakes as a percentage of total energy. This method of presentation allows meaningful comparison of the diet composition of persons with widely differing energy intakes. It can be seen as a way of comparing the 'concentration' of fat, carbohydrate or protein in different foods and diets. Quoting absolute values for intakes of these major nutrients (e.g. g/day) may be of limited usefulness and may even on occasion be misleading. For example, someone eating 4.2MJ (1000 kcal) per day and 30 g of fat will get the same proportion of their dietary energy from fat (27 per cent) as someone consuming 8.4 MJ (2000 kcal) and 60 g of fat.

As another example of the usefulness of this tool, absolute *per capita* intakes of fat (g/day) in the UK dropped sharply between 1975 and 1995. However, this reduction was almost entirely due to a reduction in total food intake and during this period the proportion of energy from fat remained almost constant. To calculate macronutrient intakes as a percentage of total energy, the energy equivalents of fat, carbohydrate and protein given in the previous section are used in the following formula:

$$\frac{\text{Nutrient consumed(g)} \times \text{energy equivalent (as in Box 6.1)}}{\text{Total energy intake}} \times 100$$

For example, to calculate the proportion of energy from fat in an 11 000 kJ diet containing 100 g of fat:

$$\frac{100 \times 37}{11000} \times 100 = \frac{3700 \times 100}{11000}$$
$$= 33.6\% \text{ of energy as fat}$$

Table 6.3 shows estimates of the contribution of the various energy-yielding nutrients to the total energy supplies of adults in the UK. This was measured directly using weighed inventories of the intakes of nationally representative samples of British adults (Gregory *et al.*, 1990; Hoare *et al.*, 2004). The energy contribution of the major macronutrients is often expressed as a percentage of food energy, i.e. excluding alcohol, and selected values from Table 6.3 are shown in this way in Table 6.4. One effect of excluding alcohol is to move the values for men and women closer together because men have higher average alcohol intakes than women.

It is clear from Tables 6.3 and 6.4 that fat and carbohydrate together provide the bulk of the food energy in Britain, almost 85 per cent of the total. This will also be true of most European and American diets and indeed it will be true for all but the most unusual or extreme diets, e.g. 'high-protein' reducing diets where almost the only foods eaten are lean meat, white fish, eggs and skimmed milk. As the bulk of any diet's energy usually comes from fat and carbohydrate, this means that as the proportion of

Table 6.3 Changes in the sources of energy in the diets of British adults expressed as percentages of total energy

Nutrient	Men		Women	
	1986/7	2000/1	1986/7	2001/1
Fat (%)	37.6	33.5	39.4	33.5
Protein (%)	14.1	15.4	15.2	15.9
Carbohydrate (%)	41.6	44.7	43.1	46.7
Sugars (%)	17.6		19.2	
Non milk extrinsic sugars (%)	16.2*	12.8	16.2*	14.6
Starches (%)	24.0		23.9	
Starches + intrinsic and milk sugars (%)	25.4	31.9	26.9	32.1
Alcohol (%)	6.9	6.5	2.3	3.9
Total (kcal/day)	2450	2321	1680	1640
(MJ/day)	10.26	9.72	7.03	6.87

* No differentiation between men and women made in the original report.
Data sources: Gregory et al. (1990) and Hoare et al. (2004).

Table 6.4 Some of the figures in Table 6.3 expressed as a percentage of food energy, i.e. excluding alcohol

Nutrient	Men		Women	
	1986/7	2000/1	1986/7	2000/1
Fat (%)	40.4	35.8	40.3	34.9
Protein (%)	15.2	16.5	15.6	16.6
Carbohydrate (%)	44.7	47.7	44.2	48.5

Data sources: Gregory et al. (1990) and Hoare et al. (2004).

one goes up so the proportion of the other tends to go down. An inverse relationship between the proportion of dietary energy derived from fat and carbohydrate is almost inevitable and could be termed a **carbohydrate–fat seesaw**. This means that that in most Western diets, there also tends to be an inverse relationship between dietary fat content and the major classes of carbohydrate, i.e. sugars, starches and NSP/dietary fibre. The consequences of the **sugar–fat seesaw** have been discussed in Chapter 4. In Chapter 9, we will also see that the inverse relationship between dietary fat and fibre makes it difficult to determine whether any proposed benefits of high-fibre (NSP) diets are because of fibre *per se* or because they also tend to be low in fat.

Tables 6.3 and 6.4 suggest that there have been significant changes in the British diet in the 14 years between the two surveys. Fat has dropped as a percentage of food and total energy by around 5 per cent and is now close to the dietary reference value (DRV) of 35 per cent of food energy. As would be expected, because of the carbohydrate–fat seesaw there has been an increase in the proportion of energy derived from carbohydrates although it is still a little way below the DRV of 47 per cent of total energy (50 per cent of food energy). There has also been an increase in the proportion of energy derived from protein of around 1 per cent partly driven by the big increase in the use of low-fat milk and milk products. The proportion of energy derived from non-milk extrinsic sugars (largely added sugars) has also fallen quite sharply especially when one considers the increase in overall carbohydrates. Despite the fall these values are still some way above the DRV of 10 per cent of total energy, especially in women.

Total recorded energy intakes dropped between the two surveys and this is consistent with the long-term decline in average energy intake since the late 1950s, indicated by household budget surveys such as the National Food Survey and its replacement Family Food and by food balance sheets (see Chapter 3). In general the changes in the macronutrient composition of the diet over the period 1986–2001 have moved them closer to the DRV for macronutrients. Perhaps the one less positive figure in Table 6.3 is the near doubling of the percentage of total energy derived from alcohol in women. While the new figure of 3.9 per cent of energy is not in itself of concern, it may indicate increased numbers of women exceeding the safe levels for alcohol intake (see Chapter 4). Table 6.5 shows the percentage of energy derived from the major macronutrients in the UK as estimated using the Household Expenditure Survey (Department for Environment, Food and Rural Affairs (DEFRA), 2006).

> ## Key points
>
> - The macronutrient content of diets and foods is often expressed as the percentage of the total energy derived from that nutrient, e.g. the percentage of energy as fat.
> - This is a measure of the 'concentration' of these nutrients in a diet.
> - In most diets, fat and carbohydrate together provide most of the food energy (approximately 85 per cent in the UK).
> - As the proportion of energy derived from fat in a diet goes up, so the proportion from carbohydrate tends to go down and vice versa – the so-called carbohydrate–fat seesaw.
> - In most Western diets there also tends to be a sugar–fat seesaw.
> - Using a weighed inventory method, in 1987 40 per cent of the food energy of the British diet was found to come from fat, 45 per cent from carbohydrate and 15 per cent from protein; by 2001 these figures were 35.5 per cent, 48 per cent and 16.5 per cent respectively.
> - The figures recorded for macronutrient breakdown of the diet in 2001 were much closer to the dietary reference value (DRV) than those of 1987, although total carbohydrate figures were still a little way below the DRV and the figures for non-milk extrinsic sugars were still some way above the DRV, especially in women.
> - There has been a marked increase in the proportion of total energy derived from alcohol in women.

Table 6.5 Percentage of energy obtained from fat, carbohydrate and protein in all food and drink purchases in the UK

	% Energy
Fat	36.4
Protein	13.7
Carbohydrate	46.5
Sugars	22.3
Non milk extrinsic sugars	14.9
Starches	24.1
Alcohol	3.4
Total energy per capita (kcal)	2239
(MJ)	9.4

Data source: Family Food 2004–5 (DEFRA, 2006).

ENERGY DENSITY

The **energy density** of a food or diet is the metabolizable energy yield per unit weight of food (e.g. kcal or kJ/100 g food). If a food is of high energy density then a little of it provides a lot of energy whereas one can eat a lot of a food of low energy density and yet obtain little energy. This is illustrated in Table 6.6 where the weights of various foods required to provide 4.2 MJ (1000 kcal) is shown. The range of energy densities in Table 6.6 is very large; just over a tenth of a kilo of vegetable oil will provide 4.2 MJ but one needs over 9 kg of boiled swede or 7 kg of lettuce. Many of the general trends illustrated by Table 6.6 are summarized here.

- As fat yields more than twice as much energy as either carbohydrate or protein, fat content must be a major factor increasing the energy density of foods or diets. High-fat foods are inevitably of high energy density (e.g. nuts, seeds and oils) whereas low-fat foods are generally of low or moderate energy density.

- Most fruits and vegetables are almost fat free and are high in water and fibre. They thus have very low energy densities (e.g. grapes and lettuce). Drying fruits (e.g. raisins) or adding sugar to them

Table 6.6 The weights of selected foods that would need to be eaten to obtain 4.2 MJ (1000 kcal)

Food	Weight (g)	Food	Weight (g)
Fruits		Doughnuts (ring)	252
Orange	5950	Pizza (cheese and tomato)	400
Banana	2280	Dairy foods	
Grapes	1667	Whole milk	1515
Raisins	368	Skimmed milk	3030
Strawberries	3704	Double cream	223
Strawberries (canned in syrup)	1538	Cheddar cheese	243
Fruit pie (individual purchased)	271	Butter	136
Vegetables		Meat, fish and products	
Lettuce	7143	Boiled egg	680
Tomato	5882	Fried egg	560
Green beans	4000	Lean boiled ham	758
Broccoli	4167	Roast chicken meat	606
Boiled swede	9091	Southern fried chicken	350
Red kidney beans (boiled)	971	Chicken nuggets	338
Soya beans (boiled)	709	Grilled rump steak (with fat)	459
Tofu (fried)	383	(trimmed)	595
Chick peas (boiled)	836	Cheeseburger	380
		Salami	204
Hummus	535	Sausage rolls	210
Starchy staples and products		Grilled pork sausage	314
Boiled potatoes	1389	Poached cod	1064
French fries	357	Cod fried in batter	503
Potato crisps (chips)	183	Steamed salmon	508
Boiled yam	752	Boiled prawns	935
Boiled sweet potato	1190	Fish fingers (fried)	429
Boiled rice	725	Fried scampi (breaded)	316
Spaghetti (boiled)	962	Nuts, seeds and oils	
Wheat bread	464	Peanuts (raw)	177
Corn grits (made with water)	1666	Walnuts	145
Porridge		Sunflower seeds	167
Made with water	2041	Margarine	136
Made with whole milk	862	Low-fat spread	256
Tortilla/chapatti (no added fat)	478	Vegetable oils	112
Cornflakes	278	Miscellaneous	
Weetabix	279	Sugar	254
Chocolate biscuits (cookies)	191	Chocolate	189
Fruit cake	282	Quiche	318

Adapted from Webb (1998).

(e.g. strawberries canned in syrup) increases their energy density. Cooking or preparing vegetables with fat or oil greatly increases their energy yield (e.g. French fried potatoes, hummus and fried tofu).

- When eaten boiled, starchy cereals and roots are low in fat and absorb substantial amounts of water. This means that despite their importance as major sources of energy in many diets, their energy density is rather modest (e.g. boiled potatoes, boiled rice and corn grits).
- Very lean meat and white fish are low in fat and so their energy density is moderate or low (e.g. roast chicken meat), especially if boiled (e.g. lean boiled ham, poached cod). The meat in our ancestors' diets (and even in a few of today's population) would have come from wild animal carcasses and this is usually low in fat.
- Many of the modern processed foods in Table 6.6 have a relatively high energy density. Many modern methods of preparing and processing foods-tends to remove water and fibre but add fat and/or sugar (e.g. fish fingers, chicken nuggets, fruit/meat pies, cornflakes, cookies and cakes).

The present day diets of affluent populations are of much higher energy density than those of our hunter–gatherer ancestors or in subsistence agricultural communities today. The cross-population changes in diet that are associated with increasing affluence also increase the energy density of the diet, i.e. the partial replacement of vegetables and starchy, fibre-rich foods, with foods rich in fats and sugars but low in fibre. These compositional changes produce diets that as well as being more energy dense are also more palatable. This combination of high palatability and high energy density may increase the likelihood of energy intake exceeding requirements and encourage weight gain. If gut-fill cues (e.g. stomach distension) play any role at all in the regulation of energy intake, one would expect high energy density of the diet to reduce the effectiveness of food-intake regulating mechanisms. This may be particularly so if there is also low energy expenditure due to inactivity. It is widely believed that a reduction in the energy density of adult diets in affluent, industrialized countries will help people to control their energy intake better and so lessen the risks of excessive weight gain.

Diets high in fat, and therefore of high energy density, have often been used to induce obesity in rodents.

According to Miller (1979), high energy density, rather than fat content *per se* is the primary obesifying influence. Varying the energy density and the proportion of fat independently (by using an inert bulking agent) produced a strong correlation between the fatness of the animals and dietary energy density but not between body fatness and dietary fat content.

At the other end of the spectrum, it is now widely believed that the low energy density of some children's diets, especially weaning diets, may be a major precipitating factor for malnutrition. Weaning diets, particularly in some developing countries, may have energy densities that are so low that, even under optimal conditions, children may have difficulty in consuming sufficient volume of food to satisfy their energy needs. Children fed these low energy diets may be in energy deficit (i.e. starved) despite apparently being fed enough to satisfy their demands. These low-energy diets are based on starchy staples, are often practically fat free and have large amounts of water added to produce a consistency considered suitable for babies and young children. Children fed such low energy density diets may need to consume anything up to eight times the weight of food that children on a typical Western weaning diet would need to obtain the same amount of energy.

Key points

- Energy density is the number of kJ/kcal per unit weight in a food or diet.
- Fat is a concentrated source of energy so high-fat foods are energy dense and adding fat (e.g. frying) to foods raises their energy density.
- Foods with high water content, such as fruits and vegetables, have very low energy density.
- Starchy foods have only modest energy density despite being the major energy source in most pre-industrial human diets.
- Modern diets of affluent populations tend to be much higher in energy density than those eaten by hunter–gatherers or subsistence farmers.
- High energy density diets probably predispose to obesity.
- Very low energy weaning diets may precipitate malnutrition because children are unable to eat enough of the dilute food to satisfy their needs.

NUTRIENT DENSITY

Nutrient density is the amount of nutrient per unit of energy in the food or diet (e.g. μg nutrient per kcal/kJ). In the diets of the affluent, nutrient density is often almost a mirror image of energy density; adding ingredients to foods or diets, which contain much energy but few nutrients (e.g. fats, sugar and alcohol), raises the energy density but reduces the overall nutrient density. Diets and foods high in nutrient density help to ensure nutritional adequacy but those low in nutrient density increase the possibility that energy requirements may be met and appetite satisfied without also fulfilling the requirements for essential nutrients. Those consuming relatively small amounts of energy (e.g. those on reducing diets or elderly, immobile people) or those requiring higher amounts of some nutrients (e.g. pregnant women) may need to take particular care to ensure that their diet is nutrient dense. It is possible to predict the likely adequacy of a combination of foods for any particular nutrient as follows:

Nutrient density × energy EAR (or RDA)

= amount of nutrient consumed
by subjects meeting their energy needs

If this figure exceeds the RNI (RDA) for that nutrient, the diet is probably adequate for that nutrient. Similar calculations are also often made for individual foods to illustrate their value as a source of particular

nutrients; some examples are shown in Table 6.7. Clearly oily French fries from a burger bar are a poor source of vitamin C. Even fresh home-made chips (fries) are much worse than boiled new potatoes. Oranges, peppers and grilled tomatoes are clearly good sources of the vitamin. Addition of sugar (canned oranges) or fat (fried tomatoes or potatoes) reduces the nutrient density because it adds energy but no more vitamin C. Avocados have relatively modest amounts of vitamin C and the nutrient density is further depressed because they are relatively high in fat and energy.

> ## Key points
>
> - Nutrient density is the amount of nutrient per kJ or kcal in a food or diet.
> - Adding sugar, alcohol or fat to foods lowers nutrient density because it adds energy but little or no nutrient.
> - A nutrient-dense diet helps to ensure nutritional adequacy but low nutrient density increases the chances that appetite can be satisfied without fulfilling all nutrient requirements.
> - People with low energy intakes especially need to ensure that their diet is nutrient dense, e.g. elderly housebound people and those on reducing diets.

Table 6.7 Amount of energy from various foods that would need to be consumed to obtain the UK adult reference nutrient intake (RNI) for vitamin C (40 mg)

Food	Amount of energy	
	kcal	kJ
New potatoes (boiled)	175	735
French fries (burger bar)	2764	11 611
(home-made UK)	840	3528
Avocado pear	1266	5317
Banana	345	1499
Orange	27	113
Mandarin oranges (canned in syrup)	139	584
Green pepper (capsicum)	5	21
Tomatoes (grilled)	45	189
Tomatoes (fried in oil)	228	958

Compare with the UK energy estimated energy requirement for a man of 10.6 MJ/day (2550 kcal/day).

THE SOURCES OF DIETARY ENERGY BY FOOD GROUPS

The same surveys that were used to estimate the contribution of the major macronutrients to energy intake in the UK can also be used to estimate the contribution that the major food groups make to energy intake. This can also be estimated using data from the family expenditure survey Family Food (DEFRA, 2006). Table 6.8 gives a summary of the food sources of dietary energy using these two approaches. Considering the very different methodologies of the two surveys used to devise Table 6.8, the two sets of results are reassuringly similar. Comparison of the results obtained by Gregory *et al.* (1990) and Hoare *et al.* (2004) also suggests that these proportions have remained fairly stable over the period 1987–2001. Some particular factors that would lead to differences between the two approaches are as follows.

Table 6.8 Percentage contribution of the major food groups to total energy intakes in the UK*

Food group	Hoare et al. (2004) (Gregory et al., 1990)	DEFRA (2006)
Cereals and cereal products	31 (30)	32
Milk and milk products (including cheese)	10 (11)	12
Meat, fish, eggs and products	21 (20)	17
Fats and sugars (including soft and alcoholic drinks and confectionery)	21 (21)	21
Fruits and vegetables (about half of this energy comes from potatoes and potato products)	16 (14)	13

DEFRA, Department for Environment, Food and Rural Affairs.
*As measured by weighed inventory (Hoare et al., 2004) and by family expenditure survey (DEFRA, 2006). Figures in brackets are from weighed inventory conducted in 1986/7 (Gregory et al., 1990).

- In the weighed inventory (Hoare *et al.*, 2004), cooking fats and oils will be incorporated into other foods whereas in the expenditure survey (DEFRA, 2006) they are measured as purchased and incorporated into the fats and sugars group.
- The weighed inventory was confined to adults aged 16–64 years but the expenditure survey includes all age groups.

Comparison of Table 6.8 with the 'ideal diets' suggested by the UK **food guide plate** (or the US **food guide pyramid**) shows that the fats and sugars seem much too prominent; these provide few nutrients but lots of energy, largely as fat and sugar. Cereals plus potatoes are the largest contributors of energy (almost 40 per cent) but a deeper analysis would indicate that highly refined products and those with considerable added fat and/or sugar are much more prominent than would be considered ideal. Fruits and vegetables (excluding potatoes) provide only around 6–7 per cent of total energy. This is lower than ideal but a very low energy yield from these foods is almost inevitable given the very low energy density of most of them.

Key points

- According to data in Family Food 2004–5 (DEFRA, 2006):
  - almost 40 per cent of the energy in the UK diet comes from the cereals and potatoes
  - 12 per cent comes from milk and milk products
  - 17 per cent comes from the meat group
  - 21 per cent comes from fats and sugars (including drinks and confectionery)
  - 6–7 per cent comes from the fruits and vegetables food group (excluding potatoes).
- These figures are quite similar to those obtained by weighed inventory using a representative sample of British adults.
- Ideally, more of the energy should come from unrefined cereals and potatoes, fruits and vegetables, slightly less from the milk and meat groups and much less from the fats and sugars group.

STARVATION

The immediate causes of starvation

For most of the world population, starvation results from local food shortages or from lack of money to buy food. It was also suggested earlier in the chapter that some children may be unwittingly starved because they are fed foods of such low energy density that they are unable to consume sufficient volume of the dilute food to meet their energy needs. Inadequate food intake usually results in hunger and, if food is available, in eating. In some circumstances, hunger may not occur or be suppressed and in some circumstances nourishment will not reach the tissues despite hunger and eating. In affluent countries, with ready availability of food of high energy density, inadequate intake may result from various causes.

- Illness, injury or therapy may result in loss of appetite.
- Infirmity may reduce the ability to eat or to obtain and prepare food, e.g. in stroke patients or elderly immobile people.
- Illness may result in hypermetabolism or loss of nutrients, e.g. the increased metabolic rate in those with overactive thyroid glands or the glucose and ketones lost in the urine of diabetics (see Chapter 16).
- Psychological state or psychological illness may result in inadequate food intake despite its ready availability, e.g. **anorexia nervosa**.
- Some diseases may result in poor digestion and absorption of nutrients, e.g. coeliac disease and cystic fibrosis (see Chapter 16).

Physiological responses and adaptations

The most obvious physiological response to starvation is wasting. If energy intake is not sufficient to cover expenditure then the deficit must be made up by burning body energy reserves. All tissues, with the exception of the brain, will waste during starvation – the most obvious wasting will be in body fat and muscle but other vital organs will also waste. After prolonged starvation, the heart may be only half its original weight and this wasting of heart muscle can lead to death from circulatory failure. The intestines of starving people will atrophy. They become thin and have greatly reduced digestive and absorptive capacity. This may cause problems in re-feeding people after prolonged starvation.

A healthy and well-nourished non-obese man should be able to lose more than 25 per cent of his initial body weight before his life is threatened. During such a 25 per cent weight loss, the man would lose around 70 per cent of his stored fat and around 25 per cent of his body protein. Total carbohydrate content of the body is small (say 500 g) even in well-fed people, and so the small loss of carbohydrate during this prolonged period of weight loss would make an insignificant contribution to total losses of body energy. The energy yield of this 25 per cent loss of body weight represents around 6–7 weeks' energy expenditure in a totally starved and sedentary man. This means that well-nourished adults can survive several weeks of total starvation and this was strikingly illustrated by the Irish Republican Army (IRA) hunger strikers in the Maze

prison in Northern Ireland during the 1980s. It took up to 2 months of total starvation for these healthy young men to reach the point of death (obese people may survive much longer). This capacity of people to survive long periods of food shortage, or even complete starvation, clearly represents a very considerable aid to the survival of the species. If there is a temporary food shortage then there is a good chance that many people will survive until food supplies are restored, e.g. a new harvest. Children are more vulnerable to starvation than adults, survival times of completely starved babies or children may be measured in days rather than weeks, depending on age.

Many cells can use either glucose or fatty acids as an energy source. As body stores of carbohydrate are minimal, during a fast such cells will increasingly switch to using fatty acids as an energy source. The cells of some tissues, including the brain and red blood cells, cannot use fatty acids directly as an alternative energy source and most tissues have a limited capacity to use fatty acids. Glucose can be manufactured in the liver from the glycerol component of stored fat and from amino acids released from the protein in muscles and vital organs but *glucose cannot be synthesized from fatty acids* (see **gluconeogenesis** in Chapter 5). This process of gluconeogenesis is energy expensive (i.e. wasteful) and supplies of amino acids are limited because they are being taken from protein in muscles and essential organs. A maximum of around 5 kg of protein is available for gluconeogenesis in a man.

It was once thought that the brain relied exclusively on glucose as its substrate for energy production. As there are negligible carbohydrate stores, this would mean that the brain would have to rely entirely on glucose produced from gluconeogenesis during prolonged fasting. The brain normally uses the equivalent of around 100 g of glucose per day and unless some adaptation occurred, use of protein in gluconeogenesis would lead to rapid depletion of body protein reserves and the size of these protein reserves would limit the duration of survival during fasting. Starving people would be likely to die from depletion of body protein reserves before body fat stores were exhausted. If nitrogen excretion (i.e. protein breakdown) during fasting is monitored it can be seen that it declines as the fast is extended and after a week or so is down to about 30 per cent of the initial rate. An important adaptation to starvation has

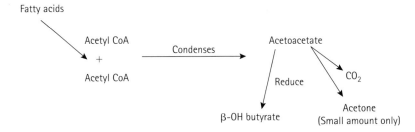

Figure 6.1 *The origins of ketone bodies.*

occurred, which preserves lean tissue during prolonged fasting. During the course of fasting, the blood levels of substances called **ketone bodies** rise as they are produced from fatty acids in the liver. After a few day of fasting, these ketone bodies become the most abundant metabolic fuel in the blood. It is now clear that they act as alternative substrates for the brain and other tissues during prolonged fasting. These ketones are synthesized in the liver from the acetyl CoA produced during the β-oxidation of fatty acids (see Figure 6.1 and Chapter 5).

After prolonged fasting, as much as three-quarters of muscle energy production and more than half of the brain's energy supply will be from β-OH butyrate and acetoacetate (acetone is produced in small amounts as a by-product of the process but is not metabolized). The brain is thus indirectly using fatty acids as an energy source. During a prolonged fast, the brain's requirement for glucose will fall from 100 g/day to 40 g/day and most of this will come from the glycerol component of stored fat. This use of ketones as a substrate thus represents a substantial brake upon the depletion of lean tissue during starvation.

For many years, these ketones were thought of solely as abnormal metabolic products produced during uncontrolled diabetes. In severe diabetes they are produced to excess and their concentration builds up to the point where they become highly toxic. They are toxic principally because they are acidic and produce a metabolic acidosis. Acetone is responsible for the 'pear drops' smell on the breath of persons in diabetic (hyperglycaemic) coma. Persons on severe reducing diets or diets in which carbohydrate intake is severely restricted will experience mild ketosis.

Another important adaptation to starvation is a reduced rate of energy expenditure. This slows the rate at which reserves are depleted and extends the survival time. Some of the very obvious reasons why energy expenditure decreases during fasting (or severe dieting) are:

- with little or no eating, there is less food to digest, absorb and assimilate. These processes each have an energy cost and eating raises resting metabolic rate
- most starving people curtail their physical activity; however, many anorexics are an exception to this generalization – they exercise to lose yet more weight
- as the body wastes, it gets smaller and so the energy costs of maintenance decrease
- the energy costs of any activity are also reduced if the body is smaller
- there is an increase in metabolic efficiency perhaps related to changes in body temperature regulation.

This means that during starvation, the rate of energy expenditure decreases and the rate at which energy stores are used up also decreases. During deliberate weight loss, the amount of energy needed to maintain body weight also declines. Many dieters find that a diet initially succeeds in achieving weight loss but then their weight sticks and they need to reduce their intake still further to get continued weight loss. Prentice *et al.* (1991) estimated that the crude reduction in energy expenditure during dieting might exceed 25 per cent but when corrected for changes in lean body mass it varies between 5 per cent and 15 per cent depending on the severity of the intake restriction.

Some adverse consequences of starvation

Some of the consequences of starvation are summarized in Box 6.2. People with anorexia nervosa (see later in the chapter) vividly illustrate these consequences in developed countries.

Box 6.2 Some consequences of starvation including the starvation associated with anorexia nervosa (after Webb, 1998)

- Wasting of lean tissue and vital organs
- Shrinkage of heart muscle, irregular heart rhythm and risk of heart failure
- Reduced digestive and absorption capability in the gut often leading to diarrhoea
- Reduced growth and development in children and young people, perhaps intellectual as well as physical development
- Depressed immune function and increased susceptibility to infections
- Delayed puberty, lack of menstruation, infertility and loss of sex drive
- Reduced bone density (osteoporosis) and increased risk of fractures, especially stress fractures in anorexic athletes
- Slow healing of wounds
- Reduced strength and physical work capacity and impaired performance in dancers and athletes
- Hypothermia
- Insomnia, changes in personality and brain function

Endocrine function becomes deranged during starvation. Pituitary gonadotrophin secretion is greatly depressed in starvation and this manifests itself outwardly in a cessation of menstruation in starving women. Puberty is delayed by malnutrition. In industrialized countries, the age of onset of menstruation has decreased markedly over the past century as children have become better nourished and grow faster. Women need a minimum threshold amount of fat to maintain their fertility and proper menstrual cycling. Underweight women may have difficulty in conceiving a child and they are more likely to have an underweight baby. The reduced secretion of sex hormones also leads to loss of bone mass. This makes fractures more likely and may, for example, predispose women who have had anorexia nervosa to osteoporosis fractures later in life.

Infection is often associated with starvation and there is said to be a cycle of infection and malnutrition:

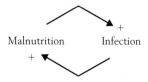

Malnutrition predisposes to infection and infection increases the severity of malnutrition or may precipitate malnutrition in areas where there is not overt food shortage. Sick children (or adults) may have reduced appetite and increased requirement for nutrients. They may also be starved or fed a very restricted diet in the belief that this is the correct way to treat sick children. Malnutrition has very profound, specific and deleterious effects on the functioning of the immune system; these are discussed at some length in Chapter 16. Cohort studies in malnourished children in which nutritional status has been related to subsequent death rate showed that the risk of dying increases exponentially as one moves from the better nourished to the mildly, moderately and severely malnourished (Waterlow, 1979).

There may also be very pronounced psychological effects and personality changes produced by starvation. During the 1940s, in Minnesota, a group of young male volunteers were subjected to a period of partial starvation that resulted in a 25 per cent body weight loss (Keys *et al.*, 1950, summarized in Gilbert, 1986). The feeding behaviour of these men changed markedly during their period of deprivation, including a dramatic decline in their speed of eating. They became preoccupied with food, it dominated their conversations, thoughts and reading. They became introverted, selfish and made irrational purchases of unwanted items. Personality tests conducted during the period of starvation showed a considerable movement towards the neurotic end of the scale as starvation occurred. Towards the end of the period of weight loss, the results from personality tests with these starved men became comparable with those of people with frank psychiatric disease.

Key points

- Worldwide, starvation is usually the result of famine or poverty but it can also be a consequence of illness or infirmity.
- During starvation the body uses stored fat and tissue protein to make up its energy deficit.
- Healthy non-obese adults can survive up to 2 months of total starvation and for much longer on restricted rations.

- During starvation, ketone bodies (β-OH butyrate and acetoacetate) produced from fat become the major body substrates.
- Ketone use reduces the need to produce glucose and spares body protein.
- More than half of even the brain's energy needs are met by ketones during prolonged starvation.
- Starvation leads to a large fall in energy expenditure (less digestion and assimilation, reduced activity, reduced tissue mass and increased metabolic efficiency).
- Adverse consequences of starvation include tissue wasting, reduced growth and healing, depressed immune function, reduced physical performance, endocrine disturbances and reproductive impairment, and psychological disturbances.

EATING DISORDERS

The term **eating disorders** is used to describe the diseases **anorexia nervosa** and **bulimia nervosa**. The term also encompasses many other people who have some symptoms of these conditions but who do not meet the formal diagnostic criteria for either condition and these are termed **EDNOS (eating disorder not otherwise specified).**

Characteristics and consequences

Anorexic people have very low energy intakes and are severely underweight, occasionally they may starve themselves to death. Anorexia nervosa is characterized by an obsessive desire to be thin and an intense fear of being fat even though the victim may be severely emaciated. The disease has significant mortality estimated at between 1 and 13 per cent. Perhaps half of patients show little improvement or make only a partial recovery; they continue to eat very restricted diets, to maintain very low body weights and females do not start menstruating. Perhaps as many as a fifth of patients continue to have severe and unremitting symptoms of the condition. The consequences of this self-starvation are essentially the same as for starvation generally (summarized in Box 6.2 in the previous section). Some symptoms are particularly associated with anorexics such as excessive growth of dry brittle facial and body hair ('lanugo hair'), constipation and peripheral oedema. Those who take purgatives or

resort to induced vomiting are also likely to have adverse consequences of these behaviours including:

- electrolyte imbalances which may lead to muscle weakness, fatigue and increased susceptibility to cardiac arrhythmias
- irritation of the throat and damage to the teeth caused by the corrosive effects of vomitus.

The diagnostic characteristics of anorexia nervosa are:

- low body weight – at least 15 per cent below expected minimum for age and height
- intense fear of gaining weight or becoming fat even though underweight
- distorted body image – seeing themselves as fat even though alarmingly emaciated to the outside observer
- lack of menstrual periods in females for 3 consecutive months.

Many anorexic people also often exhibit one or more of the following behaviours:

- frequent use of purgatives, induced vomiting or emetics
- high levels of physical activity, in contrast to most other victims of starvation.

Victims of the disease may also go to great lengths to hide their restricted food intake and their physical emaciation from relatives and friends. They may wear loose clothing, avoid social eating situations, eat very slowly, choose only foods very low in calories, conceal food that they have pretended to eat and then dispose of it, or induce vomiting after they have eaten. It is, of course, important to rule out other physical and psychological causes of undernutrition and weight loss before concluding that an underweight person is suffering from anorexia nervosa.

Bulimia nervosa is characterized by recurrent bouts of binge eating. Periods of restricted eating are interspersed with sometimes huge binges where massive quantities and bizarre mixtures of foods may be consumed in very short periods of time – the voracious eating may continue until abdominal pain, sleep or interruption trigger its end. Often the binge is followed by self-induced vomiting or purging. The morbid fear of fatness and distortion of body image seen in anorexia are also seen in this condition. A diagnosis of bulimia would be made if the following features are present in people who are not very underweight:

- recurrent bouts of binge eating in which large amounts of food are consumed and in which the person loses control of their eating
- recurrent bouts of inappropriate compensatory behaviour to prevent weight gain after binges, e.g. induced vomiting, purging, excessive exercise or fasting
- these bouts of bingeing and compensation should occur at an average rate of twice a week for 3 months to qualify for a diagnosis of bulimia
- the person's self-image is unduly dependent on their body shape and weight.

This condition can also have serious repercussions on the health of individuals with the condition, including:

- damage to the throat, teeth, oesophagus (gullet) and stomach caused by overloading or the induced vomiting with consequent risk of infection
- possible harmful side effects of any laxatives or emetics used.

Mortality associated with this condition is less than that of anorexia nervosa at between 0 and 3 per cent. If someone who is seriously underweight binge eats, they are classified as having a form of anorexia nervosa.

Incidence

Some surveys among college students and among more random samples of women in the UK and USA have suggested disturbingly high proportions of subjects exhibiting bulimic behaviour (as many as 20 per cent of sampled women in some surveys). Gilbert (1986) concluded 'that at any one time up to 2 per cent of women up to the age of forty may be experiencing problems with controlling their eating'.

Anorexia nervosa is the best known of the eating disorders. The condition was first described more than a century ago but there is general agreement that the disease has become more prevalent in recent decades. It affects less than 0.5 per cent of women. Anorexia nervosa affects mainly females, who typically are:

- white
- aged 15–19 years (about 40 per cent of cases are within this age range although it can occur at any time between 12 and 44 years)
- from middle and upper class families, well-educated and with a good knowledge of nutrition.

Cases do occur in men (less than a tenth of the frequency in women) and among other social and racial groups. As it becomes more common, so anorexia is radiating out from its traditional risk group and is being reported increasingly in Asian and African Caribbean women and in women of other social classes.

Bulimia nervosa occurs in people whose weight is within the normal range and as they are guilty and secretive about their behaviour, this makes it difficult to diagnose and difficult to make estimates of its incidence, hence the wide variability in the estimated frequency of eating disorders noted earlier. Perhaps the best estimates of frequency are about 1 per cent of adolescent girls and young women and about a tenth of this frequency among the corresponding male population. Estimates of the frequency of EDNOS is higher than for anorexia nervosa or bulimia nervosa at 2–3 per cent with a much lower female to male ratio and tending to onset later in life, often between 30 and 50 years.

Causes of eating disorders

There seems to be a general acceptance that these eating disorders have become more prevalent in recent decades, although part of this apparent increase may be due to better detection and increased awareness of these conditions. There are genetic influences on the susceptibility to an eating disorder. Close relatives of those with an eating disorder have much higher prevalence of an eating disorder than controls. Monozygotic twins have higher concordance than dizygotic twins, and twin studies suggest that heritability accounts for in excess of 50 per cent of the risk of developing an eating disorder. It is widely believed that they are triggered in genetically susceptible people by dieting and social pressures on young people to be thin, pressures that may be particularly acutely felt by young women.

Most adolescent girls have tried dieting and preoccupation with body weight and dieting has been reported in children as young as 10 years old. Many bulimic patients have a history of cycles of weight loss and regain or 'yo-yo dieting'. The average woman (and man) in most industrialized countries is getting fatter as judged by surveys of weight and height but images of the ideal woman are apparently getting thinner. Many of the models used in classical painting of the female form would be overweight by present standards and studies on American winners of beauty contests and models for men's magazines indicated that the 'ideal' body shape got thinner during the 1960s and 1970s. Almost all of the models used by fashion photographers are lean and many are frankly underweight. Young women aspire to a body shape that is unhealthy and unattainable except by the most extreme restrictive diets. These disorders do seem to occur more often in girls and women for whom thinness is a career requirement, e.g. models, ballet dancers and airline stewardesses. In male athletes and ballet dancers, eating disorders are almost as common as in women despite their general rarity in men.

Over the years, many suggestions have been made as to the individual causes of anorexia nervosa and related eating disorders – social conditions may favour increasing prevalence of the disease but what individual factors make some women develop the disease? It is likely that the cause of these diseases is multifactorial and that there is no one simple cause that applies to all who have the condition.

The effects of starvation on the men in the experiment of Keys and his colleagues in Minnesota, were discussed earlier and may be of some relevance in understanding the development of anorexic behaviour. The slowness of eating seen in these starving men is typical of anorexics. The men's unsociability, their obsessive interest in food and their curtailment of other activities are all recognized as traditional symptoms of anorexia nervosa. These men also developed personality profiles that were characteristic of people with frank psychiatric disease as they starved. During the period of re-feeding and rehabilitation of these men, many of them showed a marked tendency to binge eat, behaviour in many ways similar to that found in bulimia. Some months after the re-feeding period, a high proportion of the men had put themselves on a reducing diet; men who had previously had a normal interest in food became preoccupied with dieting after this bout of starvation.

These observations on starving individuals have encouraged the suggestion that anorexia and bulimia may be triggered by social and cultural conditions that require young women in particular to be thin. The dieting itself may, in genetically susceptible individuals, cause some of the grossly aberrant and apparently irrational behaviour characteristic of anorexia

nervosa and bulimia. Weight loss and leanness are generally admired and praised in our culture and thus the initial positive reactions to the results of anorexic behaviour may serve as powerful reinforcement or reward and thus encourage learning of anorexic behaviour. In someone whose self-esteem is low and who feels that because of their family environment they lack control over their own lives this, initially praised, ability to totally control some aspect of their lives may also act as positive reinforcement and encourage continuation and intensification of the anorexic behaviour.

Coughlin and Guarda (2006) suggest that parents' comments about weight are the most consistent factor associated with children's concerns and behaviour regarding their weight and shape. They suggest that each of the following factors relating to family life are associated with increased risk of a child developing an eating disorder:

- if the child frequently eats alone
- perception of poor family communication and caring
- low parental expectations
- having parents who are not married.

There are numerous other theories on the origins of anorexia nervosa. Some have suggested that there is some defect in the hypothalamic mechanisms regulating intake but this idea is largely discounted these days and the frequent occurrence of binge eating suggests suppression of appetite rather than lack of appetite. Some adherents to Freudian psychological theories have suggested that the subconscious goal of these women and girls is to avoid adult responsibility and sexuality by starving themselves. The cessation of menstruation, inhibition of sexual development and lack of the adult female form found in anorexic women are seen as the aims and rewards of anorexic behaviour. This theory has attracted much attention over the years and is probably the one theory about anorexia that non-specialists will have heard of. It would be fair to say that this theory has gone out of fashion as has, to some extent, the Freudian view of psychology.

Some have suggested that anorexia is a symptom of a frank affective psychiatric disorder such as clinical depression. This is supported, to some extent, by claims of successful treatment of anorexics with antidepressant drugs. One major problem of trying to investigate the psychological and physiological characteristics that bring about the disease is that by the time the disease is recognized, it will be impossible to decide which abnormalities are due to starvation and which are causes of the self-starvation. A detailed discussion of either the causes or treatment of eating disorders is beyond the scope of this book – the aim of this brief discussion has been to increase the awareness of non-specialists and to help them to recognize potential sufferers. The disease requires specialist management, the non-specialist's role can only be to be able to recognize likely sufferers, appreciate that this is a 'real' and potentially life-threatening illness and direct them towards specialist help.

The above discussion may also give those in contact with anorexic people some insight into the psychological consequences of anorexia/starvation and thus help them to deal more sympathetically with difficult and incomprehensible behaviour. A detailed and well-referenced account of eating disorders may be found in Gilbert (1986) and a shorter, more recent, summary can be found in Coughlin and Guarda (2006).

> ## Key points
>
> - The term eating disorders encompasses the two well-defined conditions anorexia nervosa and bulimia nervosa, but it could also include many other people with some features of these diseases but who fail to meet the formal diagnostic criteria referred to as EDNOS (eating disorder not otherwise specified).
> - People with anorexia nervosa starve themselves, sometimes to the point of death, because of an obsessive preoccupation with their weight and a pathological fear of fatness even when they are grossly emaciated.
> - People with bulimia nervosa are not seriously underweight but engage in recurrent bouts of bingeing followed by inappropriate compensatory behaviour to prevent weight gain, e.g. induced vomiting, purging, fasting or excessive exercise.
> - The consequences of anorexia nervosa are similar to those of starvation. In addition, people with eating disorders may have adverse consequences associated with induced vomiting, use of purgatives or emetics, and overloading of the stomach during binges.

> - Eating disorders are predominantly found in adolescent girls and young women.
> - Estimates of frequency vary widely but in the young women estimates of 0.5 per cent for anorexia and 1 per cent for bulimia may be reasonable; the frequency in men is less than a tenth of that in women.
> - Frequency of EDNOS is higher and tends to onset later in life.
> - There are many theories about the causes of these conditions but there is a widespread belief that they may be triggered in genetically susceptible people by dieting and preoccupation with being slim.
> - Family relationships are seen as important predisposing factors for eating disorders.
> - Eating disorders are more common in men and women for whom thinness is a career requirement.

CANCER CACHEXIA

Severe emaciation and malnutrition are frequently associated with terminal malignant disease and starvation may, in many cases, be the immediate cause of death. This is termed **cancer cachexia**. Several readily identifiable causes for the loss of weight may be seen in these people with cancer, e.g.:

- when malignancy affects the alimentary tract
- where the disease makes eating difficult or painful
- when appetite is depressed in patients who are in great pain or extremely distressed
- the anti-cancer treatments may themselves induce nausea and anorexia.

There are, nonetheless, occasions when patients with malignant disease may lose weight initially for no clearly apparent reason. Sometimes weight loss may be the symptom that triggers the investigation leading to the diagnosis of malignancy. Hypermetabolism (increased energy expenditure) seems to be partly responsible for such weight loss and this may be a reflection of the metabolic activity associated with rapidly dividing malignant cells. There is additionally thought to be an anorexic effect of tumour growth. The metabolic disturbance or metabolic by-products of tumour growth have a depressing effect on appetite. In simple starvation, around three-quarters of weight loss is adipose tissue but in cancer cachexia a much higher proportion of the weight loss is lean tissue. This accelerated loss of lean tissue hastens death in the cachectic patient. Increasing food intake does not always reverse the cachectic process and some studies have found that even intravenous feeding fails to stabilize weight in the long term. In the short term, intravenous feeding does seem to increase body fat but does not reverse the loss of muscle and lean tissue.

Cytokines are proteins that are secreted as part of the immune response and several cytokines are known to be produced as a response to tumour growth, e.g. **tumour necrosis factor**. These cytokines may be partly responsible for the anorexia and metabolic changes seen in malignant disease. All of the cytokines produced in cancer cause anorexia and weight loss. Once cancer is suspected or confirmed, the psychological reactions to the disease, the effects of any treatment, the pain and discomfort caused by the disease or treatment as well as the direct pathological effects of the disease will all interact to reduce appetite and hasten weight loss. A short referenced review of cancer cachexia may be found in Tisdale (1997).

Key points

- Large weight losses due to both reduced appetite and hypermetabolism are a usual feature of malignant disease – cancer cachexia.

- In cancer cachexia there is greater loss of lean tissue than in simple starvation.

- Many factors contribute to the weight loss in cancer but cytokines such as tumour necrosis factor produced as part of the immune response depress appetite and play a part in this response to malignancy.

- Neither raised food intake nor intravenous feeding seems able to correct the excess loss of lean tissue seen in cancer even if body weight is increased or maintained.

7

Energy balance and its regulation

CONCEPT OF ENERGY BALANCE

When we digest and metabolize food, the oxidation of fats, carbohydrates, protein and alcohol releases chemical energy that can be used for body functions. The first law of thermodynamics states that 'energy can neither be created nor destroyed but only changed from one form to another'. This means that all of the energy released during the oxidation of the macronutrients in food (the **metabolizable energy**) must be accounted for. It must be used to keep the body's internal systems functioning (this is ultimately lost from the body as heat energy), to do external work (e.g. move something) or be stored within the body (e.g. as fat in adipose tissue).

If an adult's energy intake (the metabolizable energy in food) exactly equals their energy expenditure (as internal and external work), they are in **energy balance** and their total body energy content (and thus their fat stores) will remain constant (see Figure 7.1). The 'energy in' is the sum of the metabolizable energy yields of all of the food and drink consumed; it will normally be influenced by only the nature and amount of food and drink consumed. The 'energy out' can be directly measured by determining heat output in a calorimeter or, as is more usual, by predicting the heat output from measurements of oxygen consumption and carbon dioxide evolution (see Chapter 3). This output figure will be influenced by several factors (see list below) that raise heat output above the resting level, i.e. factors that have a thermogenic (heat-producing) effect.

- *The thermogenic effect of exercise.* Metabolic rate rises as exercise load is increased. The sweating

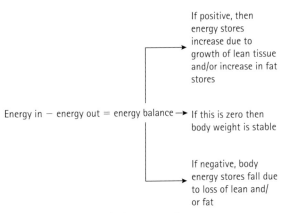

Figure 7.1 *The energy balance equation.*

and rise in skin temperature induced by exertion are obvious outward signs of this thermogenesis. Some of this extra energy output may also be used to do external work.

- *Thermoregulatory thermogenesis.* The increase in metabolic rate, and therefore heat output associated with shivering or non-shivering mechanisms used for heat generation in a cold environment. Energy expenditure also increases in a very hot environment.

- *Drug-induced thermogenesis.* The increase in heat output brought about by certain drugs (e.g. caffeine) that have a stimulating effect on metabolic rate.

- *The thermic effect of feeding* or postprandial thermogenesis. This is the increase in metabolic rate and heat output that follows feeding and is the energy expended in digesting, absorbing and assimilating the food (e.g. in the synthesis of fat and glycogen).

- *Adaptive thermogenesis.* An increase in metabolic rate as a consequence of overfeeding that is claimed to help in the maintenance of energy balance (see later in the chapter).

For a healthy adult whose weight is stable, over a period of time, the energy intake and output must be matched. There is a zero balance, i.e. the energy content of the body remains constant. There is wide variation in the energy intakes that different individuals require to maintain balance (see Chapter 6, Energy requirements). If an individual's energy intake exceeds output they are said to be in **positive energy balance**. Under these circumstances, body energy content must be increasing because 'energy cannot be destroyed'. The surplus energy is converted from chemical energy of food to chemical energy of body tissues. Increase in body energy content means either increases in lean body mass (growth) or increase in body fat deposition or both. Children, pregnant women, and those regaining weight after a period of illness or starvation would all properly be expected to show a positive balance. For most of the rest of the population, sustained positive balance means increasing fat stores, which will ultimately lead to obesity.

If an individual's energy output exceeds intake they are said to be in **negative energy balance**, and because 'energy cannot be created', the shortfall must be made up from body energy stores. Individuals in negative energy balance must be losing body energy and this will almost certainly be reflected in weight loss. It is possible that body energy content can fall without weight loss if fat loss is compensated for by increases in lean tissue and/or water content, e.g. in starvation there may be excess accumulation of tissue fluid, **oedema**. Loss of body energy may be due to loss of lean tissue (protein) or loss of fat or, as is most likely, both. Persons who are starving or successfully dieting will be in negative energy balance, as will:

- many sick or seriously injured people
- those losing large amounts of nutrients, e.g. people with uncontrolled diabetes
- those whose expenditure is particularly high, such as people with hyperactive thyroid glands or those undertaking intense physical activity for prolonged periods.

Key points

- Energy can neither be created nor destroyed, only changed from one form to another.
- If energy intake exactly equals expenditure then a person is in energy balance and their weight should remain stable.
- Energy intake is the metabolizable energy content of food and drink.
- Energy expenditure consists of basal metabolic rate (BMR) plus extra energy expended as a result of exercise, thermoregulation, drug action, feeding, etc.
- If energy intake exceeds expenditure (positive energy balance) then there must be either growth of lean tissue or extra fat accumulation.
- Growing children, pregnant women and those recuperating after illness or starvation would all be expected to show a positive energy balance.
- If expenditure exceeds intake (negative energy balance) then there must be a corresponding decrease in body energy stores.
- Negative energy balance occurs in starvation, serious illness, and in those undertaking intense physical activity. Reducing diets are intended to achieve a negative energy balance.

IS THERE PHYSIOLOGICAL REGULATION OF ENERGY BALANCE?

Many adults maintain their body weight within a very narrow range over periods of years or even decades. Let us consider a normal 65 kg man who consistently takes in 420 kJ (100 kcal) per day more than he uses. This small surplus represents only 3–4 per cent of his estimated requirements and would be equivalent in food terms to not much more than the generous layer of butter or margarine on a slice of bread. On the basis of the assumption that 1 kg of adipose tissue yields about 30 MJ (7000 kcal), if this surplus were maintained for a year it would be energetically equivalent to 5 kg of adipose tissue and in 10 years to 50 kg of adipose tissue! If we consider the opposite scenario, i.e. if the man had a similar constant daily deficit, he would lose adipose tissue at this rate and his fat stores would be totally exhausted in 1–2 years. Such calculations imply that unless there is extraordinarily precise long-term matching of energy intake to expenditure, over a period of decades massive changes in fat stores will occur. Of course, in reality these changes will tend to be self-limiting. For the man taking in the small daily surplus, the energy requirements would tend to rise in response to the constant surplus intake for the following reasons.

- Even adipose tissue uses some energy so as he gets bigger it costs more energy to maintain his bigger body – BMR increases with size.
- The energy costs of any activity are increased as he gets bigger.
- It costs energy to convert surplus food energy into stored fat, especially if the surplus is in the form of carbohydrate or protein.

These changes will tend to bring him back into balance after a modest weight gain unless he increased intake or curtailed his activity to maintain the imbalance. We saw in the previous chapter a corresponding list of changes that occur when there is an energy deficit – changes which tend to reduce energy requirements and weight loss.

Key points

- Long-term weight stability requires very accurate matching of intake and expenditure.
- Even tiny sustained imbalances can lead to massive changes in body fat stores over years or decades.
- This implies that there is regulation of energy balance.
- Weight losses or gains do tend to be self-limiting because over-consumption increases expenditure and under-consumption decreases expenditure.

'SET POINT' THEORY

According to the **'set point' theory**, body weight control mechanisms operate to maintain a fixed level of body fat stores. If volunteers are weighed accurately every day for a period of months then one finds that even though their weight may be unchanged over the period, nevertheless their day-to-day weight does tend to fluctuate and seems to oscillate around a 'set point'. This is analogous to the oscillations in temperature that occur in a room

where the temperature is controlled by a thermostat. During periods of illness or food restriction weight decreases. During times of feasting weight tends to increase. However, when normal conditions are restored, the subject's weight tends to return to the 'set point'. Similar observations have been made in animals. Even rats that have been made obese by damage to the brain centres that control energy balance seem to control their body weight to a set point, albeit a higher set point than in normal animals. Unfortunately, as we will see in Chapter 8, over the course of adulthood the set point of many people seems to drift upwards so that most middle-aged Europeans and Americans become overweight or obese.

Key points

- Physiological control mechanisms may operate to maintain a constant level of body fat stores, the 'set point' theory.
- Body weight appears to oscillate around this set point although in the long term there is often an upward drift in body fat stores with age.

IS ENERGY EXPENDITURE REGULATED?

Regulation of energy balance could be achieved by regulation of energy intake or expenditure or by a combination of the two. The sensations of hunger and satiation are universally experienced manifestations of some energy intake regulating mechanism. Traditionally, therefore, studies on the regulation of energy balance have focused on the mechanisms regulating food intake and these are discussed at length later in this chapter. The regulation of energy expenditure as a mechanism for the controlling energy balance has been a more controversial topic. We have already seen that overfeeding increases energy expenditure and that energy restriction reduces expenditure and these changes tend to restore balance. There is little doubt that an increase in 'metabolic efficiency' occurs during fasting and food restriction; BMR drops by up to 15 per cent even when one allows for any decrease in lean body mass (Prentice *et al.*, 1991). The point of controversy is whether any mechanism exists whose primary purpose is to compensate for overeating by 'burning off' surplus calories.

In 1902 the German scientist Neumann coined the term *luxoskonsumption* to describe an adaptive increase in energy expenditure in response to overfeeding. The term **adaptive thermogenesis** is often used today. Essentially, it is envisaged that some energy-wasting metabolic process is activated when people overeat and that this 'burns off' the surplus calories to restore energy balance or to reduce the imbalance.

Rats can be persuaded to overeat and become obese by the provision of a variety of varied, palatable and energy dense human foods (**cafeteria feeding**). This mode of feeding in caged animals is designed to mimic the affluent human lifestyle. Rothwell and Stock (1979) reported that some rats fed in this way stored less of the surplus food energy than they had predicted and seemed to burn off some of this extra energy. Sims *et al.* (1973) did similar experiments with young men who were persuaded to consume an extra 3000 kcal (13 MJ) per day for a period of 8 months. At the end of this period, only about 15 per cent of the surplus energy that had been eaten could be accounted for in the increased fat stores. This implied that some adaptive thermogenesis had occurred. Many subsequent shorter and less extreme overeating experiments have failed to find evidence of significant adaptive thermogenesis in human subjects. If there is any significant capacity for adaptive thermogenesis, under conditions of abundant food supply people might eat more than their bare minimum requirements and burn off some energy. The apparent increase in metabolic efficiency seen during fasting might represent a switching off of this adaptive thermogenesis, and there might be limited further capacity to increase thermogenesis under conditions of experimental overfeeding.

Rothwell and Stock (1979) proposed that in small mammals a tissue known as **brown adipose tissue (BAT)** or **brown fat** is the site of adaptive thermogenesis. Brown fat is the major site of cold-induced heat production (non-shivering thermogenesis) in small mammals and is particularly prominent in hibernators where it is important in generating heat during arousal from hibernation. The sympathetic stimulation of brown adipose tissue results in an uncoupling of oxidative phosphorylation, i.e. oxidation accelerates but does not result in ATP production. The chemical energy produced during oxidation is released as heat and this warms the body during cold

exposure. This mechanism is well established for thermoregulatory thermogenesis in small mammals (and human babies) and Rothwell and Stock (1979) suggested that this also occurs during overfeeding. The heat generated during overfeeding is then dissipated from the relatively large surface of the small animal. This theory was given added credence by evidence of abnormal thermoregulation in several animal models with inherited obesity. The most widely used of these models is the **ob/ob mouse**, which is homozygous for a mutation at a gene locus referred to as *obese*, or *ob*. These mice have low body temperature, reduced heat production and die during cold exposure. They were said to have a 'thermogenic defect' which made them prone to a metabolic obesity as they would have little capacity for adaptive thermogenesis. A similar thermogenic defect might also predispose people to obesity.

It would be unwise to be too ready to extrapolate these findings in laboratory rodents to people. Adult human beings have limited capacity for non-shivering thermogenesis and brown adipose tissue has traditionally been regarded as vestigial in adult humans. People keep warm largely by heat conservation supplemented by shivering rather than non-shivering thermogenesis. A large animal with a relatively small surface area to volume ratio is less able to dissipate large amounts of surplus heat generation; this might also make adaptive thermogenesis a less advantageous strategy for maintenance of energy balance in people. Accurate long-term measurements of metabolic rate in obese people provide no evidence for any thermogenic defect in the obese and indeed basal metabolic rates and total energy expenditure of obese people are increased because of their higher body mass (Prentice *et al.*, 1989). Drugs that are highly specific activators of the β**-3 adrenoreceptor** on brown fat (β-3 agonists) cause big increases in metabolic rate in rodents but have little effect in people.

Even in the *ob/ob* mouse the abnormal thermoregulation probably represents an adaptation rather than a defect (Webb, 1992b). If the genetic defect of these mice makes them unable to detect their large fat stores then they would respond as if being continually starved (see discussion of **leptin** later in the chapter). One of the strategies that mice employ to conserve energy during fasting is to reduce their heat output and lower their body temperature. Fasting mice can enter a state of torpor where they allow their body temperature to fall by as much as 15°C for several hours at a time (Webb *et al.*, 1982). The low body temperature of *ob/ob* mice could represent a permanent semi-torpid state, as an adaptation to perceived starvation and their poor cold tolerance might represent a form of disuse atrophy of their brown fat. Torpor is not a usual human response to starvation. Children have now been identified who have an analogous gene defect to that of the *ob/ob* mouse but these very obese children have normal body temperature and thermoregulation (Montague *et al.*, 1997). See Webb (1990, 1992b) for critical discussion of the applicability of these studies on small animal models of obesity to people.

The publication of this brown fat theory by Rothwell and Stock in 1979 generated a flurry of interest and excitement in the early 1980s. It raised the prospect that adaptive thermogenesis could represent a major component of human energy expenditure and that differences in thermogenic capacity might explain the apparent variation in the susceptibility of people to obesity. It also raised the prospect of thermogenic drugs that would specifically stimulate adaptive thermogenesis. These might offer an attractive alternative to appetite suppressants for the pharmacological treatment of obesity. β-3 Adrenoreceptor agonists that specifically stimulate brown fat thermogenesis have shown promising results in rats but not people. This is probably because of the low capacity for brown fat thermogenesis in people. It would be fair to say that the initial enthusiasm for this theory has cooled considerably over the past 20 years. There is little evidence that adaptive thermogenesis makes a major contribution to human energy balance control.

Later work has further undermined the theory that adaptive thermogenesis is a major factor in controlling body weight. Enerback *et al.* (1997) produced transgenic mice that lack the key protein required for the uncoupling of oxidation and phosphorylation in brown fat (UCP1). This protein is the key initiator of heat generation in brown fat. These mice are cold sensitive but they are not obese and their ability to regulate their body weight is normal. This work seemed to be a decisive blow against the brown fat theory of obesity. There are, however, now known to be other uncoupling proteins called UCP2 and UCP3. UCP2 is expressed not only in both white fat and brown fat but also in other tissues (Fleury *et al.*, 1997); UCP3 is found mainly in skeletal muscle (see Hirsch, 1997). The role of these other uncoupling proteins (UCP2 and UCP3) in the control of human metabolic rate is as yet unclear, but Schrauwen *et al.* (1999) suggest that they may be important. Uncoupled oxidative phosphorylation (proton leakage) may account for up to 20 per cent of the resting metabolic rate in people. Nevertheless, the idea of a thermogenic defect being a major cause of human or even mouse obesity is now largely discounted.

Key points

- It seems self-evident that food intake is regulated but do animals and people have the capacity to burn off surplus energy and thus limit weight gain as an adaptive response to overfeeding (adaptive thermogenesis)?

- Rothwell and Stock (1979) proposed that overfeeding increases sympathetic stimulation to brown fat which uncouples oxidative phosphorylation in this tissue and so increases heat generation.

- This mechanism is well established as a means of heat generation in small mammals and human babies during cold exposure (non-shivering thermogenesis).

- Rothwell and Stock also proposed that genetically obese mice (*ob/ob*) and humans might get fat because of some thermogenic defect that impaired their capacity for adaptive thermogenesis.

- Adaptive thermogenesis is not now thought to be a major component of human energy expenditure.

- There is no evidence of any thermogenic defect in most obese people and indeed the BMR and total energy expenditure of obese people tends to be higher than that of lean people.

- Transgenic mice that lack a key protein required for brown fat thermogenesis (UCP1) are hypothermic but not obese.

- Even the well-documented hypothermia of some obese mice probably represents an inappropriate energy conserving response in animals whose brains falsely perceive that their fat stores are depleted.

- The presence of other uncoupler proteins (UCP2 and UCP3) that are expressed in tissues outside brown fat may still mean that the regulated uncoupling of oxidative phosphorylation may have a role in controlling human metabolic rate.

- Up to 20 per cent of resting metabolic rate may be due to uncoupled oxidative phosphorylation (proton leakage).
- The proposal that a thermogenic defect is a major cause of human obesity is now discounted by most nutritionists and physiologists.

EXTERNAL INFLUENCES THAT AFFECT FOOD INTAKE

In the rest of this chapter I am going to consider the physiological regulation of energy intake. However, it is not only 'internal' physiological factors that influence when, what, where, and how much we eat. Eating is also a conscious voluntary act that is affected by a host of 'external' influences (see below).

- *The palatability of food and the pleasure derived from eating.* We do not have to be hungry to eat and indeed we may be persuaded to eat some delicious item even when feeling distinctly full.
- *Habit,* e.g. always eating a particular snack when reading, driving or watching a favourite TV programme.
- *Our psychological state,* eating to relieve psychological states other than hunger, e.g. to relieve anxiety, boredom or unhappiness.
- *Eating for social rather than physiological reasons,* e.g. to participate in a social 'feast' or to please someone who has offered us food.

It is perhaps only in newborn babies that eating is regulated largely by internal physiological hunger control mechanisms uncluttered by these external influences. We may, on occasion, ignore or over-ride our physiological mechanisms that control food intake and this may be one reason why we are so prone to obesity.

Key points

- Even though physiological control mechanisms affect feeding, eating is a voluntary activity that is influenced by a host of social, cultural and psychological factors.
- These external influences on feeding may reduce the effectiveness of physiological control mechanisms.

CONTROL OF ENERGY INTAKE

Early work with experimental animals

Over the past 100 years or so, there have been several reports in the medical literature of patients becoming very obese after damage to their hypothalamus caused by trauma or tumours. This pointed to a role for the hypothalamus in weight control, and it is now well established that the hypothalamus is involved in other physiological regulatory systems, such as:

- body temperature control
- control of water balance
- control of the female reproductive cycle.

Around 1940, the development of the stereotaxic apparatus allowed experimenters to make discrete and accurately located lesions deep within the brains of experimental animals. Over the next couple of decades this lesioning technique showed that damage to certain areas of the hypothalamus could profoundly affect a rat's eating and drinking behaviour. Damage to the ventromedial region of the hypothalamus in many mammalian species, ranging from mice to monkeys, produced a period of massive overeating and weight gain, leading to severe and permanent obesity. The weight of rats with such lesions stabilized at a much higher level than that of unoperated rats and their food intake returned to a level that maintained this 'new set point'. If these rats were slimmed down they went through a second bout of overeating and seemed to defend their new set point. It was also found that lesions in the lateral part of the hypothalamus completely abolished eating and drinking behaviour in rats, and they died unless tube fed.

As a result of such observations, a simple theory of food intake regulation was proposed, the **dual-centre hypothesis** (see Figure 7.2). A spontaneously active feeding centre that initiates food seeking and eating behaviour was envisaged as being located in the lateral hypothalamus. Its destruction by lateral hypothalamic lesions would result in a cessation of eating behaviour. This feeding centre was periodically inhibited by a satiety centre located in the ventromedial region of the hypothalamus. This satiety centre would become active in response to certain **satiety signals**, which strengthen after feeding; it would then inhibit the feeding centre and produce satiation. As time after feeding elapsed, one would

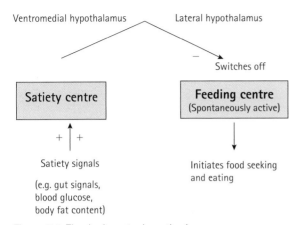

Figure 7.2 *The dual-centre hypothesis.*

envisage these satiety signals dying away, the satiety centre would become quiescent, allowing the feeding centre to become active again and producing hunger. Destruction of this satiety centre would reduce satiation and result in excessive food consumption and obesity. The hypothalamus was thus envisaged as acting like a meter or 'appestat' that adjusts the feeding drive in response to a variety of physiological signals that reflect the short- and long-term energy status of the body – energy intake is thus matched to output and energy balance is maintained.

The dual–centre hypothesis: a more recent perspective

The dual-centre hypothesis has had enormous influence on thinking about control of energy balance and body weight. It was prominent in many textbooks published in the 1960s and 1970s, and it may still be found in some modern texts. It is now regarded as a rather simplistic model of a complex process. Since these early studies, much detailed work has been done in trying to identify hypothalamic and extra-hypothalamic brain areas that are involved in the control of feeding and body weight. A detailed discussion of the anatomical locations and interconnections of neural centres controlling energy balance is beyond the scope of this book but several hypothalamic and other brain areas are known to have a role. I will generally use the term **appestat** (*cf.* thermostat) as a term to collectively describe the centres in the hypothalamus that control energy balance. References to the early experimental work on the hypothalamic

mechanisms regulating food intake have been excluded. Interested readers will find detailed and well-referenced accounts of this work in editions of many texts published during the 1960s and 1970s or by reference to Mayer (1956, 1968), Kennedy (1966) or Brobeck (1974), three of the most prolific and influential researchers in this field.

Despite nowadays being regarded as simplistic, the dual-centre hypothesis does have the three basic elements that any system for controlling food intake must have (Figure 7.3):

- a series of physiological inputs to the appestat that provide information about the feeding status and the level of body energy stores, so-called **satiety signals**
- areas within the brain that integrate information about feeding status and level of body energy stores – the **appestat**
- a hunger drive that can be modified by the appestat in response to the information received from the satiety inputs (also mechanisms for controlling energy expenditure).

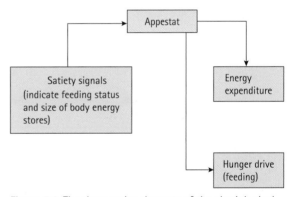

Figure 7.3 *The three major elements of the physiological control of energy balance.*

The arcuate nucleus of the hypothalamus seems to have a key role in receiving and responding to both short- and long-term signals that reflect the body's feeding and nutritional status and thus control body weight. Circulating factors can interact directly with neurones of the arcuate nucleus because it is incompletely separated from the general circulation by the blood–brain barrier. Within the arcuate nucleus are subpopulations of neurones involved in food intake regulation; some are appetite inhibiting and some are appetite stimulating. These neurones release peptides such as neuropeptide Y (NPY) and Agouti-related peptide (AgRP), which bind to receptors within the central nervous system to produce appetite stimulation while α-melanocyte-stimulating hormone (α-MSH) causes an anorectic response (see Murphy and Bloom, 2004).

Various satiety signals have been proposed and investigated over the years. These fall into three major categories.

- Signals emanating from the alimentary tract and transmitted via sensory nerves or hormones released from the gut. These provide information about the amount and the nature of food in the gut.
- Blood substrate levels. After eating, the blood concentration of substrates such as glucose and amino acids rises as they are absorbed from the gut. These concentrations fall in the post-absorptive state. If we eat three meals per day and they each take around 4 hours to digest and absorb, then for most of our waking hours we are absorbing food. The notion that blood glucose concentration or the rate of glucose utilization is a major satiety signal has historically been very popular – the **glucostatic theory**.
- Signals that emanate from adipose tissue and indicate the level of body fat stores – the **lipostat theory**.

Gut–fill cues

We all experience the feeling of stomach fullness that occurs after a meal and the feeling of stomach emptiness and hunger contractions that occur after fasting. Feeding normally finishes before there have been detectable changes in blood substrate levels (or changes in blood leptin levels – see later in chapter). These observations suggest that signals from the alimentary tract play some part in signalling satiation and have some role in short-term appetite regulation. The signals could be mediated either through sensory nerves in the gut directly affecting the appestat or perhaps through hormones released from the gut by the presence of food.

The energy density of the diets of laboratory rats can be greatly altered by the use of an inert bulking agent (e.g. methylcellulose) or by the addition of energy-rich fat. Rats fed diluted diets are able to maintain their body weights and compensate for

the dilution by increasing the volume of food they eat. However, long-term feeding with diets of high energy density causes obesity in rats, which suggests that over-concentration of the diet may reduce the effectiveness of feeding control mechanisms. It is widely believed that reducing the energy density of human diets will help to prevent excessive weight, which implies widespread acceptance of the belief that dietary bulk has some modulating effect on appetite. One could, for example, envisage alimentary signals having an important role in signalling satiety at the end of a meal but when food is very dilute, being over-ridden or dampened by other physiological signals indicating the need for energy intake. The mechanisms regulating energy balance are generally more effective in preventing under- rather than over-consumption (see Chapter 8).

The hormone **cholecystokinin (CCK)** is released from the intestine when food is present and it induces satiety and reduces feeding and pre-prandial administration of substances that block the CCK receptor leads to increases in meal size in animals and people. It was the first gut hormone identified as playing a part in the control of appetite. It is said to act by activating sensory branches of the vagus nerve in the gut and these relay the information to the appestat. Prolonged administration of CCK to animals leads to rapid diminution in its anorectic effect and animals that have been bred with no CCK receptors have normal food intake and body weight. Animals adapt to oversupply of CCK and also adapt to an absence of the CCK response.

A recently discovered hormone **ghrelin** is the only peripherally produced hormone that has an appetite-stimulating effect. It is a small peptide (28 amino acids) produced mainly in the stomach. Plasma ghrelin levels are inversely correlated with body weight and they rise during fasting and weight loss and they fall rapidly after a meal. It has been suggested that ghrelin may have a role in meal initiation. Peripherally administered ghrelin binds to appetite stimulating cells in the arcuate nucleus of the hypothalamus and this leads to increased production and release of appetite-stimulating peptides within the hypothalamus. Chronic administration of ghrelin leads to overeating and weight gain in rats whereas anti-ghrelin antibodies lead to a reduction in the amount of food consumed after fasting.

Pancreatic peptide (PP) and polypeptide YY (PYY) are two appetite-suppressing hormones produced in the gut that are both structurally related to the appetite-inhibiting brain peptide NPY. Pancreatic peptide is produced in the pancreas and when administered peripherally to rats it reduces food intake and slows stomach emptying; it also suppresses food intake in humans. Increases in blood levels of PP lead to increases in hypothalamic levels of NPY. PYY is produced by endocrine cells within the gut and levels in the blood rise after eating. When PYY is administered to rats or people in amounts that mimic the normal postprandial levels in the blood, it leads to activation of appetite-suppressing neurones in the arcuate nucleus and markedly reduces food intake.

Glucagon-like peptide 1 (GLP-1) and oxyntomodulin (Oxm) are peptides that are produced in the small intestine and colon and released into the blood after eating. They both have appetite-suppressing effects. GLP-1 receptors are found in the arcuate nucleus and in other parts of the brain and administration of GLP-1 to rats or people inhibits food intake. Oxm has similar anorectic effects and it may act via GLP-1 receptors.

Murphy and Bloom (2004; http://ep.physoc.org/cgi/content/full/89/5/507) and Druce et al. (2004; http://endo.endojournals.org/cgi/content/full/145/6/2660) have written concise referenced reviews of the role of the gut in regulating appetite and both reviews can be accessed free online.

The glucostatic theory

This theory envisages that there are glucose receptors or sensors in the appestat and perhaps elsewhere that respond to blood glucose concentration (Mayer, 1956). These glucose receptors induce satiety when blood glucose concentration is high and induce hunger when it is low. The occurrence of both high blood glucose and hunger in uncontrolled diabetes was explained by the suggestion that the glucoreceptor cells needed insulin for glucose entry in the same way as say resting muscle cells do. In the absence of insulin (i.e. in diabetes), despite a high blood glucose concentration, the glucoreceptor cells are deprived of glucose resulting in hunger. As the brain was regarded at this time as being exclusively dependent on a supply of glucose in the blood, hypothalamic glucoreceptors sensitive to fluctuations in blood glucose concentration seemed a logical homeostatic device.

The glucostatic theory was given an important boost in the 1950s by work that showed that a glucose derivative, **gold thioglucose**, produced both obesity and lesions in the ventromedial region of the hypothalamus of mice. No other gold thio compounds produced this effect; the glucose moiety appeared to be essential. This supported the proposal that there are glucoreceptors in this region that bind the gold thioglucose, leading to accumulation of neurotoxic concentrations of gold in their vicinity (reviewed by Debons et al., 1977). Later versions of this theory suggested that a high rate of glucose metabolism produces satiation rather than high blood concentration per se. Satiation correlates very well with the difference between arterial and venous blood glucose concentration, which is a measure of the rate of glucose utilization.

When the rate of glucose metabolism is high, fat use is low. In healthy people, this high glucose–low fat usage occurs after eating carbohydrate and produces satiation. When glucose metabolism is low, metabolism of fat is high and this results in hunger. High fat–low glucose utilization occurs:

- during fasting
- in the absence of insulin (uncontrolled diabetes)
- if meals with little or no carbohydrate are eaten.

Insulin, when released after a meal, causes glucose to be taken up and metabolized by the cells and this leads to satiation. Use of fat in metabolism is associated with hunger. Carbohydrate intake increases use of carbohydrate and reduces use of fat, but fat intake has little effect on either fat or carbohydrate metabolism (Schutz et al., 1989). As fat is absorbed, much of it is shunted directly into our fat stores. This may help explain why high-fat diets may be less satiating than high-carbohydrate diets and why high-fat diets seem to predispose to weight gain and obesity (see Chapter 8).

The evidence that some glucostat mechanism has an important role in the short-term control of appetite is very persuasive (see the more recent review by Penicaud et al., 2002).

The lipostat or adipostat theory

It is difficult to see how short-term satiety signals such as gut-fill, blood glucose concentration or even the rate of glucose utilization could produce long-term weight stability, i.e. over a period of months, years or decades. They are more likely to fulfil functions such as:

- limiting the size of meals to prevent overload of the gut and the body's metabolic processes for assimilating nutrients
- ensuring a regular flow of energy and nutrients to maintain optimal metabolic functioning even when body fat stores are substantial and so reducing the need for regular and prolonged activation of starvation mechanisms (note that the need to avoid excessive fat stores may have played a relatively minor role in shaping our physiology – see chapter 8).

This **lipostat** or adipostat theory was used to explain how body energy stores (i.e. fat) could be regulated in the long term by regulation of apparently short-term phenomena such as hunger and satiety. It was first proposed by Gordon Kennedy in the 1950s (see Kennedy, 1966). It is envisaged that some appetite-regulating chemical (a satiety factor or satiety hormone) is released from adipose tissue so that its concentration in blood indicates to the appestat the total amount of stored fat. This would allow total amount of body fat to have a modulating effect on appetite and would offer a relatively simple mechanism for long-term control of energy balance. This lipostat theory would fit well with the notion of a set point for body weight discussed earlier in the chapter.

Some very persuasive but indirect evidence for the existence of such a satiety hormone (now called **leptin**) came from the work of Coleman (1978) using two types of genetically obese mice. *Obese* (*ob/ob*) and *diabetes* (*db/db*) are two forms of genetic obesity in mice. Both *ob/ob* and *db/db* mice inherit a very severe obesity associated with diabetes. On a similar genetic background the two syndromes are practically identical and yet are caused by mutations at different gene loci. Coleman proposed that in the *ob/ob* mouse the genetic defect is in the leptin (satiety hormone) gene leaving them unable to produce this satiety hormone (leptin) and making their appestat unable to detect any fat stores. As a consequence of this they overeat and get very fat. He suggested that in the *db/db* mouse, the abnormal protein is one that allows the appestat to respond to leptin (the leptin receptor). *db/db* rats would thus produce lots of leptin because they have lots of fat in their adipose tissue. However, without any leptin receptor their appestat cannot detect the leptin and so once again they cannot sense any fat stores and so they overeat. At this time, leptin had not been discovered and was a purely hypothetical hormone. These suggestions were the result of an ingenious series of parabiosis experiments; these are experiments where pairs of animals are surgically linked together so that hormones and other substances can pass between their blood systems. The results obtained from four of these parabiotic pairings are explained in Table 7.1.

Table 7.1 Results of parabiotic pairings of lean and obese rodents

Pairing	A normal animal paired with one that has had its ventromedial hypothalamus (part of the appestat) destroyed	A normal and an ob/ob mouse	A normal and and a db/db mouse	An ob/ob mouse and a db/db mouse
Result	The animal with the damaged hypothalamus overeats and gains weight as expected; the normal animal eats less and loses weight	The ob/ob mouse eats less and loses weight	The normal mouse stops eating and starves	The ob/ob mouse eats less and loses weight
Explanation	The animal with its hypothalamus damaged gets fat because the area where the leptin acts in the brain has been destroyed and so it cannot respond to leptin. As this lesioned animal gets fatter, its adipose tissue produces large amounts of leptin. This extra leptin enters the blood of the normal animal and this animal's appestat responds by reducing food intake	The ob/ob mouse cannot produce its own leptin, but it can respond to leptin produced by its lean partner, so eats less and loses weight	The db/db mouse cannot respond to leptin and so gets fat and produces excess leptin. This leptin enters the blood of the normal mouse and acts on this animal's appestat to suppress food intake	The ob/ob mouse is responding to the excess leptin produced by its db/db partner

Key points

- The hypothalamus plays a major part in the control of feeding and experimental lesions in the hypothalamus profoundly affect feeding behaviour.
- The hypothalamic 'appestat' receives input of satiety signals that indicate the feeding state and level of body fat stores.
- The hypothalamus alters the feeding drive and rate of energy expenditure in response to these satiety inputs.
- Satiety signals relay information to the appestat about the amount and nature of food in the gut, the level or rate of usage of blood substrates and the amount of fat stored in adipose tissue.
- Sensory nerves in the gut and hormones released from the gut indicate the nature and amount of gut contents.
- In the glucostat theory it is envisaged that information from glucose sensors in the hypothalamus and elsewhere have a major role in the short-term control of feeding.
- In the lipostat theory, Kennedy proposed that some satiety factor (leptin) is released from adipose tissue in proportion to the amount of stored fat. This would enable the appestat to regulate feeding and energy expenditure to maintain a constant level of these stores.
- Indirect evidence suggested that obese mice with mutations at the *obese* locus (*ob/ob*) do not produce this satiety factor whereas mice with mutations at the *diabetes* locus (*db/db*) do not respond to it.

The leptin story

It is a bit of a cliché that scientific books may become out of date before they are published. Nonetheless, a paper was published just after the manuscript of the first edition of this book was finished which radically changed scientific thinking about the physiological mechanisms that control energy balance. In 1994, Zhang *et al.* identified the *obese* (*ob*) gene and the protein that is produced by it in healthy lean mice. The *obese* gene produces a secretory protein of 167 amino acids that seemed to be produced exclusively in adipose tissue and has been named leptin (note that later studies have

shown that it is also produced in the placenta and stomach). It seems to have all the characteristics of the hypothetical satiety factor from adipose tissue that was proposed in the lipostat theory of weight control. In normal mice, leptin production falls during starvation and it increases in environmentally induced obesity. Leptin production seems to be proportional to the mass of adipose tissue. In genetically obese, *ob/ob*, mice a mutation in the *obese* gene results in the production of a shorter, inactive protein that is not secreted. This leaves the appestat of *ob/ob* mice with no input from adipose tissue. The appestat perceives this as absence of fat stores and so initiates appropriate starvation responses.

Leptin administration to *ob/ob* mice causes weight loss, normalization of body composition and corrects all of the other metabolic and hormonal abnormalities of these mice. Leptin also causes reduced food intake, increased energy expenditure and loss of body fat when it is administered to normal mice. Leptin administration has no effect in the *db/db* mouse, an observation that is entirely consistent with the earlier suggestion of Coleman (1978) that the genetic defect in these mice was in a gene that codes for the system that senses the then hypothetical satiety factor (i.e. the leptin receptor). In 1995, Tartaglia *et al.* were able to identify and characterize the leptin receptor. They confirmed that the mutation in *db/db* mice leads to abnormalities in the leptin receptor. The leptin receptor can be detected in all the areas of the hypothalamus known to be involved in control of energy balance and in the vascular region where leptin is conducted across the blood–brain barrier (the choroid plexus).

Leptin seems to have a central role in the long-term regulation of energy balance (Figure 7.4). During starvation and weight loss, leptin production from adipose tissue decreases. This decrease in leptin is detected by the hypothalamic appestat which then triggers the normal responses to starvation that are seen at their most extreme in the *ob/ob* mouse, such as:

- increased food intake if food is available
- reduced activity and resting energy expenditure, including reduced body temperature and the permanent semi-torpid state of *ob/ob* mice
- reduced production of hormones in the pituitary gland (gonadotrophins) that leads to delayed puberty and infertility

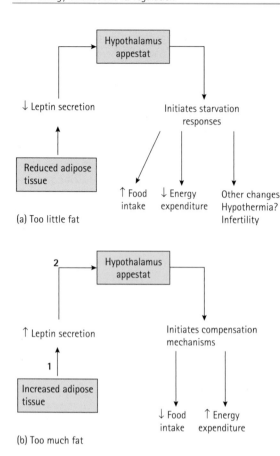

(a) Too little fat

(b) Too much fat

1 If production of leptin is absent (*ob/ob* mice) or insufficient, obesity will result

2 If leptin sensing is absent (*db/db* mice) or reduced (mice fed high-fat diets), obesity will result

Figure 7.4a,b *Role of leptin in responses of mice to excess or inadequate fat stores.*

body's weight control mechanism seems to be much more geared to preventing underweight and maintaining adequate fat stores (the evolutionary priority) than preventing excessive weight gain (see Chapter 8 for further discussion of this point). Nevertheless, obesity would theoretically occur under either of the following circumstances:

• complete failure of leptin production (as in *ob/ob* mice) or inadequate leptin production, i.e. a failure to produce sufficient leptin to reflect the level of fat stores to the hypothalamus
• a complete lack of response to leptin (as in *db/db* mice) or a reduced response to leptin.

The observation that leptin levels are high in most induced animal obesities suggests that reduced leptin sensitivity is the scenario in most obesity. Increasing the fatness of animals by feeding them a high-fat diet does indeed lead to a decrease in their sensitivity to leptin. There is thus a complete spectrum of leptin sensitivity in mice, from the high sensitivity of *ob/ob* mice through to the complete insensitivity of *db/db* mice (Figure 7.5). Normal mice lie between these two extremes but inducing obesity by dietary means reduces leptin sensitivity. There is a clear precedent for diet and lifestyle causing increased production and declining sensitivity to a hormone. The commonest and mildest form of diabetes begins in middle or old age and does not normally require insulin injections (**type 2 diabetes**). In type 2 diabetes there is no primary failure of the pancreas to produce insulin as there is in the severe

• other changes in the secretion of hormones from the pituitary, which in turn regulate most of the other endocrine glands. The output of pituitary hormones is controlled by the hypothalamus.

During weight gain, as the fat content of adipose tissue increases so increasing leptin production should act via the hypothalamus to reduce food intake and increase energy expenditure. However, it does seem that although the absence of leptin in the circulation caused by depletion of adipose tissue or genetic defect has profound effects on appetite, fat storage and fertility, the effects of raised leptin levels are much less dramatic. This may be just another manifestation of the general observation that the

Leptin

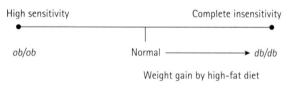

Insulin

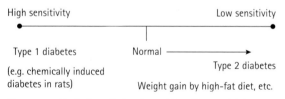

Figure 7.5 *Variations in leptin and insulin sensitivity.*

form of the disease that starts in childhood and requires regular insulin injections for survival (**type 1 diabetes**). In type 2 diabetes, an affluent Western lifestyle (inactivity, high-fat diet and excessive weight gain) triggers a progressive decrease in the sensitivity to insulin, probably as a response to high insulin secretion. In genetically susceptible people, this eventually leads to symptoms of diabetes. In a recent review, Zhang and Scarpace (2006) discussed results from several studies which suggested that as with the insulin-type 2 diabetes analogy, high circulating leptin levels lead directly to reduced leptin sensitivity by reducing the number of leptin receptors in the hypothalamus and reducing the signalling efficiency of these receptors. They argue that the increased leptin production associated with increased adipose tissue mass directly contributes to leptin resistance and thus promotes further weight gain leading to a vicious cycle of:

Weight gain → elevated blood leptin → leptin resistance → weight gain → obesity

Leptin appears to have a key role in long-term energy balance control even though other factors such as blood glucose and gut-fill cues seem to control meal spacing and the short-term control of hunger and satiety. Leptin levels do not rise noticeably after a meal, and it is not thought to immediately induce satiety during feeding and signal the end of a meal. However, the observation that some leptin is produced in the stomachs of rats and that it is released during feeding may herald some role for leptin in short-term hunger and satiety control. Administration of the hormone cholecystokinin also causes release of leptin from the stomach (Bado *et al.*, 1998). Cholecystokinin is released from the gut during feeding and like several other gut hormones is known to induce satiety or in the case of ghrelin increase appetite (see Gut-fill cues, p. 180).

So far, this discussion has been largely confined to studies in experimental animals – what is the relevance of this work to people and more especially, what future role can leptin play in human obesity therapy? In their original leptin paper, Zhang *et al.* (1994) identified a human version of leptin produced in human adipose tissue. Measurements of serum leptin concentrations in people with varying levels of fatness suggest that leptin concentration rises in proportion to the adipose tissue mass. This means that, in general, leptin levels are higher in obese people than in lean people. For example, in a large sample of Polynesian men and women, Zimmet *et al.* (1996) found a very high correlation ($r = 0.8$) between serum leptin concentration and body mass index (i.e. body fat content).

In 1997 the first two cases of people with obesity caused by mutations in their leptin genes were identified; two British cousins of Pakistani origin. These are the apparent human equivalents of *ob/ob* mice. These two children were extremely obese, at 8 years the girl weighed 86 kg whereas the boy weighed 29 kg at 2 years (Montague *et al.*, 1997). There are technical reasons why one would expect that this mutation (analogous to the *ob* mutation in *ob/ob* mice) would be extremely rare in humans (Sorensen *et al.*, 1996). It is thus no coincidence that these children were from a close-knit immigrant community with a history of consanguineous marriage, which increases the chances of people being homozygous for any rare harmful recessive trait and thus having a genetic disease. According to Friedman and Halaas (1998) only about 5–10 per cent of obese humans may have relatively low leptin levels. One group that is particularly prone to obesity, the Pima Indians, tends to have low leptin levels which may explain their extreme propensity to obesity. The first identified cases of people who are obese because they have a mutation in their leptin receptor gene, the human equivalent of *db/db* mice (Clement *et al.*, 1998) were of three members of a French immigrant family.

When humans with leptin or leptin receptor mutations reach the normal age for puberty, they show similar reproductive abnormalities to *ob/ob* and *db/db* mice, they do not go through normal pubertal changes and the females do not menstruate. Studies such as these provide confirmation that leptin has a similar role in the regulation of energy balance in mice and humans (see Figure 7.4). However, as noted earlier both types of obese people, unlike their mouse equivalents, have apparently normal thermoregulation and there is no suggestion that their obesity is caused by any thermogenic defect.

When the discovery of leptin was first announced, an American pharmaceutical company paid millions of dollars for the patent on the leptin gene. Leptin seemed to offer the prospect of a major advance in the treatment of obesity, even though most obesity seems to be associated with leptin resistance rather than reduced leptin production. Leptin is a protein that needs to be administered by injection, a major drawback to its potential therapeutic usage. Early trials of leptin injections in obese people suggest that even though it does produce a small average weight loss over a month of use, the individual response is variable and in general its efficacy as an anti-obesity 'drug' is limited. As with *ob/ob* mice, leptin has proved to be effective in human patients who have a congenital leptin deficiency (Murphy and Bloom, 2004). For a fully referenced review of the first few years of leptin developments, see Friedman and Halaas (1998).

Key points

- In 1994 the protein produced from the *obese* gene in healthy mice and people was identified and characterized.
- The *obese* gene product is a secreted protein called leptin that is mainly produced in adipose tissue.
- Leptin seems to be the hypothetical satiety factor from adipose tissue that was predicted in the lipostat theory of weight control.
- In general, leptin concentration in blood is proportional to the amount of stored fat.
- Obesity could result from inadequate leptin production or inadequate response to leptin as this would cause the appestat to 'underestimate' the fat content of adipose tissue.
- In general, low blood leptin caused by congenital deficiency or adipose tissue depletion seems to have more profound effects than high blood leptin levels.
- The leptin system, like other regulatory mechanisms, seems to more geared towards maintaining adequate fat stores than preventing excessive accumulation of fat and obesity.
- Obese mice with mutations at the *obese* locus (*ob/ob*) do not produce functional leptin and mice with mutations at the *diabetes* locus (*db/db*) do not respond to leptin because they have a defective receptor protein.
- A few very obese children have been identified with mutations at the leptin gene locus (analogous to *ob/ob* mice) and at the leptin receptor locus (analogous to *db/db* mice).
- Only a small proportion of obese people have low leptin levels, most have high leptin levels that reflect their large amounts of stored fat.
- Most human obesity is probably due to an environmentally induced reduction in sensitivity or response to leptin. By analogy, most human diabetes is due to reduced insulin sensitivity.
- In experimental animals, leptin sensitivity declines if they are made obese by environmental means, e.g. feeding a high-fat diet.
- High leptin secretion caused by excessive weight gain causes leptin insensitivity which predisposes to further weight gain.
- Leptin is effective in treating *ob/ob* mice and in treating humans with congenital leptin deficiency but has low efficacy in other obese people.

8

Obesity

DEFINING OBESITY

Obesity strictly refers to an excess accumulation of body fat but as we saw in Chapter 3, body fat content is difficult to measure quickly and accurately in people. For this reason, the **body mass index (BMI)** is now widely used to determine whether someone is excessively fat (see Chapter 3 for a critical discussion of the use of BMI for this purpose). The BMI classification system in Table 8.1 is now used internationally and the **World Health Organization (WHO)** defines clinical obesity as a BMI of over 30 kg/m². This classification is a simple one because it uses:

- a small number of ranges
- mainly whole round numbers
- the same cut-off points for men and women.

Table 8.1 The internationally recognized classification of people according to their body mass index (BMI)*

BMI range (kg/m²)	Classification
Under 18.5	Underweight
18.5–25	Ideal range
25–30	Overweight
Over 30	Obese
Over 40	Severely obese

*BMI = weight (kg) ÷ height² (m)

This simplicity must have a cost in terms of accuracy and sensitivity and so these ranges should be used as a general guide rather than absolute cut-off points. A small difference in BMI is still small even

if one value is above and one below a barrier. Note that 20–25 kg/m² was for some time used as the normal range and some data sources used in this book still use this range for normality. However at the upper end, the cut-off points for the definitions of overweight and obese have remained constant and in this book, **overweight** always refers to a BMI in excess of 25 kg/m² and **obese** to a BMI of over 30 kg/m² unless otherwise specified.

> ## Key points
>
> - BMI, body mass index, is the standard way of classifying people according to fatness.
> - BMI = weight (kg) ÷ height² (m).
> - 18.5–25 kg/m² is taken as the ideal range for BMI in adults.
> - People below the ideal range are classified as underweight and those above it overweight.
> - A BMI of over 30 kg/m² is taken as the definition of clinical obesity.

PREVALENCE OF OBESITY

There is little doubt that overweight and obesity are more common in the UK and USA than in previous generations and that the prevalence is still rising. There have been particularly rapid increases in prevalence since the start of the 1980s in both countries. Around 60 per cent of English adults are currently overweight or obese (i.e. BMI 25+) and over

22 per cent are clinically obese (i.e. BMI 30+). Figure 8.1 shows the proportion of English adults in various BMI categories. (Most of the data for English adults quoted in this chapter is from the health survey for England (e.g. Sproston and Primatesta, 2004).) In America, the situation is even worse with around two-thirds of adults having BMI that is above $25 \, \text{kg/m}^2$ and over 30 per cent classified as obese.

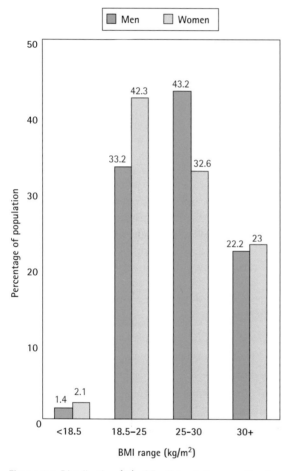

Figure 8.1 *Distribution (%) of English adults according to body mass index (BMI) category.*

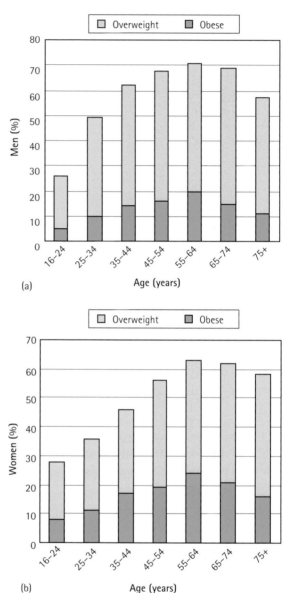

(a)

(b)

Figure 8.2a,b *Effect of age on the percentage of English men (a) and women (b) who are overweight or obese.*

Even the high frequency of obesity indicated in Figure 8.1 somewhat understates the problem in middle-aged people. Figure 8.2 (a,b) shows how the proportion of people who are overweight or obese changes with age among English adults. The proportion of people who are overweight and obese rises steeply throughout early adulthood and middle age, only in the over 75s do the proportions start to fall back slightly. In the 45–64-year-old age band, about 70 per cent of adults are either overweight or obese. Essentially similar age-related changes in prevalence are seen in the USA and Figure 8.3 shows the prevalence of obesity in various age groups of men and women in 2000. Obesity peaks in American adults in the 60–69 year age group where 40 per cent of adults are classified as obese. Note also the substantial fall in obesity prevalence in old age especially in the over 85s; many people tend to lose weight at the end of their life, or perhaps the increased mortality of the obese is selectively removing them from the population and so decreasing the prevalence of obesity in the older age groups. Note than in Chapter 14

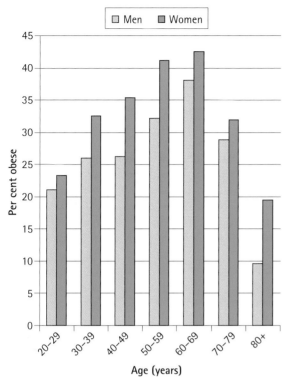

Figure 8.3 *Percentage of obesity in American men and women in different age groups (2000).*

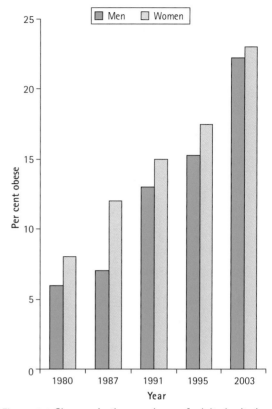

Figure 8.4 *Changes in the prevalence of adult obesity in England (1980–2003).*

evidence will be presented which suggests that in older age groups, excess weight seems to be associated with reduced mortality, i.e. an apparent protective effect of extra fat stores in old age.

Figure 8.4 shows changes in the estimated prevalence of obesity in England; obesity prevalence has trebled since 1980. In 1992, the British government set a target of reducing clinical obesity prevalence in England to no more than 6 per cent of men and 8 per cent of women by the year 2005 (Department of Health (DH), 1992). Even at the time they were set, these seemed to be very ambitious targets, and they now seem to have been totally unrealistic, yet these targets represent the estimated prevalence of obesity in 1980. This target date of 2005 has now passed and obesity prevalence is around three times the target values and still seems to be rising.

Flegal *et al.* (2006) have reported similar rapid increases in obesity prevalence in the USA. Between 1960 and 1980 the prevalence of adult obesity in the USA rose slowly from 13.5 per cent to 15 per cent of adults aged 20–74 years. However between 1980 and the end of the millennium US rates of adult obesity doubled to 31 per cent (see Figure 8.5).

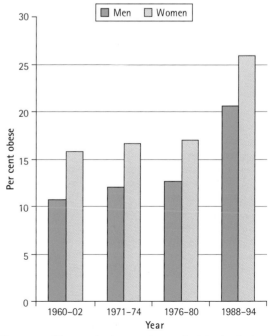

Figure 8.5 *Changes in the prevalence of adult obesity in the USA (1960–94).*

The stated aim of the American government in 1992 (DHHS, 1992) was that by the year 2000 no more than 20 per cent of Americans should have a BMI that exceed 27.8 kg/m² for men and 27.3 kg/m² for women (these cut-off points were widely used in the USA at that time). The number of people exceeding these thresholds in 2000 was at least twice this 20 per cent target value.

A worldwide perspective

The prevalence of obesity is rising not just in Britain and America but throughout the industrialized world. According to the WHO (2006) more than a billion adults around the world are overweight and at least 300 million of them are clinically obese (BMI 30+) and given the rapid rates of increase these figures will no doubt be out of date before this edition is published. The WHO suggests that as in Britain and the USA, obesity rates have also trebled since

1980 in eastern Europe, the Middle East, the Pacific Islands, Australasia and China. The epidemic of obesity is not just confined to industrialized countries but is also affecting many developing countries. The rate of increase in some of these developing countries is even higher than that in the industrialized world. In some developing countries there is widespread obesity in some parts of the country (often urban areas) or in some affluent sectors of the population whereas in other areas or in the poorer sectors of society there may be widespread under-nutrition.

Figure 8.6(a–d) shows WHO estimates of prevalence of obesity and overweight in 10 selected European countries and 10 countries outside Europe. Figure 8.6a shows that in the each country in the European sample, 35 per cent or more of adults are classified as overweight. The prevalence of obesity in these same European countries is shown in Figure 8.6b and the rate of obesity varies from around 10 per cent or less in France, the Netherlands

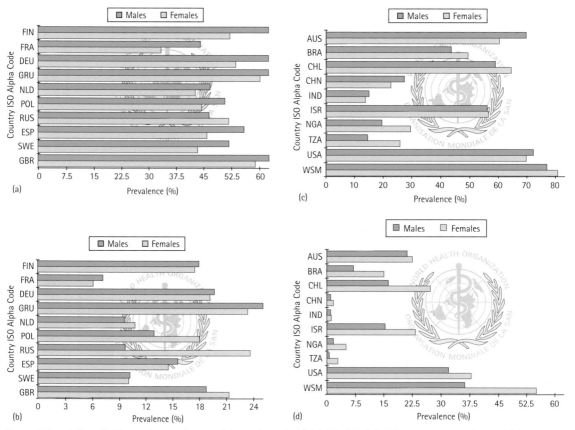

Figure 8.6a–d *Year 2000 prevalence of overweight and obesity (BMI 25+) in (a) 10 European countries and (c) 10 countries outside of Europe. Year 2000 prevalence of obesity (BMI 30+) in (b) 10 European countries and (d) 10 countries outside of Europe. Source: World Health Organization.*

and Sweden to around 20 per cent or even more in Greece, the UK, Germany and Finland. The data for the Russian Federation show a very large sex difference with less than 10 per cent of Russian men classified as obese but approaching 25 per cent of Russian women. Data supplied by the Obesity Research Information Centre, London, at the time of the previous edition did suggest that rates of increase in Sweden, the Netherlands and Denmark were either very slow and in some instances appeared to be stabilizing or even falling slightly.

Figures 8.6c and 8.6d show rates of overweight and obesity in the 10 selected non-European countries. The variation in prevalence is much greater than with the European countries because this sample includes countries at varying stages of industrial development. In the most industrialized countries like Australia, Israel and the USA, rates are similar to those seen in Europe but rates are much lower in China, Nigeria, Tanzania and India. The data for Samoa (WSM) are particularly striking and almost 80 per cent of Samoan adults are overweight and over 45 per cent obese (around 54 per cent of Samoan women are obese). Hodge *et al.* (1994) reported that in urban areas of then Western Samoa 60 per cent of men and 75 per cent were obese and less than 10 per cent were not overweight. Hodge *et al.* (1994) also reported large increases in obesity rates in all regions of Western Samoa over the period 1978–91 but increases in the rural areas were particularly dramatic, e.g. in men in the rural Tuasivi region, obesity rates quadrupled in 13 years. In 1978 there was a large urban–rural difference in obesity rates in Western Samoa. Obesity rates were much higher in the urban areas where many people were employed in sedentary jobs and had ready access to imported Western foods but less prevalent in the rural areas where the diet and lifestyle was more traditional. With increasing development and industrialization, the rural populations are rapidly becoming as obese as their urban neighbours (see sample figures in Table 8.2).

The four graphs that make up Figure 8.6 have been produced using a WHO website (http://infobase.who.int). This website allows one to choose up to 10 countries from an extensive list and generate a graphical comparison of chosen health parameters in these countries using a pre-programmed template. This site can also be used to compare in countries of one's choice, blood pressure, blood cholesterol

Table 8.2 Changes in the prevalence of obesity (% with BMI 30+) in selected areas of (Western) Samoa*

Region	1978	1991
Apia (urban)		
Men	38.7	58.5
Women	61.2	77.7
Tuasivi (rural)		
Men	9.9	39.3
Women	26.6	57.2

*Data of Hodge et al. (1994).

concentration, mortality and, as in Figure 8.6, the percentage of adults who are overweight or obese.

Effects of ethnicity and social status on prevalence of obesity

In the UK and USA, there are marked differences in the prevalence of obesity between different socioeconomic and ethnic groups. In the USA, obesity (and **type 2 diabetes**) is much more prevalent among certain Native American tribes such as the Pima of Arizona than it is in the white population. Table 8.3 shows the prevalence of overweight (BMI 25+) and obesity (BMI 30+) in the three major ethnic groupings in the USA. Rates of obesity in American men do not vary greatly between the three groupings although if one looks at figures for both overweight and obese then these do suggest an excess adiposity in Mexican Americans. The data for women in Table 8.3 show a substantially higher prevalence of overweight and obesity in both Black American and Mexican American women than in the white female population. In Britain, obesity is also more common

Table 8.3 Ethnic differences in prevalence of overweight and obesity in the USA*

	BMI 25+ (%)	BMI 30+ (%)
Men		
White	67.4	27.3
Black	60.7	28.1
Mexican American	74.7	28.9
Women		
White	57.3	30.1
Black	77.3	49.7
Mexican American	71.9	39.7

*Data from Flegal et al. 2006.

in black women and people of south Asian origin; this latter group are particularly prone to abdominal obesity. An English survey (Prescott-Clarke and Primatesta, 1998) found that 45 per cent of middle-aged black women were obese compared with 28 per cent and 21 per cent, respectively, of middle-aged Indian and white women (unpublished statement by Primatesta). In the industrialized countries, obesity is more prevalent in the lower socioeconomic groups and among the less well educated. Table 8.4 shows a pronounced trend for increased prevalence of obesity in English women as one goes down the socioeconomic scale (Sproston and Primatesta, 2004). This class-related pattern of obesity is less clear in English men although rates in the two highest social categories are significantly lower than those in the lower three (see Table 8.4).

Table 8.4 The percentage of English adults who are obese (BMI 30+) in different socioeconomic groupings*

Grouping[†]	Men	Women
Managerial/professional	20.9	18.7
Intermediate	19.7	18.7
Small employers and own account workers	26.7	20.5
Lower supervisory and technical	24.9	28.8
Semi-routine and routine	21.6	29.1

*Data from Sproston and Primatesta (2004).
[†]This socioeconomic classification is based on the current or former occupation of the household reference person.

There is a strong inverse correlation between level of educational attainment and obesity; those with higher levels of education are less likely to become obese than those with more limited education. Molarius et al. (2000) related BMI to educational attainment in 26 populations around the world using WHO data. They found that lower educational attainment was associated with higher BMI in almost all the 26 female populations and in about half of the male populations. They also found that these differences between BMI in groups with different levels of educational attainment had widened over a 10-year period. Sobal and Stunkard (1989) reviewed the influence of socioeconomic status on obesity around the world. They concluded that in industrialized countries, obesity tends to be more prevalent among the lower socioeconomic groups, whereas in poorer

countries it is more common in the upper social groups because only the relatively affluent have the opportunity to get fat. This is most obviously seen in countries where obesity and under-nutrition coexist in different sections of the population; one of the major factors leading to obesity in such countries is a relatively affluent urban lifestyle.

Overweight and obesity in children

One problem with estimating the prevalence of overweight and obesity in children has been the lack of agreed international standards of classification. In Chapter 3, a set of international standards devised by Cole et al. (2000) were discussed which estimated the BMI of girls and boys at various ages that are equivalent to the cut-off values for overweight (BMI $25 \, kg/m^2$) and obesity ($30 \, kg/m^2$). Sample numerical values were given in Chapter 3 and these standards are shown in graphical format in Figure 8.7. Where numerical values for obesity prevalence are given in this section, they are based on these international standards.

Not many years ago, I was able to confidently write in another book that, although rising, obesity in children was still relatively uncommon. In a recent WHO fact sheet (2006) it was stated that childhood obesity is now epidemic in some parts of the world and rising in other areas. The International Obesity Task Force (IOTF, 2004) recently estimated that about 10 per cent of school-aged children are overweight (155 million) and 30–40 million of these are classified as obese, i.e. 2–3 per cent of all the world's children aged 5–17 years. In addition somewhere around 22 million children aged under 5 years are estimated to be overweight.

In the UK 22 per cent of boys and 27.5 per cent of girls aged 2–15 years were estimated to be overweight in 2002 and this includes 5.5 per cent of boys and 7.2 per cent of girls classified as obese. These percentages translate into somewhere around 2.4 million British children being overweight and 700 000 of these being obese. The trends for overweight and obesity in UK children are very like those already described for adults with levels of overweight rising from around 7 per cent of children being overweight and only around 1 per cent being obese in the mid-1970s to an estimated 27 per cent and 7 per cent, respectively, in 2002. Rates of increase have been particularly high in children in

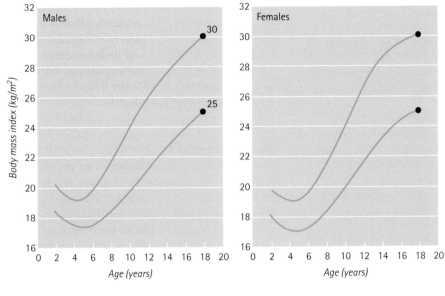

Figure 8.7 *The body mass index (BMI) that corresponds to adult values of 25 kg/m² and 30 kg/m² in children at different ages. Redrawn from Cole* et al. *(2000) by kind permission of BMJ Publishing Group.*

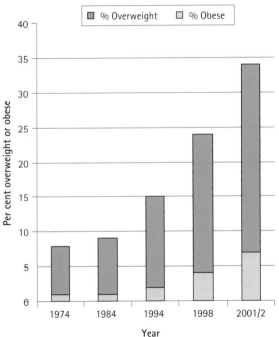

Figure 8.8 *Changes in prevalence of overweight and obesity in English children aged 7–11 years (1974–2002).*

the 7–11 years age band and Figure 8.8 shows changes in the prevalence of overweight and obesity in this age group over a 25-year period. Similar trends to those in the UK have been documented in American children, where the number of overweight children (6–11 years) has more than doubled since 1980 and the number of overweight

adolescents (12–17 years) has trebled over the same period. Rates of increase have been particularly high in black and Mexican American children. Numerical values for American children along with graphical analysis may be found in Ogden *et al.* (2002) or summarized on the website of the National Centre for Health Statistics (www.cdc.gov/nchs/). (Numerical values have not been given here because they have been calculated using American standards, not those of Cole *et al.*, 2000.)

Key points

- Obesity rates are rising rapidly in most industrialized countries and in many developing countries.
- In England in 2002, 23 per cent of adults were obese and a further 43 per cent of men and 33 per cent of women were overweight.
- Two-thirds of American adults have a body mass index (BMI) of over 25 kg/m² and more than 30 per cent are classified as obese.
- In 1980 it was estimated that only 6 per cent of English men and 8 per cent of women were obese.
- The proportion of people who are overweight or obese rises steeply throughout early adulthood and middle age, so that by middle age over two-thirds of English people have a BMI of over 25 kg/m².
- In the USA, 40 per cent of adults aged 60–69 years are obese.

- In the USA, obesity is much more prevalent among certain tribes of Native Americans, Mexican Americans and black American women than it is in white Americans.
- In Britain, south Asians and African Caribbean women are more likely to be obese than white women.
- In industrialized countries, obesity is more prevalent in the lower socioeconomic groups and less well-educated sectors of the population. In England, this trend is particularly pronounced in women.
- Internationally there is a marked tendency for BMI to be higher in those with the lowest educational attainment.
- In developing countries, obesity may be more prevalent in the upper socioeconomic grouping because it is only these groups that have the opportunity to get fat by overeating and being sedentary.
- Overweight and obesity in children is also rising rapidly with perhaps 10 per cent of the world's school age children overweight and 2–3 per cent obese.
- A quarter of UK children (aged 2–15 years) are overweight and 7 per cent of them are obese using international standards.
- In the UK and USA rates of childhood obesity and overweight have shown similar dramatic increases since 1980 to those detailed for adults although the baseline starting values were much lower in children.

CONSEQUENCES OF OBESITY

Relationship between BMI and life expectancy

Studies conducted by life insurance companies since early in the twentieth century have found that being overweight or obese is associated with excess mortality and that mortality rises steeply when BMI is over $30\,\text{kg/m}^2$; mortality ratio is doubled at a BMI of around $35\,\text{kg/m}^2$. In a study of 200 morbidly obese American men, death rates were 12 times higher than normal in those aged 25–34 and still three times higher than normal in the 45–54-year age group when the total number of deaths is much higher (Drenick et al.,1980).

According to life insurance studies, the health effects of obesity seem to be greater in men than in women. Such studies usually show some increase in mortality in those who are underweight as well as in those who are overweight, i.e. there is a so-called J curve when mortality is plotted against BMI. This idea of a J curve in the relationship between BMI and mortality is now generally accepted (Hill et al., 2006). The higher death rate at low BMI has usually been explained by suggesting that being underweight is often an indicator of poor health, or the result of smoking or of alcohol or drug misuse. Smoking, for example, is known to depress body weight and is also a cause of much ill health and many premature deaths. Figure 8.9 uses data from the Nurses' Health Study discussed in Chapter 3 and shows a typical J curve of mortality against BMI. The figure also shows the results from this study when the following 'corrections' were made:

- those who died within the first 4 years were excluded (i.e. already in poor health when the study started?)
- when only those whose weight was stable at the start of the study were included (recent unintentional weight loss may be an indicator of existing ill-health)

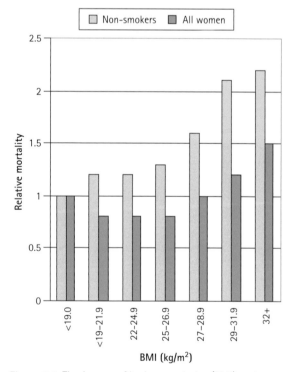

Figure 8.9 *The J curve of body mass index (BMI) and mortality and the effects of smoking (see text for details). Data source: Manson* et al. *(1995).*

- when only women who had never smoked were included (smoking damages health and lowers body weight).

The J-curve disappears when these women are excluded. The increase in death rate with increasing BMI is also more pronounced. These data suggest that raised mortality among smokers and women whose weight is depressed by poor health tend to obscure the strength and steepness of the association between BMI and mortality.

The mortality risk associated with being overweight or obese seems to be greater in young people. Andres *et al.* (1985) used life insurance data to calculate the BMI associated with the lowest risk of dying during the follow-up period in various age bands. This analysis is summarized in Figure 8.10 and it seems to indicate that the 'ideal BMI' (the one associated with lowest mortality risk) seems to rise progressively with age. Although the data used to construct Figure 8.10 is now more than 20 years old, more recent evidence will be presented in Chapter 15 which indicates an apparent protective effect of overweight in elderly and very elderly people.

Box 8.1 shows a list of conditions that are associated with high BMI and which are probably caused or worsened by obesity. Increased numbers of

premature deaths from some of these conditions are largely responsible for the increased mortality and reduced life expectancy of obese people. Death rates from strokes, coronary heart disease, type 2 diabetes, diseases of the liver and digestive system and certain cancers in women are particularly high in the obese.

Box 8.1 Some conditions which are thought to be caused by obesity or worsened by it

Heart and circulatory system

- Coronary heart disease
- Stroke
- Hypertension
- Angina pectoris
- Sudden death due to ventricular arrhythmia (abnormal heart rhythm)
- Congestive heart failure
- Varicose veins, haemorrhoids, swollen ankles, and venous thrombosis.

Joints

- Osteoarthritis – knees

Endocrine/metabolic

- Type 2 diabetes (maturity-onset diabetes)
- Gout
- Gallstones

Cancer

- In women, increased risk of cancer of the ovary, cervix (neck of the womb), breast and endometrium (lining of the womb)
- In men, increased risk of prostate cancer and cancers of the colon and rectum

Other

- Increased risk of pregnancy complications
- Reduced fertility
- Menstrual irregularities
- Increased risk during anaesthesia and surgery
- Reduced mobility, agility and increased risk of accidents
- Adverse psychological, social and economic consequences (see later in the chapter)

Risk factors

- Raised blood lipids including blood cholesterol
- Raised blood uric acid levels
- Elevation of blood pressure
- Insulin resistance
- Increased plasma fibrinogen concentration

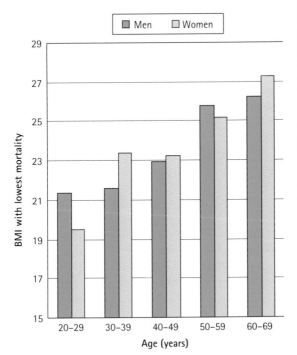

Figure 8.10 *Effect of age on the apparent 'ideal' body mass index (BMI). Data source: Andres* et al. *(1985).*

The WHO has suggested that approximately 58 per cent of diabetes, 21 per cent of ischaemic heart disease and 8–42 per cent of cancers in the world are attributable to a BMI in excess of $21\,kg/m^2$.

Obesity and the quality of life

Some of the conditions listed in Box 8.1 may cause ill health and disability even if they are unlikely to be a primary cause of death, e.g. gout and arthritis. Type 2 diabetes increases the risk of cardiovascular disease and strokes and also leads to many problems that are disabling even though not necessarily acutely fatal, e.g. blindness, peripheral neuropathy, gangrene and progressive renal failure (see Chapter 16). One Finnish study (Rissanen et al., 1990) found that overweight people were much more likely to claim a disability pension than normal weight people. The authors concluded that being overweight is a major cause of disability in Finland. This effect of overweight on disability seemed to start at relatively low BMI where the effect on mortality is normally small or non-existent (25+ for women and 27+ for men). The effect of overweight on disability also seemed to be more pronounced in women than in men. Being overweight or obese not only shortens life but also reduces the proportion of life that is spent free of major illness and disability. In the USA, it has also been reported that obese workers take increased amounts of sick leave and have higher numbers of disability claims. The direct medical costs of obesity in the USA were estimated to represent more than 7 per cent of the total healthcare budget in 1995 and the costs of higher rates of sick leave and disability claims were estimated to cost American businesses more than $3 billion at 1996 prices.

Box 8.1 also shows several **risk factors** for heart disease that are raised in the obese. Risk factors are parameters that predict the risk of developing or dying of particular diseases and in many cases are assumed to contribute to the cause of the disease. It is the increases in these risk factors that probably lead to much of the excess mortality of obese people. In a large survey of English adults, Bennett et al. (1995) found the following examples of associations between BMI and cardiovascular risk factors.

- Overweight and obese people have high blood pressure. In this survey, people with a BMI of over 30 had double the risk of **hypertension** compared

with people with a BMI in the 20–$25\,kg/m^2$ range. Blood pressure rose with increasing BMI in all age and sex groups. More recently, Sproston and Primatesta (2004) have confirmed a progressive increase in systolic blood pressure in both men and women in England as one goes up the standard BMI categories shown in Table 8.1.

- Overweight and obese people have reduced insulin sensitivity and high average blood glucose concentrations (early indications of the onset of type 2 diabetes). **Glycosylated haemoglobin** concentration in blood tends to rise with average blood glucose concentration and so it is used as a marker for high blood glucose concentration. In this survey, obese people had the highest levels of glycosylated haemoglobin and those with a BMI of less than $20\,kg/m^2$ had the lowest levels.
- People who are overweight or obese tend to have the highest blood cholesterol levels. In this survey there was a clear tendency for blood cholesterol to rise with increasing BMI.
- Obese people in this survey tended to have increased plasma uric acid levels.
- Plasma fibrinogen concentration is used as an indicator of the blood's tendency to clot and form thromboses. Plasma fibrinogen concentration tended to rise with increasing BMI in this survey.

In general, these risk factors tend to rise during weight gain and they tend to fall during weight reduction and this indicates that weight gain, per se, or the behaviours that lead to weight gain, are the direct cause of these elevated risk factor levels. Type 2 diabetes seems to be triggered by a decline in target tissue sensitivity to insulin (insulin resistance) rather than a primary failure of insulin secretion. In experimental studies, deliberate overfeeding and weight gain reduces insulin sensitivity in animals and people; insulin sensitivity increases during weight loss (e.g. Sims et al., 1973). Weight loss is known to lessen the symptoms of type 2 diabetes. For men in their forties, being moderately obese (BMI $31\,kg/m^2$) increases the risk of developing type 2 diabetes by 10-fold and in those with a BMI of over $35\,kg/m^2$ the risk is 77 times higher (Chan et al., 1994). Type 2 diabetes has until recently been almost exclusively confined to older adults but more recently the disease has started to affect obese children even before they reach the age of puberty.

Weight loss is also an accepted part of the treatment for hypertension and gout. Gout is the painful joint condition caused by crystals of uric acid forming in the joints when blood uric acid levels are elevated.

In addition to higher morbidity and mortality, there are major social and economic disadvantages to being overweight. In some cultures, obesity may be admired as a symbol of wealth and success and fatness regarded as physically attractive. In most Western countries, however, the obese have long been poorly regarded and discriminated against. In his book on obesity, Mayer (1968) devotes a whole chapter to largely literary examples of hostility towards the obese and Gilbert (1986) also includes a short, referenced review of negative attitudes towards the obese. Several studies have been conducted in which children have been asked to rate the likability of other children from pictures and to assign various character traits to them. They consistently rate the obese children in these pictures as less likeable than the lean and, in some studies, even less likeable than children with physical deformities such as missing limbs or facial disfigurement. They attribute unpleasant characteristics to the obese children in the pictures – comments such as they are 'lazy', 'dirty', 'stupid', 'ugly' and that they are 'cheats' and 'liars'. Similar attitudes are also widespread among adults of all social classes. Even among those professionally involved in the treatment of obesity, the obese may be seen as self-indulgent people who lack willpower and overeat to compensate for their emotional problems (these early studies are reviewed and referenced in Wadden and Stunkard, 1985).

Obese people are subject to practical discrimination as well; they are less likely to be accepted for university education and for employment. Gortmaker *et al.* (1993) did a 7-year follow-up study of 10 000 young people in Boston, who were aged 16–24 years at the start of the study. They found that, particularly among women, there were substantial social and economic disadvantages to being obese. After 7 years, those women who were obese at the start of the study:

- had completed fewer years at school
- had lower household incomes and were more likely to be below the poverty line
- were less likely to be married (another study has reported that obese lower class women are much less likely to marry men of higher social class than lean lower class women).

Similar trends were seen in the men but the magnitude of the disadvantages attributed to being obese were substantially smaller. The investigators concluded that prejudice and discrimination were the main causes of these socioeconomic disadvantages of being obese. They were not due to differences in the socioeconomic status of the obese subjects at the start of the study nor to differences in levels of ability as measured by initial performance of the young people on intelligence and aptitude tests. This conclusion was also supported by their finding that there was no evidence of similar reduced socioeconomic prospects for those subjects who at the start of the study had a chronic physical condition such as asthma, diabetes or a musculoskeletal problem. Such conditions could well have reduced physical performance but being obese was more of a socioeconomic handicap over this 7-year period than having a chronic condition. It was noted earlier in this chapter that in industrialized countries, obesity, especially among women, is more common in those with the lowest socioeconomic status and the least well educated groups (see Table 8.4). This is usually presented as low educational attainment and low social status being risk factors for obesity but these observations also suggest that perhaps obesity may restrict educational opportunities and lower social status.

These negative attitudes to the obese may well be rooted in the historically assumed association between overweight, excessive food intake and inactivity, i.e. obesity is widely assumed to be due to greed and laziness. The obese are seen as responsible for their own condition due to the presence of these two undesirable personality traits.

Is all body fat equally bad?

Studies in the early 1980s indicated that the **waist-to-hip ratio (WHR)** was an important determinant of the health risks associated with obesity. This measure is the circumference of the body at the waist divided by that around the hips and it is used as a simple indicator of body fat distribution. The health risks seem to be greater if the obesity is associated with a high WHR. Such people are sometimes called 'apple-shaped' and this is the typically male (ovoid) pattern of fat distribution. There is much less risk if the obesity is associated with a low WHR. This is termed 'pear-shaped' or gynoid and is the typically female pattern (reviewed by Seidell, 2000).

Inactivity, smoking and high alcohol consumption seem to be associated with high WHR and **hormone replacement therapy** in post-menopausal women seems to reduce central fat deposition (see Samaras and Campbell, 1997).

As one would expect, average WHR is higher in men than in women and it tends to rise with age in both sexes, i.e. people tend to thicken around the waist as they get older 'middle-aged spread'. Figure 8.11 shows how average WHR rises with age in English men and women. Note that the values used to construct Figure 8.11 are on average approximately 2 per cent higher in men and 3 per cent in women than equivalent data collected a decade previously; not only is average BMI rising but so is average WHR. A raised WHR is defined as 0.95 or more in men or 0.85 or more in women. Waist circumference is also used as an even simpler indication of abdominal obesity and a raised waist circumference is defined as 102 cm or more in men and 88 cm or more in women. Simple measures of fat distribution like WHR and waist circumference are being increasingly used to gauge the magnitude of risk associated with a particular level of overweight or obesity and thus the priority that should be given to weight reduction (see Ashwell, 1994 for a review of these measures). A BMI of 27 kg/m^2 in a person with a high WHR seems to carry more health risk than a BMI of 30 kg/m^2 in someone with a low WHR.

Table 8.5 shows the percentage of English men and women at different ages who are over the threshold values for WHR and waist circumference. Over a third of all English adults are above these thresholds with substantially higher proportions in middle-aged and elderly people.

Table 8.5 The percentage of English men and women by age above the threshold values indicative of raised waist-to-hip ratio WHR (0.95 men/0.85 women) and raised waist circumference (102 cm men/88 cm women)

Age (years)	Waist-to-hip ratio		Waist circumference	
	Men	Women	Men	Women
16–24	4	11	9	21
25–34	14	18	20	30
35–44	32	26	30	37
45–54	41	28	38	42
55–64	54	42	41	51
65–74	57	45	49	61
75+	51	54	31	41
All ages	33	30	31	41

Date source: Sproston and Primatesta (2004).

This research on WHR and related measures suggests that fat deposited in the abdominal cavity may be largely responsible for the detrimental health consequences of being overweight or obese. Large amounts of abdominal fat seem to predispose people to diabetes and heart disease. The increase in heart disease may be largely a consequence of the predisposition to diabetes. South Asians seem to be particularly prone to diabetes and heart disease and have higher WHRs than Caucasians at any given BMI (see Chapter 17).

The fat cells in the abdominal cavity have different metabolic characteristics and hormone receptor profiles to those of fat cells taken from subcutaneous sites. The abdominal fat cells of obese women have fewer insulin receptors and the receptors have lower affinity for insulin compared to fat cells taken from a subcutaneous site in the same women. Thus high levels of abdominal obesity predispose individuals to type 2 diabetes and the other adverse health consequences of abdominal obesity are probably secondary to this increased risk of diabetes (Bolinder et al., 1983).

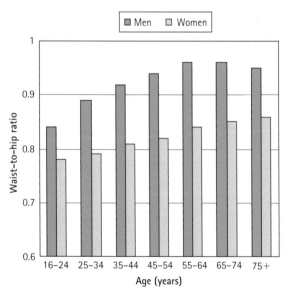

Figure 8.11 *Rise in average waist-to-hip ratio with age. Data source: Sproston and Primatesta (2004).*

Weight cycling

In line with the high prevalence of obesity, there is also a high prevalence of weight dissatisfaction and dieting, particularly among women. At any one time, perhaps a third of American women are dieting and studies in England and Ireland have found that most adolescent girls have tried to lose weight (see Ryan *et al.*, 1998). Many dieters fail to lose significant amounts of weight but many others do achieve substantial short-term weight losses only to regain this weight once their diet is relaxed. This cycle of weight loss and regain has been termed **weight cycling** or **yo-yo dieting**.

It is a common perception that people find it increasingly difficult to lose weight after previous cycles of weight loss and regain. One obvious explanation for this observation is simply that it becomes increasingly difficult for people to summon up the effort and willpower to stick to a weight reduction programme after being dispirited by previous experience of rapid weight regain soon wiping out any hard-won weight losses. It has also been suggested that cycles of weight loss and regain might lower metabolic rate and so predispose people to weight gain because of the replacement of lean tissue by fat during these cycles of loss and regain. Those studies that have attempted to test this hypothesis with animals or people have generally not found evidence to support it (e.g. Jebb *et al.*, 1991).

Weight fluctuation is also associated with increased mortality risk, leading to speculation that yo-yo dieting might have detrimental health effects *per se*. One large American study did indeed find that men who had experienced weight loss or weight fluctuation had an elevated mortality risk. However, when smokers and those with existing ill health were excluded from the analysis then this association between weight fluctuation and elevated mortality risk disappeared. This led the authors to conclude that any association between weight fluctuation and elevated mortality is due to the effects of pre-existing illness and smoking and that weight cycling is not, in itself, directly harmful to health (Iribarren *et al.*, 1995). Note, however, that many patients with eating disorders do have a history of yo-yo dieting.

Does high BMI directly cause an increase in mortality?

The earlier observation that risk factors (e.g. blood pressure and insulin resistance) tend to rise and fall with induced changes in body weight provides persuasive support for the belief that the association between BMI and mortality is a cause and effect relationship. There are two probable scenarios:

- *either* the presence of excessive amounts of body fat directly hastens death via development of the diseases shown in Box 8.1
- *or* the behaviours that cause people to gain weight also increase the risk of ill health.

Such a subtle distinction might seem to be pedantic because in either case changes in behaviour that prevent or reduce obesity should lead to corresponding improvements in health and longevity. Some work by Lee *et al.* (1998) suggests that this may be a significant distinction. They related measured fitness to all-cause mortality in a large sample of men divided into strata on the basis of their BMI. They found, as one might expect, that in each BMI strata, mortality was inversely related to fitness (i.e. the fit were less likely to die). More surprisingly, they also found that men in the high and moderate fitness categories had similar death rates irrespective of BMI category (even those in the BMI 30+ category) and that men in the unfit category had high death rates again irrespective of their BMI category. This suggests that men with high BMI have high mortality because they are much more likely to be inactive and unfit – the inactivity and lack of fitness is the common cause of both their high BMI and high mortality risk. More encouragingly, this would also suggest that increasing activity and improving fitness could substantially reduce the health consequence of overweight and obesity even if it does not lead to substantial weight loss. This lends support to the suggestion in an editorial in the influential *New England Journal of Medicine* (Byers, 1995) that the emphasis of research and health education should be shifted away from body weight *per se* and focus more on the behaviours that lead to excessive weight gain. Rather than focusing on body weight reduction, we should concentrate more on encouraging healthier food choices and increased physical activity, and on reducing the behavioural and cultural barriers that prevent people from adopting this lifestyle pattern.

This is an important point for those working in health education and health promotion to take on board. Huge numbers of people go on diets and spend lots of money on a variety of books and products to try, usually unsuccessfully, to achieve an 'ideal' body shape. The severe social and psychological consequences of being obese mean that very few people are content to be obese and many people are desperate to become or remain lean and are willing to adopt desperate measures to achieve this. Despite this, obesity rates continue to increase. The work of Harris (1983) exemplifies this almost universal wish to be lean. She asked Australian psychology students how they would feel about being obese themselves. All of the students gave negative responses to this question and 60 per cent chose the highest level of negative response offered. Studies with teenage girls in Britain and Ireland have found a high level of dissatisfaction with their body weight. For example, Ryan *et al.* (1998) found that 60 per cent of a sample of 15-year-old Dublin schoolgirls wanted to be slimmer and 68 per cent had tried to lose weight. Most worryingly, many normal-weight and even underweight girls also expressed this wish to be thinner. Many of these girls reported using a variety of unhealthy practices to try to lose weight including purging, smoking, periodic fasting and avoidance of staple foods. Health promotion campaigns that focus on body fat *per se* are, at best, probably pointless because most people already desperately want to become or remain lean. At worst, they may increase the prejudice and discrimination against obese people and push some impressionable young people into trying to lose weight when it is inappropriate, using methods that are harmful.

Key points

- A raised body mass index (BMI) is associated with reduced life expectancy, increased risk of illness and disability, and increased levels of cardiovascular risk factors.

- Increased prevalence of childhood obesity means that type 2 diabetes, once a disease confined to older adults, is now being recorded in obese pre-pubertal children.

- The health consequences of obesity are greater in the young and probably greater in men.

- Low BMI is also associated with reduced life expectancy but this is probably because of an excess of smokers and those with existing ill health in this category.

- Obesity has adverse social and economic consequences for the individual; obese people, especially women, are the subject of widespread prejudice and discrimination.

- Obesity that is associated with a high WHR or a high waist circumference is more harmful than if the WHR is low; excess fat stored in the abdominal cavity is largely responsible for the adverse health consequences of obesity.

- Abdominal fat cells from obese subjects have fewer insulin receptors and these receptors have lower affinity for insulin than those taken from subcutaneous sites.

- Increased predisposition to type 2 diabetes caused by high levels of abdominal fat is probably responsible for the adverse health consequences of abdominal obesity.

- There is no convincing evidence that cycles of weight loss and regain (yo-yo dieting) are directly harmful to health or have physiological consequences that predispose to obesity.

- Any excess mortality attributed to yo-yo dieting (weight fluctuation) is probably due to the weight instability of many smokers and those with existing ill health.

- Cardiovascular risk factor levels (e.g. insulin resistance and blood pressure) tend to rise and fall with weight gain and loss. This suggests that the relationships are probably causal, i.e. either weight gain *per se* or the behaviours that cause weight gain are responsible for the elevated risk factor levels.

- Some evidence suggests that the inactivity and low physical fitness of many obese people may be largely responsible for both their obesity and their reduced health prospects.

- Health promotion should concentrate on encouraging and enabling people to increase their activity and fitness and to eat a healthy low-fat diet.

- Most people already desperately want to become or remain lean so health promotion campaigns that focus on body weight *per se* may achieve little. They may simply:
  - increase prejudice and discrimination against the obese
  - increase the dissatisfaction of overweight people
  - encourage some young people to aim for an inappropriately low body weight and adopt harmful strategies to achieve it.

THE METABOLIC SYNDROME OR 'SYNDROME X'

Type 2 diabetes accounts for over 90 per cent of all diabetes in the UK and is by far the most common endocrine disorder. This type of diabetes is now known to be caused by insulin resistance rather than a primary failure of insulin supply. In type 2 diabetes, lifestyle factors like inactivity, high food intake, obesity (particularly abdominal obesity) and high-fat diet lead to insulin resistance. Those people who develop type 2 diabetes cannot produce sufficient insulin to compensate for the decline in sensitivity and so there is a progressive shortfall in insulin supply leading to gradually increasing symptoms of diabetes. Many people with insulin resistance can compensate by raising their insulin production and thus are able to avoid the immediate symptoms of diabetes such as severe hyperglycaemia, glucose in the urine, high urine flow and excessive thirst and drinking. These non-diabetic but insulin resistant individuals are, however, subject to other metabolic consequences of insulin resistance such as:

- hyperinsulinaemia
- moderate glucose intolerance
- hypertension
- raised plasma triacylglycerol levels
- lowered plasma high-density lipoproteins (HDL) levels.

This myriad of metabolic consequences of insulin resistance are termed the **metabolic syndrome** or sometimes 'syndrome X'. Although people with this syndrome do not have the acute symptoms of diabetes, their condition does nevertheless predispose them to cardiovascular disease in just the same way as having overt type 2 diabetes. Many people with syndrome X will go on to develop overt type 2 diabetes. Any individual who meets three of the following criteria would be classified as syndrome X:

- high waist circumference
- moderate fasting hyperglycaemia
- raised blood pressure
- raised blood triacylglycerol levels
- low plasma HDL levels.

Numerical thresholds for the above criteria have been suggested by an American expert panel (see Reaven, 2006).

Key points

- Insulin resistance in the absence of overt type 2 diabetes still leads to hypertension, high blood triacylglycerol levels, reduced high-density lipoprotein levels and some degree of hyperglycaemia.
- These metabolic consequences of insulin resistance are called the metabolic syndrome or syndrome X.
- Some people with syndrome X will develop diabetes and all of them will be predisposed to cardiovascular disease by their metabolic abnormalities.

CAUSES OF OBESITY

During the course of human evolution, intermittent food shortages and an active lifestyle would have been the norm. The assured availability of a varied, highly palatable and energy dense diet coupled with a negligible requirement for physical work would not have been a general experience. The reality would often have been a general state of food shortage or insecurity interspersed with occasional gluts of food. Those best equipped to cope with limited rations and to survive prolonged bouts of severe food shortage would be the most likely to survive, reproduce and pass on their genes. Some deposition of extra fat reserves during periods of abundance to act as a buffer during the almost inevitable periods of food shortage would have been a considerable aid to survival. Permanent and severe obesity is unlikely under these circumstances because, as we saw in Chapter 7, energy expenditure tends to rise under conditions of energy surplus and this tends to restore energy balance. The monotony, low palatability and low energy density of primitive diets would have tended to limit excess consumption. Overweight and obese people may also have been at a disadvantage in the competition for food. Only where people have an unlimited supply of palatable, varied and energy dense food and where they can curtail their activity as they gain weight would obesity be likely to be prevalent, progressive and often severe. The struggle to ensure energy adequacy and security would have been major selection pressures shaping our mechanisms of energy balance control. The need to prevent excess fat accumulation would have been a more minor influence.

Given these selection pressures, one would expect our regulatory mechanisms to be more efficient at preventing energy deficit rather than preventing energy surplus. Those best equipped to cope with periods of famine and shortage would be more likely to survive and reproduce whereas those best equipped for conditions of continual plenty and inactivity would tend to be selected out during times of famine. It is therefore not too surprising that under conditions of affluence and plenty that many people store more body fat than is desirable for their long-term health prospects. Some populations seem to be even more prone to obesity than Europeans and their descendants, e.g. the Polynesian people of Samoa and some Native American tribes such as the Pima Indians of southern Arizona, where the majority of the adult populations are clinically obese. Often populations that have recently adopted Western dietary and lifestyle habits and are historically accustomed to a harsher energy supply environment seem to be particularly prone to obesity and diabetes. They may have evolved a 'thrifty' genotype that makes them better able to survive such conditions. There is also some evidence that a period of food shortage in early life (or other adverse circumstances like cold exposure) may programme people to become obese in later life if environmental conditions allow it.

Nature or nurture?

Both genetic and environmental influences must be involved in the genesis of obesity, only the relative contribution of nature and nurture is disputed. As we saw in Chapter 7, certain relatively uncommon genetic defects can cause profound obesity in animals and people. It is also possible to selectively breed animals for leanness or fatness. Dietary and environmental changes can also markedly affect the degree of fatness of laboratory or farm animals, e.g. offering rats a varied, palatable and energy-rich diet when confined in cages (cafeteria-feeding) causes them to get fat. The situation of the cafeteria-fed rat seems to mimic the situation of many affluent humans.

There is a strong correlation between the fatness levels of parents and their children and between the fatness levels of siblings but it is difficult to dissect out how much of this is due to common environmental factors and how much to shared genes. Several lines of inquiry point towards a considerable genetic component in this tendency of obesity to run in families.

- There is a much higher correlation between the fatness of monozygotic (identical) twins than between dizygotic (non-identical) twins when they share the same environment. The fatness levels of the monozygotic twins are closer because they share more common genes.
- When monozygotic twins are adopted and reared apart, their fatness levels are still very similar. Despite their differing environments, their identical genes mean that they show similar levels of fatness.
- Large studies on adopted children in Denmark suggest that correlations between the BMI of adopted children and their natural first-degree relatives (parents and siblings) are similar to those in natural families – suggesting that family resemblances in adiposity are mostly due to genetic factors. Of course the environmental and dietary variation between Danish families may be relatively small and this will tend to exaggerate the prominence of genetic factors in determining obesity levels. See Sorensen (1992) for a referenced review of these genetic aspects of obesity.

Although the papers on which the above bullet point statements are based are now more than 15 years old, Hill *et al.* (2006) have quoted a series of more recent papers that essentially repeat and confirm the above findings. Hill *et al.* also conclude that perhaps 40 per cent of the variation in BMI is explained by genetic factors.

Clearly, certain environmental conditions are necessary for the expression of any genetic tendency to obesity but equally some individuals and some populations like the Samoans and Pima Indians, do seem to be more susceptible than others. The widespread use of animal models with some inherited or induced lesion that produces extreme obesity may have encouraged the view that obese and lean are two distinct categories. In reality, there will be a continuum of genetic susceptibility to obesity in people, ranging from very resistant to very susceptible. As the conditions in affluent countries have increasingly favoured the development of obesity so more and more people's 'threshold of susceptibility' has been reached, and so the number of overweight and obese people has risen. The recent large rises in the prevalence of obesity in many populations cannot be due to genetic change; they must be caused by lifestyle changes. The increase in obesity as one goes down the socioeconomic classes is also unlikely to be due primarily to genetics, particularly as it is much less obvious in men than women. The relatively low rates of obesity in some affluent European countries and the low rates of increase suggest that very high rates of obesity and rapid increases in its prevalence are not an inevitable consequence of affluence. That obesity rates in England in 1980 were less than a third of current levels confirms that this change must be the result of dietary and/or lifestyle changes. If English people reversed some of the lifestyle and dietary changes of the past 25 years then there would be corresponding falls in the levels of obesity.

Studies on the Pima Indians provide striking evidence of the need for environmental triggers to produce widespread obesity even in a population considered genetically susceptible to obesity. Several centuries ago, one group of Pima Indians settled in southern Arizona while another group settled in the mountains of Mexico. These two groups remain genetically very similar. Present day Mexican Pimas do not have widespread obesity; they are subsistence farmers who spend many hours each week in hard physical labour and still eat a fairly traditional low-fat, high-carbohydrate diet. In contrast, the Arizona Pimas have ceased to be subsistence farmers, they are now a sedentary population, and they eat a typical high-fat American diet, consequently, they have one of the highest rates of obesity in the world (see Gibbs, 1996).

A weakening link between hunger and eating? The internal/external hypothesis and behaviour therapy

Hunger is the drive or need to eat food that is initiated by the **appestat** in response to internal physiological signals such as absence of food in the gut, low blood glucose concentration or depleted fat stores. As noted in Chapter 7, many 'external' factors, in addition to physiological need, determine when, where, what and how much we eat. **Appetite**, the desire to eat palatable food, may persist even after hunger has been quenched. Social convention, emotional state or just the hedonistic pleasure of eating may cause us to eat in the absence of hunger. Hunger will usually drive us to eat but absence of hunger will not necessarily prevent us from eating. By analogy, we do not have to be thirsty to make a cup of tea or to accept the offer of a social drink. Thirst will cause us to drink but we may drink for pleasure or to be sociable when we are not thirsty. We can easily excrete excess fluid but we are less well equipped to burn off surplus calories notwithstanding the discussion of adaptive thermogenesis in Chapter 7. Perhaps modern diets and lifestyles weaken the link between hunger and eating and make us more prone to excess consumption and weight gain. For most people in affluent populations:

- food is more consistently abundant than it has ever been
- there is less effort required to prepare food and more encouragement to consume it (e.g. advertizing) than ever before
- food is more varied, palatable and energy dense than it has ever been
- the requirement for food has never been lower because of our inactive lifestyles and the high energy density of our diets.

Schachter (1968) proposed that lean people regulate their food intake primarily in response to their internal physiological hunger mechanisms whereas obese people are much more responsive to external, non-physiological influences on their feeding behaviour. Schachter and Rodin (1974) identified certain behavioural characteristics of obese rats and then, in an ingenious series of experiments, demonstrated very similar behavioural characteristics in obese people (see the examples below).

- Obese rats and people consumed more food than leans when it was readily available but less than leans when they were required to work for the food. Obese rats generally ate more than lean ones but if they were required to run through a maze to obtain food then the lean ate more than the obese. In another experiment, lean and fat people were offered nuts to eat in a disguised situation. If these nuts were opened and easy to eat, the obese subjects ate many more than the lean ones but when the subjects had to crack them open for themselves the obese ate far fewer nuts than the lean!

- Obese rats and people consumed more than leans when the food was palatable but less when it was made unpalatable, e.g. by the addition of bitter-tasting quinine. They were more finicky.
- The feeding behaviour of obese rats and people was more affected by their anxiety state than was that of the lean.

Schachter and Rodin (1974) concluded that the feeding behaviour of obese rats and obese people was motivated primarily by appetite (the learned, hedonistic desire to eat food) rather than by hunger (the physiological need to eat food). The lean appeared to be driven to eat by hunger but the obese were persuaded to eat by ease of access, high palatability and for emotional comfort. This theory has lost favour in recent years – external orientation of food regulation is not confined to the obese. Nevertheless, it has had a great practical influence on the treatment of obesity. Much of the behavioural treatment of obesity is based on this concept of external orientation of food intake regulation in obese people.

Behaviour is envisaged as being initiated by certain cues or antecedents and then if the behaviour results in pleasure that acts as a reward or reinforcement and that behaviour is learned. If the behaviour has unpleasant consequences then this acts as negative reinforcement and discourages repetition of the behaviour (see Figure 8.12). Thus obese people are triggered into inappropriate eating behaviour by certain circumstances or cues and their inappropriate behaviour is rewarded, and thus learned, because of the pleasure or relief of anxiety that results from the inappropriate eating behaviour. **Behaviour therapy** seeks to identify the cues or antecedents to inappropriate behaviour (e.g. eating high-energy foods). It then involves devising ways of avoiding these cues and ways of reinforcing or rewarding appropriate behaviours (e.g. taking exercise or achieving weight loss targets) so that they are 'learned'.

To identify the antecedents or cues that trigger inappropriate eating behaviour, patients are often asked to keep a diary of when and what they eat, and in what circumstances they eat it. They are then encouraged to modify their habits and environment to reduce these cues using techniques such as:

- they may be encouraged to avoid the temptation to buy high-energy foods on impulse by shopping strictly from a list
- they may reduce casual, impulse consumption of high-energy snacks by making them less accessible, e.g. keeping them on a high shelf or in a locked cabinet so that this snacking has to be a premeditated act
- they may reduce the temptation to pick at food they are preparing by encouraging other family members to prepare their own snacks
- they can reduce the temptation to eat leftovers by throwing them away immediately.

They may be encouraged to modify the process of eating using techniques such as:

- always using utensils and never eating with fingers
- slowing down the eating process by chewing food thoroughly, using a smaller spoon, pausing between mouthfuls or introducing a short gap in the meal
- never eating alone but always with other family members
- leaving some food on their plate at the end of a meal.

They are also encouraged to increase the cues to appropriate behaviour, e.g.:

- keeping walking shoes and equipment for active pursuits in easily accessible and visible locations
- keeping low-energy snacks ready prepared and in a prominent place in the refrigerator.

Most therapists avoid the use of active 'punishment' in their schemes. Patients are encouraged to eat with others and therapists will praise and encourage appropriate behaviour but pointedly ignore inappropriate behaviour and simply withhold praise. Scolding is seen as attention giving and thus a form of reward, whereas withholding of attention is seen as punishment. In the past, some behaviour therapists have used punishment as an active part of their programme – so-called aversion therapy. Patients were shown images of problems foods followed by painful electric shocks or some other unpleasant image in the hope that they would learn to associate these foods with unpleasant sensations

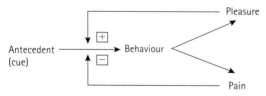

Figure 8.12 *Pain or pleasure elicited by an action encourages learning and repetition of that action.*

and so avoid them! A thorough and referenced review of the behavioural methods employed to treat obesity may be found in Gilbert (1986).

Variety of food and sensory-specific satiety

Rolls *et al.* (1982) reviewed a series of experiments which suggested that increasing food variety may encourage increased consumption. Volunteers were asked to rate the pleasantness of different foods after eating various foods. Previous consumption of a food reduced its pleasantness rating and the desire to consume more of it, but had little effect on that of other foods – they termed this phenomenon '**sensory-specific satiety**'. When people ate sausages then their rating for sausages was reduced but the pleasantness rating for other foods, e.g. fruit or cookies was largely unaffected by eating sausages. Subjects offered successive plates of sandwiches ate more if the sandwiches contained different fillings than if they were all the same. More surprisingly, subjects offered successive plates of pasta ate more if the pasta shape was varied than if the shape was the same. Variation in taste or appearance increased the amount eaten. If a diet is monotonous then we are less likely to overeat than if it is varied. This is not too surprising a conclusion – most of us can usually be persuaded to accept a little dessert even when satiated by earlier courses of the meal. Even laboratory rats eat much more when they are offered a variety of foods (**cafeteria feeding**).

Sensory-specific satiety should increase the range of foods that people eat and limit the consumption of any single food. It should therefore decrease the likelihood of nutritional inadequacies because they are unlikely if the diet is varied. It would also reduce the likelihood that any of the toxins found in small amounts in many foods would be consumed in sufficient quantities to be hazardous. In an affluent population, nutrient deficiencies are unlikely, food is always plentiful and its variety appears almost limitless. Under such conditions, sensory-specific satiety probably encourages overeating and excessive weight gain.

Since these early studies, the concept of sensory-specific satiety has become widely accepted. A decline in sensory specific-satiety with age may explain why elderly people consume a more monotonous diet and may have a role in the decline in appetite frequently reported in older people

(Rolls, 1993). Other studies have shown formally that increased variety leads to increase in food and energy intake and may lead to positive energy balance in the short to medium term (sensory influences on food intakes are reviewed by Sorensen *et al.*, 2003). For example, McCrory *et al.* (1999) found that with each of 10 food groups, energy intake was positively associated with variety. They suggested that increased variety within certain food groups was positively associated with body fatness, e.g. sweets, snacks, condiments, entrees and carbohydrates, and that increased variety from vegetables was negatively associated with body fatness.

> ## Key points
>
> - Evolutionary pressures may have caused the mechanisms that regulate energy balance to be relatively ineffective at preventing excess energy storage.
> - Some populations (e.g. the Pima Indians and Samoans) are extremely prone to obesity; a harsh environment in the past may have caused them to evolve with a 'thrifty' genotype.
> - Studies with twins and adopted children suggest that much of the family resemblance in fatness levels is due to genetic factors.
> - Clearly, both environmental and genetic influences determine an individual's or a population's fatness.
> - Certain environmental conditions are necessary before any inherited predisposition to obesity is expressed.
> - Recent changes in obesity prevalence must be due to lifestyle changes.
> - Even in those groups with an extreme propensity to obesity (such as the Pima Indians), it only becomes prevalent when environmental conditions are conducive to obesity.
> - Hunger will drive us to eat during fasting or fat store depletion but absence of hunger will not always prevent us from eating.
> - 'External' influences such as pleasure of eating, habit, social pressures or anxiety may cause us to eat in the absence of hunger.
> - The feeding of obese people is said to be more influenced by external factors than that of lean people who are thought to be more responsive to their internal regulatory mechanisms.

- Behavioural therapy is based on the notion of external orientation of feeding control in obese people.
- In behaviour therapy obese people are encouraged to identify and avoid the external cues that trigger inappropriate eating and to facilitate and reward appropriate behaviour (e.g. taking exercise).
- Wide variety of food encourages higher consumption. As one food is eaten, so satiation for that food develops but the desire to eat other foods is much less affected – sensory-specific satiety.
- Increased variety within some food groups encourages over-consumption of food energy and weight gain.

Is fat more fattening than carbohydrate?

This topic was reviewed by Livingstone (1996) and some of the uncited references are listed here. For many years, it was very widely held that carbohydrates, and especially sugar, were the most fattening components of the diet. This notion was reinforced by a string of popular diet books that promoted a variety of low-carbohydrate diets as the best diets for weight loss. These popular diet books included one written by an eminent British professor of nutrition (John Yudkin – *This slimming business*). In his book, Yudkin made the point that severe restriction of dietary carbohydrate would not only affect the carbohydrate foods that provided a high proportion of the dietary energy but would also indirectly reduce the fat that is normally consumed with these foods. He expected that on his diet, fat consumption would either drop or stay the same. Thus bread, sugary foods and drinks, breakfast cereals, rice, pasta, potatoes, cakes, biscuits, etc. are deliberately restricted but so indirectly are, for example, butter/margarine that is spread on bread, fat used to fry potatoes, rice or other carbohydrate foods, the fat in battered or bread-crumbed fish or meat, the fat in pies. Low-carbohydrate diets may also include milk (especially low-fat milk!) on the prohibited or restricted list because of its lactose content. Under these circumstances it is difficult to make up the lost carbohydrate calories by replacing them with fat because concentrated fat is nauseating. The net result would often be a reduction in total energy intake and this accounts for the frequent short-term successes of currently fashionable low-carbohydrate diets such as the Atkins diet.

Current wisdom and advice is the opposite to these earlier views; fat is now regarded as more fattening than carbohydrate and the current consensus among nutritionists is that diets that are rich in starch and fibre but low in fat are most likely to prevent excessive weight gain and achieve long-term weight control. There are, of course, other important reasons for moderating fat intake as discussed in Chapter 11. In cross-sectional studies of populations, dietary and anthropometric data are collected from large samples of people. It is often found in such studies that there is a positive correlation between the proportion of energy that is derived from fat and BMI; those who get the highest proportion of their energy from fat are the most likely to be fat. Given the **carbohydrate–fat** and **sugar–fat see-saws** discussed in Chapter 6, it almost inevitably follows that as the proportion of energy from carbohydrate or even sugar increases so BMI tends to fall; those who get more of their energy from carbohydrate or sugar tend to be leaner. In one study of over 11 500 Scots, Bolton-Smith and Woodward (1996) found that the prevalence of overweight and obesity decreased with an increase in the proportion of energy derived from carbohydrate or from sugar but increased with increases in the proportion of energy that came from fat. In the 20 per cent of the men in this Scottish population who had the highest fat-to-sugar ratios, rates of obesity were 3.5 times higher than in the 20 per cent with the lowest ratios (double in women).

There is evidence that very-low-fat diets (say under 20 per cent of energy from fat) are associated with weight loss even when total energy intake is not restricted. High-fat diets on the other hand lead to over-consumption of energy (positive energy balance) in animal studies and those using free-living human subjects. Lissner *et al.* (2000) discuss data obtained from a prospective study of middle-aged and elderly Swedish women which indicate that increases in dietary fat content predict the long-term development of central obesity as measured by WHR. They concluded that their data 'may reflect a causal role for total fat intake in the development of central adiposity'. Astrup *et al.* (2000) did a meta-analysis of studies that had used *ad libitum* (i.e. not calorie restricted) low-fat diets in intervention trials. Their analysis indicated that low-fat diets prevented weight gain in normal weight individuals and led to modest weight loss in overweight and obese subjects. The magnitude of weight loss in these studies was greatest in those who were most overweight at the start of the trial. Effective population-based messages aimed at reducing the proportion of dietary calories derived from fat may achieve some weight loss but the greatest benefit is likely to be in preventing excess weight gain in the first place.

There may well be an interaction between activity and dietary fat content in their effects on energy balance control. In one study the proportion of energy from fat was varied (20 per cent, 40 per cent or 60 per cent of energy from fat) in active and sedentary men. The active men were in negative energy balance on the 20 per cent fat diet and still in slight negative balance at 40 per cent but had a small positive balance when fat was raised to 60 per cent of energy. The inactive men, however, only achieved balance on the 20 per cent fat diet and were in substantial positive balance on the other two diets. These observations suggest that in sedentary populations, diets with fat contents typically found in Western industrialized societies are likely to promote positive energy balance and weight gain. As we become more sedentary so our high-fat diets will make us increasingly susceptible to obesity.

These are several theoretical reasons why one might expect fat to be more fattening than carbohydrate.

- Fat is energy dense. It yields more than twice as much energy as the same weight of carbohydrate or protein. This means that high-fat diets are inevitably energy dense. This may be the predominant reason why high-fat diets encourage over-consumption in free-living situations (see discussion of energy density in Chapter 6).
- Fat increases the palatability of food and this will tend to encourage over-consumption especially if it replaces bland starch. Overweight and obese people seem to have an increased preference for high-fat foods.
- The conversion of excess dietary fat to body fat is a very efficient process and only about 4 per cent of the energy is wasted in the conversion process. In contrast, the conversion of dietary carbohydrate to fat leads to the loss of about 25 per cent of the energy in the conversion process. The

conversion of dietary protein into fat is even more wasteful. In practice, on normal, high-fat Western diets, there is very little conversion of dietary carbohydrate to fat and most carbohydrate is either used directly as an energy source or converted to **glycogen**.

- Calorie-for-calorie, fat seems to be less satiating than carbohydrate. Numerous experiments have been performed in which subjects are given iso-energetic preloads of varying composition and the effect on their subsequent hunger ratings and the amount consumed at a subsequent meal are compared. These studies consistently suggest that fat is slightly less satiating than carbohydrate (usually sugar) and that this difference is more pronounced in obese than in lean subjects.
- Consumption of carbohydrate leads to an accelerated use of glucose in metabolism and a reduction in fat oxidation – conditions that are associated with satiation. Consumption of fat has little effect on the metabolism of fat or carbohydrate.

Key points

- Obesity was at one time widely blamed on high-carbohydrate and especially high-sugar diets.
- Low-carbohydrate diets have been widely recommended for weight reduction and often achieve short-term success because they reduce total energy intake and tend also to reduce total fat consumption.
- In cross-population studies, people who get the highest proportion of their energy from fat tend to have the highest body mass index (BMI) whereas those who obtain the highest proportion from carbohydrate or even sugar tend to have the lowest BMI.
- An increase in dietary fat content may be a causal factor in the development of central obesity.
- Very-low-fat diets are associated with weight loss even when total intake is not restricted whereas high-fat diets encourage weight gain.
- Active people may be able to tolerate medium- and high-fat diets without weight gain but in inactive people they lead to weight gain.
- High fat intake encourages weight gain because fat is energy dense, palatable, less satiating than carbohydrate and more efficiently converted to storage fat.

Inactivity as a cause of obesity

The decline in the requirement for physical activity is strongly implicated as an important cause of the rapid increases in the number of overweight and obese people in Europe, America and elsewhere (Prentice and Jebb, 1995). Car ownership, together with automation in the home, garden and workplace have all combined to substantially reduce our mandatory energy expenditure, i.e. the energy we must expend each day to accomplish the tasks of everyday life. Few people in the USA and western Europe now have jobs that are physically demanding. Some people have increased their leisure-time activities to compensate, e.g. recreational walking, jogging, exercise classes, participation in sports, active games. However, for most people any increase in recreational activity does not compensate for the decline in mandatory activity.

There is persuasive evidence that, *per capita*, energy intakes have dropped substantially in Britain in recent decades. According to Durnin (1992) average energy intakes of teenagers were up to a third higher in the 1930s than they were in the 1990s. According to the old National Food Survey, *per capita* household food consumption in Britain dropped by more than a quarter between 1950 and 1992; a similar trend is seen using wider measures of energy consumption (see Figure 8.13). The 2004–5 Expenditure and Food Survey which has replaced the National Food Survey (see Chapter 3) reports that average energy intake in 2004–5 was 1.8 per cent lower than in the previous year, and the long-term trend of a gradual fall in energy intake was continuing. This fall in energy intake has corresponded with the very large increases in the number of people who are overweight and obese, detailed earlier in the chapter; i.e. we are eating less but getting fatter. The only obvious explanation for these opposing trends is that activity levels have declined sharply. The fall in intake has lagged behind the fall in expenditure resulting in an increasingly positive population energy balance that has led to a fattening of the population.

Prentice and Jebb (1995) have reported that increases in obesity prevalence in Britain since 1950 have tended to mirror increases in car ownership and the number of hours that Britons spend in watching television. Large cross-sectional surveys in both the USA and in Britain have found that those who report

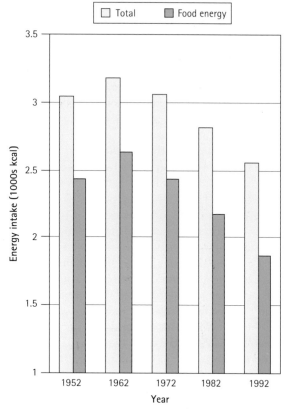

Figure 8.13 *Apparent decline in average energy intake in the UK. Principal data source: COMA (1984).*

being the least active are the most likely to be overweight or obese. Bennett *et al.* (1995) recorded BMI and assessed activity by questionnaire in a large representative sample of English adults. In both men and women, obesity was more than twice as common in the lowest activity band compared to the highest. Information on physical activity was collected by questionnaire in the Health Survey for England 2003 (Sproston and Primatesta, 2004); this found that only 37 per cent of men and 24 per cent of women were meeting the current recommended target of at least 30 minutes of activity of at least moderate intensity on at least five occasions per week. In men the proportion who met this recommended level declined sharply with age whereas in women in remained fairly stable until around 55 years of age and then declined. This survey, as in previous years, found a strong inverse relationship between reported physical activity and BMI. Participants were classified as having high, medium or low activity and the proportion of those with high activity declined as BMI rose whereas the proportion of those classified as low activity rose with increasing BMI category. Figure 8.14 shows the odds ratio (relative risk) of having a BMI of over 25 kg/m^2 or over 30 kg/m^2 in the three different activity categories. The chances of having a BMI of over 25 kg/m^2 declines highly significantly with increasing activity and this trends is even more pronounced for a BMI of over 30 kg/m^2.

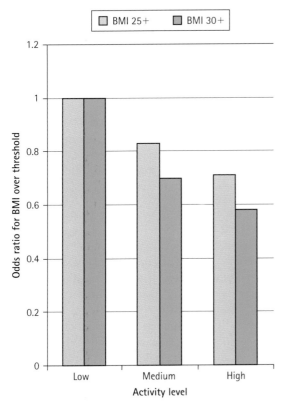

Figure 8.14 *The risk of being overweight or obese according to activity level. BMI, body mass index (kg/m^2).*

In women there is a very pronounced class variation in obesity prevalence. Prentice and Jebb (1995) showed that hours of television viewing, number of people reporting being inactive and obesity rates all rise as one goes down the social classes. Gregory *et al.* (1990) reported that BMI increased with declining social class but that recorded energy intake was also lower in the lower social classes. Women in the lower classes were fatter but reported eating less, again an indication of reduced activity in the most overweight categories. One note of caution must

be sounded about all of these studies. Both food consumption and activity level are self-reported in most studies and there is persuasive evidence that food intake tends to be under-recorded and activity level overestimated in such studies. This tendency to be over-optimistic about activity levels and energy intakes is probably more pronounced in the obese.

Television viewing is now the most popular recreational activity in most industrialized countries. The average Briton now spends twice as much time watching television as they did in 1960 and the average American child watches 28 hours of television each week. Many people now spend more time watching television each week than they do at work or at school. Dietz and Gortmaker (1985) analysed data on television viewing in American children when they were aged 6–11 years and again when they were aged 12–17 years. When they divided the children according to the number of hours of television watched, they found that at both times the prevalence of obesity rose with increased television viewing hours. This trend was most marked in adolescence, and at this stage there was a 2 per cent rise in obesity prevalence for every extra hour of television viewing. They also found that the number of hours of television watching in the 6–11-year-olds was significantly correlated with the prevalence of obesity 6 years later. Those 6–11-year-olds who watched the most television were the most likely to be obese when they reached adolescence, a strong indication that the relationship is a cause and effect one. This study is now more than 20 years old but numerous studies since 1985 have generally confirmed its findings. Thus Jago *et al.* (2005) in the USA conducted a longitudinal study of girls and found that those who watched more than the recommended 2 hours per day when younger were 13.2 times more likely to be overweight at the age of 11 years than those who watched less than 2 hours per day. Viner and Cole (2005) in the UK found that a higher number of hours of weekend television viewing at the age of 5 years predicted a higher BMI at 30 years of age. Each additional hour of television viewing at age 5 increased the risk of being obese at 30 years by 7 per cent. Finally Hancox *et al.* (2004), in a 26-year follow-up of 1000 New Zealand children, found that average weeknight television viewing between the ages of 5 and 15 years was associated with a higher BMI at

26 years and was associated with other adverse health indicators.

Of course, even strong and consistent associations between obesity and inactivity in a variety of studies does not prove that inactivity causes obesity. Apart from the difficulty of measuring activity level, it is also likely that excess weight gain reduces fitness and exercise tolerance and this discourages activity, i.e. an effect and cause relationship. There is almost certainly a large element of truth in both of these suggestions and so a dangerous obesity–inactivity cycle is created (Figure 8.15).

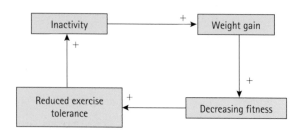

Figure 8.15 *The inactivity–obesity cycle*

Key points

- Reduced requirement for activity to travel and to accomplish household and occupational tasks has led to a general decline in energy expenditure.
- Average energy intake in Britain has fallen substantially in the past 50 years and yet levels of fatness have also increased markedly.
- Energy intake has fallen more slowly than energy expenditure leading to increased levels of fat stores in the population.
- Indirect measures of population inactivity in Britain, such as amount of television viewing and car ownership, have mirrored increases in obesity rates.
- There is persuasive evidence in children that amount of television viewing is positively linked to the risk of obesity.
- Inactivity is a major factor in recent increases in the prevalence of overweight and obesity.
- Inactivity encourages weight gain and weight gain probably discourages activity, leading to a cycle of inactivity and weight gain.

PREVENTION AND TREATMENT OF OBESITY IN POPULATIONS

Adopting a 'low-risk' lifestyle

For effective, long-term weight control one needs to identify dietary and lifestyle patterns that are associated with low risk of obesity without the need for continual restraint on food consumption and calorie counting. From the earlier discussion on the causes of obesity, there seem to be two changes that would lessen an individual's risk of becoming overweight (see below). If these were generally adopted this would lead to a levelling off and eventually a fall in the population prevalence of overweight and obesity. These changes are:

- an increase in activity and fitness levels of the population (or perhaps just a reduction in inactivity)
- a reduction in the proportion of dietary energy that is derived from fat.

Both of these changes would also be likely to have substantial health benefits over and above their effects on body weight. High-fat diets are implicated in the genesis of cardiovascular disease, cancer and perhaps diabetes. The many health benefits of regular exercise are detailed in Chapter 17.

The most obvious way of increasing activity and fitness is by participation in active games, sports or formal exercise sessions and, of course, these need to be encouraged and facilitated. However, the major reason why affluent populations are now so inactive is because mandatory activity has been almost eliminated from everyday life for many people. In order to bring about a substantial increase in the weekly energy expenditure of most people, we also need to find ways of incorporating more activity into everyday living such as in the examples below.

- Making more journeys on foot or bicycle rather than by car. In Britain, journeys of less than a mile account for a third of all car journeys and these have been growing rapidly as a proportion of the total. More of these short journeys need to be made on foot or bicycle.
- Making more use of stairs rather than always taking lifts (elevators) or escalators.
- Becoming less reliant on labour-saving gadgets and doing some tasks by hand.

- Engaging in more leisure-time pursuits that, although not formally exercise, do have a physical activity element, e.g. gardening, home improvement/maintenance, playing with children or walking pets.
- Limiting the time that is spent in totally passive pursuits like watching television or playing computer games. Such pursuits demand physical inactivity and studies with obese children have found that simply reducing access to these sedentary activities was more effective in long-term weight control than programmes involving strenuous exercise sessions. See above for evidence that children who watch the most television have the highest risk of becoming obese in adolescence or even in adulthood.

Health promotion campaigns that are aiming to improve population weight control need to concentrate on:

- making it clear that the priorities for improving weight control are increased activity and a reduction in dietary fat
- educating people about the ways in which they can achieve these objectives, e.g. the sources of fat in the diet and dietary choices that would reduce fat consumption (see Chapter 11), how more activity can be incorporated into everyday living, as well as encouraging participation in formal exercise sessions
- identifying and then looking for ways to minimize the barriers that make it difficult for people to be active and consume less fat.

It must be said that personal choice is a major reason why people are inactive and eat high-fat diets. High fat and sugar content makes food more palatable and so affluent populations tend to consume diets that are high in fat and sugar. Many affluent people have no necessity to be active and indeed their sedentary occupations may force them to be inactive during long working and commuting hours. To fill their leisure-time they have access to pleasurable and almost addictive pursuits that are also totally inactive. It is therefore not surprising that many people chose to be very inactive under these circumstances. Health promoters can only try to encourage people to go against their natural inclinations and adopt healthier lifestyle patterns. However, there may also be circumstances that encourage

unhealthy lifestyles or barriers that prevent people adopting healthier lifestyles. Some barriers to being more active are as follows.

- A lack of access to sports facilities or just to safe, attractive open space, e.g. no local facilities, inconvenient opening hours, high cost of entry or membership fees, lack of money to buy sports clothing or equipment.
- Real or perceived danger when walking or cycling, e.g. vulnerability to injury by motor vehicles, fear of mugging or molestation, the noise and pollution caused by motor vehicles.
- Town planning decisions that assume that the car is the only mode of transport and make no provision for pedestrians or cyclists.
- Long hours spent in the workplace, in sedentary jobs in an environment that discourages physical activity and with no opportunity to do anything active.

Some barriers to reducing fat consumption are listed below.

- Low-fat diets tend to be less palatable than high-fat diets.
- Lack of availability of low-fat foods. In fact the availability of low- or reduced-fat foods has increased in line with consumer demand for these products. Low-fat spreads, reduced-fat cheddar cheese, low-fat milk and yoghurt, reduced-fat crisps (chips) and savoury snacks, extra lean meat, reduced-fat French fries, low-fat cakes and biscuits (cookies) and reduced-fat ready meals are all readily available now. Note that some of the products listed still contain substantial amounts of fat and/or sugar even though their fat content is lower than the standard product, e.g. reduced-fat crisps and savoury snacks, reduced-fat cheddar cheese. Until recently the food provided in restaurants and some fast food outlets usually had much more limited low-fat options although this is starting to change and even some of the large fast food chains are introducing 'healthier ranges'.
- The increased cost of a diet that is both lower in fat and still palatable. Starchy foods are cheap but rather bland. Many low or reduced fat products carry a price premium over the standard product and almost all do if one expresses cost as calories (or joules) per penny. Fruits and vegetables, lean

meat, white fish are all relatively expensive using this criterion. These extra costs may be significant for those on low incomes.

- Lack of knowledge about the sources of dietary fat.

Suggesting measures to reduce these barriers takes us firmly into the political arena and so I am not going to attempt to suggest detailed solutions. An increased risk of obesity is just one of many health consequences of poverty and poor educational attainment. If we are to substantially increase activity levels in the population as a whole then the safety and comfort of pedestrians and cyclists needs to be given a higher priority by politicians, town planners, property developers and law enforcement agencies. This may have to include active measures to discourage car usage, especially for short urban journeys.

Targeting anti-obesity measures or campaigns

Is it possible to identify an age groups where intervention to prevent or reduce obesity is likely to be most effective? Intuitively, childhood would seem to be a crucial time because this is when good dietary and lifestyle patterns can be set for the rest of life and this would seem like a better option than trying to change bad habits later in life. Most obese adults were not obese as children but the two-thirds of obese children do become obese adults and it may well be bad habits learned earlier in life that are responsible for much adult-onset obesity. The observations noted earlier that hours of television viewing in early childhood predicts BMI in adulthood supports this intuitive belief. Some possible measures that could be directed towards children are listed below.

- Giving proper weighting to food and nutrition, including food preparation skills, in the school curriculum. If people are advised to reduce their fat consumption they must have a clear idea of where our dietary fat comes from and what practical measures would reduce fat consumption. They should have the skills and confidence to prepare appealing healthy dishes.
- Recognition of the importance of physical education to the long-term well-being of children. It should not be sacrificed to make room for more academic work in the school timetable.

- Games teaching should seek to involve all children, not just the talented minority. There should also be more emphasis on those activities that are more likely to be continued into adulthood. We would think poorly of a school that concentrated all of its academic efforts onto the brightest pupils and on subjects that were unlikely to be used in later life. It may require considerable innovation and ingenuity to engage some of the less athletically minded pupils with physical education programmes that they will enjoy and willingly participate in.
- Trying to limit the time spent in watching television and playing computer games. Ideally this should be by persuasion rather than coercion, e.g. by offering children more attention and more opportunities to spend some of their leisure time in enjoyable alternative activities.
- Every effort should be made to facilitate activity in children, e.g. by ensuring that they can walk or cycle to school safely. One can try to change the **subjective norm** by making activity more fashionable, e.g. by emphasizing the environmental benefits of walking to school.

At one time, the **fat cell theory** (Hirsch and Han, 1969) gave a formal theoretical basis for this belief that childhood was the best time to act. Hirsch and Han suggested that early overfeeding permanently increased the number of fat cells and thus predisposed children to obesity in later life. This theory was based on some dubious extrapolation of experiments with rats to people. In the first few weeks of life, Hirsch and Han suggested that rat adipose tissue grew by both cell division increasing the number of fat cells and by increases in fat cell size. According to this theory, at about 6 weeks old the number of fat cells in the rat was fixed and any increases in adipose tissue in adult rats could only occur by increases in the size of existing fat cells. Overfeeding before 6 weeks of age permanently increased rats' numbers of fat cells and so might have permanently increased their susceptibility to obesity. Pond (1987) provided very persuasive arguments for not applying these ideas to people. Pond had found that fat cell numbers could be increased throughout life in primates and that the capacity of primate fat cells to increase by expansion alone was rather limited compared with the rat. She suggested that the key premise of this fat cell theory was false.

It has also been suggested earlier that a period of deprivation in early life may programme people to become obese in later life if conditions allow it.

OBESITY TREATMENT IN INDIVIDUALS

Realistic rates of weight loss

To lose substantial amounts of weight, energy expenditure must exceed energy intake for a considerable length of time. A moderately low-fat diet and a reasonably active lifestyle may be effective in preventing much excess weight gain. However, to lose fat that has already accumulated within a reasonable time-scale will probably require a period of deliberate and uncomfortable food restriction (dieting). Most treatments for obesity represent different strategies for making this dieting easier, more effective and more acceptable. This applies even to most anti-obesity drugs and surgical treatments for obesity.

If one assumes that 1 kg of adipose tissue yields about 29 MJ (7000 kcal) then even a daily deficit of 4.2 MJ (1000 kcal) will only result in the loss of 1 kg of adipose tissue per week. This is probably the most that can be hoped for from conventional dieting and for small women or inactive people then perhaps as little as half of this may be a more realistic target. During the first week of a diet or in severe dieting, weight loss may be much faster than this because of loss of glycogen reserves and protein (lean tissue). Every 1 kg of body glycogen or protein is associated with $\geq$3 kg of water, so to lose 1 kg via these routes requires an energy deficit of only about 4.2 MJ (1000 kcal). However, body glycogen reserves are limited and loss of lean tissue is not the aim of dieting. Any weight lost via these routes can be rapidly regained once the diet is relaxed. It also takes significantly more than 29 MJ (7000 kcal) to synthesize 1 kg of adipose tissue and so on a more positive note, an occasional lapse in an otherwise successful diet (say two chocolate bars at 1 MJ (250 kcal) each is not going to undo weeks of hard won losses.

The aim of dieting is to lose fat but to minimize losses of muscle and other metabolically active lean tissue. It is inevitable and proper that some of the weight lost during slimming is lean tissue because obese people have more lean tissue as well as more fat and even adipose tissue has a cellular, protein, component. A ratio of about three-quarters fat to one-quarter lean may be a reasonable rule of thumb for planned weight loss. Extreme dieting and very rapid weight loss increases the proportion of lean that is lost while exercise seems to protect against lean tissue loss during dieting (reviewed by Prentice et al., 1991).

As we saw in Chapter 6, starvation reduces resting metabolic rate (RMR) and this conservation of energy during starvation is an aid to survival during food shortage. It will also tend to thwart the efforts of the dieter. This decline in RMR remains even after correcting for changes in lean body mass and is rapid. It can be detected within 24 hours of the start of dieting and a rise in RMR occurs within 24 hours of the return to normal eating (Prentice *et al.*, 1991). The magnitude of this protective response to dieting is not so large as to present an insurmountable barrier to successful weight loss. According to Prentice *et al.* (1991), even in severe dieting (say under 3 MJ or 700 kcal per day) the decline in RMR per unit of lean body mass rarely exceeds 15 per cent and in more moderate dieting (over 5 MJ or 1200 kcal per day) it is only about 5 per cent.

The reducing diet

The diet should aim to produce a daily energy deficit of 2–4 MJ (500–1000 kcal). It should achieve this by selectively restricting fat, added sugars and alcohol. Such measures will drastically reduce the energy density of the diet but will actually increase the nutrient density, which makes nutrient deficiencies unlikely despite the reduced energy intake. As we saw in Chapter 7, most fruits and vegetables have extremely low energy yields and so can be eaten in large quantities without adding much energy to the diet. Starchy foods like potatoes and cereals are relatively low in energy density and whole grain cereals have the added advantage of high amounts of dietary fibre (**non-starch polysaccharide**) which may increase their satiation value (see Chapter 9). Low-fat milk, very lean meat, white fish, pulses or the vegetarian options in the meat group will also be essential components of a healthy reducing diet. Foods from the fats and sugars group of the food plate (or pyramid), high-fat meats and dairy products, fried foods and other foods with added fats and sugars are the prime candidates for reduction in a healthy reducing diet.

Alternative diets

Numerous alternative diets are presented in popular books, often employing strategies and recommendations that seem totally at odds with the low-fat, low-sugar diet with low energy density but high nutrient density recommended in this book and by the bulk of orthodox nutritionists and dieticians. Many of these books offer some new gimmick that will allow the dieter to achieve large and rapid weight losses with relatively little inconvenience. They often contain impressive case histories of people who have lost large amounts of weight using the author's plan

or an account of how the author stumbled upon this new diet and how it transformed their lives. If all of these diets are so successful then why, despite the publication of dozens of new 'spectacularly successful' diet books each year, do rates of obesity and overweight spiral ever upwards? In practice, these diet books usually employ one or more strategies that will tend to reduce energy intake if the reader sticks to the rules. Take, for example, the currently fashionable low-carbohydrate diets which forbid consumption of foods that normally provide the bulk of our daily energy intake. Cereal products, potato products, milk and milk products, sugar, sweets, soft drinks, many sauces, coated meat and fish products, pies, etc. are all excluded from the acceptable foods and yet these normally account for well over 70 per cent of our energy intake. Exclusion of these foods will also limit the consumption of fats that are normally eaten with carbohydrates such as spreading and cooking fats. It is not surprising that total energy intake tends to fall if people stick to this very restrictive and monotonous diet which may become nauseating after a short while. Some other strategies employed in these books are listed below.

- Making the diet monotonous and reducing its palatability. Obese people may be particularly sensitive to reductions in palatability. Remember that rats giving access to a variety of palatability and energy-dense foods tend to gain weight like people; some of these diets seem to be aiming to almost reverse this process and persuade people to eat the human equivalent of the rat's pellet diet.
- Giving unlimited access to low-energy foods like certain fruits and vegetables. Conventional diets also do this.
- Making eating hard work or expensive. For example, certain so-called 'food-combining diets' forbid the mixing together within a meal of foods that are high in protein and those that are high in carbohydrate as well as other restrictions. This theory is based on a book written in the early twentieth century which falsely suggested that the gut is incapable of digesting carbohydrates and proteins at the same time because different conditions are required for their digestion. This diet excludes many of the culturally normal meals such as:
  - cereal with milk
  - cheese, meat, egg or fish sandwiches
  - pasta with meat, fish or cheese sauce

- potatoes or rice with meat, fish, eggs or cheese
- pizza
- a hamburger.

The role of exercise

The evidence that inactivity is strongly implicated as a cause of obesity seems very persuasive. This would also mean that regular exercise should be of major importance in preventing excess weight gain. However, evidence that exercise has a major impact on rates of weight loss during dieting is less persuasive. Most studies that have looked at the contribution of exercise to weight loss programmes have concluded that the exercise has led to only a modest increase in weight loss as compared with dieting alone. However, when long-term outcome has been assessed, the evidence is that an exercise component increases the chances of long-term success, i.e. it helps to prevent rapid regain of lost weight. These conclusions were those made in the previous edition of this book but more recently Wadden *et al.* (2006) made similar conclusions, i.e. that exercise in the absence of dieting produces very little weight loss in the short- or medium-term and that the benefits of exercise are to prevent weight gain, maintain weight losses and to improve health rather than induce weight loss.

It takes a long time to walk off 2–4 MJ (500–1000 kcal), say 2–6+ hours depending on speed and the person's size. Very few people have this much time to devote to formal exercise. Many very overweight people will have a low exercise tolerance and so the amount of energy that can be consumed in a formal exercise session will be small. These observations highlight the need to incorporate more activity into everyday living as well as in formal exercise sessions. Earlier in the chapter it was suggested that inactivity and weight gain become part of a vicious cycle (see Figure 8.15). Increased activity should break this cycle and create a virtuous cycle – exercise improves tolerance and so enables more exercise to be taken (see Figure 8.16).

The energy expenditure and energy requirements of an individual are determined by their basal metabolic rate (BMR) and their physical activity level (PAL) (see Chapter 6). The PAL is the factor that BMR is multiplied by to allow for the increase in energy expenditure caused by all activities:

$$\text{Energy expenditure} = \text{BMR} \times \text{PAL}$$

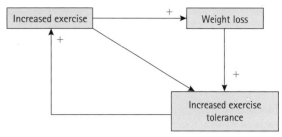

Figure 8.16 *The hoped for virtuous cycle of increased activity and weight loss.*

Table 8.6 shows how the energy a woman needs to achieve balance and to produce a 2.1–4.2 MJ (500–1000 kcal) deficit increases with the PAL multiple.

A sedentary, largely housebound woman with a PAL multiple of 1.3 can eat less than 3.4 MJ (800 kcal) per day if she is aiming for a 4.2 MJ (1000 kcal) daily energy deficit. As the PAL multiple

Table 8.6 The energy needs of a 65 kg woman at various physical activity levels (PALs) to achieve energy balance and a 500 kcal (2.1 MJ) or 1000 kcal (4.2 MJ) deficit*

Energy needed:	PAL multiple[†]					
	1.0	1.3	1.5	1.7	2.0	2.2
For balance						
kcal	1375	1788	2063	2338	2750	3025
MJ	5.78	7.51	8.66	9.82	11.55	12.71
500 kcal (2.1 MJ) deficit						
kcal	875	1288	1563	1838	2250	2525
MJ	3.68	5.41	6.56	7.72	9.45	10.61
1000 kcal (4.2 MJ) deficit						
kcal	375	788	1063	1338	1750	2025
MJ	1.58	3.31	4.46	5.62	7.35	8.51

*Modified from Webb (1998).
[†] *1.3 represents an extremely inactive person, e.g. a largely housebound elderly person.*
1.5 represents someone like a teacher who walks around quite a bit while they are working.
1.7 represents a person who walks around quite a bit at work and also takes part in some regular leisure-time physical activity, e.g. jogs several times a week.
2.0 represents someone whose job involves a lot of heavy manual work and probably also takes part in regular vigorous leisure-time pursuits.
2.2+ represents a serious athlete during training.
Note that a brisk 30–40 minute walk would increase the PAL by around 0.1 on that day.

rises so the amount that can be eaten and still achieve this deficit rises, so a woman with a PAL multiple of 1.7 could eat over 5.5 MJ (1300 kcal) and still achieve this deficit. A higher PAL multiple increases the amount that can be eaten while maintaining an energy deficit and this also reduces the likelihood that dieting will lead to inadequate intakes of other nutrients. About 4 hours walking per week increases the PAL multiple by 0.1.

These calculations suggest that achieving and maintaining long-term energy deficits of the required magnitude may be much easier in people who are active and may be quite impractical in people who are very inactive. It should also be borne in mind that exercise may protect against lean tissue loss during diet and so increase the quality of weight loss.

Are obese people less 'vigilant'?

In 1992, Garrow suggested that one major reason why some people remain relatively lean while others get very fat, is that the lean are more vigilant. Lean people monitor their body weight more closely and take steps to correct any weight gain (i.e. eating less and exercising more) before it has become a major problem. He argued that obese people, on the other hand, are less vigilant and therefore do not initiate corrective steps until the condition has progressed to the point where the person cannot cope with the magnitude of weight loss that is required to restore normal body weight. This has been used to explain the social class and educational influences on obesity prevalence; perhaps those in the lowest socioeconomic or educational groups are less vigilant in monitoring their body weight and this is why they are more prone to becoming obese. This class/educational difference in body weight vigilance would be consistent with the general trend for the upper social groups and better educated to be more health aware. They are, for example, more likely to choose foods with 'healthy images' and more likely to take dietary supplements. Similar lack of vigilance, it has been argued, allows regain of weight after successful slimming – the weight creeps back on unnoticed by the person until it is not readily correctable. Once the weight loss or re-loss required is high, the person feels unable to control the situation, becomes disheartened and no longer makes any sustained effort to reduce or even to maintain body weight.

Garrow (1992) reported the use of an adjustable weight cord to increase the vigilance of his patients – the patient is only able to adjust the length of this cord by an amount that allows for normal day to day fluctuations in waist size. Any increase in waist size above the adjustable range would make the cord uncomfortable to the patient and immediately signal the need for corrective measures. He has used such a cord to reduce the risk of weight regain during and after slimming. The cord is shortened by the doctor as slimming proceeds. It could also be used as a preventive measure. A cherished or expensive item of clothing that becomes uncomfortably tight may serve as a similar early warning signal for many of us who struggle to keep our weight within certain tolerance limits.

Key points

- Substantial weight loss will require a sustained period of dieting and negative energy balance.
- A daily deficit of 4.2 MJ (1000 kcal) is equivalent to a weekly loss of 1 kg of adipose tissue; this is around the realistic maximum for conventional dieting.
- It is inevitable that both fat and lean are lost during slimming and a ratio of three-quarters fat to one-quarter lean is a realistic guideline figure.
- Extreme energy restriction increases the proportion of lean that is lost while exercise reduces lean tissue losses.
- Resting metabolic rate (RMR) falls during dieting and rises when the diet is relaxed. In severe dieting, the RMR per unit of lean body mass may fall by up to 15 per cent but only by about 5 per cent in moderate dieting.
- The reducing diet should selectively restrict fat, added sugars and alcohol, which will reduce the energy density of the diet but increase its nutrient density.
- Exercise has only a modest direct effect on rates of weight loss in most studies but programmes that include an exercise element seem to have better long-term success rates.
- It takes a long time to expend 2–4 MJ (500–1000 kcal) in a formal exercise session. This highlights the need to incorporate more activity into everyday life.
- Many overweight and obese people will have limited exercise tolerance but increased activity

should increase tolerance and create a virtuous cycle.

- An active lifestyle increases the amount of food that can be consumed while still achieving the target energy deficit. It may be impractical for inactive people to aim for an energy deficit of 4.2 MJ (1000 kcal) with a conventional diet.

- A moderate diet increases the quality of weight gain (more of it is fat) and causes a smaller decrease in RMR.

- Obese people may be less vigilant in monitoring their body weight. Lean people are thus able to initiate corrective measures early while the obese may not start them until the magnitude of weight loss required is large and very difficult to achieve.

MORE 'AGGRESSIVE' TREATMENTS FOR OBESITY

Drug therapy

There are a number of potential therapeutic approaches to the pharmacological treatment of obesity and these are briefly outlined in the following sections. Some of these have resulted in licensed drugs whereas others are still only approaches that may have long-term potential.

Appetite suppressants

Appetite suppressants are drugs that affect appetite usually by affecting neurotransmission in the brain centres that regulate feeding. When noradrenaline (norepinephrine) is injected into the brains of experimental animals it reduces hunger and food intake and also stimulates the sympathetic nervous system. Amphetamine has a noradrenaline-like effect and was the first appetite suppressant to be widely used. Amphetamine itself also increases the activity of the nerve transmitter dopamine and this produces a potentially addictive euphoric effect. Modified amphetamines maintain the noradrenaline-like effect but the addictive dopamine-like effect is minimized. They have been widely used in the USA because until 1996 they were the only appetite suppressants approved by the US Food and Drug Administration (FDA). In controlled trials they produce only modest extra weight loss as compared to placebos and then only in the first few weeks of treatment.

Up until 1997 **fenfluramine** and **dexfenfluramine** were the most widely used anti-obesity drugs in the UK and Europe. They act to increase the activity of the nerve transmitter serotonin or 5-HT (5-hyrdoxytryptamine) in the brain. They block the re-uptake of serotonin which is the normal mechanism for inactivation of this transmitter after its release. When serotonin (5-HT) is injected into the brains of animals it also decreases feeding. These drugs mimic the actions of serotonin but do not have the addictive dopamine-like effects of the amphetamines. They act not by reducing the desire to eat but by causing the patient to feel full or satiated earlier. Fenfluramine was in use for about 30 years and tens of millions of Europeans have taken these drugs over that period (over 60 000 Britons in 1996 alone). In 1996, they were finally approved by the FDA for use in the USA. Long-term studies of over a year have reported significantly greater weight loss in people treated with drug and diet as compared to diet and placebo. Rare but potentially fatal side effects of these drugs have been known for some time (pulmonary hypertension) and there have been suggestions from animal experiments that they may damage serotonin-producing brain cells. However in 1997 new evidence was produced in the USA suggesting that they might cause damage to heart valves. This led to both drugs being withdrawn from the market in both Europe and the USA.

A newly licensed drug available in both the UK and USA called **sibutramine** has combined noradrenaline and serotonin effects. Large controlled trials of sibutramine in association with a reducing diet show that sibutramine does increase weight losses compared to diet alone and substantially increases the proportion of obese patients who maintain most of their weight loss after 2 years (James *et al.*, 2000). The sibutramine group in this trial also showed significant improvements in blood high-density lipoprotein (HDL) and very-low-density lipoprotein (VLDL) concentrations and some other risk factors but also showed some increases in blood pressure and heart rate and some patients from the sibutramine group were withdrawn because of increases in their blood pressure. High blood pressure would thus be a contraindication for sibutramine use and blood pressure should be regularly monitored in patients receiving this drug. It is also not suitable for patients taking the most popular antidepressant (selective serotonin re-uptake inhibitors, SSRI).

It is interesting to look at the detailed numbers in the trial of James *et al.* (2000). Initially 605 obese patients were selected from several centres and given individual weight loss programmes based on a 600 kcal/day energy deficit. After 6 months 467 patients (77 per cent) had lost more than 5 per cent of their initial weight and were then entered in the second stage of the study with 352 receiving sibutramine with their diet and 115 the placebo. After another 18 months, 204 patients remained on sibutramine treatment and 57 in the placebo group. In the sibutramine group, 89 patients (43 per cent) retained 80 per cent or more of their initial weight loss but only 9 (16 per cent) of the placebo group. This dramatically demonstrates the earlier observation that even those obese patients who lose weight initially rarely retain their initial weight losses, perhaps only 8 per cent of the original placebo group despite an individualized programme and regular monitoring. The figures for the sibutramine group were substantially higher with at least 19 per cent maintaining most of their initial weight loss. Nevertheless even with an individually tailored weight reduction programme and labour intensive monitoring as follow-up, the vast majority of patients did not maintain their initial weight loss and although pharmacotherapy helped it did not change this qualitative summary. It still requires great motivation and will power for obese individuals to lose substantial amounts of weight and maintain that weight loss even in the medium term.

Rimonabant is a totally new type of anti-obesity agent that has recently been licensed for use in the UK. This compound blocks the endocannabinoid receptors in the brain where the active ingredient of cannabis binds and where endogenously produced cannabinoids bind. Endogenous cannabinoids and those taken in the form of cannabis are known to increased appetite – the increased appetite associated with cannabis use is sometimes referred to as 'the munchies'. This drug was licensed in 2006 in the UK after successful clinical trials in the USA and in Europe.

Drugs that block digestion

Orlistat is a drug that blocks pancreatic lipase and this results in up to 30 per cent of dietary fat not being digested and passing through the gut into the faeces. This drug has been approved for use in the UK, USA and several other countries. This compound irreversibly and selectively inhibits gut lipase by modifying a serine residue at the active site of lipase. At therapeutic doses it blocks the absorption of about a third of the fat in a meal which then passes into the faeces. People taking this drug need to eat a low-fat diet because if they eat a lot of fat it produces adverse symptoms due to the high fat entry into the large bowel such as oily stools, anal leakage, urgency of defecation and increased intestinal gas production. These adverse symptoms of eating too much fat may help to encourage people to stick to a low-fat diet, which may also help them to lose weight. The increased faecal loss of fat may decrease absorption of fat-soluble vitamins and so supplements are advised. Long-term trials do suggest that orlistat in combination with a low-fat diet leads to modest but significant and clinically useful extra loss of weight compared with diet alone (see Wadden *et al.*, 2006).

Olestra is a synthetic fat that is not digested in the gut and so it passes out through the faeces. It has the palatability benefits of fat but yields no calories. Its use is permitted in the USA in savoury snacks such as potato crisps (chips) but not in the European Union. Compounds like olestra are being promoted as potentially able to replace up to 30 g of fat per day in the diet. In the short term, they can cause problems because of the entry of indigestible fatty material into the large bowel, e.g. diarrhoea, bowel urgency, anal 'leakage', abdominal cramps, greasy staining of toilets and underwear. They also reduce the absorption of fat-soluble substances including fat-soluble vitamins and cholesterol. In the USA, foods containing olestra have to be fortified with fat-soluble vitamins to compensate for their reduced absorption. Olestra is currently restricted to use in savoury snacks in the USA on the grounds that these foods are not usually eaten with meals and so the olestra will not interfere with the absorption of vitamins in normal meals.

Drugs based on gut hormones

In Chapter 7, several gut hormones were noted as having appetite-suppressing effects and so drugs that mimic the actions of these hormones might have potential as anti-obesity agents. Cholecystokinin (CCK) is a gut hormone released during feeding that causes satiety and it is also a transmitter in the brain where it seems to depress feeding. Despite early promise, CCK has limited potential as an obesity agent because animals rapidly adapt to excess CCK and become tolerant to it and even when animals are produced who lack CCK receptors they are still able to regulate their body weight normally (Murphy and Bloom, 2004). Some preliminary experiments suggest that another gut hormone discussed in Chapter 7, oxyntomodulin, may have potential as an anti-obesity agent although the research is still in its early stages. In small-scale trials it caused decreased body weight in obese people by both reducing energy intake and also increasing activity-related energy expenditure (Wynne *et al.*, 2006).

Drugs that increase energy expenditure

In the early 1980s drugs that increase energy expenditure or 'thermogenic agents' were considered to have major potential for the treatment of human obesity. At this time the 'brown fat theory' was at its height, i.e. the belief that adaptive thermogenesis in brown fat could have a major effect on human energy expenditure and protect against obesity when people overeat. Drugs that stimulate the rat β_3-adrenergic receptor and lead to uncoupling of oxidative phosphorylation in rat brown fat have been developed but these have limited effects in people. It would be fair to say that few nutritionists now believe that brown fat thermogenesis plays a major role in any human adaptive thermogenic response to overfeeding and so the theoretical basis for this approach to obesity treatment has weakened substantially.

Leptin and leptin analogues

Early trials of recombinant leptin in obese people have been disappointing as it was only associated with modest weight loss, so that according to Wadden *et al.* (2006) the manufacturer is unlikely to seek FDA approval for its use in the USA. Leptin is a protein and so it needs to be administered frequently by injection. In the long-term, perhaps orally active agents may be found that mimic or potentiate the actions of leptin. The fact that most human obesity seems to be associated with leptin resistance weakens the theoretical basis for this approach.

Surgical treatment for obesity

Surgery is a last resort treatment for severe and intractable obesity. All surgical procedures carry some risks and these are much higher in obese people. Surgical treatment does seem to offer some help

in losing weight to severely obese people and it may even be the most effective treatment for this extreme group judged purely on the basis of weight lost.

Several surgical treatments have been used in the treatment of obesity and are summarized below.

- *Gastric stapling or gastric banding.* These procedures involve reducing the capacity of the stomach by surgically stapling off a large part of it or by using an adjustable silicone band. This small pouch may only have a capacity of 30 mL which means that the patient can only eat small meals, if they eat too much then this may cause them to vomit. This is the most common surgical approach in Europe and it has low mortality of less that 0.1 per cent.
- *Gastric bypass.* This is the most common procedure used in the USA with around 125 000 operations in 2004. A small pouch is created at the base of the oesophagus and this is then linked directly to a part of the jejunum thus bypassing the stomach and the duodenum. The mortality from this procedure in the month after surgery is 0.5–1 per cent, but many patients have several side effects in the months after surgery including vomiting, nausea, bloating and extreme diarrhoea. Patients may need iron and vitamin B_{12} supplements.

Weight losses of up to 30 per cent have been reported for both of these procedures with associated improvements in other risk factors (see Wadden *et al.*, 2006).

- *Jaw wiring.* Wiring the jaws restricts intake of solid food although the intake of liquids is relatively unhindered. This procedure is often effective in producing short-term weight loss while the jaws are actually wired but patients usually regain the weight once the wires are removed. It may be useful for achieving short-term weight loss prior to surgery.
- *Fat removal.* This can be achieved by cutting or by **liposuction** (literally sucking out areas of adipose tissue). This unpleasant procedure may be judged by some people to be worthwhile for its short-term, localized, cosmetic effects.
- *Intestinal bypass.* This procedure involves surgically bypassing a large section of the small intestine and shunting food past most of it. This hinders digestion and absorption. Patients often have

chronic diarrhoea and nutrient deficiencies and may also develop liver and kidney damage. This risky procedure has now been largely superseded by gastric banding or gastric bypass.

Very-low-energy diets (VLEDs)

Very-low-energy diets are commercial products that are formulated to contain all of the essential vitamins and minerals but provide only 1.6–3.2 MJ (400–800 kcal) per day. The product is consumed as a flavoured drink and is used to replace normal food. It is very difficult, using normal food, to provide all of the essential nutrients with such a low energy intake. Sometimes a cheaper 'milk diet' is used as an alternative to these commercial products, i.e. skimmed or semi-skimmed milk plus a multivitamin and mineral supplement. The attraction for dieters is that they are absolved of all responsibility for food choice – the regimen is very clearly prescribed, significant mistakes are not possible and weight loss must occur if one sticks to the regimen. These regimens must produce substantial and rapid weight loss in people complying with these regimens. Some of the disadvantages of VLEDs are listed below.

- The patient gets no experience of eating a real diet that is capable of maintaining any short-term weight losses induced by this 'controlled starvation'– they are likely to regain any weight as soon as control of their eating is returned to them. It has been argued that this could be viewed as an advantage of these products because it minimizes contact with food and breaks bad eating habits. In practice, maintenance of weight loss after use of a VLED is poor (Wadden *et al.*, 2006).
- The rapid weight loss leads to high loss of lean tissue. It is difficult to measure this change in body composition accurately and some advocates of these products claim that this problem has been exaggerated.
- The energy deficit is so severe that **ketosis** occurs.
- Might this 'controlled starvation' risk precipitating an eating disorder?
- They are potentially dangerous, especially if used for prolonged periods without proper supervision.

Despite these problems some nutritionists do consider that these products may have a role in the supervised treatment of people with moderate or severe obesity (BMI well in excess of 30 kg/m²) that poses a larger threat to health. In a similar vein, there are many 'meal replacement' products on the market that are designed to replace one or more meals each day with a drink or snack. These products have a clearly defined energy yield and so are supposed to make it easy for dieters to control their energy intake. Often these products are nutrient enriched but in some cases have similar energy yields to much cheaper conventional equivalents.

Use of these more extreme treatments

All drugs have potential side effects, all surgical procedures entail some risk and prolonged use of VLEDs may also have adverse consequences. They are relatively extreme measures that are inappropriate for people who are only moderately overweight and even more inappropriate for normal-weight people who wish to be thinner to enhance their self-esteem. The commercial motivation may persuade some unscrupulous 'counsellors' and even doctors to recommend them to people who are not even overweight. The health and other consequences of obesity may justify their use if there is some reasonable prospect that they are likely to be effective. This must be a matter for individual clinical judgement. As a general guide, surgical treatment should normally be reserved for people with a BMI in excess of 40 kg/m² although the presence of other risk factors such as high blood pressure and glucose intolerance may lower this threshold to patients with a BMI of over 35 kg/m². Pharmacotherapy would normally be considered for those who are clinically obese (BMI >30 kg/m²) but once again the presence of other risk factors might lower this threshold and patients and the upper end of the overweight range might be considered suitable for drug treatment.

Wadden *et al.* (2006) suggest the following guidelines for selection of obesity treatment:

- BMI 25–27 kg/m² – treat with diet and exercise if other risk factors are present
- BMI 27–30 kg/m² – use diet and exercise treatment but consider pharmacotherapy if other risk factors are present
- BMI 30–35 kg/m² – use diet and exercise treatment together with anti-obesity drugs
- BMI 35–40 kg/m² – as 30–35 kg/m² but consider surgery if other risk factors are present

- BMI $40+\,kg/m^2$ – consider all available options including surgery.

These more extreme treatments are not alternatives to diet and exercise. In most cases their aim is to make it easier for people to comply with their weight-loss programmes. Appetite suppressants may reduce hunger during dieting, psychotherapy may help people to control their hunger, and dietary changes may maximize the satiating value of each food calorie. Despite this, dieting will inevitably involve a considerable period of discomfort and the dieter will have to exercise a considerable degree of sustained willpower to achieve substantial weight loss. A VLED will not produce weight loss if it is supplemented by other eating, an appetite suppressant will only produce weight loss if food intake is actually reduced. Some patients who have had their stomach capacity reduced by 90 per cent by surgical stapling still manage to consume enough to prevent weight loss.

Key points

- Drugs can combat obesity by interfering with the digestion and absorption of food, by decreasing appetite or by increasing energy expenditure.
- Amphetamines suppress appetite by increasing the activity of noradrenaline (norepinephrine) in the brain. Their effects on appetite diminish after a few weeks.
- The appetite suppressants fenfluramine and dexfenfluramine suppress appetite by increasing the activity of the transmitter serotonin in the brain.
- These were the most commonly used anti-obesity drugs in Europe and had been available for 30 years prior to their withdrawal from sale in 1997 after new doubts were raised about their safety.
- Sibutramine is a newly licensed drug in both the UK and USA that increases the effects of both noradrenaline and serotonin in the brain.
- Rimonabant has recently been licensed for use as an appetite suppressant in the UK. It blocks receptors in the brain that are normally involved in the response to endogenous cannabinoids and those from the drug cannabis.
- Several gut hormones and their analogues bring about satiety, and preliminary data suggest that oxyntomodulin may have potential in obesity treatment.

- Orlistat interferes with fat digestion by blocking pancreatic lipase and has been approved for use in the UK and the USA.
- Gastric reduction in Europe and gastric bypass in the USA are the most popular surgical treatments for obesity.
- Jaw wiring, intestinal bypass and lipid reduction are some of the other surgical treatments that have been used to treat obesity.
- Gastric reduction involves reducing the stomach capacity by stapling or banding off a large part of it and thus severely limiting meal size in the patient.
- Very-low-energy diets are liquid formulas designed to provide all of the essential nutrients but only a very low energy yield, 1.6–3.2 MJ (400–800 kcal) per day. They are either used to replace all solid food or perhaps just some meals.
- These more severe measures inevitably carry some risks which makes them suitable only as treatments of last resort for people in whom the risks of their obesity is likely to outweigh any risks of therapy.
- These treatments are adjuncts to conventional dieting rather than substitutes for it, i.e. they make it easier for the patient to maintain an energy deficit and only work if it is maintained.

PART THREE

THE NUTRIENTS

9

Carbohydrates

INTRODUCTION

Carbohydrates have traditionally supplied the bulk of the energy in most human diets. They still provide the bulk of the energy intake for most of the world population, whose diets are based on cereals or starchy roots. Dietary carbohydrates are almost exclusively derived from the vegetable kingdom and the carbohydrate content of most foods of animal origin is dietetically insignificant. The only major exception is lactose or milk sugar, which provides around 40 per cent of the energy in human milk and 30 per cent of the energy in cow milk. It is usually only in populations consuming large amounts of meat, oily fish and dairy produce that fat challenges carbohydrates as the principal source of dietary energy. Some affluent vegetarian populations may derive a high proportion of their dietary energy from fat in the form of extracted vegetable oils and margarine.

In some developing countries, over 75 per cent of dietary energy is derived from carbohydrate which is predominantly starch. In the affluent countries of western Europe, Australasia and North America, carbohydrates are likely to provide only around 45 per cent of total dietary energy and close to half of this in the form of simple sugars in some instances. These affluent populations are currently being advised to increase the proportion of their energy derived from carbohydrates to 50–60 per cent of the total and yet, at the same time, to substantially reduce their consumption of simple sugars, perhaps limiting 'extracted' sugars to no more than 10 per cent of the total energy intake.

Key points

- Historically, carbohydrates have provided most of the energy in human diets.
- Carbohydrates, principally starch, still provide as much as 75 per cent of the energy in many developing diets.
- In many affluent countries only around 45 per cent of dietary energy comes from carbohydrate and close to half of this may be in the form of simple sugars.
- Almost all dietary carbohydrate is from plant foods except for the lactose in milk.
- In populations consuming large amounts of animal foods and/or extracted vegetable oils then fat will threaten carbohydrate as the major energy source.
- Western consumers are advised to take 50–60 per cent of their energy as carbohydrate but ideally with less than 10 per cent coming from added sugars.

NATURE AND CLASSIFICATION OF CARBOHYDRATES

Carbohydrates are monomers or polymers of simple sugar units or saccharides. Carbohydrates may be described according to the number of saccharide units they contain, i.e. the **monosaccharides** (one), the **disaccharides** (two), the **oligosaccharides** (a few), and the **polysaccharides** (many). Although a range of monosaccharides are present in human diets, three of them make up the bulk of the monosaccharide that is released for absorption and utilization during the digestion of most diets, namely glucose, galactose and fructose. These three monosaccharides each contain six carbon atoms and are therefore termed **hexoses**. The two five-carbon sugars (pentoses), ribose and deoxyribose are released from the digestion of the nucleic acids DNA and RNA in food.

Carbohydrates must be broken down (digested) to their component monosaccharide units before they can be absorbed in the small intestine. Saliva and pancreatic juice contain an enzyme known as **alpha (α)-amylase** that breaks up digestible polysaccharides (starches) into oligosaccharides and disaccharides. The enzymes maltase and isomaltase, which are localized on the absorptive surface of the small intestine, complete starch digestion by cleaving the products of the partial digestion by α-amylase into glucose. The enzymes lactase and sucrase, which are also located on the absorptive surface of the small intestine, digest any of the disaccharides lactose and sucrose present in the diet.

Dietary carbohydrates are usually classified into three major subdivisions – the **sugars**, the **starches** and the **non-starch polysaccharides (NSP)** (Figure 9.1). Sugars and starches are readily digested and absorbed in the human small intestine, they thus clearly serve as a source of dietary energy and are sometimes termed the available carbohydrates; they all yield around 3.75 kcal (16 kJ) per gram. The NSPs are resistant to digestion by human gut enzymes and are thus referred to as the unavailable carbohydrate although they may yield up to

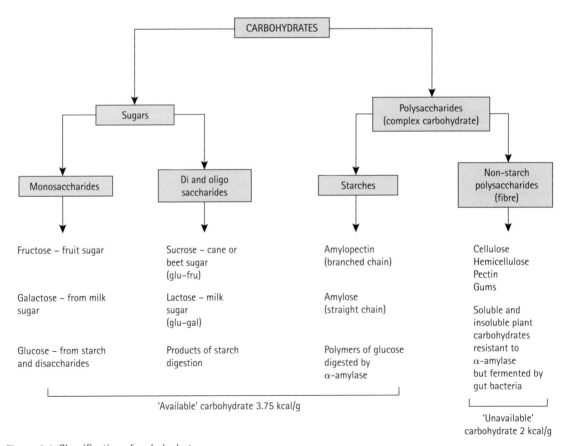

Figure 9.1 *Classification of carbohydrates.*

2 kcal/g (8 kJ/g) if they are fermented by bacteria in the large intestine. This fermentation yields volatile fatty acids (e.g. propionate, butyrate and acetate) which can be absorbed and metabolized.

Key points

- Carbohydrates may be monosaccharides (one sugar unit), disaccharides (two), oligosaccharides (a few) or polysaccharides (many).
- Only monosaccharides can be absorbed from the gut.
- α-Amylase in saliva and pancreatic juice cleaves polysaccharides to di- and oligosaccharides. Other enzymes on the surface of the small intestine complete the digestion of carbohydrates to monosaccharides.
- Sugars, starches and non-starch polysaccharides (NSPs) are the major subdivisions of the carbohydrates.
- Sugars and starches are digested and absorbed in the small intestine.
- NSPs are indigestible and enter the colon undigested but may be fermented by bacteria in the colon.

DIETARY SOURCES OF CARBOHYDRATE

The UK's household expenditure survey Family Food 2004–5 (DEFRA, 2006) indicates that carbohydrates provide around 48 per cent of food energy (excluding alcohol), with 23 per cent coming from simple sugars (15.5 per cent from non-milk extrinsic sugars) and 25 per cent from starch. Using a weighed inventory of food as eaten, the Dietary and Nutritional Survey of British Adults (Hoare *et al.*, 2004) reported that 48 per cent of food energy came from carbohydrates with 12.8 per cent from non-milk extrinsic sugars. According to the National Food Survey, between 1952 and 1996 the carbohydrate content of household food fell from 324 g/day to 228 g/day, i.e. from 53 per cent of food energy in 1952 to 46 per cent in 1996. The figures for both years exclude alcohol, soft drinks and confectionery because these were not recorded in 1952 and the current values expressed in the same way are approximately 230 g/day and 43 per cent (estimated from data in DEFRA, 2006).

Around 75 per cent of the starch in British household food comes from cereals and cereal products and about 20 per cent from vegetables (mostly from potatoes). About 4 per cent of the starch comes from cereals added to meat and fish products, e.g. breadcrumb coatings. Just under half of the NSP in British diets comes from fruit and vegetables and most of the rest comes from cereal foods. Table 9.1 shows the sources of total sugars in the British diet as estimated in the previous edition from the Ministry of Agriculture, Fisheries and Food (MAFF) (1997); for comparison more recent estimates for the food sources of non-milk extrinsic sugars have been added. Clearly foods in the sugars and fats group of the **food guide plate** or **pyramid** (see Chapter 4) are the major sources of added sugars in the British and other Western diets. Most of the sugar in the milk group and in fruits and vegetables is sugar that is naturally present in the food.

Table 9.1 The estimated contribution of food groups to the total sugars (MAFF, 1997) and non-milk extrinsic sugars (NMES) (DEFRA, 2006) in the average British diet

Food	Total sugars (%)	NMES (%)
Milk and milk products including cheese	*16*	*5*
Sugar, preserves, confectionery, soft and alcoholic drinks	*39*	*64*
Vegetables	*6*	*1*
Fruit including fruit juices	*14*	*7*
All cereals	*18*	*17*
(cakes, pastries and biscuits)	*10*	*10*

Key points

- Carbohydrates provide about 48 per cent of food energy in Britain and around 50–55 per cent per cent of this carbohydrate is starch.
- The carbohydrate content of British diets has fallen since the 1950s both in absolute terms and as a proportion of food energy.
- Around 90 per cent of the starch in British diets comes from cereal foods and potatoes.
- The non-starch polysaccharide in British diets is derived roughly equally from cereal foods and from fruits and vegetables.

- Almost two-thirds of the non-milk extrinsic sugars in British diets comes from sweetened drinks, sweets, preserves and sugar itself.
- Sweetened cereal products, including cakes and biscuits, are another major source of added sugars.

SUGARS

Sugars may be monosaccharides, disaccharides or oligosaccharides; they are characteristically soluble in water and have a sweet taste. The monosaccharides glucose and fructose are present in some fruits and vegetables and in honey. Fructose is three times as sweet as glucose and is largely responsible for the sweet taste of fruits and some vegetables. Sucrose (relative sweetness 100) is used as the standard against which the sweetness of other sugars and also of artificial sweeteners is measured. The relative sweetness of the other major dietary sugars is: lactose 30; glucose 50; fructose 170.

Lactose or milk sugar

Lactose is a disaccharide found exclusively in milk and is the least sweet of the major dietary sugars. It comprises one unit of glucose and one of galactose. Lactose is the only significant source of galactose in the diet. Galactose is essential in several synthetic pathways but can be readily synthesized from glucose and so it is not an essential nutrient. On rare occasions, babies may inherit an enzyme deficiency that renders them unable to metabolize dietary galactose. If such babies are fed with breast milk or lactose-containing infant formula then galactose accumulates in their blood (**galactosaemia**). This galactosaemia results in a range of symptoms (e.g. vomiting, weight loss and jaundice) and if untreated it may result in death or permanent disability (e.g. cataracts, retarded physical and mental development). Infants with this condition must be fed on a lactose-free formula and will need to continue to avoid milk and milk-containing foods after weaning.

Some babies are born deficient in the enzyme **lactase** that cleaves lactose into its component monosaccharides in the small intestine (congenital lactase deficiency). This deficiency results in a failure to digest and absorb dietary lactose. Such infants will fail to thrive. They have diarrhoea because of the osmotic effect of undigested lactose causing retention of water within the gut and bloating because of fermentation of lactose by intestinal bacteria causing gas production. These infants also need to be fed on a lactose-free formula.

In most human populations (and other mammals) lactase activity in the small intestine declines with age after about 4 years of age. This reduces the capacity of the gut to digest and absorb lactose in older children and adults (primary lactase non-persistence). This decline in lactase activity is genetically determined; it is not prevented by continued consumption of lactose and is exhibited to some degree by up to two-thirds of the world population. Lactase activity does not usually decline with age in the white populations of North America and northern Europe. People who exhibit primary lactase non-persistence are termed **lactose intolerant** and they experience symptoms of diarrhoea and bloating when challenged with a high dose of lactose. Lactose intolerance may also occur as a secondary consequence of intestinal infection, inflammatory gut diseases and parasitic infestations of the gut (secondary lactase deficiency). The high prevalence of lactose intolerance has led to suggestions that milk and milk products are inappropriate for use in nutritional support programmes in many countries. In a detailed review, Rosado (1997) confirmed that many adults and older children in developing countries are indeed intolerant to the 50 g of lactose (equivalent to 1.5 L of milk) used in standard lactose tolerance tests. However, he suggested that only about 30 per cent of these people are intolerant of the smaller amounts of lactose that are likely to be consumed, e.g. in a glass of milk. Even this 30 per cent, whom he termed lactose maldigesters, can tolerate smaller amounts of milk without symptoms and their colon metabolism will adapt to regular milk intake to eliminate symptoms. He suggested that the problem of primary lactase non-persistence does not warrant elimination or severe restriction of milk intake in developing countries.

Sucrose

Sucrose is a disaccharide composed of one unit of glucose and a unit of fructose and it is digested by the enzyme sucrase, which is located on the absorptive surface of the small intestine. Sucrose is found in several fruits and vegetables and is present in large quantities in sugar beet and sugar cane from which it is extracted and purified on a vast industrial scale. Sucrose is readily available in highly purified or partly purified forms (e.g. white sugar, brown sugars, treacle or syrup). It is also very widely used by food processors to sweeten, preserve and to texturize a variety of foods. The terms sucrose and sugar are often used as if they are synonymous.

High sucrose consumption has, at one time or another, been blamed for many of the illnesses that afflict affluent populations. The poor health image of sucrose was encapsulated in the phrase 'pure, white and deadly'. Its poor health image has led many food manufacturers to use other sugars, or sugar-containing extracts, in their products so that they can imply in advertising claims that their product is 'healthier' because it has reduced levels of sucrose. The term **extrinsic non-milk sugar** has been used to cover all of the dietary sugars (still principally sucrose) that are not present as natural components of the fruit, vegetables and milk in the diet. Conversely, sugars that are naturally present within the cell walls of plants are termed **intrinsic sugars**; note that the sugars in fruit juice are classified as part of the extrinsic non-milk sugars.

Sucrose is a natural plant sugar. It happens to be present in large enough amounts in readily cultivatable plants to make it convenient for extraction in industrial quantities. It seems reasonable to suppose that if sucrose is indeed innately harmful, as it is used in affluent countries, then other sugars used in the same ways and quantities are also likely to be harmful. Substitution of sucrose by other extracted sugars that have not yet acquired the poor health image of sucrose does not appear to offer a high probability of dietary 'improvement'. Extrinsic non-milk sugars provide between about 10 and 20 per cent of the total energy intake in most affluent populations.

Sucrose and other sugars have a very high, almost addictive, sensory appeal and this might be expected to encourage over-consumption of food energy and thus predispose to obesity. Providing sugared drinking water to rats and mice has been used as an experimental means of inducing obesity. In these experiments with rodents, increasing sugar consumption depresses intake of solid food (and therefore also nutrient intake) but not by enough to fully compensate for the extra energy in the sugar (e.g. Kanarek and Hirsch, 1977). However, as we saw in Chapter 8, most of the epidemiological evidence suggests that those people who take in a high proportion of their

energy as sugar are less likely to be obese than those who consume a lower-sugar diet. The proportion of energy derived from fat and sugar tends to be inversely correlated in Western diets (the **sugar–fat seesaw**) and there are good reasons to expect fat to be more fattening than carbohydrates including sugar. There is thus no convincing evidence to link high sugar intake to increased risk of obesity.

There is little convincing evidence that, at levels typical of UK and US diets, added sugars are directly implicated in the aetiology of cardiovascular diseases, diabetes or hypertension. There is convincing evidence to link some dietary fats to these conditions and the sugar–fat seesaw means that high sugar consumers will often consume less of these fats. At very high intakes, 30 per cent or more of total calories, they may raise serum cholesterol levels and lead to insulin resistance, which is important in the aetiology of the maturity-onset form of diabetes (Committee on the Medical Aspects of Food (COMA), 1991). In an invited review, Bruckdorfer (1992) presented the case against the current consensus view that sugar is a relatively benign factor in the aetiology of obesity, cardiovascular disease and type 2 diabetes.

When extracted sugars are added to foods, they add energy but no nutrients. They reduce the nutrient density of the diet and the phrase 'empty calories' has been coined. The significance of this reduction in nutrient density will depend on the general level of nutrient adequacy. In populations or individuals with high nutrient intakes, it will be of less significance than those whose nutrient intakes are more marginal. Some nutrient-rich foods may only become palatable if sugar is added, e.g. some sour fruits. In groups such as the elderly, where high nutrient density is considered a nutritional priority (COMA, 1992) moderation of added sugar to no more than 10 per cent of total energy should help to achieve high nutrient density. However, when appetite is poor, then any reduction in dietary palatability resulting from reduction in sugar intakes may simply depress both energy and nutrient intake.

Key points

- Sugars have a sweet taste and are soluble in water.
- The relative sweetness of sugars and artificial sweeteners is graded in relation to sucrose

(relative sweetness 100). Fructose is the sweetest dietary sugar (170) and lactose the least sweet (30).

- Lactose is a disaccharide of glucose and galactose that is found exclusively in milk.
- Babies with congenital galactosaemia are unable to metabolize galactose and those with congenital lactase deficiency are unable to digest and absorb lactose. These infants need a lactose-free formula.
- In most non-European populations, lactose activity in the gut declines after early childhood causing them to become lactose intolerant (primary lactase non-persistence).
- Most lactose intolerant people can tolerate moderate amounts of milk and so lactose intolerance does not warrant the elimination of milk from developing countries' diets.
- Lactose intolerance may also occur as a secondary consequence of gut disease.
- Sucrose is a disaccharide of glucose and fructose and is the major added sugar in the diet.
- The term non-milk extrinsic sugars covers all sugars (largely sucrose) that are not present naturally in the fruit, vegetables and milk that we eat; it includes the sugar in fruit juice.
- Sugars contained within the cell walls of plants are termed intrinsic sugars.
- There is little evidence that high sugar intake is causally linked to diabetes, heart disease or obesity.
- The proportion of energy derived from fats and sugars tends to be inversely correlated – the sugar–fat seesaw.
- Low-fat diets, which because of the sugar–fat seesaw tend to be high in sugar, are associated with reduced risk of obesity.
- High sugar consumption does reduce the nutrient density of diets and this may be particularly important in groups such as the very elderly with marginal intakes of essential nutrients.

ARTIFICIAL SWEETENERS

Artificial sweeteners have been developed and manufactured to satisfy our craving for sweetness without the necessity to consume sugars (e.g. saccharin, aspartame and acesulphame K). These substances are not sugars or carbohydrates and are essentially calorie free. They are also intensely sweet; these examples are typically 200–300 times as sweet as sucrose and so very small quantities are needed to replace the sweetness normally provided by sugar. Their use is particularly prominent in drinks. Low-calorie soft drinks containing artificial sweeteners account for around 40 per cent of the soft drinks consumed by British adults (Hoare *et al.*, 2004). There is a marked difference between the sexes in their choice of soft drinks; in women about half of the soft drink they consume is low in calories but in men it is only just over a third of the total.

Saccharin was the first of these artificial sweeteners and has been in use for much of this century. Saccharin is absorbed and excreted unchanged in the urine. Very large intakes have been reported to increase the incidence of bladder tumours in rats; despite this, it is still a permitted sweetener in most countries including the USA and UK because at practical intake levels it is not thought to represent a significant hazard. Saccharin has a bitter aftertaste and is destroyed by heating which means that saccharin cannot be used as a substitute for sugar in cooking; this limits its usefulness to food manufacturers. Aspartame is a more recent addition to the sweetener range; it is a dipeptide made up of the amino acids aspartic acid and phenylalanine. Despite being digested to its constituent amino acids and absorbed, it has a negligible calorific yield because so little is used. In the rare inherited condition, **phenylketonuria (PKU)**, there is an inability to metabolize dietary phenylalanine and so it can accumulate in the blood causing severe brain damage and learning disabilities in affected children (see Chapter 16). Obviously people with PKU should avoid aspartame but there have been some largely unsubstantiated suggestions that consuming large amounts of phenylalanine in the form of aspartame might also cause brain damage in non-PKU sufferers. Sucralose is the most recent addition to the list of approved sweeteners; it was licensed for use in the USA in 1998 and in 2002 for UK use. Sucralose is made from cane sugar; three of the hydroxyl groups of sucrose are replaced by chlorine atoms and taste tests suggest that it is perceived to taste very much like sugar. The chemical modification of sucrose produces a compound that is 600 times as sweet as sucrose but is not metabolized to yield energy and most of it passes through the gut unchanged. A major advantage of sucralose is its stability; it is heat resistant and so unlike the other major sweeteners can be used in cooked and baked goods. It is also retains its stability and sweetness at low pH. Although these intense sweeteners mimic the sweetness of sugar they do not have the preservative or textural effects of sugar; this means that even with sucralose recipes need to be modified if the sugar is serving other functions besides just adding sweetness.

Artificial sweeteners would seem to offer great potential benefits, especially in those people who are trying to lose weight. If a glass of regular cola is replaced by a 'diet' version sweetened with one of these sweeteners then this would reduce energy intake by 75 kcal (300 kJ). If a sweetener is used to replace two spoonfuls of sugar in a cup of tea or coffee then this saves 40 kcal (150 kJ) each time. Consumption of these artificial sweeteners is equivalent to billions of sugar calories in Europe and America each year and this saved energy is equivalent to several kilograms of theoretically prevented weight gain for every European and American. However, the massive growth in the use of these products has not been accompanied by corresponding reductions in sugar use and it has coincided with a large rise in the prevalence of obesity.

These intense sweeteners do not provide energy but neither do they have the satiating effect of sugar. This means that unless users are consciously restricting their energy intake, i.e. dieting, then they will tend to replace any lost sugar calories with more of their usual mixed food. The net effect is that there tends to be some replacement of carbohydrate calories (sugar) by fat calories and so the proportion of energy derived from fat tends to rise. Given the arguments about the greater fattening effects of fat compared with carbohydrate in Chapter 8, this would not be a desirable outcome for improving weight control. Data from the USA show that there has been no significant decline in sugar use to parallel the growth in sales of intense sweeteners – are they really substituting for sugar or are they largely an addition to the usual diet? Of course these sweeteners may be helpful to those who are consciously dieting but who do not want give up sweet drinks and other sweet products. They may also have benefits for dental health and nutrient density if they really reduce sugar consumption. The effects of sugar substitutes on food choice and dietary composition have been reviewed by Mela (1997).

Sugar replacers

More recently, there has been a growth in the use of bulk sweeteners or **sugar replacers** that have a similar sweetness to sucrose on a weight-for-weight basis (typically 40–90 per cent of the sweetness of sucrose). These compounds are mostly sugar alcohols (e.g. xylitol, sorbitol and isomalt) that yield fewer calories than sugar because they are incompletely absorbed or metabolized; they typically yield 40–60 per cent of the energy of an equivalent weight of sucrose. They can be used in similar amounts to sugar in some food products and they add not just sweetness but also the textural and mouth-feel properties of sugar. They may be used in combination with intense artificial sweeteners to boost their sweetness. These sugar replacers do not promote dental caries and because they are only slowly and partially absorbed, they do not cause the same large rises in blood glucose and insulin that sugar does, which may be particularly useful for people with diabetes. However, if they are eaten in large amounts then because of their limited absorption, large amounts of carbohydrate may enter the large bowel. This can have an osmotic effect and increase bacterial fermentation leading to diarrhoea and flatulence. Sugar replacers have been reviewed by McNutt (1998).

Key points

- Artificial sweeteners such as saccharin and aspartame are intensely sweet and so only need to be used in minute amounts; they are essentially calorie free.
- Saccharin and aspartame are destroyed during cooking but sucralose is a recent addition to the sweetener range that is stable when heated and retains its sweetness at low pH.
- Aspartame is a source of phenylalanine and so must be avoided by those with phenylketonuria.
- These sweeteners do not have the preservative or textural effects of sugar and this limits their usefulness in cooking and food processing.
- Artificial sweeteners can cut total energy intake if they replace sugar in a calorie-controlled diet.
- Sweeteners do not have the satiating effect of sugar and so in unregulated diets any 'saved'

sugar calories are likely to be replaced by calories from other foods.

- If sweeteners really replace sugar then they will have benefits for dental health and should improve the nutrient density of the diet.
- Sugar replacers are mostly sugar alcohols like sorbitol that have similar sweetness to sugar but yield less energy because they are incompletely absorbed and metabolized.
- Sugar replacers provide similar textural effects to sugar in food processing.
- Sugar replacers do not promote dental caries and may be useful for people with diabetes because their slower absorption means they cause smaller rises in blood sugar and insulin release than sugar.
- In large doses, sugar replacers spill into the large bowel and can cause flatulence and diarrhoea.

DIET AND DENTAL HEALTH

COMA (1989a) and Binns (1992) have given referenced reviews of the role of sugars in the aetiology of dental caries. Moynihan (1995) reviewed the relationship between all aspects of diet and dental health. Most of the uncited references used in this section are listed in these reviews.

The notion that sugar is implicated in the aetiology of dental caries (tooth decay) stretches back to the Ancient Greeks. The evidence that sugars, and sucrose in particular, have some effect on the development of dental caries is overwhelming; only the relative importance of sugar compared with other factors, such as fluoride intake and individual susceptibility, is really disputed. There is a strong correlation across populations between average sugar consumption and the number of **decayed, missing and filled (DMF)** teeth in children. In populations with low sugar consumption (less than 10 per cent of energy intake) dental caries is uncommon. Observations in island populations and other isolated communities have shown a strong correlation between changes in the sugar supply and changes in the rates of tooth decay. In Britain, during World War II, the rates of tooth decay fell when sugar was rationed. Low rates of tooth decay have been found in diabetic children living in institutions whose sugar intake would have been kept very low as part of their diabetic management. Studies of other groups

of people with habitually low sugar intakes have also found low levels of dental caries, e.g. children living in children's homes, Seventh Day Adventists and children of dentists. Conversely, groups with high habitual sugar intakes have high rates of caries, e.g. sugarcane cutters and those working in factories producing confectionery.

In a study conducted almost 50 years ago in Swedish mental hospitals, the Vipeholm study, groups of patients were exposed to not only differing levels of sugar intake but also differences in the form and frequency of that sugar intake. The amount of sugar was important in determining rates of tooth decay and its form and frequency had an even greater impact.

- Sugar taken between meals was found to be the most cariogenic.
- Frequent consumption of small amounts of sugar was more harmful than the same amount consumed in large infrequent doses.
- The most cariogenic foods were those where the sugar was in a sticky form that adhered to the teeth, e.g. toffees.

Studies with animals have also found that:

- the presence of sugar in the mouth is required for caries to occur
- all common dietary sugars are cariogenic to some extent
- increased frequency and duration of eating sugar-containing foods increases the risk of caries production.

The key event in the development of dental caries is the production of acid by the bacteria *Streptococcus mutans* in dental **plaque** – the sticky mixture of food residue, bacteria and bacterial polysaccharides that adheres to teeth. These bacteria produce acid by fermenting carbohydrates, particularly sugars, in foods. When the mouth becomes acidic enough (i.e. pH drops below 5.2) this causes demineralization of the teeth. This can lead to holes in the hard outer enamel layer of the tooth, exposing the softer under layers of dentine, and thus enabling the decay to proceed rapidly throughout the tooth. This is not a one-way process. Between periods of demineralization, there will be phases of remineralization or repair; it is the balance between these two processes that will determine susceptibility to decay.

The key role of oral bacteria in the development of caries is highlighted by experiments with germ-free animals; rats born by caesarean section into a sterile environment and maintained germ free throughout their lives do not develop dental caries even when their diets are high in sucrose. Tooth decay could be considered a bacterial disease that is promoted by dietary sugar. Sugars are ideal substrates for the acid-producing bacteria of the plaque. When sugars are consumed as part of a meal, other constituents of the food can act as buffers that 'soak up' the acid and limit the effects on mouth pH of any acid produced. High saliva production also reduces acid attack by buffering and diluting the acid. The more frequently that sugar-containing snacks or drinks are consumed, and the longer that sugar remains in the mouth, the longer is the period that the overall pH of the mouth is below the level at which demineralization occurs. In the UK, there is a target for reducing extrinsic non-milk sugars to around half of current intakes. Reducing between-meal sugar in drinks and sugary snacks is regarded as the priority in the prevention of dental caries. Prolonged sucking of sugary drinks through a teat by infants and young children is particularly damaging to teeth and manufacturers of such drinks recommend that they be consumed from a cup. Some foods contain factors that protect against caries, particularly milk and cheese. Despite containing large amounts of lactose, milk is regarded as non-cariogenic. Chocolate may also contain factors that protect against caries but this is counterbalanced by its high sugar content.

In a review of the role of sugars in caries induction from the sugar industry viewpoint, Binns (1992) emphasized the importance of other factors in determining caries frequency. Binns gave evidence of a substantial reduction in caries frequency in industrialized countries between 1967 and 1983 (Table 9.2). During the period covered in Table 9.2 sugar consumption did not change substantially and Binns suggests that consumption of sugary snacks between meals may even have increased. Moynihan (1995) summarizes more recent UK data suggesting that between 1983 and 1993 the number of 15-year-old children who were free of caries rose from 7 per cent to 37 per cent and the average DMF fell from 6 to 2.5. There have been similar improvements in the dental health of adults; between 1968 and 1988 the number of Britons aged 65–74 years

who had no natural teeth dropped from three-quarters to under half.

Table 9.2 Changes in the average number of decayed, missing and filled (DMF) teeth in 12-year-old children in 1967 and 1983*

Country	1967	1983
Australia	4.8	2.8
Denmark	6.3	4.7
Finland	7.2	4.1
Netherlands	7.5	3.9
New Zealand	9.0	3.3
Norway	10.1	4.4
Sweden	4.8	3.4
UK	4.7	3.0
USA	3.8	2.6

*Data source: Binns (1992).

The decline in the prevalence of caries in British children and other industrialized countries may be attributed in large part to the effect of increased fluoride intake. In some places, water supplies have been fluoridated, some parents give children fluoride supplements and, most significantly, almost all toothpaste is now fluoridated. The evidence that fluoride has a protective effect against the development of dental caries is very strong. There is an inverse epidemiological association between the fluoride content of drinking water and DMF rates in the children. These epidemiological comparisons suggest that an optimal level of fluoride in drinking water is around 1 part per million (1 mg/L). At this level, there seems to be good protection against tooth decay without the risk of the mottling of teeth that is increasingly associated with levels much above this. Intervention studies where the water supply has been fluoridated (see example in Chapter 3) and studies using fluoridated milk and salt have also confirmed the protective effects of fluoride.

The major effect of fluoride in preventing tooth decay is thought to be by its incorporation into the mineral matter of the tooth enamel; incorporation of fluoride into the calcium/phosphate compound **hydroxyapatite** to give **fluorapatite** renders the tooth enamel more resistant to demineralization. This means that fluoride is most effective in preventing dental caries when administered to young children (under 5s) during the period of tooth formation. Fluoride in relatively high doses also inhibits bacterial acid production and inhibits bacterial growth; it may concentrate in plaque to produce these effects even at normal intake levels (Binns, 1992). Fluoride in the mouth assists in the remineralization process, the more soluble hydroxyapatite dissolves when the mouth is acid and is replaced by the more acid-resistant fluorapatite. Several expert committees have made specific recommendations to ensure adequate intakes of fluoride, especially in young children (e.g. COMA (1991) and National Research Council (NRC) (1989a)). COMA (1991) give a 'safe intake' of fluoride for infants only, NRC (1989a) give a range of safe intakes for all age groups – details of quantitative fluoride recommendations are given in Chapter 14.

Despite the very strong evidence for a beneficial effect of fluoride on dental health, there has been limited fluoridation of water supplies in the UK in contrast with the USA where water fluoridation is widespread. Only around 12 per cent of England has optimally fluoridated water even though water companies have had the power to add fluoride to drinking water at the request of the Health Authority since the passage of the Water (Fluoridation) Act in 1985. This is because of strong opposition from some pressure groups. Opposition to fluoridation has been partly on the grounds that addition of fluoride to the public water supply amounts to mass medication without individual consent. There have also been persistent concerns expressed about the long-term safety of this level of fluoride consumption; it is very difficult, for example, to prove beyond any doubt that there is no increased cancer risk associated with lifetime consumption. The consensus is that fluoride in drinking water at optimal levels for dental health is not associated with any increase in risk of cancer or other diseases. The difference between the therapeutic levels proposed and the dose associated with early signs of fluoride overload (mottling of the teeth) is also relatively small (twofold to threefold). There may also be a relatively small number of people who are fluoride sensitive. Once the Water Act 2003 comes fully into force then water companies will be required to fluoridate their water supplies if requested to do so by the local health authority. A map showing current levels of natural and artificial fluoride in drinking water in England and Wales can be found at the DEFRA website (http://www.defra.gov.uk/environment/statistics/inlwater/iwfluoride.htm).

Dental caries is not the only cause of tooth loss. In adults, gum disease (periodontal disease) is the most frequent cause of tooth loss. **Gingivitis** is an inflammation of the gums caused by the presence of plaque. It can lead to receding of the gums which exposes the roots of the teeth to decay and eventually may lead to loosening and loss of teeth. As with caries, sugar is a major causative factor for gum disease but Moynihan (1995) suggests that practically attainable reductions in sugar consumption are unlikely to have much impact on this condition. Improved oral hygiene may be the most effective way of controlling this condition: regular brushing, flossing and attention from a professional dental hygienist. There is some speculation whether the antioxidant vitamins, e.g. vitamins C and E, might protect against gum disease. Certainly, deficiencies of vitamins A, C, E and folic acid have detrimental effects on gum health.

Key points

- Cross-cultural comparisons, time trends and observations in groups with high or low sugar intakes all suggest that high sugar intake promotes dental caries.
- Sugar is most damaging to teeth when it is taken frequently, between meals and in a form that adheres to the teeth.
- Bacteria in the mouth ferment carbohydrates in food, especially sugars, to produce acid and this acidity leads to demineralization of teeth making them prone to decay.
- Germ-free animals do not get dental caries.
- When sugar is taken as part of a meal, other components of the meal may buffer any acid produced. Saliva also buffers and dilutes mouth acid.
- Some foods contain factors that protect against dental caries including milk, cheese and chocolate.
- A reduction in the consumption of added sugar with a particular emphasis on reducing sugary snacks and drinks between meals is recommended to improve dental health.
- Infants should not be allowed to suck sugary drinks slowly through a teat.
- Rates of dental caries in children have fallen in recent decades in many countries and this has been largely attributed to higher fluoride

intakes, particularly the use of fluoridated toothpaste.

- In areas with naturally high fluoride content in drinking water of 1 mg/L, rates of child dental disease are low and there are no indications of any adverse effects.

- Fluoride is incorporated into the tooth enamel in young children and makes teeth more resistant to acid demineralization. It may also protect the teeth in other ways.

- Expert committees in both the USA and UK have recommended that adequate intakes of fluoride should be ensured, especially in infants and young children.

- Some areas have artificially fluoridated their water up to a level of 1 mg/L, but there has been considerable resistance to widespread fluoridation largely because of unsubstantiated concerns about the long-term safety of this level of fluoride intake.

- In adults, gum disease is the most frequent cause of tooth loss.

- Gum disease is also promoted by sugar, but improved dental hygiene may be the most effective way of reducing tooth loss by this route.

STARCHES

Plants use starches as a store of energy in their roots and seeds. Animals also manufacture and store a form of starch, **glycogen**, in their muscles and livers but the amounts present in most flesh foods are dietetically insignificant. The amount of energy that animals and people store as glycogen is very small. Total glycogen stores of people amount to only a few hours' energy expenditure. Glycogen is an inefficient bulk energy store because it yields only around 4 kcal(16 kJ) per gram and because it holds with it somewhere around four times its own weight of water. Fat on the other hand yields 9 kcal (37 kJ) per gram and does not hold water. Glycogen serves as a store of carbohydrate that can maintain blood glucose concentration during normal inter-meal intervals.

Starches are polymers of glucose; the glucose may be arranged in predominantly straight chains (**amylose**) or, more frequently, in highly branched chains (**amylopectin**). The glucose residues in starches are joined together by linkages that can be broken (hydrolysed) by human digestive enzymes. These linkages are mainly $\alpha 1$–4 linkages with some $\alpha 1$–6 linkages that cause the branching of the glucose chain; amylose has few $\alpha 1$–6 linkages whereas amylopectin has many and the latter's extensively branched structure has been likened to a bunch of grapes (Figure 9.2). The dimers and trimers of glucose that are produced as a result of digestion by α-amylase are then finally cleaved by enzymes on the mucosal surface of the small intestine to yield glucose. The enzyme maltase breaks $\alpha 1$–4 linkages in these dimers and trimers and the enzyme isomaltase breaks $\alpha 1$–6 linkages.

Starches provide approximately the same energy yield as sugars, i.e. 3.75 kcal/g (16 kJ/g). They have low solubility in water and they do not have a sweet taste. As starches are bland, starchy foods also tend to be bland. This is one reason why affluent populations take the opportunity to select foods with more sensory appeal and tend to reduce the proportion of their dietary energy that is supplied by starch and replace it with fats and sugars. To reduce both sugar and fat intakes in line with the recommendations discussed in Chapter 4, a large increase in starch consumption is inevitable, perhaps a doubling of current intakes. Something like 90 per cent of the starch in the British diet comes from cereals and potatoes, and so any major increase in starch consumption must mean eating more potatoes, bread and other cereals.

Key points

- Animals store a form of starch, glycogen, in their livers and muscles but the starch content of meat is insignificant.

- Glycogen is an inefficient bulk energy store for animals because it has a lower energy yield than fat and also holds large amounts of water.

- Starches are polymers of glucose.

- Amylose is starch in which the glucose residues are joined in long straight chains by α-1–4 links.

- In amylopectin there is considerable branching of the glucose chain caused by the presence of α-1–6 links.

- The enzyme α-amylase in saliva and pancreatic juice cleaves starches to dimers and trimers of glucose by hydrolysing α-1–4 links.

Glucose

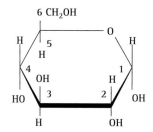

Maltose
Glucose joined by α 1–4 link

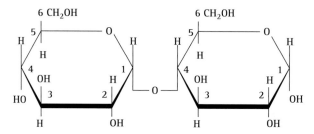

Amylose
Long chains of glucose residues joined by α 1–4 links

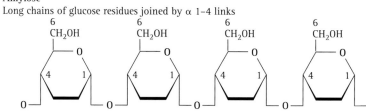

Amylopectin
A branch point in amylopectin due to an α 1–6 link

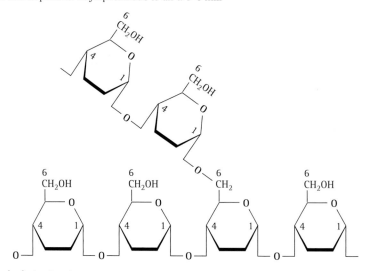

Figure 9.2 *Some carbohydrate structures.*

- The enzymes maltase and isomaltase located on the surface of the small intestine complete the digestion of starch to glucose.

- Starches are insoluble in water and are bland so affluent populations tend to replace much of the starch that predominates in peasant diets with fats and sugars.

- Reducing fat and sugar intakes to recommended levels will mean large increases in starch consumption, which means eating more potatoes, bread and other cereals.

NON-STARCH POLYSACCHARIDE

Halliday and Ashwell (1991a) have written a concise, referenced review of this topic; many of the uncited references used for this discussion are listed here. Non-starch polysaccharides are structural components of plant cell walls (cellulose and hemicellulose) and viscous soluble substances found in cell sap (pectin and gums). They are resistant to digestion by human gut enzymes. Animal-derived foods can be regarded for dietetic purposes as containing no NSP. Non-starch polysaccharide contains numerous different sugar residues but it passes through the small intestine and into the large bowel undigested. The term is used interchangeably with the term **dietary fibre** although the latter also includes **lignin** and **resistant starch** (see later). Lignin is an insoluble, chemically complex material that is not carbohydrate. It is found in wood and is the woody component of cell walls. Dietary lignin comes from mature root vegetables, wheat bran and the seeds of fruits such as strawberries.

Americans and Britons are currently being advised to substantially increase their consumption of NSP or fibre – current recommendations suggest increases over current intakes of 50–100 per cent. Non-starch polysaccharide and starches are usually found within the same foods particularly in cereals and starchy vegetables such as potatoes. This means that increasing NSP and starch intakes are likely to go hand in hand. The milling of cereals so that all or part of the indigestible outer layers of the cereal grains (**bran**) is removed, substantially reduces the NSP and micronutrient content of the end product, but without removing significant amounts of starch. Wholegrain cereals therefore contain substantially more NSP than refined cereals (Box 9.1).

Box 9.1   NSP content g/100g

- Wholemeal bread – 5.8
- White bread – 1.5
- Brown rice – 0.8
- White rice – 0.2

Current average intakes of NSP in the UK are around 14 g/day with a wide individual variation and this compares with the dietary reference value of 18 g/day; around 72 per cent of men and 87 per cent of women take in less than the 18 g/day target value. Non-starch polysaccharide is frequently categorized into two major fractions: the soluble substances that form gums and gels when mixed with water (the gums and pectins plus some hemicellulose) and the water-insoluble fraction (cellulose and some hemicellulose). The NSP in the UK diet is made up of similar proportions of **soluble** and **insoluble NSP**. The insoluble forms of NSP predominate in the bran of wheat, rice and maize but oats, rye and barley contain higher proportions of soluble NSP. The proportions of soluble and insoluble NSP in fruit and vegetables varies but they generally contain a substantially higher proportion of soluble NSP than wheat fibre, the principal cereal NSP in the British diet. Table 9.3 shows the total NSP content of several common foods and the proportion of the NSP that is soluble.

Table 9.3 The soluble non-sugar polysaccharide (NSP) content of some common foods*

Food(g/100 g)	Total NSP	% Soluble NSP
Wholemeal bread	5.8	17
Brown rice	0.8	12
Oatmeal (raw)	7.0	60
'All-bran'	24.5	17
Cornflakes	0.9	44
Potatoes	1.2	58
Apples	1.6	38
Oranges	2.1	66
Bananas	1.1	64
Carrots	2.5	56
Peas	2.9	28
Sprouts	4.8	52
Cabbage	3.2	50
Baked beans	3.5	60
Roasted peanuts	6.2	31

*Data source: Halliday and Ashwell (1991a).

Although NSP is resistant to digestion by human gut enzymes and passes through the small intestine largely intact, in the large intestine, most of the components of NSP are fermented to variable extents by gut bacteria. The pectins are very readily fermentable but cellulose remains largely unfermented in the human colon and in general soluble NSP is more fermented than insoluble NSP. Non-starch polysaccharide thus acts as a substrate for bacterial growth within the large intestine; the by-products of this fermentation are intestinal gases and short-chain fatty acids (acetate, butyrate and propionate). The short-chain fatty acids thus produced can be absorbed from the gut and can serve as a human energy source so that the typical mix of NSP in British and American diets may contribute as much as 2 kcal (8 kJ)/g to dietary energy. (Note that in ruminating animals like sheep and cattle, the short-chain fatty acids produced by the fermentation of starches and NSP by microbes in the rumen are the animal's principal energy source. Even in pigs, whose gastrointestinal physiology is much more like that of humans, such fermentation in the large intestine, and the resulting short-chain fatty acids, can make up a substantial proportion of the total dietary energy.)

Increasing levels of NSP in the diet can be convincingly shown to have a number of physiological effects in the short term.

- Increased NSP content of foods slows down the rate of glucose absorption from the gut and thus reduces the postprandial peak concentrations of glucose and insulin in blood. This effect is attributed to the soluble components of NSP and it is thought to be partly due to the mechanical effect of the viscous NSP components in reducing the contact of dissolved glucose with the absorptive surface of the intestinal epithelium. Soluble NSP may also slow down the mixing of gut contents with digestive enzymes and so slow the digestive process. Guar gum (a soluble NSP that forms a viscous solution when mixed with water) has been shown to reduce the outflow of dissolved glucose even *in vitro* experiments using a dialysis bag made from synthetic materials. The NSP can only produce this effect if taken with the glucose or digestible carbohydrate – it cannot work if taken a few hours before or after the ingested glucose.

Increased intakes of dietary fibre have been shown to improve glucose tolerance; people with diabetes, in particular, may benefit from this improvement. Dietary guidelines for people with diabetes now include a recommendation to ensure good intakes of high NSP foods.

- Increased intakes of NSP increase the volume of stools produced and reduces the **transit time** (i.e. the time it takes for an ingested marker to pass out in the faeces). The fermentable components of NSP lead to increased proliferation of intestinal bacteria and thus increase the bacterial mass in the stools. The short-chain fatty acids produced during fermentation also tend to acidify the colonic contents and act as substrates for the intestinal cells and this may increase gut motility. The unfermented components of NSP hold water and thus they also increase the stool bulk and make the stools softer and easier to pass. The increased bulk and softness of stools, together with more direct effects on gut motility produced by the products of fermentation, combine to accelerate the passage of faeces through the colon. These effects of fibre/NSP on the gut are often presented as being only relatively recently recognized but they do in fact have a very long history. The following quotes are from a booklet published by the Kellogg Company in 1934.

> It is imperative that proper bulk be included in the foods that are served. Otherwise, the system fails to eliminate regularly. Common constipation, with its attendant evils, sets in.
> This bulk is the cellulose or fibre content in certain natural foods.
> Within the body, it [bran] ... absorbs moisture and forms a soft mass which gently helps to clear the intestines of wastes.

Even back in the 1880s, Dr Thomas Allinson was championing the cause of wholemeal bread. He suggested many benefits of wholemeal over white bread (i.e. of bran) that are widely accepted today, e.g. prevention of constipation and the prevention of minor bowel disorders like haemorrhoids (piles).

- NSP and some of the substances associated with it (e.g. phytate) tend to bind or chelate minerals and probably also vitamins and thus may hinder their absorption. In compensation, foods rich in NSP tend also to have higher levels of micronutrients than refined foods. If the NSP is fermented in the colon then this releases bound minerals. At intakes of NSP likely to be consumed by most Britons or Americans, this is thought unlikely to pose a significant threat to micronutrient supply.

- In recent years, there has been considerable interest in the possible effects that increased intakes of soluble NSP may have in reducing the serum cholesterol concentration. A number of controlled studies have indicated that consumption of relatively large quantities of oats, which are rich in soluble NSP, can have a significant cholesterol-lowering effect in subjects with either elevated or normal cholesterol levels. The most widely promulgated explanation for this effect is that the soluble NSP binds or chelates both dietary cholesterol and bile acids (produced from cholesterol) and this reduces their absorption or reabsorption in the small intestine and thus increases the rate of faecal cholesterol loss. Most of the considerable quantity of bile acids and cholesterol secreted in the bile each day are reabsorbed and recycled (see entero-hepatic recycling of bile acids in Chapter 11); high NSP intake may interfere with this process.

- High fibre diets tend to be high in starch and low in fat and thus the energy density of such diets tends to be low. There is a widespread belief that such dietary bulking may contribute to maintaining energy balance and thus to reducing overweight and obesity. Blundell and Burley (1987) reviewed evidence that NSP may also have a satiating effect and thus may be a useful aid to regulate energy balance in those prone to overweight and obesity (another effect of bran proposed by Allinson in the 1880s). Some possible reasons why high-NSP foods could be more satiating are:
  - they reduce eating speed because they require increased chewing (this also stimulates saliva production and may be beneficial to dental health)
  - soluble NSP slows gastric emptying and may contribute to feelings of fullness
  - NSP slows down the absorption of glucose and other nutrients and reduces the insulin response to absorbed nutrients. A large insulin response to absorbed nutrients may cause blood glucose concentration to fall below resting levels (the rebound effect), triggering feelings of hunger.

Key points

- Non-starch polysaccharides (NSPs) are carbohydrates such as cellulose, hemicellulose, pectin and some gums that are all resistant to digestion by α-amylase.

- NSPs pass into the large bowel undigested.

- The term dietary fibre includes not only NSP but also lignin, a complex, woody material that is not carbohydrate, and also starch that resists digestion by α-amylase.

- UK and US consumers should increase their fibre/NSP intakes by 50–100 per cent.

- Most of the NSP in cereal grains is in the bran layer and so milling cereals to remove the bran removes much of their NSP.

- Wholegrain cereals contain much more fibre/NSP than refined cereals.

- Some components of NSP are soluble and form gels when mixed with water whereas other components are insoluble.

- Insoluble NSP predominates in wheat, rice and maize bran but other cereals (e.g. oats) and most fruits and vegetables contain higher proportions of soluble NSP.

- In the bowel, most components of NSP are fermented to some extent by bacteria to yield short-chain fatty acids.

- These short-chain fatty acids can be absorbed and may yield significant amounts of metabolizable energy.

- Soluble NSP slows glucose absorption and reduces the postprandial peaks of glucose and insulin.

- NSP increases the volume of stools and reduces transit time. Stools have an increased bacterial mass and higher water content.

- NSP may bind vitamins and minerals and hinder their absorption. However, many high-NSP foods are relatively rich in micronutrients and any bound nutrients will be released if the NSP is fermented.

- Soluble fibre has a lowering effect on plasma cholesterol. One proposed mechanism is that it hinders the recycling of bile acids and so increases faecal losses of cholesterol.

- High-fibre foods may help in the regulation of energy intake because:
  - they reduce eating speed
  - NSP slows gastric emptying
  - NSP slows glucose absorption and may help to prevent rebound hypoglycaemia caused by a large insulin response to a rapid absorption of glucose.

RESISTANT STARCH

Many starchy foods such as bread, cornflakes and boiled potatoes, contain starch that is resistant to digestion by α-amylase *in vitro*. If resistance to α-amylase digestion is used in the chemical determination of NSP in food then this **resistant starch** would be classified as part of the NSP. Studies in patients with ileostomies (patients whose small intestine has been surgically modified so that they drain externally into a bag rather than into the large intestine) show that this resistant starch also resists digestion by gut enzymes *in vivo*. Like NSP, resistant starch enters the large intestine undigested. It acts as a substrate for bacteria in the large bowel and this affects bowel function. There is some debate whether resistant starch should be regarded as part of the 'dietary fibre' with similar health benefits to NSP.

Starch that is within starch granules is in a partial crystalline form that is insoluble and relatively resistant to α-amylase digestion. During cooking (heating with moisture) this crystalline starch is disrupted (gelatinized) and this renders it much more digestible. During cooling, the starch starts to recrystallize (retrogradation) which reduces its digestibility. There are essentially three reasons why starch may be resistant to digestion in the gut:

- it may be inaccessible to digestive enzymes because it is enclosed within unbroken cell walls or in partly milled grains or seeds
- some forms of raw crystalline starch, e.g. in raw potatoes and green bananas, are resistant to α-amylase digestion
- retrograded starch in food that has been cooked and cooled is indigestible.

This resistant starch is usually a small component of total starch in any food. However, it may make a considerable contribution to the apparent NSP content of some foods. For example, resistant starch would represent around 30 per cent of the apparent NSP in white bread, 33 per cent in boiled potatoes and 80 per cent in boiled white rice. The amount of resistant starch in any given food may vary quite a lot depending on slight differences in preparation. In freshly cooked potatoes around 3–5 per cent of the starch is not digested in the small intestine but this rises to 12 per cent when potatoes are cooked and cooled before being eaten; in greenish under-ripe bananas as much as 70 per cent of the starch reaches the large intestine. It has been estimated that average intake of resistant starch in Europe is around 4 g/day. If it were considered desirable it would be possible to alter the resistant starch content of processed food considerably by manipulating the choice of raw materials and the processing conditions.

Resistant starch is just one of a number of factors that complicate the measurement of dietary fibre intakes of a population. Englyst and Kingman (1993) gave values for the estimates of fibre intake in several foods, which vary by as much 100 per cent, depending upon the analytical methods used to estimate it. This clearly represents a major hindrance to epidemiological investigations of the effects of NSP/fibre on health. For example, several oriental populations with rice-based diets have lower fibre intakes than the British because of the very low NSP content of white rice. These oriental diets are, however, often high in starch and inclusion of resistant starch with NSP would significantly change the fibre position of these diets. The Englyst method specifically measures the NSP content of food. Starch is completely removed by enzyme hydrolysis and then the amount of sugars released by acid hydrolysis of the food is determined and used as the measure of NSP content. Resistant starch has been reviewed by Asp *et al.* (1996).

Key points

- Some starch resists digestion by α-amylase and enters the large bowel undigested, the resistant starch.
- Resistant starch is fermented in the large bowel and behaves like a fermentable component of NSP.
- Some starch resists digestion because it is inaccessible to gut enzymes, e.g. it is within cell walls.

- Raw crystalline starch is resistant to α-amylase, e.g. the starch in raw potatoes.
- When crystalline starch is cooked, it gelatinizes and becomes digestible but during cooling some of it recrystallizes (retrogradation) and becomes indigestible again.
- The way in which foods are processed can have a big influence on the resistant starch content, e.g. cooling boiled rice and potatoes greatly increases their resistant starch content.
- White rice has very little NSP but does contain significant amounts of resistant starch. This could make a significant difference to the functional NSP content of the diets of several oriental populations that are based on white rice.

THE GLYCAEMIC INDEX

Ingested carbohydrate foods differ markedly in the way they affect blood glucose. If pure glucose is ingested it is absorbed rapidly and causes a rapid large rise in blood glucose which in turn stimulates a large release of the hormone insulin which rapidly brings the blood glucose down again and the blood glucose concentration often falls below the starting level (**rebound hypoglycaemia**). Other foods such as oat-based breakfast cereals are absorbed more slowly and produce a smaller rise in blood glucose concentration and a smaller insulin response without the rebound effects often seen with glucose or rapidly absorbed carbohydrates. Jenkins *et al.* (1981) coined the term **glycaemic index (GI)** to describe in a quantitative way the rise in blood glucose that different carbohydrate foods produce. Time course curves of blood glucose concentration are plotted in the 2 hours after consumption of matched amounts of carbohydrate (usually 50 g) contained within different foods. The area under the time course curve for each food is then expressed as a percentage of that induced by the same amount of pure glucose (note that 50 g of carbohydrate contained in white bread is sometimes used as the standard). Foods can be classified as having a high, medium or lower GI:

- High GI – 90 per cent or more of the area under the glucose curve – includes foods such as white bread and rice, boiled old potatoes, cornflakes, most cakes, pancakes and crackers made from white flour

- Medium GI–70–90 per cent – includes wholemeal bread, boiled new potatoes and sweetcorn
- Lower GI – less than 70 per cent – includes dried beans and peas, most pasta, all-bran, porridge (oatmeal), muesli and German black bread (pumpernickel).

Some factors that affect the GI of an isolated food are:

- the speed of digestion of the carbohydrate – the slower the digestion, the lower the GI
- the amount and type of dietary fibre – dietary fibre, especially soluble fibre, delays gastric emptying and slows absorption and so lowers the glycaemic response to a food or meal
- presence of monosaccharides such as fructose which are slowly absorbed from the gut and thus lower GI
- ripeness of a fruit.

The presence of other foods in a meal will also modify the glycaemic response to a food so the glycaemic response to a meal may be difficult to predict from the GIs of foods measured individually. It is generally accepted that foods with low GI would be beneficial for glycaemic control in diabetes management. Manipulation of GI has been generally regarded as too complex to be usefully incorporate into formal individual dietary advice for people with diabetes. However, a popular book (Leeds *et al.*, 1998) has sought to increase popular awareness and to encourage the use of this concept in food selection for better weight control, diabetic management and for general healthy eating. For example, it suggests that low-GI foods/meals will have a more sustained satiating effect that high-GI foods and thus aid in control of appetite and thus in obesity management.

DOES DIETARY FIBRE/NON-STARCH POLYSACCHARIDE PROTECT AGAINST BOWEL CANCER AND HEART DISEASE?

The recent preoccupation with the protective effects of dietary fibre against bowel problems such as constipation, diverticular disease, appendicitis, haemorrhoids and perhaps cancer of the colon and rectum, can be traced back to the work of Burkitt, Trowell, Painter and others in the 1960s and 1970s. These workers noted the rarity of bowel diseases in rural

African populations consuming high-fibre diets and their much greater frequency in populations consuming the 'Western' low-fibre diet. Burkitt (1971) suggested that dietary fibre might protect against bowel cancer by diluting potential carcinogens in faeces and speeding their elimination so that the intestine is exposed to them for less time.

As a general rule, populations with high rates of coronary heart disease also tend to have high incidence of bowel cancer. This means that much of the evidence that implicates any dietary factor in the aetiology of coronary heart disease could also be used to implicate that factor in the aetiology of bowel cancer. This link between bowel cancer and coronary heart disease is not inevitable. There are populations such as the British Asians that have high rates of coronary heart disease and low rates of bowel cancer. The modern Japanese population has a relatively high rate of bowel cancer but still has a relatively low rate of coronary heart disease. Bingham (1996) reviewed the role of NSP and other dietary factors in the aetiology of bowel cancer and Halliday and Ashwell (1991a) have written a general review of NSP and uncited references published prior to 1996 may be found in one of these reviews.

Descriptive epidemiology

In the UK, the bowel is the second most common site for cancer in both men (after lung cancer) and women (after breast cancer). Age-standardized rates for bowel cancer are even higher in the USA than in Britain. There are very large international variations in the incidence of bowel cancer, with generally high rates in the USA, Australasia and northern Europe but low rates in, for example, India, China and rural Africa. Bingham (1996) suggests that age-standardized rates of bowel cancer may vary among countries by as much as 15-fold. These large international variations in bowel cancer could be the result of genetic differences between populations or could be due to dietary and other environmental differences between them. Migration studies, together with time trends for populations such as the Japanese, clearly indicate the predominance of environmental factors in the aetiology of bowel cancer which also means that bowel cancer is a potentially preventable disease. Rates of bowel cancer have increased amongst migrants and their

descendants who have moved from low to high bowel cancer areas, e.g. Japanese migrants to Hawaii in the late nineteenth and early twentieth centuries. Over the past 40 years there have been marked changes in the diets of people living in Japan, and this has been accompanied by major increases in the incidence of colon cancer. In 1960, age-standardized rates of bowel cancer in Japan were about a third of those in the UK whereas they are now similar.

Naturally high-fibre diets tend to be low in fat and low-fibre diets tend to be high in fat. This means that much of the evidence linking low-fibre diets to increased risk of bowel cancer could equally well be used to implicate high-fat diets. This is another example of the recurring problem of confounding variables that plagues the epidemiologist. Cross-cultural comparisons indicate that populations with diets high in meat and fat but low in NSP, starch and vegetables are at high risk of bowel cancer. There is thus a general trend for populations with high fibre intakes to have low rates of bowel cancer but the negative relationship between fibre intake and incidence of bowel cancer is very sharply reduced when this relationship is corrected for differences in fat and meat consumption. Vegetarian groups, such as Seventh Day Adventists in the USA, have lower rates of bowel cancer than other Americans and they also have higher intakes of dietary NSP. Once again low meat and fat intakes or even high intakes of antioxidant vitamins in fruits and vegetables make it impossible to finally attribute these low cancer rates to a direct protective effect of dietary NSP. According to Bingham (1996), the cross-cultural data suggest that high meat and fat intakes are prerequisites for a population to have high incidence of bowel cancer but that in such populations high intakes of NSP seem to exert a protective effect. High starch and vegetable intakes may also be protective; high vegetable intake would mean a high intake of the antioxidant vitamins (e.g. β-carotene, vitamin E and vitamin C) and high starch intake probably also means high intake of resistant starch.

As already noted there has been a threefold rise in incidence of bowel cancer in Japan since 1960. During this period there has been no significant change in overall NSP intakes but major increases in consumption of meat, dairy produce and wheat and a large decrease in rice consumption. Even though fibre intakes have not changed over this period, there has been a substantial decline in the proportion of calories derived from starch and most of the functional dietary fibre in white rice is resistant starch. Measures of the fibre intake that have taken no account of residual starch may thus be misleading. The reduction in the amount of carbohydrate in the Japanese diet over this period has been offset by increased fat consumption; consumption of animal fat has more than doubled over this period.

Case–control and cohort studies

According to Bingham (1990) a large majority of case–control studies indicate that people with bowel cancer ate less vegetable fibre than controls. According to Willett *et al.* (1990) most case–control studies also indicate a significant positive association between total fat intake and bowel cancer. Bingham (1996) concluded that these studies have indicated similar trends to those found in cross-cultural studies, i.e. that individuals with high intakes of fat and meat but low intakes of fibre and vegetables are at increased risk of bowel cancer. The limitations of case–control studies have been discussed in Chapter 3. As Bingham (1996) points out, diseases of the large bowel produce pain and altered bowel function and so one of the effects of bowel disease may be to make patients change their diets to avoid the symptoms. The low fibre intakes of the cases in these case–control studies might be a consequence of the disease rather than an indication of its cause. Note that many studies do attempt to address this problem by asking cases about their past diets but other studies suggest that recall of past diet is strongly influenced by current diet.

Willett *et al.* (1990) have reported results from a 6-year follow-up using a cohort of almost 90 000 American nurses. They found no significant association between total fibre intake and risk of developing colon cancer over the 6-year period. They also found no significant associations when they used subdivisions of the fibre from different food sources, i.e. vegetable, fruit or cereal fibre (although there was a non-significant trend with fruit fibre). They did find significant positive associations between total fat intake and colon cancer risk and an even stronger association with animal fat intake (illustrated in Chapter 3, Figure 3.9, p. 109); 'red meat' (beef, pork and lamb) consumption was also positively associated with bowel cancer risk. They

confirmed the expected negative association between fibre intake and animal fat intake in their population; this perhaps explains the apparent contradiction between these results and the fibre results from case–control studies. Their results provide rather weak support for the proposition that low intakes of fruit fibre might contribute to the risk of colon cancer but stronger evidence in favour of the proposition that high animal fat intake is linked to increased risk of colon cancer. It should nonetheless be borne in mind that despite the apparently very large sample size, the analysis is based on only 150 total cases and only 103 cases when those developing cancer within the first 2 years of follow-up were excluded.

In an overall assessment of all of the cohort studies published up to 1996, Bingham (1996) concluded that there is only weak evidence for a slightly increased risk for high meat and fat consumers and for a slightly decreased risk in those with high vegetable and NSP intakes. All of the cohort studies published prior to 1996 had major drawbacks such as:

- poor dietary assessment methodology
- sample populations that had too narrow a range of dietary habits.

Bingham suggested that good additional data from large and well-designed cohort studies using large populations with very diverse dietary habits would not become available until well into the new millennium. One of those large cohort studies was the European Prospective Investigation of Cancer and Nutrition (EPIC), which had a cohort of over half a million individuals from 10 different European countries with diverse dietary habits and lifestyles (brief details of this study are given in Chapter 3 along with the official EPIC website address). Bingham *et al.* (2003) published data from this study which found that there was a 40 per cent lower risk of bowel cancer in those with the highest quintile of fibre intake compared with those in the lowest quintile. In the following months and years several other authors have criticized these data because Bingham did not correct for physical activity, alcohol intake, smoking, red and processed meat consumption and especially for consumption of folate. The folate issue and to an extent these other potentially confounding variables are addressed in a review by Bingham (2006). She discussed cases of bowel cancer that have occurred since the data set on which the 2003 paper was based and concluded that correcting the results for folate intake did not materially affect the inverse relationship between fibre intake and bowel cancer risk. She reported that incidence of bowel cancer decreased by around 9 per cent for each quintile increase in dietary fibre intake. She also concluded that although there is a negative association in other published studies between folate intake from food and risk of bowel cancer this does not apply to folate taken as supplements, i.e. suggesting that it is not a direct effect of folate but of those foods which contain folate (and also contain dietary fibre). She suggested that correcting for other confounding variables confirmed the association between fibre and reduced bowel cancer risk. The EPIC study also suggests that consumption of red and processed meats increases the risk of bowel cancer and that this increase is most pronounced in those who consume little fibre – fibre protects against the cancer inducing effects of a high-meat diet? In those people with high fibre intake (>28 g/day) colon cancer risk was lower at all levels of meat intake than in those in the low meat/low fibre intake category. This latter observation seems to be contrary to Bingham's (1996) suggestion that high intake of red meat is a prerequisite for high bowel cancer incidence.

Assessment of the evidence

The overall conclusion from the current evidence is that there is strong support for the proposition that a diet higher in fibre/NSP containing foods (cereals, vegetables and fruit) will reduce the incidence of bowel cancer in countries such as the UK and USA. Such dietary changes are consistent with current nutrition education guidelines. The resulting diets would not only have more fibre than current diets but would also have less fat, less animal fat, less meat protein, more starch and more antioxidant vitamins. The evidence supporting a direct protective effect of dietary fibre, or any individual component of the NSPs, is weaker than the evidence supporting this more generalized change although the results of the EPIC study so far published add considerable weight to the argument that dietary fibre has a direct protective effect (see Bingham, 2006). The current evidence may be interpreted in several ways.

- High dietary NSP/fibre intake directly protects against bowel cancer.
- High dietary fat/animal fat promotes bowel cancer and any apparent protective effect of high intake of complex carbohydrates is an artefact due to the inverse relationship between fat and complex carbohydrate intakes.
- NSP protects against the cancer promoting effects of high dietary fat (or meat protein) in the bowel. The data from the EPIC trial support the notion that high meat intake increases bowel cancer risk and that fibre is strongly protective against this effect.
- High fruit and vegetable intake protect against bowel cancer because of their high content of antioxidants such as vitamin E, vitamin C and β-carotene.
- High intake of meat protein increases the risk of bowel cancer.

It is quite possible that several of these statements are true and that several dietary factors promote and help prevent bowel cancer.

As with the link between NSP and bowel cancer, the evidence supporting the beneficial effects of dietary changes that would increase NSP intake on risk of coronary heart disease is very much stronger than the evidence for a direct link between NSP intake and coronary heart disease. These conclusions mean that the consumption of more foods naturally rich in complex carbohydrates has a much higher probability of reducing the risk of these diseases than adding extracted fibre to foods or the use of foods in which the fibre content has been greatly 'amplified' by food manufacturers.

Key points

- High fibre diets have long been thought to protect against bowel cancer as well as alleviate other bowel problems such as constipation, diverticular disease and haemorrhoids.
- Bowel cancer is the second most common site for cancer in the UK for men and women.
- High rates of bowel cancer and high rates of coronary heart disease tend to go together although there are exceptions, e.g. British

Asians and the present-day Japanese population.

- Internationally, rates of bowel cancer vary by 15-fold with high rates in the USA, Australasia and northern Europe but low rates in India, China and rural Africa.

- Migration studies and recent changes in bowel cancer frequency in Japan show that environmental factors are largely responsible for the variations in bowel cancer incidence.

- Vegetarian groups and populations with diets low in meat and fat but high in NSP and vegetables have low rates of bowel cancer.

- At both the individual and population level, intakes of fat and NSP tend to be inversely correlated.

- It is difficult to differentiate the contributions of high meat, high fat, low NSP and low vegetable intakes to the aetiology of bowel cancer.

- Bingham (1996) suggested that high meat and fat intakes are prerequisites for high population rates of bowel cancer and that NSP is protective in these circumstances.

- Most case–control studies indicate higher fat and/or lower NSP intakes in bowel cancer cases. The diets of those who have colon cancer may reflect their disease rather than indicate its cause.

- Cohort studies published prior to 1996 provide weak evidence for a slightly increased bowel cancer risk in high fat and meat consumers and a slightly decreased risk in those with high vegetable and NSP intakes.

- Most cohort studies published before1996 used subjects with a narrow range of dietary habits and/or used inadequate means for assessing dietary intake.

- Evidence that naturally high-fibre diets are associated with low bowel cancer risk is much stronger than evidence for a specific protective effect of NSP.

- Naturally high-fibre diets tend to be low in meat and fat but high in vegetables and antioxidants.

- The EPIC study has enrolled over half a million subjects with diverse European dietary and lifestyle practices.

- Data from EPIC suggest that for each quintile of rise in dietary fibre intake the incidence of bowel cancer drops by around 9 per cent, i.e. it is more that 40 per cent lower in the highest compared to the lowest fibre quintile.

- EPIC data also show an increase in bowel cancer risk associated with increasing red meat consumption and that high fibre intake seems to reduce this effect of meat.

- The relationship between colon cancer risk and dietary fibre intake is not diminished by correction for many confounders including folate intake.

POSSIBLE MECHANISMS BY WHICH DIET MAY INFLUENCE THE RISK OF BOWEL CANCER AND HEART DISEASE

Human faeces contain substances that induce mutation in bacteria (mutagens). Such mutagens are known to be likely carcinogens in animals and people. Some of these mutagens are:

- bile acid breakdown products
- nitrosamines from cured meats and beer
- heterocyclic amines present in cooked meat and fish – more of these are produced if the food is fried, grilled or barbecued than if it is stewed or microwaved.

High-fat and/or high-meat diets may increase the mutagenicity of faeces. A high-fat diet increases the production of bile acids and these may be converted to mutagenic derivatives within the gut. High consumption of meat protein increases the intake of carcinogenic heterocyclic amines and increases the production of nitrosamines and other nitrogen-containing carcinogens within the large bowel. Mechanisms that have been used to explain how high intakes of NSP and resistant starch could help protect against bowel cancer are:

- NSP and resistant starch increase the weight and water content of stools and thus would tend to dilute any potential carcinogens in stools
- they decrease transit time and thus reduce the time that the gut cells are exposed to these faecal carcinogens
- the short-chain fatty acids produced during fermentation of NSP and resistant starch in the

colon act as substrates for the epithelial cells of the gut. Butyrate in particular may inhibit the proliferation of mutated cells into cancerous tumours. The acid environment they produce in the bowel may reduce the conversion of bile acids to their mutagenic derivatives.

In controlled experimental studies in which animals are exposed to known chemical carcinogens, bran has been consistently reported to reduce the number of tumours. Bran appears to protect against these chemically initiated cancers. In other experimental studies, bran fibre has been reported to reduce the mutagenicity of faeces produced by human subjects (see Bingham, 1990, 1996).

Some of the possible mechanisms by which NSP might have a specific influence on coronary heart disease risk are listed below.

- Soluble NSP may help to lower the plasma cholesterol concentration, e.g. by interfering with the entero-hepatic recycling of cholesterol and bile acids.
- A high intake of NSP, particularly soluble NSP, improves glucose tolerance and reduces insulin secretion (diabetes greatly increases the risk of coronary heart disease); it would decrease the GI of a meal.
- High NSP intake may act indirectly to reduce coronary heart disease by reducing the risk of obesity, e.g. because it reduces the energy density of the diet and increases satiety by slowing gastric emptying and absorption of the products of digestion (and thus decreasing GI).

Key points

- Human faeces contains carcinogenic substances including bile acid derivatives, nitrosamines from cured meats and beer and heterocyclic amines from cooked meat and fish.
- High meat and fat consumption increases the carcinogenicity of faeces.
- Fat increases bile acid production.
- Non-starch polysaccharide (NSP) could protect against bowel cancer by causing dilution and more rapid elimination of faecal carcinogens.
- Increased production of butyrate from the fermentation of NSP and resistant starch may inhibit the proliferation of mutated cells into tumours and reduce the conversion of bile acids to their carcinogenic derivatives.
- Naturally high-fibre diets (low in fat and saturated fat) are also associated with reduced rates of coronary heart disease.
- NSP might reduce the risk of coronary heart disease by:
  - reducing the reabsorption of bile acids and lowering plasma cholesterol
  - improving glucose tolerance
  - indirectly by helping to prevent excessive weight gain
  - decreasing the glycaemic index of the diet.
- Choosing a diet that is high in natural fibre/NSP is more likely to reduce the risk of bowel cancer or coronary heart disease than artificially enhancing the fibre content of existing diets.

10

Protein and amino acids

TRADITIONAL SCIENTIFIC ASPECTS OF PROTEIN NUTRITION

Experiments stretching back over the past two centuries have demonstrated the principle that all animals require an exogenous supply of protein. In humans, and in other non-ruminating mammals, this protein must be present in the food that they eat. (Note that some ruminants can survive without dietary protein if their diet contains alternative sources of nitrogen. This is because bacteria in the rumen can make protein from non-protein nitrogen sources such as urea and the animals can digest and absorb this bacterial protein.) In the early 1800s, Francois Magendie fed dogs with single foods that were regarded as highly nutritious but lacked any nitrogen (e.g. sugar, olive oil or butter). These unfortunate dogs survived much longer than if they had been completely starved but they lost weight, their muscles wasted dramatically and they all died within 40 days. Several modern writers, including myself, have assumed that Magendie completed the cycle of evidence by showing that the dogs recovered when nitrogen-containing foods were added back to their diets. In his excellent book on the history of protein nutrition, Carpenter (1994) points out that Magendie did not actually do these positive controls. Despite this he is still usually credited with the discovery that nitrogen-containing foods are essential in the diet. In later years it became clear that Magendie's initial conclusions were in fact correct, i.e. that adequate amounts of nitrogen-containing foods were essential to allow growth and even survival in experimental animals. Such experiments demonstrated the need for nitrogen-containing foods (i.e. protein) even before the chemical nature of dietary protein was known.

> ## Key points
>
> - Protein is an essential nutrient for all animals.
> - Even before protein was chemically characterized it was clear that animals needed foods that contain nitrogen.

Chemistry and digestion

Protein is the only major nitrogen-containing component of the diet. It is composed of long chains of 20 different **amino acids** that are linked together by **peptide bonds**. Figure 10.1 illustrates the chemical nature of amino acids and proteins. The amino acid side chain (the R-group in Figure 10.1) is the group that varies between amino acids and some examples of the R-groups in particular amino acids are shown in Figure 10.1. Amino acids are usually classified into groups according to the nature of the side chain or R-group. These side chains vary in size shape, charge, hydrogen-bonding capacity, affinity for water and reactivity; these properties determine the three dimensional structure of any given protein. The groupings are:

- glycine has just a hydrogen atom (H) as its side chain and is the only amino acid without two optical isomers
- those with aliphatic (hydrocarbon) side chains – alanine, valine, leucine and isoleucine

Generalized chemical formula of amino acids

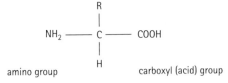

amino group   carboxyl (acid) group

Examples of amino acid side chains

R = H	amino acid = glycine
R = CH$_3$	amino acid = alanine
R = CH$_2$SH	amino acid = cysteine
R = (CH$_2$)$_4$NH$_2$	amino acid = lysine
R = CH$_2$OH	amino acid = serine

Two amino acids linked by a peptide bond

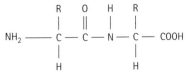

Diagrammatic representation of a protein

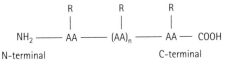

N-terminal   C-terminal

Figure 10.1 *The chemical nature of proteins and amino acids.*

- those with hydroxyl aliphatic side chains, i.e. containing an OH group – serine and threonine
- proline is an aliphatic amino acid but in this case it has a ring structure because the amino group binds to the terminal methyl group of the side chain (it is a secondary amine)
- those with aromatic side chains, i.e. with aromatic or benzene ring – phenylalanine, tyrosine and tryptophan
- amino acids which have basic side chains due the presence of an amino group in the side chain and these are positively charged at neutral pH – lysine, arginine and histidine
- those with carboxyl groups in the side chain and these are negatively charged at neutral pH – glutamic and aspartic acids
- those with sulphur-containing side chains – cysteine and methionine
- those with amide groups (CONH$_2$) in their side chains – glutamine and asparagine.

Note than some amino acids may be modified after they have been incorporated into a protein, e.g. the proline in collagen is hydroxylated to hydroxyproline (this reaction requires vitamin C) and the glutamate in prothrombin and other clotting proteins is carboxylated (this reaction requires vitamin K).

The way in which amino acids are linked together by peptide bonds is also illustrated in Figure 10.1. The nitrogen atom in the **amino group** of one amino acid is linked to the carbon atom of the **carboxyl group** in the adjacent amino acid. A protein may be comprised of hundreds of amino acids linked together in this way; each protein will have a free amino group at one end (the **N-terminal**) and a free carboxyl group at the opposite end (the **C-terminal**).

Dietary proteins are digested to their constituent amino acids prior to absorption in the small intestine. Significant amounts of dipeptides and other small peptide fragments may also be absorbed. (It is also clear that small amounts of intact protein can also be absorbed, e.g. some bacterial toxins and IgG antibodies from milk in many newborn mammals.) Peptidase enzymes in gastric and pancreatic juice break (hydrolyse) the peptide bonds between specific amino acids in dietary proteins yielding small peptides, dipeptides and free amino acids. Other peptidase enzymes located on the mucosal surface of the small intestine continue the digestion of these small protein fragments. Some peptidases are classified as endopeptidases because they hydrolyse the bonds between certain amino acids within the protein or peptide molecule. The major endopeptidases in the gut are:

- pepsin in gastric juice
- trypsin in pancreatic juice
- chymotrypsin in pancreatic juice
- collagenase (which breaks down collagen) and elastase are other endopeptidases in pancreatic juice.

The peptidases that break off one of the amino acids at the end of the peptide chain are termed exopeptidases. These are:

- carboxypeptidases in pancreatic juice break off the C-terminal amino acid
- aminopeptidases located on the surface of the small intestine break off the N-terminal amino acid.

Also located on the surface of the small intestine are dipeptidases and tripetidases, which break down dipeptides and tripeptides. Dipeptidases and tripeptidases within the cells complete the digestion of any dipeptides and tripeptides that are absorbed intact into the intestinal cells.

Key points

- Protein is made up of 20 different amino acids joined together in long chains by peptide bonds.
- The 20 amino acids used in protein synthesis can be classified according to the nature of their side chains.
- The amino acid side chains differ in size, charge, ability to form hydrogen bonds, reactivity and affinity for water, and these largely determine the three-dimensional shape of a protein.
- Protein is largely digested to its constituent amino acids in the gut by peptidase enzymes although some peptide fragments and even some intact protein is absorbed.
- Endopeptidases such as pepsin, trypsin and chymotrypsin in gastric and pancreatic juice break proteins into peptide fragments by breaking peptide bonds within the protein chain.
- Carboxypeptidases (cleave the C-terminal amino acid), aminopeptidases (cleave the N-terminal amino acid) and a range of dipeptidases and tripeptidases complete the digestion of dietary protein.

Intakes, dietary standards and food sources

Table 10.1 shows the reference nutrient intake (RNI) for protein of selected population groups expressed both as an absolute value and as a percentage of dietary energy. The values for all adults are based on a notional 0.75 g/kg body weight/day while values for children are set at a higher value per kg body weight to reflect the extra protein requirements for growth with maximum value being 1.65 g/kg body weight/day in 4–6-month-old children (this issue is addressed more fully later in the chapter). Hoare *et al.* (2004) found that average adult intakes of protein in the UK were around 150 per cent of the RNI and contributed about 16.5 per cent of the food energy. Intakes of protein were lower in the younger age groups but average intakes did not drop below 130 per cent of the RNI in any age group. Less than

Table 10.1 Some UK reference nutrient intakes (RNIs) for protein expressed in absolute terms and as a percentage of average energy requirements*

Age (years)	RNI g/day	% Energy
1–3	*14.5*	*4.7*
7–10	*28.3*	*5.7*
Male		
11–14	*42.1*	*7.7*
19–50	*55.5*	*8.7*
65–74	*53.3*	*9.2*
Female		
11–14	*41.2*	*8.9*
19–50	*45.0*	*9.3*
Pregnancy	*+6[†]*	*9.5–10.5[†]*
Lactation	*+11[†]*	*8.9–9.4[†]*

*Data source: COMA (1991).
[†] Additional to that of non-pregnant or lactating woman.
[†] Varies as the energy estimated average requirement (EAR) varies during pregnancy and lactation.

3 per cent of adults had a protein intake that was below the estimated average requirement (EAR) (45 g/day for men and 33 g/day for women). If one assumed a lower RNI (LRNI) that was set two standard deviations below the EAR then no healthy individuals would be likely to fall below this level. Intakes of essential amino acids (see later in the chapter) are not considered as a specific issue because the Committee on the Medical Aspects of Food (COMA) (1991) concluded that any group in the UK that is consuming food supplying sufficient energy and sufficient protein would be very unlikely to contain insufficient amounts of the essential amino acids; similar conclusions have been made in the USA. Almost no individuals would be consuming more than twice their RNI, which is the guideline upper limit suggested in both the UK (COMA, 1991) and the USA (National Research Council (NRC), 1989a). The main food sources of protein for UK adults are:

- cereals and cereal products – 23 per cent
- milk and milk products – 16 per cent
- meat and meat products – 37 per cent
- fish and fish dishes – 7 per cent
- eggs and egg dishes – 3 per cent
- vegetables including potatoes – 9 per cent.

The categories have been chosen partly to reflect the effect of different types of vegetarian diets but bear in mind that although a vegan would exclude foods that normally provide two-thirds of the daily protein they would consume much larger amounts of other foods with relatively high protein contents, e.g. pulses, soya milk, nuts, cereals and possibly vegetarian meat substitutes.

Key points

- The protein RNI for adults is set at a notional 0.75 g/kg body weight/ day.
- The RNI for children ranges up to 1.65 g/kg body weight/day and reflects the extra requirements for growth.
- Average adult protein intakes are 1.5 times the RNI and probably no healthy person in the UK is at risk of primary protein deficiency.
- Anyone in the UK consuming sufficient energy and sufficient protein will almost certainly get enough of all the essential amino acids.
- Foods from the meat and milk groups provide around 63 per cent of average adult protein intakes but vegans and other vegetarians will inevitable consume larger amounts of other protein-containing foods.

Nitrogen balance

Estimation of protein content

Early in the nineteenth century, the German chemist, Liebig, noted that proteins from different sources all contained approximately 16 per cent by weight of nitrogen. This observation remains the basis of estimating the protein content of foods. The nitrogen content is determined by a relatively simple chemical analysis (the Kjeldahl method) and then multiplied by 6.25 (i.e. 100/16) and this gives an estimate of the protein content. (In the Kjeldahl method, the food is boiled with concentrated sulphuric acid and a catalyst, which converts the nitrogen into ammonium sulphate. Alkali is then added to the digest and liberated ammonia is distilled into acid and the amount of ammonia liberated is determined by titration.)

Weight of protein = weight of nitrogen × 6.25

This figure of 6.25 is an approximation and more precise values may be used for some foods. Some foods may contain non-protein nitrogen but in most

this is largely amino acid and so would not produce any dietetic error. The Kjeldahl method can also be used to estimate the nitrogen content of urine and if this is multiplied by 6.25 it indicates how much protein has been broken down to produce this amount of nitrogen. Sweat and faeces can also be analysed for nitrogen to give a complete picture of protein losses by catabolism or direct protein loss in faeces.

Key points

- All proteins contain about 16 per cent nitrogen by weight.
- Protein content of food can be estimated from its nitrogen content and the rate of protein catabolism can be estimated from the nitrogen loss in urine.
- Nitrogen can be estimated using the Kjeldahl method.

Concept of nitrogen balance

Intakes and losses of nitrogen are used as the measure of protein intake and protein breakdown, respectively, and the difference between intake and total losses is the **nitrogen balance**.

$$\text{Nitrogen balance} = \text{nitrogen input} - \text{nitrogen losses}$$

The nitrogen input is from food protein. Nitrogen losses arise from the breakdown of dietary and body protein. Most nitrogen is lost in the urine but with small amounts also lost in faeces and via the skin. If the nitrogen balance is zero then this means that intakes completely offset losses and that the body protein content (lean mass) remains constant.

Negative nitrogen balance

A negative balance indicates that body protein is being depleted because more nitrogen is being lost than is taken in the diet. Injury, illness, starvation (including dieting) or inadequate protein intake *per se* may lead to negative nitrogen balance. The minimum amount of protein, in an otherwise complete diet, that enables an adult to achieve balance indicates the minimum requirement for protein. A deficit in energy supplies would be expected to lead to negative nitrogen balance for two reasons.

- A diet that that has insufficient energy will also tend to have a low protein content.

- During energy deficit, the protein that is present will tend to be used as a source of energy rather than being used for protein synthesis.

Requirements for balance

The protein requirement of an adult is the minimum intake that results in nitrogen balance. When adults are put onto a protein-free, but otherwise complete diet, their rate of nitrogen loss drops during the first few days as they adapt to this situation. Even after adaptation they excrete a low and relatively constant amount of nitrogen – this is termed the **obligatory nitrogen loss** and represents the minimum replacement requirement. Studies using radioactively labelled amino acids indicate that about 300 g of protein is normally broken down and re-synthesized in the body each day, the **protein turnover**. Most of the amino acids released during the breakdown of body protein can re-enter the body amino acid pool and be recycled into new protein synthesis, but a proportion (say 10 per cent) cannot be recycled and becomes the obligatory nitrogen loss. Several amino acids have additional functions to that of protein building and are irreversibly lost from the body amino acid pool, e.g. for synthesis of non-protein substances such as pigments or transmitters, to maintain acid–base balance, and for conjugation with substances to facilitate their excretion. When amino acids are lost from the pool for such reasons, then some other amino acids have to be broken down to retain the balance of the body's pool of amino acids. Some protein will also be lost as hair, skin, sloughed epithelial cells and mucus, etc. Such obligatory losses explain why adults have a requirement for dietary protein even though their total body protein content remains constant.

Positive nitrogen balance

A positive nitrogen balance indicates a net accumulation of body protein. Healthy adults do not go into sustained positive nitrogen balance if dietary protein intake is stepped up but use the excess protein as an energy source and excrete the associated nitrogen as urea. Growing children would be expected to be in positive nitrogen balance, as would pregnant women, those recovering after illness, injury or starvation, and those actively accumulating extra muscle, such as body builders. One would expect these groups, particularly rapidly growing children, to have a relatively higher protein requirement than other adults, i.e. they would be expected to require more protein per kilogram of body weight. Lactating women would be expected to have a higher protein requirement because they are secreting protein in their milk. Note that the daily positive nitrogen balance in body builders is very small and would not indicate a significant increase in their protein requirements.

Dietary adequacy for protein is not a major issue

Table 10.1 shows some of the current UK reference nutrient intakes for protein; in addition to the absolute values, the energy yield of the protein RNI is also calculated as a percentage of the EAR for energy. To put these values into context, the average UK diet has around 16.5 per cent of the energy as protein compared with the 5–10 per cent of energy as protein indicated as maximum requirements in Table 10.1. Note that the RNI is a generous estimate of protein requirement in those who need most whereas the EAR is a less generous estimate of average requirement. This suggests that primary protein deficiency is highly improbable in the UK and indeed in other industrialized countries.

To give the values in Table 10.1 an international perspective, rice has around 8 per cent of energy as protein and hard wheat around 17 per cent whereas most other major cereal staples lie between these two extremes; only finger millet (*Eleusine corocana*) is below this range (7 per cent). Some starchy roots, which are important staples, do fall substantially below this range for cereals, e.g.:

- cassava – 3 per cent energy as protein
- plantains (cooked bananas) – 4 per cent
- yam – 7 per cent
- sweet potato – 4 per cent.

Table 10.2 shows the protein content of some common foods. Note that only three of the foods on this list have crude protein contents that are less than that in human milk and most have more than 10 per cent of their energy as protein. A comparison of these values with those in Table 10.1 suggests that people meeting their energy needs and eating a varied diet, even a varied vegetarian diet, would seem to run little practical risk of protein deficiency. This is generally true even though fats, oils, alcoholic drinks, soft drinks and sugar-based snacks provide additional

Table 10.2 The protein content of some foods expressed in absolute terms and as a percentage of energy. Values are generally for raw food

Food	g Protein/ 100 g food	Protein (% energy)
Whole milk	3.3	20.3
Skimmed milk	3.4	41.2
Cheddar cheese	26.0	25.6
Human milk	1.3	7.5
Egg	12.3	33.5
Wholemeal bread	8.8	16.3
Sweetcorn	4.1	12.9
Cornflakes	8.6	9.3
Beef (lean)	20.3	66.0
Pork (lean)	20.7	56.3
Chicken (meat)	20.5	67.8
Cod	17.4	91.6
Herring	16.8	28.7
Shrimps	23.8	81.4
Peas	5.8	34.6
Broad beans	4.1	34.2
Baked beans (can)	5.1	31.0
Lentils	23.8	31.3
Potatoes	2.1	9.7
Mushrooms	1.8	55.4
Broccoli	3.3	57.4
Carrots	0.7	12.2
Peanuts	24.3	17.1
Peanut butter	22.4	14.5
Almonds	16.9	12.0
Apple	0.3	2.6
Banana	1.1	5.6
Orange	0.8	9.1
Dried dates	2.0	3.2

energy but little protein so they reduce the nutrient density for protein. Of course, this conclusion might be altered by variations in the quality of different proteins and this is discussed in the next section.

Key points

- The nitrogen balance is the difference between nitrogen intake from food and nitrogen losses.
- Positive nitrogen balance indicates a net increase in body protein (e.g. during growth) and a negative nitrogen balance indicates a net loss of body protein (e.g. in starvation).
- Adults require protein to replace that lost from the body pool each day.

- Even under conditions of maximal conservation after adaptation to a protein-free diet, there is still an obligatory nitrogen loss.
- When the RNI for protein is expressed as a percentage of the EAR for energy, values of 5–10 per cent energy as protein are obtained for all age groups.
- Diets in industrialized countries typically contain around 15 per cent or more of the energy as protein, which makes protein deficiency improbable.
- Only a few staple foods contain low enough levels of protein to make primary protein deficiency even a theoretical prospect and in most Third World diets, protein is not the limiting nutrient.

Protein quality

The observation that all proteins contain approximately 16 per cent by weight of nitrogen enabled early workers not only to measure the protein contents of diets but also to match then for crude protein content by matching them for nitrogen content. Using such nitrogen-matched diets it soon became clear that all proteins were not of equal nutritional value, i.e. that both the amount and the quality of protein in different foods was variable. For example, pigs fed on diets based on lentil protein grew faster than those fed barley-based diets even though the diets were matched for crude protein (nitrogen) content; lentil protein was apparently of higher nutritional quality than barley protein.

Essential amino acids

It is now known that quality differences between individual proteins arise because of variations in their content of certain of the amino acids. To synthesize body protein, an animal or person must have all 20 amino acids available. If one or more amino acids is unavailable, or in short supply, then the ability to synthesize protein is generally compromised irrespective of the supply of the others. Proteins cannot be synthesized leaving gaps or using substitutes for the deficient amino acids. Each body protein is synthesized with a genetically determined and unalterable, precise sequence of particular amino acids.

About half of the amino acids have carbon skeletons that can be synthesized by people and these amino acids can therefore be synthesized by transferring amino groups from other surplus amino acids, **transamination** (see Chapter 5). The remaining amino acids have carbon skeletons that cannot be synthesized by people and they cannot, therefore, be made by transamination. These latter amino acids are termed the **essential amino acids** and have to be obtained preformed from the diet. The protein gelatine is lacking in the essential amino acid tryptophan and so dogs fed on gelatine, as their sole nitrogen source, do not fare much better than those fed on a protein-free diet. Despite a surplus of the other amino acids, the dog cannot use them for protein synthesis because one amino acid is unavailable. Under these circumstances, the amino acids in the gelatine will be used as an energy source and their nitrogen excreted as urea. The essential amino acids for humans are:

- histidine (in children)
- isoleucine
- leucine
- lysine
- methionine
- phenylalanine
- threonine
- tryptophan
- valine.

The amino acids cysteine and tyrosine are classified as non-essential even though their carbon skeletons cannot be synthesized. This is because they can be made from methionine and phenylalanine, respectively. They may be conditionally essential in premature babies because the enzymes required for their synthesis do not normally develop until late in gestation and they may also be conditionally essential in patients with liver disease because the ability to synthesize these amino acids in the liver may be compromised. In the hereditary condition phenylketonuria the enzyme phenylalanine hydroxylase that converts phenylalanine to tyrosine is defective and so tyrosine becomes an essential amino acid (see Chapter 16).

Establishing the essential amino acids and quantifying requirements

Young rats have been shown to grow normally if synthetic mixtures of the 20 amino acids are given as their sole source of dietary protein. Growth is not affected if one of the non-essential amino acids is left out of the mixture because the rats are able to make this missing amino acid by transamination. Growth ceases, however, if one of the essential ones is left out. In this way the essential amino acids for the rat have been identified and the amount of each one that is required to allow normal growth (when all of the others are in excess) has also been determined.

Such experiments with children have been ruled out on ethical grounds. However, adults have been shown to maintain nitrogen balance if fed mixtures of the 20 amino acids and like the rats can cope with removal of certain amino acids and still maintain this balance; these are the non-essential amino acids. When one of the essential amino acids is left out then there is a net loss of body nitrogen, i.e. a depletion of body protein. The requirement for each of the essential amino acids has been estimated from the minimum amount that is necessary to maintain nitrogen balance when the other amino acids are present in excess. The range and relative needs of the essential amino acids in rats and people are found to be similar and the rat has been widely used as a model for humans in biological assessments of protein quality.

Limiting amino acid

In any given dietary protein, one of the essential amino acids will be present in the lowest amount relative to human requirements, i.e. a given amount of the protein will contain a lower proportion of the requirement for this essential amino acid than for any of the others. The availability of this amino acid will 'limit' the extent to which the others can be used if that particular protein is fed alone and in amounts that do not fully supply the need for the amino acid. This amino acid is called the **limiting amino acid**. The amino acid is limiting because if supplies of this essential amino acid are insufficient, the use of the others for protein synthesis will be limited by its availability – protein cannot be made leaving gaps where this missing amino acid should be. For example, if only half of the requirement for the limiting amino acid is supplied then, in effect, only about half of the protein requirement is being supplied; surpluses of the others will be used as energy sources and their nitrogen excreted. In many cereals the limiting amino acid is lysine, in maize it is tryptophan and in beef and milk it is the sulphur-containing amino acids; one of these is the limiting amino acid in most dietary proteins. In the past, lysine supplementation of cereal-based diets or developing 'high-lysine' strains of cereals have been widely advocated, and sometimes used, as means of improving the protein quality of diets based on cereals.

First and second class proteins

Whatever measure of protein quality is used then most proteins of animal origin have high values. Meat, fish, egg and milk proteins contain all of the essential amino acids in good quantities; they have been termed **first class proteins** or complete proteins. Many proteins of vegetable origin, however, have low measured quality; this is true of many staple cereals and starchy roots; they have been termed **second class** or incomplete proteins because they have a relatively low amount of one or more of the essential amino acids. Pulses (peas and beans) are a major exception to this general rule and have good amounts of high-quality protein. Some examples of the relative quality values of common dietary proteins are shown in Table 10.3.

Table 10.3 The relative qualities (NPU, net protein utilization) of some dietary proteins

	Protein quality (NPU %)
Maize	36
Millet	43
Wheat	49
Rice	63
Soya	67
Cow milk	81
Egg	87
Human milk	94

Mutual supplementation of protein

The concept of a limiting amino acid producing large variations in protein quality may have limited practical relevance in human nutrition, especially in affluent countries, for two reasons.

- First, the human requirement for protein is low. This is true both in comparison to other species and in comparison to the protein content of many dietary staples.
- Second, affluent people seldom eat just single proteins; rather they eat diets containing mixtures of several different proteins. The probability is that the different proteins consumed, over a period of time, will have differing limiting amino acids and thus that any deficiency of an essential amino acid

in one protein will be compensated for by a relative surplus of that amino acid in another. Thus the quality of the total protein in different human diets will tend to equalize even though the nature and quality of the individual proteins in those diets may vary very considerably. This is called **mutual supplementation of proteins**, and it means that any measure of protein quality of mixed human diets tends to yield a fairly consistent value.

Measurement of protein quality

The simplest method of assessing the quality of a protein is to chemically compare its limiting amino acid content with that of a high-quality reference protein; this is called the **chemical score**. Egg protein has traditionally been used as the reference protein in human nutrition but breast milk protein is another possible reference protein. In the protein under test, the limiting amino acid is identified and the amount of this amino acid in a gram of test protein is expressed as a percentage of that found in a gram of egg protein.

$$\text{Chemical score} = \frac{\substack{\text{mg of limiting} \\ \text{amino acid in } 1\,\text{g} \\ \text{of test protein}}}{\substack{\text{mg of this amino} \\ \text{acid in } 1\,\text{g of egg} \\ \text{protein}}} \times 100$$

This chemical score does not necessarily give an accurate guide to the biological availability of the amino acids in the protein. Thus, for example, if a protein is poorly digested then the chemical score could greatly overestimate the real biological quality of the protein.

Net protein utilization (NPU) is a widely used biological measure of protein quality. It is a particularly important measure in agricultural nutrition but is nowadays considered to be of much less significance in human nutrition. To measure NPU the protein to be tested is fed as the sole nitrogen source at a level below the minimum requirement for growth of the animal (usually weaning rats). The amount of nitrogen retained under these circumstances is corrected for the nitrogen losses that occur even on a protein-free diet and then expressed as a percentage of the intake. Net protein utilization can be directly assessed in human adults using nitrogen balance measurements.

$$NPU = \frac{\text{amount of retained nitrogen}}{\text{nitrogen intake}} \times 100$$

Retained nitrogen = intake
− (loss − loss on protein-free diet)

The NPU values for some proteins are shown above in Table 10.3. The NPU of diets as well as those of individual proteins may be determined, and because of the mutual supplementation effect then the NPU of most human diets comes out within a relatively narrow range even though the qualities of the individual constituent proteins may vary widely. An NPU of around 70 would be typical of many human diets and would be not greatly affected by, for instance, the proportion of animal protein in the diet. The NPU is only likely to be of significance in human nutrition if a single staple with low amounts of poor-quality protein makes up the bulk of the diet and is the source of most of the dietary protein.

- Proteins that are low in one or more essential amino acid are termed second class proteins, e.g. gelatine, cereal proteins and most proteins from starchy root staples.
- When mixtures of proteins are eaten, deficits of essential amino acids in individual proteins will usually be compensated for by relative surpluses in others, i.e. mutual supplementation.
- The protein quality of human diets tends to equalize towards the mean because of mutual supplementation.
- The chemical score is a measure of protein quality and is the amount of the limiting amino acid in a gram of the protein expressed as a percentage of that found in a gram of a high-quality reference protein such as egg.
- NPU is a biological measure of protein quality and is the percentage of the protein that growing animals can retain under conditions where protein intake is limited.

Key points

- Feeding trials using nitrogen-matched diets indicated that proteins vary in their nutritional quality.
- Variation in protein quality is due to variation in their complement of essential amino acids.
- Essential amino acids cannot be made in the body but non-essential amino acids can be made by transamination.
- Animals can grow and adults can maintain nitrogen balance if provided with complete amino acid mixtures but not if one of the essential ones is missing from the mixture.
- The limiting amino acid is the one present in a food in the lowest amount relative to how much is needed.
- When one essential amino acid is taken in insufficient quantities it limits the extent to which the others can be used for protein synthesis.
- Lysine is the limiting amino acid in most cereals and lysine, tryptophan or sulphur-containing amino acids are the limiting amino acids in most foods.
- Proteins containing good amounts of all essential amino acids are termed first class proteins, e.g. meat, fish, egg and pulse proteins.

SIGNIFICANCE OF PROTEIN IN HUMAN NUTRITION

The change in attitude to protein deficiency as a suspected key cause of human malnutrition represents one of the most striking changes in human nutrition over the past 50 years.

The author has previously reviewed this topic (Webb, 1989) and the book by Carpenter (1994) contains a detailed and thorough review of both the discovery of protein and changing attitudes to protein in nutrition. The following discussion is a development of my earlier review. This topic can serve as a case study to illustrate the three important general points that have been discussed earlier in the book (see below).

- The potential costs of premature and ineffective 'health promotion' intervention. These costs may be very real and substantial even if an unhelpful intervention does not do direct physiological harm (Chapter 1). The financial and time costs of all the measures to solve the illusory 'world protein crisis' were enormous and this meant that other more real problems were ignored or deprived of funding.
- The potential dangers of overestimating dietary standards by 'erring on the safe side' (Chapter 3).

The 'world protein crisis' seems to have been precipitated by a massive overestimation of the protein needs of children.

- The dangers of hasty and ill-considered extrapolation of results obtained in animal experiments to people (Chapter 3). Observations of very high protein requirements in rapidly growing young animals was probably a factor in creating the illusory belief that the protein needs of children were also very high.

It is largely because it illustrates these points so well that I have given a topic dealing with an historical and primarily developing world issue such prominence in a book whose main focus is on nutrition for promoting health in industrialized countries. These issues are very current in relation to nutrition for health promotion.

> ## Key point
>
> Changes in the importance attached to protein illustrate the potential costs of unwarranted health promotion initiatives, the dangers of overestimating dietary standards and the potential problems of carelessly extrapolating results obtained from laboratory animal studies to people.

Historical overview

For more than two decades (the 1950s and the 1960s) the belief that primary protein deficiency was 'the most serious and widespread dietary deficiency in the world' (Waterlow *et al.*, 1960) dominated nutrition research and education. The consensus of nutrition opinion considered it likely that 'in many parts of the world the majority of young children suffered some protein malnutrition' (Trowell, 1954). The relative protein requirements of young children compared with adults were generally considered to be very high, perhaps five times higher on a weight-for-weight basis. Even where diets contained apparently adequate amounts of total protein it was believed that protein availability might still be inadequate unless some high-quality protein (usually animal or pulse protein) was taken with each meal. Calculations of the amount of protein required by the world population when compared with estimates of protein availability gave the impression of a large and increasing shortfall in world

protein supplies – **the protein gap.** Jones (1974) suggested that an extra 20 million tons of protein were required each year and this figure implied that many hundreds of millions of people were protein deficient. This protein gap was so large that a whole new field of research was initiated to try to close it, namely the mass production of protein-rich foods from novel sources such as fishmeal and microbes. An agency of the United Nations (UN) the 'Protein Advisory Group' was set up specifically to oversee these developments. As late as 1972 the chairman's opening address to an international scientific conference contained the following statements:

> Every doctor, nutritionist or political leader concerned with the problem of world hunger, has now concluded that the major problem is one of protein malnutrition.
> The calorie supply [of developing countries] tends to be more or less satisfactory, but what is lacking is protein, and especially protein containing the essential amino acids.
>
> *Gounelle de Pontanel, 1972*

As estimates of human protein requirements were revised downwards then this protein gap disappeared 'at the stroke of a pen' with no significant change in protein supplies. The above quotations from Gounelle de Pontanel contrast very sharply with the conclusions of Miller and Payne (1969) that almost all dietary staples contain sufficient protein to meet human needs and that even diets based on very low protein staples are unlikely to be specifically protein deficient. In the decades since 1969 this latter view has become the nutritional consensus. Despite this revolutionary change of mind, the greatly reduced emphasis on protein in human nutrition was slow to permeate beyond the ranks of the specialists. Even among nutrition educators some ambivalence towards protein persisted well into the 1990s. The following quotations from a 1991 edition of a well-respected American nutrition text seems to sum up that ambivalence.

> Most people in the United States and Canada would find it almost impossible not to meet their protein requirements
> Protein is at the heart of a good diet. Menu planners build their meals around the RDA for protein.
>
> *Hamilton et al., 1991*

This exaggerated importance attached to protein in the past led to a huge concentration of research effort, physical resources, educational effort and political priority into protein nutrition and into efforts to close the protein gap. It now seems almost certain that much of this effort was wasted and directed towards solving an illusory problem. McClaren (1974), Webb (1989) and Carpenter (1994) have discussed some of these costs of exaggerating human protein needs and McClaren was moved to entitle his historically important article 'The great protein fiasco'. Some of the measures taken to try to solve the apparently false protein crisis are summarized below (further extensive details may be found in Carpenter, 1994).

- In 1955, the UN set up the Protein Advisory Group to 'advise on the safety and suitability of new protein-rich food preparations'. This group held regular meetings and produced various reports until it was finally terminated in 1977.
- In 1957, UN experts suggested that there was an urgent need to develop cheap, locally produced, high-protein foods that would be safe, palatable and easy to incorporate into existing diets from things such as fishmeal, soybeans, peanuts, coconut, sesame and cotton seed. To this was added in the late 1960s, the development of protein from yeasts and bacteria (single cell protein (SCP)), the production of genetically improved plants and the use of synthetic amino acids to boost the quality of dietary proteins.
- In 1970, the UN approved a programme to implement these recommendations despite initial costs estimated at $75 million (at 1970 prices!).
- Numerous problems delayed and increased the development costs of high-protein foods from existing raw materials such as:
  - the need to remove lipids from fishmeal to make it palatable and improve its storage
  - the presence of 'unhygienic' intestinal contents in meal made from small whole fish
  - the presence of fungal toxins in peanut products
  - rising market prices of some of the raw materials.

Ultimately no cheap and widely used product emerged from these expensive undertakings. The poor did not eat the few products that got beyond the trial stage to full marketing.

- Many expensive projects to produce single cell proteins were begun but most failed to produce products that were safe and acceptable for human consumption. One fungal product (Quorn) did emerge from these efforts but it is now marketed as a meat substitute for affluent vegetarians rather than a high-protein food for needy children in developing countries.
- Decades of expensive research did produce high protein quality strains of corn but these have never been widely grown.
- Chemical production of synthetic lysine for food supplementation was tried but proved ineffective in improving nutritional status in human field trials.
- The total costs of these largely unsuccessful and seemingly unnecessary programmes and initiatives must amount to billions of dollars at today's prices.

> ## Key points
>
> - In 1960, protein deficiency was widely regarded as the most serious and widespread form of malnutrition and the majority of children in many developing countries were believed to be protein deficient.
> - In 1960, estimates of protein needs greatly exceeded protein supplies and indicated a large and increasing shortfall in world protein supplies – the protein gap.
> - As estimates of children's protein needs decreased so the concept of a protein gap became discredited.
> - The current consensus is that few diets are specifically protein deficient and that if children eat enough food for their energy needs, they will probably get enough protein.
> - During the 'protein gap era' huge amounts of time and money were wasted on projects to solve the protein crisis, e.g. the production of high-protein foods from fishmeal, peanuts and microbes, the development of genetically enhanced plants, and programmes to supplement cereals with synthetic amino acids.

Origins of the 'protein gap'

The three assumptions listed below seem to have been critical in creating the illusion of a massive world protein shortage.

- The belief that children required a high protein concentration in their diets, i.e. that the proportion

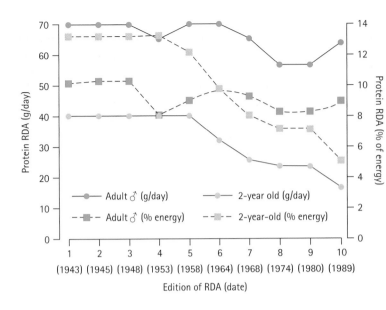

Figure 10.2 *Changes in the American recommended dietary allowance (RDA) for protein for a man and a 2-year-old child over 10 editions (1943–89). Expressed both in absolute terms and as a percentage of the energy RDA. Source: Webb (1994).*

of total dietary energy derived from protein should be substantially higher in children than in adults.

- The assumption that the nutritional disease known as **kwashiorkor** was due to primary protein deficiency, i.e. due to a diet in which the proportion of energy derived from protein was too low.
- The belief that kwashiorkor was the most prevalent form of malnutrition in the world and that cases of frank clinical kwashiorkor represented only the 'tip of the iceberg' with many more children impaired to some extent by lack of protein.

There are now good grounds for suggesting that each of these assumptions is either dubious or improbable.

Past exaggeration of protein requirements?

Figure 10.2 illustrates the changes in the American recommended dietary allowances (RDAs) for protein since 1943. In 1943, the protein RDA for a 2-year-old child was substantially more than double its current value (also more than double the current UK RNI). When expressed as a proportion of the energy allowance, the child's protein RNI was well above the adult value in 1943 but is now well below the adult value (see numerical values in Table 10.4).

The more recent values given above suggest that children can manage on a lower minimum protein concentration in their diets than adults can. This conclusion seems at first sight to be inconsistent with the notion that growing children have higher relative protein needs than adults. It has been and still is

Table 10.4 Changing American estimates of protein needs

	1943	1989
g/day		
Man	70	65
2-year-old child	40	18
% Energy		
Man	10	8
2-year-old child	13	5

assumed that children need more protein on a weight-for-weight basis than do adults, only the assumed scale of this difference has declined. In the past, figures of up to five times higher weight-for-weight requirements in children have been suggested (e.g. Waterlow *et al.*, 1960), nowadays a figure of around double is considered more reasonable. Table 10.5 shows why this higher relative requirement is not inconsistent with need for a lower dietary protein concentration as suggested by Figure 10.2. Children not only require relatively more protein than adults but also more energy. Table 10.5 shows the current UK RNIs for protein and the EARs for energy as a multiple of the standard adult value when expressed on a weight-for-weight basis (i.e. expressed per kilogram of body weight). A 2-year old child requires almost three times as much energy as an adult per kilogram of body weight but only

Table 10.5 Weight-for-weight energy estimated average requirements (EARs) and protein reference nutrient intakes (RNIs) as a multiple of the standard adult value at various ages. Calculated from data in COMA (1991)

Age	Energy EAR	Protein RNI
0–3 months	2.7	2.9
4–6 months	2.7	2.2
7–9 months	2.7	2.1
10–12 months	2.8	2.0
1–3 years	2.9	1.5
4–6 years	2.8	1.5
7–10 years	2.1	1.3
11–14 years	1.5	1.3
15–18 years	1.3	1.2
19–50 years	1.0	1.0
75 + years	0.9	1.0

about one and a half times as much protein. The need for increased energy intake (i.e. total food intake) is far greater than the increased relative need for protein. For all ages of children the increased energy needs cancel out or, in most cases, greatly exceed the increased need for protein. The 2-year-old child may need 1.5 times as much protein as an adult but needs to eat three times as much food; any diet with enough protein for an adult should therefore provide enough for the child if they can eat enough of it to satisfy their energy requirements.

Inappropriate extrapolation from animal experiments to humans may have encouraged inflated estimates of protein requirements in children. Primates have slower growth rates than most animals and much lower rates than most common laboratory animals (see Table 10.6). The relative protein requirements

Table 10.6 Growth rates and milk composition of seven species

Species	Days to double birth weight	Protein in milk (g/L)	Energy as protein (%)
Man	120–180	1.1	6
Calf	47	3.2	19
Sheep	10	6.5	24
Cat	7	10.6	27
Rat	6	8.1	25
Mouse	5	9.0	21
Chimp	100	1.2	7

Simplified after Webb (1989).

of these rapidly growing species are thus likely to be higher than those of human infants and children and this seems to be borne out by the comparison of milk composition of the species also shown in Table 10.6. Up to 80 per cent of the nitrogen requirements of a growing rat are for growth (Altschul, 1965). Rats were widely used to model humans in protein experiments and so this probably encouraged the belief that children's relative protein requirements were up to five times those of adults. As four-fifths of the requirement of young rats is for growth and only one-fifth for maintenance, by direct analogy it might well suggest a fivefold difference in the requirements of children (for growth and maintenance) and adults (for maintenance only).

Animal experiments also probably played their part in exaggerating the importance of low protein quality as a practical problem in human nutrition. When a diet containing 10 per cent egg protein as the sole nitrogen source is fed to growing rats under test conditions, 1 g of egg protein will bring about an increase in weight of 3.8 g in the animals. Egg protein is said to have a protein efficiency ratio of 3.8. Around 80 per cent of the consumed protein is retained as body protein. Wheat protein has a protein efficiency ratio of only 1 and just 20 per cent of the wheat protein would be retained as body protein (Altschul, 1965). Under the same test conditions 1 g of wheat protein results in only 1 g of weight gain in the rats. Such experimental demonstrations of the low quality of many cereal and vegetable proteins suggest that unless some high-quality protein was present, the protein deficiency seems almost inevitable – 4 g of wheat protein is only equivalent to 1 g of egg protein in growing rats. Of course, most human diets are mixtures of proteins and mutual supplementation can occur. It was for some time thought, however, that this mutual supplementation could only occur within a meal but it is now thought that such supplementation can occur over an extended time scale. If a meal lacking in one amino acid is consumed then the liver will donate the deficient amino acid to allow protein synthesis to continue and will replenish its complement of this amino acid at a later meal. Note also the much faster growth rates and thus higher protein and amino acid requirements of young rats compared with children. This makes it rather unlikely that protein deficiency will occur due to unbalanced amino acid composition except under very particular conditions.

Low concentration of dietary protein causes kwashiorkor?

The nutritional disease kwashiorkor was first described in the medical literature in the 1930s and a very tentative suggestion made that it might be due to dietary protein deficiency. Over the next 35 years it became generally accepted that two diseases known as **kwashiorkor** and **marasmus** represented different clinical manifestations of malnutrition in children, with differing aetiologies. Marasmus was attributed to simple energy deficit (starvation) whereas kwashiorkor was attributed to primary protein deficiency. Children with marasmus are severely wasted and stunted and the clinical picture is generally consistent with what might be expected in simple starvation. Several of the clinical features of kwashiorkor, however, are not superficially consistent with simple starvation but are consistent with protein deficiency (Table 10.7). Many children develop a mixture of these two diseases and the two conditions are thus said to represent opposite extremes of a spectrum of diseases with the precise clinical picture depending on the precise levels of protein and energy deficit. The general term **protein-energy malnutrition (PEM)** has been used to describe this spectrum of diseases.

Table 10.7 Clinical features of kwashiorkor that are consistent with primary protein deficiency

Symptom	Rationale
Oedema – excess tissue fluid	Lack of plasma proteins?
Hepatomegaly – liver swollen with fat	Lack of protein to transport fat?
'Flaky paint syndrome' – depigmented and peeling skin	Lack of amino acids for skin protein and pigment production?
Mental changes – anorexia and apathy	Lack of amino acids for transmitter synthesis?
Subcutaneous fat still present	Inconsistent with simple energy deficit?
Changes in colour and texture of hair	Similar causes to skin changes?

Many studies over the past 25 years have seriously challenged the assumption that kwashiorkor is necessarily due to primary protein deficiency. When protein needs of children were thought to be high, the protein deficit in the diets of many children in developing countries seemed to be much greater than any energy deficit. When the estimated protein needs of children were reduced then protein no longer appeared to be the limiting factor in these diets and energy deficits exceeded any protein deficits. Comparisons of the diets of children developing kwashiorkor or marasmus have reported no difference in their protein concentrations. Detailed analyses of the diets of children in developing countries have indicated that primary deficiency of protein is uncommon and that protein deficiency is usually a secondary consequence of low total food intake (Waterlow and Payne, 1975).

The symptoms of kwashiorkor listed in Table 10.7 are nonetheless persuasively consistent with protein deficiency rather that energy deficit. Acute shortage of energy would, however, lead to use of protein as an energy source. Thus dietary energy deficit could well precipitate a physiological deficit of amino acids for protein synthesis and to fulfil other amino acid functions. Symptoms of protein deficiency might be triggered by energy deficit. Why starvation should sometimes result in marasmus and sometimes kwashiorkor is, as yet, still unclear. Some more recent theories have suggested that the symptoms of kwashiorkor may be triggered in an undernourished child by:

- mineral or vitamin deficiencies
- essential fatty acid deficiencies
- infection
- inadequate antioxidant response (e.g. due to lack of antioxidant vitamins and minerals) to oxidative stress (e.g. exacerbated by infection, toxins, sunlight).

Kwashiorkor – the most common nutritional disease in the world?

McClaren (1974) suggested that the widespread assumption that kwashiorkor was the most prevalent manifestation of PEM was caused by faulty extrapolation from a World Health Organization survey of rural Africa in 1952. He argued that marasmus was a much more widespread problem than kwashiorkor and that marasmus was becoming increasingly common as breastfeeding declined (marasmus is associated with early weaning). In 1974, even one of the authors of the 1952 WHO report (J F Brock) conceded that there had been a relative neglect of marasmus which was very prevalent even in rural Africa (see Carpenter, 1994).

Key points

- The protein gap originated because protein needs were exaggerated and because kwashiorkor was assumed to be both the most prevalent form of protein energy malnutrition and the result of a primary deficiency of protein.

- Estimated protein needs of children are now less than half what they were in the 1940s.

- Children were thought to need a much higher proportion of their energy as protein than adults but not now.

- Children were thought to need five times more protein per kilogram of body weight than adults but today's figure is less than twice as much.

- Young children require three times more energy per kilogram than adults and so if they get enough energy then any diet with enough protein for an adult should provide enough for a child.

- Most non-primate animals grow much faster than human babies and so require much more protein and this is reflected in much higher protein content in their milk.

- Around four-fifths of a young rat's protein requirement is for growth and this may indicate the origin of the belief that human babies require five times more protein per kilogram than adults.

- Laboratory experiments with rats suggested that many cereal and vegetable proteins were inferior to animal proteins in supporting growth and this probably exaggerated the importance attached to protein quality in human nutrition.

- Many of the symptoms of kwashiorkor are consistent with primary protein deficiency (see Table 10.7) yet there was never any hard evidence to support the belief that kwashiorkor is due to primary protein deficiency.

- Current estimates of protein and energy needs suggest that protein is rarely the limiting nutrient in Third World diets.

- Protein deficiency is usually a secondary consequence of inadequate food intake.

- It is now generally accepted that marasmus, not kwashiorkor, is the most prevalent form of protein energy malnutrition.

CONCLUDING REMARKS

Over the past 50 years, opinions as to the significance of protein in human nutrition have undergone some dramatic changes. For a time, protein adequacy was top of the list of international nutritional priorities. Nowadays primary protein deficiency is generally considered to be a relatively uncommon occurrence, not because of an improved supply, but rather because of a change of nutritional opinion. In both the UK and US dietary standards (COMA, 1991 and NRC, 1989a, respectively) there is even concern voiced about the possible health risks of high protein intakes. It has been suggested, for example, that prolonged excess protein intakes may predispose to renal failure in later life. Both of these panels suggested that it would be prudent to regard a value of twice the RNI/RDA as the safe upper limit for protein intake.

Fat

NATURE OF DIETARY FAT

Around 95 per cent of dietary fats and oils are in the form of **triacylglycerol** (note that the alternative term **triglyceride** is still widely used). Most of the storage fat in the body is also in the form of triacylglycerol. Triacylglycerols are composed of three **fatty acids** linked to the simple three-carbon molecule glycerol. Glycerol is a carbohydrate moiety which is called a tri-alcohol and has one hydroxyl (alcohol) group on each of its three carbons (propane n-1,2,3-triol in formal chemical nomenclature). Each of these alcohol groups in glycerol can form an ester linkage with the carboxyl (acid) group of a fatty acid. The three fatty acids in a triacylglycerol can be the same (simple triacylglycerol) or different (mixed triacyl-glycerol). A triacylglycerol molecule is represented diagrammatically in Figure 11.1a. Note that the term 'fat' is often used to imply a solid substance but oils and solid fats are collectively termed fats in this book.

When the third (bottom) fatty acid in Figure 11.1a is replaced by a phosphate group, this compound is known as phosphatidic acid, the parent compound for a group of compounds known as **phospholipids**. Phospholipids make up most of the dietary lipid that is not triacylglycerol and they have important physiological functions as components of membranes and in the synthesis of a range of important regulatory molecules called the **eicosanoids** (e.g. **prostaglandins**). The phosphate group of phosphatidic acid can link with various other compounds to produce a series of these phospholipids, e.g. phosphatidyl choline (lecithin), phosphatidyl inositol and phosphatidyl serine.

Lipids are usually defined on the basis of their solubility, i.e. those components of the body or food that are insoluble in water but soluble in organic solvents such as chloroform or ether. On the basis of this definition, the term lipids encompasses not only triacylglycerols and phospholipids but also the sterols (e.g. cholesterol) and waxes. Waxes are esters of monohydroxyl alcohols (one –OH group) and a long-chain saturated fatty acid; they are insoluble and inert chemically, e.g. beeswax and carnauba wax from a South American pine tree.

> ## Key points
>
> - Lipids are organic materials that are insoluble in water but soluble in organic solvents and include triacylglycerols, phospholipids, sterols and waxes.
> - 95 per cent of dietary fat (including oils) is triacylglycerol and most of the rest is phospholipid.
> - Triacylglycerol consists of three fatty acids attached by ester linkages to glycerol.
> - If one fatty acid of triacylglycerol is replaced by a phosphate-containing moiety this becomes a phospholipid.

(a) Schematic representation of a triacylglycerol

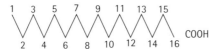

glycerol

(b) General chemical formula of a saturated fatty acid

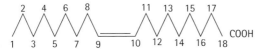

(c) Diagrammatic representation of a saturated fatty acid (palmitic acid −16:0)

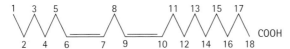

(d) Diagrammatic representation of a monounsaturated fatty acid (oleic acid − 18:1$_{\omega-9}$)

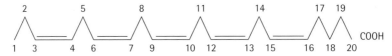

(e) Diagrammatic representation of linoleic acid (18:2$_{\omega-6}$)

(f) Diagrammatic representation of eicosapentaenoic acid (EPA, 20:5$_{\omega-3}$)

(g) Diagram to illustrate the *cis* and *trans* configurations of unsaturated fatty acids

cis configuration   *trans* configuration

Figure 11.1a–g *The chemical nature of fats.*

TYPES OF FATTY ACIDS

Fatty acids are of three major types – **saturated**, **monounsaturated** and **polyunsaturated fatty acids**. All fatty acids comprise a hydrocarbon chain of varying length with a carboxyl or acid group at one end. The only difference between these three types of fatty acids is in the number of carbon–carbon double bonds present in the hydrocarbon chain.

Saturated fatty acids

Carbon atoms have the potential to each form four bonds (i.e. they have a valency of four). In saturated fatty acids, all of the carbon atoms in the hydrocarbon chain are joined together by single bonds and all of the remaining valencies (bonds) of the carbon atoms are occupied by bonding to hydrogen atoms (Figure 11.1b). These fatty acids are termed saturated because all of the available bonds of the carbon atoms are occupied or 'saturated' with hydrogen atoms. No more hydrogen atoms can be added to this hydrocarbon chain.

The chemical structure of fatty acids is often represented schematically as shown in Figure 11.1c. Each angle represents a carbon atom. The carbon atoms in this book are numbered starting with the carbon furthest away from the carboxyl or acid group. The fatty acid depicted in this diagram is called palmitic acid – it has 16 carbon atoms and no double bonds and therefore it can be written in shorthand notation as 16:0.

Monounsaturated fatty acids

Monounsaturated fatty acids have a single point of unsaturation, i.e. two of the carbons in the chain are joined together by a double bond and thus there are two fewer hydrogen atoms than in a saturated fatty acid of the same length. Oleic acid is depicted in Figure 11.1d; it is an 18-carbon monounsaturated fatty acid that is widely found in nature both in animals and plants (it is the principal acid in olive oil). The double bond in oleic acid is between carbons 9 and 10 in the sequence – the shorthand notation for this acid is $18:1_{\omega-9}$ (i.e. 18 carbons; 1 double bond; and, ω-9, the double bond is between carbons 9 and 10). The Greek letter omega is sometimes replaced by 'n' so that oleic acid becomes 18:1n-9.

Polyunsaturated fatty acids

Polyunsaturated fatty acids have two or more double bonds in the carbon chain, i.e. they have more than one point of unsaturation. Figure 11.1e shows linoleic acid, which has 18 carbons, two double bonds and the first of these double bonds is between carbons 6 and 7 and thus its shorthand notation is $18:2_{\omega-6}$. Knowing the position of the first double bond makes it possible to predict the position of any further double bonds because they are normally separated by a single saturated carbon atom (i.e. are methylene interrupted). In linoleic acid, the first double bond is between carbons 6 and 7, carbon 8 is saturated and the second double bond lies between carbons 9 and 10. Figure 11.1f shows a slightly more complicated example: eicosapentaenoic acid (EPA) has 20 carbons, five double bonds and the first double bond is between carbons 3 and 4 hence its

shorthand notation is $20:5_{\omega-3}$. In EPA, carbon five is saturated and the second double bond is between carbons 6 and 7, carbon 8 is saturated and the third double bond is between 9 and 10, the fourth between 12 and 13 and the fifth between 15 and 16 (Figure 11.1f). Each of the double bonds in EPA is separated by a single saturated carbon atom and so knowing the position of the first double bond (given by the 'ω' or 'n' notation) one can predict the position of all of the others. Note that there is an alternative numbering system for fatty acids in which the carbons are counted from the carboxyl end of the molecule (the Δ or delta system). This is used more often by biochemists and chemists working with fatty acids rather than the 'ω' or 'n' system used throughout in this book. Thus, the enzymes described later in the chapter which insert double bonds into fatty acids are termed Δ-6, Δ-5 and Δ-4 desaturases because they insert double bonds at positions 6, 5, or 4 carbons counting from the carboxyl end of the molecule – using this technically correct nomenclature, eicosapentaenoic acid $(20:5_{\omega-3})$ in Figure 11.1f has double bonds at (Δ) positions 5, 8, 11, 14 and 17.

Cis/trans isomerization

Different positional isomers (as shown in Figure 11.1g) are possible wherever a fatty acid has a carbon–carbon double bond. When represented in two dimensions, then either both hydrogen atoms can be on the same side, the *cis* form, or the hydrogen atoms can be on opposite sides, the *trans* form. Most naturally occurring fats contain almost exclusively *cis* isomers although small amounts of ***trans fatty acids*** are found in butter (4–8 per cent) and other natural fats, especially those from ruminating animals in whom they are produced by bacteria in the animal's rumen. Whether a double bond is in the *cis* or *trans* configuration makes a considerable difference to the three-dimensional shape of the molecule. A *cis* double bond causes the molecule to bend back on itself into a U-shape whereas a *trans* double bond remains in the more linear form characteristic of saturated fatty acids.

It is possible to chemically convert unsaturated fatty acids to saturated ones if the fat is reacted with hydrogen in the presence of an activating agent or catalyst. This process is called hydrogenation and it causes oils to solidify. Partial hydrogenation was the traditional method used in the production of margarine and solid vegetable shortening, i.e. **hydrogenated vegetable oils** or hydrogenated fish oil. The process of hydrogenation can result in the production of relatively large amounts of *trans* fatty acids in the final product. Many of the early, cheap, 'hard' margarines were made from hydrogenated fish oil and were particularly high in *trans* fatty acids (up to 30 per cent of fatty acids) but these have been superseded by soft margarines made from vegetable oil which are low in trans fatty acids. Heating of cooking oils also produces some *trans* isomers and they accumulate if the oil is used repeatedly, e.g. to cook multiple batches of chips (French fries).

Effects of chain length and degree of unsaturation on fatty acid melting points

The chain length and degree of unsaturation of fatty acids affects their melting points. In general, the longer the chain length of a saturated fatty acid the higher is the melting point. The more unsaturated a fatty acid is (i.e. the more *cis* double bonds it has) the lower will be its melting point. The following examples illustrate these points:

- lauric acid (12:0) – melting point 44°C
- palmitic acid (16:0) – 63°C
- stearic acid (18:0) – 70°C
- lignoceric acid (24:0) – 84°C
- oleic acid ($18:1_{\omega-9}$) – 13°C
- elaidic acid (*trans* oleic acid) – 45°C
- linoleic acid ($18:2_{\omega-6}$) – −5°C
- linolenic acid ($18:3_{\omega-3}$) – −10°C
- arachidonic acid (20:0) – 75°C
- arachidonic acid ($20:4_{\omega-6}$) – −49°C
- eicosapentaenoic acid ($20:5_{\omega-3}$) – −54°C.

The first four fatty acids on the list are all saturated and the melting point increases with the increasing chain length – all of these are solids at room temperature. The four 18-carbon acids, stearic, oleic, linoleic and linolenic have no, one, two and three *cis* double bonds, respectively. Their melting point decreases with each double bond and all three of the unsaturated fatty acids are liquids at room temperature. The *trans* form of oleic acid (elaidic acid) has a much higher melting point than oleic itself. It is a solid at room temperature, illustrating the earlier point that *trans* fatty acids are closer in their three-dimensional configuration to saturated fatty acids.

Eicosapentaenoic acid ($20:5_{\omega-3}$) has a lower melting point than arachidonic acid the corresponding acid in the ω-6 series. In Figure 11.2 (see p. 275) every fatty acid in the ω-3 series has a lower melting point than the corresponding ω-6 acid because of the extra double bond. This also means that melting point and physical form of triacylglycerols depends on their fatty acid profiles. Triacylglycerols with lots of saturated and monounsaturated fatty acids tend to be solids at room temperature (e.g. butter and lard) whereas those with high levels of polyunsaturated fatty acids are liquid oils (e.g. corn oil, sunflower oil and fish oil).

Conjugated linoleic acid

Conjugated linoleic acid (CLA) is the collective name given to a group of isomers of linoleic acid found principally in dairy fat and meat fat, especially in meat from ruminants. In CLA the double bonds are contiguous (not separated by a methylene group) and they can be either in the *cis* or *trans* configuration. The two most prevalent acids that make up 80–90 per cent of the dietary CLA are (using the ω numbering system, counting from the end furthest from the carboxyl group) *trans* 7 *cis* 9 CLA and *cis* 6 *trans* 8 CLA. (Using the standard and more usual Δ nomenclature, counting from the carboxyl end, these are designated *cis* 9 *trans* 11 CLA and *trans* 10 *cis* 11 CLA, respectively.) Conjugated linoleic acid is produced from linoleic acid by bacteria in the rumen of cattle and other ruminants hence its presence in dairy fat and beef fat. Cattle that graze upon pasture have higher amounts of CLA in their meat milk than those that are fed on grain and commercial cattle foods. Average intakes of CLA by an omnivorous man in the UK was estimated at 150 mg/day in 1995 and more than two-thirds of this comes from dairy fat.

Conjugated linoleic acid has been marketed as a dietary supplement; it is argued that because of modern animal husbandry practices, the amounts of CLA in our diets has decreased; decreased consumption of dairy and meat fat would also decrease intakes. Studies using animals and *in vitro* systems have given rise to a number of claims for potential benefits from consuming supplemental amounts of CLA. Some of these are listed below.

- CLA has anti-mutagenic properties in bacterial tests and may reduce the formation of chemically induced experimental tumours in laboratory animals.

- It has been claimed that it moderates the inflammatory response and could thus have beneficial effects in treating chronic inflammatory conditions.
- It may have beneficial effects on blood lipoprotein profiles.
- It may increase lean body mass and reduce body fat content.

The animal studies that have led to most of these claims have used large amounts of CLA which are way beyond those that would be consumed in any normal diet, the equivalent of several grams per day (*cf.* the average 150 mg/day consumed by an omnivorous man). Roche *et al.* (2001) reviewed several relatively short-term trials (up to 2 months) that had tested the effects of doses of around 3 g/day of CLA and found that these failed to consistently produce the effects on weight, body composition and lipoprotein profiles that might have been predicted from the animal trials. They suggested that even these doses of around 20 times usual intake of male omnivores may be insufficient to produce significant effects. One relatively recent long-term placebo-controlled trial (Gaullier *et al.*, 2004) used up to 4.5 g/day of CLA for a year in 180 mainly female subjects who were overweight but not obese. The authors reported that the CLA group lost an average of 2 kg over the year and that they had lost significant amounts of fat compared with no significant changes in the placebo group. Some very small adverse effects on blood lipoprotein levels were recorded in the CLA group. Even if these results are confirmed, the effects are relatively modest and have taken a year of using a very large dose of CLA; there is as yet no clear mechanistic explanation for the proposed effects of CLA. Under such circumstances the prolonged use of pharmacological doses of a substance without any clear idea of how it might act seems at best imprudent. It should also be borne in mind that high intakes of dairy fat and meat fat are usually associated with negative health implications.

Distribution of fatty acid types in dietary fat

All fat sources contain mixtures of saturated, monounsaturated and polyunsaturated fatty acids but the proportions vary considerably from fat to fat. Table 11.1 shows the variation in proportion of these three types of fatty acids in several common dietary fats. The two animal fats in Table 11.1 are high in saturates and low in polyunsaturates and this is typical of fat from farm animals. Fat from ruminating animals (e.g. milk, beef and lamb) is the most saturated and the least amenable to manipulation by alterations in the diet of the animal. The fatty acid composition of the fat from other animals (e.g. pigs) can be manipulated more readily by altering their diets although this may affect the palatability and the texture of the meat.

Soya oil and sunflower oil are two vegetable oils that are typical of many vegetable oils in that they are low in saturates and high in polyunsaturated fatty acids. In most vegetable oils, the ω-6 **polyunsaturated fatty acids** predominate. Olive oil and rapeseed (canola) oil are the most widely eaten examples of fats that are particularly high in monounsaturates and low in saturates. Rapeseed oil also has a relatively high proportion of ω-3 polyunsaturated acids. The composition of the two tropical oils shown in Table 11.1 (coconut and palm oil) illustrates that there are exceptions to the general observation that vegetable oils are low in saturates and high in unsaturated fatty acids. On the simple basis of the proportions of the three main types of fatty acids, palm oil is quite similar in its make-up to lard. Coconut oil contains a particularly high proportion (around 78 per cent) of medium-chain saturated fatty acids (fewer than 16 carbons) that make up only a small proportion of the fatty acids in most fats. Palmitic acid (16:0) is the dominant saturated fatty acid in most types of fat.

The two fish oils shown in Table 11.1 are typical of oil in most fish, shellfish and even the fat of marine mammals such as seals and whales. These marine oils are relatively high in polyunsaturates, low in saturates and are particularly rich in ω-3 **polyunsaturated fatty acids**. Fish oils are the principal dietary source of ω-3 polyunsaturated fatty acids that contain 20 or more carbon atoms (long-chain ω-3 polyunsaturates), especially EPA and docosahexaenoic acid (DHA). Docosahexaenoic acid is also found in the lecithin present in egg yolks and in the phospholipids present in muscle meat and particularly in organ meat like liver and brain. When fish are farmed then there may be some differences in the fatty acid composition of their oil compared

Table 11.1 Typical proportions (%) of saturated (S) monounsaturated (M) and polyunsaturated (P) fatty acids in several dietary fats

Fat	% S	% M	% P	P:S ratio
Butter	64	33	3	0.05
Lard	47	44	9	0.2
Sunflower oil	14	34	53	4
Soybean oil	15	26	59	4
Rapeseed (canola)	7	60	33	5
Olive oil	15	73	13	0.8
Coconut oil	91*	7	2	0.02
Palm oil	48	44	8	0.2
Oil in salmon	28	42	30	1
Oil in mackerel	27	43	30	1

*Includes large amount of medium chain saturates (less than 16 carbons)

with wild fish and this reflects the quite different diets of farmed and wild fish.

P:S ratio

The P:S ratio of a fat is the ratio of polyunsaturated to saturated fatty acids. In the examples shown in Table 11.1, this ratio ranges from 0.02 in coconut oil to around 5 in rapeseed (canola) oil. The P:S ratio has traditionally been used as a shorthand guide to the likely effect of a fat or a diet on the plasma cholesterol

concentration. For many years it has been generally accepted that saturated fatty acids tended to raise and polyunsaturates to lower plasma cholesterol concentration. This suggests that fats and diets with higher P:S ratios have the most favourable (lowering) effects on plasma cholesterol. Current views on the effects of various fatty acid fractions on plasma cholesterol are more complex; this is discussed later in the chapter. Despite this, the simple P:S ratio is still a useful practical indicator of the likely effect of a fat or diet on plasma cholesterol level.

Key points

- Fatty acids are composed of a hydrocarbon chain with a single carboxyl (COOH) or acid group at one end.

- Fatty acids in biological systems usually have between 2 and 22 carbon atoms. In this book the carbons are numbered from the end furthest from the carboxyl group.

- Note that chemists and biochemists use an alternative Δ numbering system counting carbons from the carboxyl end of the molecule.

- In saturated fatty acids, all of the carbons in the hydrocarbon chain are joined by single bonds.

- Monounsaturated fatty acids have a single carbon–carbon double bond in the hydrocarbon chain.

- Polyunsaturated fatty acids have between two and six double bonds.

- The ω-3 or n-3 series of polyunsaturated fatty acids have their first double bond between carbons 3 and 4 whereas the ω-6 or n-6 series their first double bond between carbons 6 and 7.

- A single saturated carbon atom (methylene group) separates each double bond in a polyunsaturated fatty acid.

- The shorthand notation for fatty acids indicates the number of carbons, the number of double bonds and the position of the first double bond. Thus $18:2_{\omega-6}$ (or 18:2n-6) has 18 carbons, two double bonds and the first double bond is between carbons 6 and 7.

- Trans fatty acids are those in which the hydrogen atoms at either end of a carbon–carbon double bond are on opposite sides whereas in cis fatty acids they are on the same side.

- In most natural fats, the *cis* configuration predominates but butter, hydrogenated oils, and heated oils contain significant amounts of *trans* fatty acids.

- The presence of a *cis* double bond alters the three dimensional shape of a fatty acid and causes the carbon chain to bend back on itself whereas *trans* fatty acids have a linear configuration that is closer to saturated fatty acids.

- In general, the longer the chain length of a fatty acid, the higher is its melting point and the presence of *cis* double bonds greatly lowers the melting point. *Trans* double bonds have a much smaller effect on melting point.

- The presence of *cis* double bonds increases the fluidity of fats.

- Fats with lots of saturated fatty acids tend to be solids at room temperature, e.g. butter and lard, but those with lots of polyunsaturated fatty acids tend to be liquid oils, such as sunflower oil and corn oil.

- Conjugated linoleic acids are a group of isomers of linoleic acid which have double bonds that are contiguous and may be either in the *cis* or *trans* configuration.

- Conjugated linoleic acids are taken as supplements although most of the evidence supporting their use comes from studies in animals that have used doses many times that which could be consumed in a normal diet.

- All dietary fats contain a mixture of saturated, monounsaturated and polyunsaturated fatty acids but the proportions vary enormously.

- Meat and milk fat is usually high in saturates and low in polyunsaturates.

- Many vegetable oils are low in saturates but high in polyunsaturates and the ω-6 series of polyunsaturates tend to predominate.

- Olive oil and rapeseed oil are particularly high in monounsaturates.

- Tropical oils such as palm oil and coconut oil are high in saturates and low in polyunsaturates.

- Fish oil is low in saturates and high in polyunsaturates and the ω-3 series tend to predominate.

- Fish oil is the major dietary source of the long chain ω-3 polyunsaturates (i.e. those with 20 or 22 carbons) but docosahexaenoic acid is also found in egg yolk lecithin, muscle meat phospholipids and especially in phospholipids from organ meat such as liver and brain.

- The P:S ratio of a fat is the ratio of polyunsaturated to saturated fatty acids in it.

- P:S ratio is a useful guide to the likely effect of a fat on plasma cholesterol concentration; those with a high ratio tend to lower it whereas those with a low ratio tend to raise it.

SOURCES OF FAT IN THE DIET

There are four principal sources of fat in the human diet.

- *Milk fat.* This is found in whole milk and yoghurt, cream, butter and cheese. This fat is almost inevitably highly saturated, because it is difficult to manipulate the fatty acid content of cow milk by manipulating the cow's diet. The fatty acid profiles of foods made from milk fat are sometimes altered by blending it with polyunsaturated oil, e.g. to produce a softer butter that is easier to spread.

- *Meat fat.* This includes not only carcass meat but also (often especially) meat products such as sausages and burgers and cooking fats of animal origin such as lard and beef tallow. This fat also tends to be highly saturated especially that from ruminating animals, e.g. beef and mutton. Note

that although animal fats are usually referred to as saturated fats they do contain large amounts of monounsaturated fatty acids (44 per cent in lard) particularly oleic acid.

- *Seeds and nuts.* These contain fat/oil, which provides a concentrated source of energy for germination. These fats and oils are prominent in many diets because they are the source of the vegetable oils and most margarine. They usually have a relatively high P:S ratio and most of the polyunsaturated fatty acids are predominantly of the ω-6 type in many of the most widely used vegetable oils. The tropical oils are clearly an exception to these generalities and have P:S ratios that are typical of those found in meat fat (see Table 11.1).

- *Fish oil.* This comes from the flesh of oily fish such as mackerel, herring, trout, mullet and salmon. The flesh of white fish (e.g. cod and haddock) is low in fat although considerable amounts of fat may be stored in the liver of such fish (hence cod liver oil). Fish oils tend to have a high P:S ratio, the ω-3 acids are generally abundant and they are the only major dietary source of the long-chain ω-3 polyunsaturated fatty acids. Partially hydrogenated fish oil was widely used to make margarine, it was low in DHA and EPA but contained large amounts of *trans* fatty acids. It has been superseded by soft margarine made from vegetable oils, that are high in polyunsaturated fatty acids and very low in *trans* fatty acids.

Any food that contains any of the above as an ingredient will also contain fat. Fat is a major ingredient of cakes, pastries, biscuits (cookies), and chocolate, and thus these foods contribute significantly to total fat intake. Any foods cooked with the fats listed above will also be rich in fat. Thus, potatoes and most other vegetables contain almost no fat but when fried or roasted with fat they absorb substantial amounts of the cooking fat.

UK fat intakes and their food sources

Table 11.2 shows the sources of fat and of saturated fat in UK diets as recorded in a weighed inventory (National Diet and Nutrition Survey (NDNS) survey) by a representative sample of adults (Henderson *et al.*, 2003). Where foods contribute relatively more to the fat and saturated fat columns than to the energy column then these are rich sources of dietary fat. Thus food in the milk group provides only 10 per cent of total energy but 24 per cent of the saturated

fat; fat spreads provided only 4 per cent of total energy but 12 per cent of the fat; and saturated fat and foods in the meat group provided 16 per cent of the energy but 24 per cent of the fat and saturated fat. Conversely, the cereals group provided 31 per cent of the total energy but only 19 per cent of the fat, and foods in the sugar, confectionery and drinks category provided 17 per cent of the energy but only 3 per cent of the fat.

Most dairy fat can be avoided by choosing products made from low-fat milk. Likewise with carcass meat, much of the obvious fat can be removed although in many meat products such as sausages, burgers and pies it is not possible to selectively remove the fat. Cereal foods, normally classified as starchy foods, provide a surprisingly high proportion of both fat and saturated fat and much of this comes from products such as cakes, pastries, biscuits (cookies) and pizzas.

Up until the middle part of the 1990s, the data from the National Food Survey suggested that the contribution of fat to the UK household diet rose during the 1950s and early 1960s as post-wartime shortages eased and rationing was removed. However, since around 1975 it had remained practically constant for more than two decades at around 40 per cent of total energy (e.g. Chesher, 1990; Ministry of Agriculture, Fisheries and Food (MAFF), 1993). Absolute fat consumption did drop very substantially during this latter period but only in proportion to the decline in total energy intake that occurred over this period, leaving the proportion of fat unaltered. As discussed in Chapter 4 there were great changes in the types of fat consumed in

Table 11.2 The percentage contribution of various foods to the energy, fat and saturated fat content of UK diets*

Food group	% Energy	% Total fat	% Saturated fat
Cereals and cereal products	31	19	18
Milk and milk products (including cheese)	10	14	24
Fat spreads	4	12	12
Egg and egg dishes	2	4	3
Meat and products	16	24	24
Fish and fish dishes	3	3	2
Vegetables (excluding potatoes)	4	4	2
Potatoes and savoury snacks	9	10	7
Fruit and nuts	3	2	1
Sugar, confectionery, preserves, drinks including alcohol	17	3	6

*Data source: Henderson et al. (2003).

Britain over this period. In 1959, the P:S ratio of the British diet was 0.17, still only 0.23 in 1979 but by 1996 it had risen to 0.47, which is about where it was in 2004–05. This change in P:S ratio has been brought about principally by replacement of butter, hard margarine and animal-based cooking fats by soft margarine and vegetable oils. There has also been a huge decrease in the consumption of whole-fat milk, which now represents only about a quarter of total milk sales compared with almost 100 per cent of the total in 1975. It is estimated that saturated fat now provides around 14.8 per cent of the energy in household food purchases whereas in 1975 it was around 20 per cent. Data from household expenditure surveys also suggest that between 1994 and 2000 the contribution of fat to the energy in household food dropped from 38.8 to 36.9 per cent but has remained fairly stable since then; it was estimated at 37.6 per cent of food energy in 2004–05.

Table 11.3 compares results from the NDNS adult surveys conducted in 1986–07 and 2000–01 which used a weighed inventory of food as eaten rather than household budget surveys (like the National Food Survey and its replacement Family Food) which measure what people buy rather than what they eat. These two consumption surveys show a big drop in the percentage of food energy derived from fat from over 40 per cent to close to the target figure of 35 per cent. There was also a 3 per cent drop in the percentage of food energy derived from saturated fatty acids. Table 11.4 compares average intakes of fat and selected fat fractions recorded in the 2000–01 NDNS and compares these with the dietary reference values (DRVs) set by the Committee on the Medical Aspects of Food (COMA, 1991). This table suggests that average intakes of total fat are close to the DRV; slightly above it for men and just below it for women. The proportions of fat and saturated fat recorded in this survey were fairly consistent in different age groups of adults. Intakes of saturated fatty acids, despite being much lower than recorded in earlier surveys, were still significantly above the DRV

Table 11.3 Changes in fat and selected fat fractions as a percentage of food energy in the British diet between 1986–87 and 2000–01[*]

Fat fraction	Men		Women	
	1986–87	2000–01	1986–87	2000–01
Total fat	40.4	35.8	40.3	34.9
Saturated fatty acids	16.5	13.4	17.0	13.2
Trans fatty acids	2.2	1.2	2.2	1.2

[*]Data source: Henderson et al. (2003).

Table 11.4 The percentage of food energy from various fat fractions compared with the dietary reference value (DRV) and the percentage of subjects meeting the DRV*

Fat fraction	DRV (% of food energy)	Average (% of food energy)		% meeting DRV	
		Men	Women	Men	Women
Total fat	35	35.8	34.9	43	50
Saturated fatty acids	11	13.4	13.2	Approximately 20	Approximately 20
Trans fatty acids	2	1.2	1.2	Approximately 98	Approximately 98
Cis n-3		1.0	1.0	All above minimum	
Cis n-6		5.4	5.3	All above minimum	
Cholesterol (mg/day)	300	304	213	56	83

Note that in approximately 20 per cent of all subjects fat contributed above 40 per cent of food energy.
Individual intakes of cis n-6 polyunsaturates did not exceed 10 per cent of food energy in any subjects (the individual maximum set by COMA, 1991).
*Data source: Henderson et al. (2003).

and only about 20 per cent of adults were at or below the DRV of saturated fat representing 11 per cent of food energy. All individuals met the very low minimum requirements for ω-3 (0.2 per cent of food energy) and ω-6 (1 per cent of food energy) polyunsaturated fatty acids and no individual exceeded the recommendation that not more than 10 per cent of an individual's food energy should come from ω-6 polyunsaturated fatty acids.

Trans fatty acid intakes have been declining for several decades as the hard margarines with their high levels of *trans* fats have been phased out. In 1982 average intakes of *trans* fatty acids in the UK were around 7 g/day and in 1986–87 this had declined to 5.6 g/day for men and 4 g/day for women and in the latest NDNS survey (Henderson *et al.*, 2003) this was down to 2.9 g/day for men and 2 g/day for women. COMA (1991) suggested that there was wide variation in individual intake of *trans* fatty acids despite the declining average intake. However, Table 11.4 shows that 98 per cent of men and women had intakes that were below the 2 per cent of food energy recommended by COMA (1991) and that intakes had almost halved between 1986–87 and 2000–01.

Key points

- Most dietary fat originates from meat, milk, fish, nuts and seeds or from any food that contains these as an ingredient.

- Nuts and seeds are the source of most cooking oils and margarine.

- Variation in the fatty acid profiles of dietary fats was discussed in the previous section.

- Table 11.2 shows the contribution of the major food groups to total fat and saturated fat intake in the UK.

- Until the mid-1990s, the proportion of household food energy obtained from fat remained at around 40 per cent for 20 years but has fallen since then.

- Between 1986–87 and 2000–01 the proportion of food energy derived from fat in Britain fell by about 5 per cent.

- Highly polyunsaturated oils and margarine have largely replaced butter, lard and beef tallow in the British diet and full fat milk has been largely replaced by lower fat milk.

- The P:S ratio of the British diet has approximately trebled since 1960.

- The proportion of food energy derived from saturated fat has been falling for over 30 years and is now around 13 per cent compared to peak values back in the 1970s of around 20 per cent.

- Intakes of *trans* fatty acids have been in long-term decline and had reached just 1.2 per cent of food energy in 2000–01 with 98 per cent of people below the DRV of no more than 2 per cent of food energy.

ROLES OF FAT IN THE DIET

Fat as an energy source

A gram of fat yields more than twice as much metabolizable energy as a gram of either carbohydrate or protein. Vegetable oils and animal-derived cooking fats are almost 100 per cent fat and so yield around the theoretical maximum metabolizable energy of any food, i.e. 9 kcal (36 kJ) per gram. This compares with less than 4 kcal (16 kJ) per gram for pure sugar, which is the most concentrated form of carbohydrate and is generally regarded as an energy-rich food.

Altering the fat content of foods profoundly affects their **energy density**. Table 11.5 shows some examples of how adding relatively small amounts of fat to portions of food produces disproportionately large increases in the energy yield of the food.

- Adding 8 g of butter or margarine to a slice of bread increases the energy content by around 80 per cent
- Adding a 35 g portion of double cream to a slice of fruit pie increases the energy content of the dish by 70 per cent
- Adding 20 g of mayonnaise to a 210 g mixed salad results in a 500 per cent rise in the energy yield.

Even in the fat-enriched foods in Table 11.5, fat still accounts for a relatively small proportion of the food's weight and yet in most cases it accounts for a high proportion of the energy yield. Thus fat accounts for:

- 4 per cent of the weight of whole milk but over half the energy
- 6 per cent of the weight of the salad and mayonnaise but over 80 per cent of the energy
- 6 per cent of the weight of the lean pork chop but well over 40 per cent of the energy

Table 11.5 The effect of adding typical portions of fats to typical portions of some foods. Portion sizes and composition are from Davies and Dickerson (1991)

Food	kJ	% Increase	% Fat by weight	% Energy as fat
Slice bread	315		2.5	11
+ butter or margarine	563	80	17	61
Jacket potato	617		Trace	0.5
+ butter or margarine	928	50	5.5	34
Boiled potatoes	504		Trace	1.5
Chips (French fries)	1592	215	11	39
Pork chop – lean only	756		6.5	43
Lean and fat	1462	95	19	66
Skimmed milk	267		Trace	3
Whole milk	542	100	4	53
Chicken – meat only	508		4	25
Meat and skin	773	50	23	58
Fruit pie	937		8	38
+ double cream	1596	70	17	62
Mixed salad	118		Trace	3
+ oil and vinegar	365	210	5	70
Mixed salad	118		Trace	3
+ mayonnaise	697	500	6.5	82.5

- 11 per cent of the weight of the chips (French fries) but about 40 per cent of the energy
- 17 per cent of the weight of the buttered bread but about 60 per cent of the energy.

Consumers should be wary of claims that a product is low fat simply because the percentage of fat by weight is low. A 90 per cent fat-free product has 10 per cent of fat by weight and this may still account for a high proportion of the food's energy. One could, for example, accurately describe whole milk as 96 per cent fat-free despite the fact that more than half its energy comes from fat.

Altering the fat content of a diet profoundly affects its energy density. A high-fat diet is a concentrated diet and a low-fat diet inevitably bulkier. It may be desirable for people expending lots of energy in prolonged heavy physical work to eat a reasonably concentrated diet so that they do not have to eat inordinate quantities of food (particularly people such as explorers who also have to carry their food). For relatively sedentary adults low-fat, low energy density diets are considered desirable because they may reduce the risk of excessive weight gain (see Chapter 8). Very-low-fat and low energy density weaning diets are on the other hand considered

undesirable because they may precipitate **protein energy malnutrition** because children cannot eat enough of the dilute food to meet their energy needs.

Palatability

Fat increases the sensory appeal of foods; it enhances the flavour, colour, texture and smell of food. Many volatile flavour compounds are soluble in fat and so are concentrated in the fat fraction of unprocessed foods. Flavour compounds develop when food is cooked in fats and oils even though some processed oils may be devoid of any inherent flavour. Fat also changes the texture of solid foods and the viscosity of liquids; butter or margarine spread onto bread not only changes the taste but also the texture; full-fat milk has a higher viscosity than low-fat milk that is readily discernible to the human palate. Fat also affects the appearance of some foods, e.g. skimmed milk has noticeably less colour than whole milk and less whitening effect when used in tea or coffee. Volatile, fat-soluble materials contribute to the smell of food as well as its taste. In the foods in Table 11.5, the addition of fat generally increases the sensory appeal of a food as well as the energy yield. Boiled potatoes are essentially bland whereas chips (French fries) have much more sensory appeal to most people. Adding butter to boiled mashed potatoes enhances their flavour, texture, smell and appearance. Adding oily dressings to salads or cream to fruit pie are usually considered to enhance the sensory appeal of these foods. Although some people find the concentrated surface fat on meat nauseating, a moderate amount of intrinsic fat greatly improves the taste and texture of meat, e.g. connoisseurs of beef look for meat with some fat marbled into the flesh.

The effects of fat on the palatability of food means that as populations become richer they tend to increase the proportion of their dietary energy that is derived from fat. When affluence increases the availability of fatty foods, people tend to consume them in amounts that are probably detrimental to their long-term health prospects. This effect of fat on palatability also explains why it proved difficult to persuade affluent populations to reduce the proportion of fat in their diets. Despite intensifying health education exhortations to reduce fat intake that began well over three decades ago, changes in the proportion of energy derived from fat have only changed significantly since the mid-1990s.

Fat is important in the production of weaning foods of appropriate viscosity for young children (Church, 1979). Children require food of appropriate viscosity for their stage of development. In the immediate postnatal period they require a liquid feed, then after weaning (say 6–12 months) they need to be fed with a semi-solid gruel followed by a gradual transition to a standard adult diet (note that they may require a lower viscosity when ill). After cooking, large amounts of water needs to be added to low-fat, starchy, staple foods to produce foods of suitable viscosity for newly weaned children. They may only become edible if 70–80 per cent of their total weight is water and they may require 95 per cent water to make them liquid. Their viscosity may increase sharply as they cool. Thus thick family pap made from maize may yield 1000 kcal (4.2 MJ) per kilogram but as much as 4 kg of a typical maize gruel suitable for a newly weaned child might be required to supply the same amount of energy. Fat not only adds concentrated energy to weaning foods but also affects their viscosity, such that they become palatable to young children over a wider range of water contents. For example, milk remains drinkable even when evaporated to only 20 per cent water.

Satiation

It has traditionally been said that fat delays stomach emptying and so extends the period of satiation after consumption of the meal. Many more recent studies suggest that, in fact, quite the opposite seems to be true, i.e. that carbohydrate rather than fat may have the greater satiating effect. Not only does fat increase the palatability and energy density of the diet but calorie for calorie fat may also have less satiating effect than carbohydrate thus favouring weight gain and obesity still further (see Chapter 8 for further discussion of this issue).

Fat-soluble vitamins

The fat-soluble vitamins (A, D, E and K) are found mainly in the lipid fraction of fat-containing foods and they are also absorbed along with dietary fat in the gut. Dietary deficiency of vitamin A is a major international nutritional problem even today (see Chapter 13). Vitamin A, **retinol**, is found only in certain fats of animal origin although humans can convert the pigment **β-carotene**, from brightly coloured fruits and vegetables, into retinol. Dietary fat facilitates the absorption of carotene and so extreme fat deprivation increases the risk of vitamin A deficiency in children even when the diet contains marginally adequate amounts of carotene. Medical conditions that lead to impaired fat digestion or absorption can precipitate fat-soluble vitamin deficiencies (see Chapter 13).

Essential fatty acids

In the 1920s, a deficiency disease was induced in rats by feeding them a fat-free diet and this disease was cured by the addition of small amounts of fat to the rats' diets. Fatty acids of the linoleic acid series (ω-6) cured all of the symptoms of this deficiency disease whereas those of the linolenic acid series (ω-3) gave only partial relief of symptoms. Saturated and monounsaturated fatty acids are not effective in relieving the symptoms of this deficiency disease. The symptoms of this deficiency disease are scaly dermatitis, poor growth, increased food intake and reduced immune responses. We now know that there is an essential dietary requirement for polyunsaturated fatty acids – the **essential fatty acids**. These essential fatty acids have certain structural functions (e.g. in membranes) and they are necessary for the synthesis of a key group of regulatory molecules, the **eicosanoids**, which include the **prostaglandins**, thromboxanes and leukotrienes. Although we can synthesize fatty acids from other substrates we do not have the biochemical capability to insert double bonds between any of the first seven carbons of fatty acid molecules. Thus we can neither synthesize linoleic acid or α-linolenic acid, nor can we inter-convert acids of the ω-3 and ω-6 series. The minimum human requirement for these essential fatty acids is extremely small (around 1 per cent of energy) and it has not been possible to reproduce the symptoms of this deficiency disease of rats in deprivation studies with human volunteers. The practical risk of overt fatty acid deficiency in humans is usually remote; COMA (1991) recommend that to prevent essential fatty acid deficiency linoleic acid ($18:2_{\omega-6}$) should provide at least 1 per cent of dietary energy and that α-linolenic acid ($18:3_{\omega-3}$) should provide at least 0.2 per cent of dietary energy for all age groups.

The extremely low requirement for these essential fatty acids, the presence of considerable reserves of polyunsaturated fatty acids in body fat and the diffi-culty of eliminating all traces of fat from the diet, compound to make this disease difficult to induce experimentally in people. Even fruits, vegetable and cereals regarded as essentially fat free do contain small amounts of polyunsaturated fat. There have, however, been some reports of essential fatty acid deficiency in humans. In the 1950s, some low birth weight babies fed on skimmed milk developed eczema and other symptoms of essential fatty acid deficiency that were cured by small amounts of essential fatty acids. In the 1970s dermatitis caused by essential fatty acid defi-ciency was reported in several patients maintained on intravenous fat-free nutrition (Rivers and Frankel, 1981). The inability to safely infuse a source of fat hindered the development of long-term **total par-enteral nutrition (TPN)** (see Chapter 16). It took more than four decades after the first demonstration in the rat to demonstrate essential fatty acid defi-ciency in an adult human being and then only under unusual circumstances.

Fatty acids of both the ω-6 and ω-3 series may be metabolized to longer chain and more highly polyun-saturated acids (see Figure 11.2). Linoleic acid ($18:2_{\omega-6}$) or linolenic acid ($18:3_{\omega-3}$) first has a double bond inserted at the carboxyl end of the existing sequence of double bonds by an enzyme known as a desaturase. The product of this desaturation reaction

then has an extra two-carbon acetate unit added to the carboxyl end by an enzyme system known as an elongase. The rest of the pathway consists of two more desaturation reactions (i.e. insertion of two more double bonds) and one more elongation, i.e. addition of another two-carbon unit. The fatty acids at the end of these sequences in Figure 11.2 are essential components of cell membranes.

The EPA and DHA of the ω-3 series predominate in the membranes in the brain and retina whereas ω-6 fatty acids predominate in the membranes of liver cells and platelets. Their concentration in brain and retinal membrane phospholipids is one reason why ω-3 acids are essential in very small quantities in their own right and not just as partial substitutes for ω-6 acids. Abnormal electroencephalogram (EEG) read-ings and retinal activity have been reported in animals with lowered levels of ω-3 fatty acids in these tissues. Adequate availability of ω-3 fatty acids is probably critical for brain development in infants. The presence of ω-3 fatty acids in the diet is certainly considered to be nutritionally desirable. The major dietary source of the long-chain ω-3 fatty acids EPA and DHA is from fish oil or in some populations from the fat of marine mammals. In theory these long-chain ω-3 acids can be made from α-linolenic acid ($18:3_{\omega-3}$) it is, however,

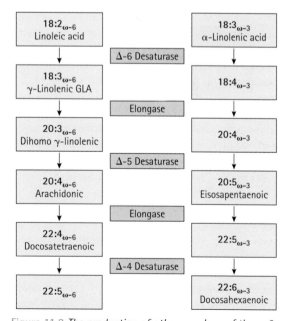

Figure 11.2 *The production of other members of the ω-6 and ω-3 series of fatty acids from linoleic acid ($18:2\omega-6$) and α-linolenic acid ($18:3\omega-3$).*

now clear that in humans there is only limited conversion of α-linolenic acid to EPA and very little conversion to DHA (Burdge, 2004). Very high intakes of ω-6 acids will tend to competitively inhibit the conversion of shorter-chain ω-3 acids to their longer-chain derivatives and vice versa. More than 20 years ago Sanders *et al.* (1984) showed that high intakes of ω-6 fatty acid reduce the amount of EPA and DHA in rat cell membranes despite the presence of significant amounts of linolenic acid in the diet. This might be of particular significance in vegans consuming large amounts of ω-6 polyunsaturates (e.g. from soft margarine and sunflower oil) because, as was noted earlier, long-chain ω-3 acids are not found in plant foods.

The growth in the use of vegetable oils for cooking and soft margarines and other vegetable-based spreading fats means that current US and UK diets have at least 10 times more ω-6 fatty acids than ω-3 and this ratio may be as high as 30 times in some instances. This compares with a ω-6 to ω-3 ratio of more like 2–4:1 in hunter–gatherer societies. Most authorities agree that the current ω-6 to ω-3 ratio is too high although opinions vary about the optimum level; it should be less than 10:1, and a very tentative optimal ratio of 4–5:1 has been suggested. Not only is rapeseed oil high in monounsaturated fatty acids but it has a relatively high ω-3 to ω-6 ratio for a vegetable oil. A number of natural oils are marketed as dietary supplements on the basis of their high concentration of particular polyunsaturated fatty acids. Some are listed below.

- Fish oil and fish liver oil are rich source of ω-3 polyunsaturated fatty acids including EPA and DHA, the long-chain derivatives (note that fish liver oils contain high concentrations of vitamins A and D which may be toxic if the recommended dose is exceeded and these should be avoided by pregnant women because high doses of vitamin A can cause birth defects).
- Evening primrose oil, starflower oil and blackcurrant seed oil are marketed as rich sources of γ-linolenic acid ($18:3_{\omega-6}$) the second fatty acid on the ω-6 pathway in Figure 11.2.
- Flaxseed oil is a rich source of α-linolenic acid ($18:3_{\omega-3}$), the parent compound of the ω-3 series. It is marketed as a rich source of ω-3 fatty acids that is suitable for vegetarians but as noted earlier there is limited conversion of this to EPA and little conversion to DHA in humans.

- Algal extracts containing significant amounts of DHA are marketed as a source of DHA that is available to vegetarians.

Essential fatty acids and eicosanoid production

The eicosanoids are a range of regulatory molecules that take part in the regulation of most physiological processes, e.g. in the initiation of labour, blood platelet aggregation, blood vessel constriction/dilation, inflammation and many secretory processes. They are often referred to as 'local hormones' because they act close to or on the cells that produce them. The prefix 'eico' is derived from the Greek for 20, and these eicosanoids are made from ω-6 and ω-3 polyunsaturated fatty acids that have 20 carbon atoms, i.e. dihomo γ-linolenic acid (DGLA, $20:3_{\omega-6}$), arachidonic acid ($20:4_{\omega-6}$) and eicosapentaenoic acid (EPA, $20:5_{\omega-3}$). In general those produced from arachidonic acid are the most potent.

Figure 11.3 illustrates the origins of the different eicosanoids produced from the three fatty acid precursors. As noted earlier, the enzymes involved in the elongation and desaturation of fatty acids are common to the ω-3 and ω-6 pathways, so there is competition between ω-3 and ω-6 substrates for these enzymes. Likewise, the eicosanoid precursors also compete for the lipoxygenase and cyclo-oxygenase pathways shown in Figure 11.3. This means that altering the availability of the precursor fatty acids will change the balance of eicosanoid production and thus affect the processes regulated by these eicosanoids. High intakes of ω-3 fatty acids would be expected to increase the production of the EPA derived eicosanoids and decrease the production of those from the ω-6 precursors and especially from arachidonic acid; remember, however, that there is only limited conversion of α-linolenic acid to EPA in humans and so, for example, flaxseed oil (rich in α-linolenic acid) will have much less effect than fish oil supplements which contain preformed EPA.

Certain oils such as evening primrose oil and starflower oil and are rich in γ-linolenic acid ($20:3_{\omega-6}$) and this favours the production of eicosanoids made from DGLA. Note that relatively little γ-linolenic acid is synthesized from most human diets because they contain high levels of arachidonic acid (e.g. from meat) and this inhibits the Δ6 desaturase that converts linoleic acid to γ-linolenic acid.

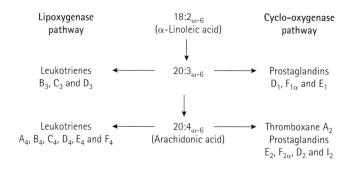

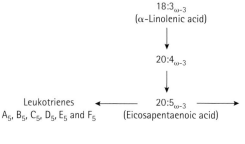

Figure 11.3 *Production of eicosanoids from 'essential' ω-6 and ω-3 polyunsaturated fatty acids.*

Key points

- Fat is the most concentrated source of dietary energy.

- Adding relatively small amounts of fat to a food can produce a disproportionately large rise in energy yield.

- Claims that a food has a low percentage of fat by weight may disguise the very large proportion of the energy yield from the fat.

- A relatively high-fat, high energy density diet may be necessary for those expending very large amounts of energy and for active and rapidly growing babies and children.

- For sedentary adults, a high-fat diet probably encourages excessive weight gain and obesity.

- Fat improves the palatability of food and this encourages affluent populations to eat more fat than is good for their long-term health and makes it difficult to persuade them to eat less fat.

- Very-low-fat weaning foods may be of such low energy density that babies cannot eat enough of them to meet their energy needs.

- Fat is a concentrated source of energy for weaning foods and produces a suitable viscosity at relatively low water content.

- Calorie for calorie fat is probably less satiating than carbohydrate.

- Impaired fat absorption or extreme low-fat diets may precipitate fat-soluble deficiencies (especially vitamin A).

- Polyunsaturated fatty acids are essential nutrients; they have structural functions and are precursors of prostaglandins and other eicosanoids.

- The requirement for essential fatty acids is small and it is difficult to induce overt deficiency in human volunteers.

- The parent compound of the ω-6 series of polyunsaturated fatty acids is linoleic acid ($18:2_{\omega-6}$) and that of the ω-3 series is α-linolenic acid ($18:3_{\omega-3}$).

- Linoleic and linolenic acid undergo a series of desaturation and elongation reactions to produce two series of ω-6 and ω-3 polyunsaturated fatty acids with the end products of these sequences being $22:5_{\omega-6}$ and $22:6_{\omega-3}$, respectively.

- Small amounts of ω-3 polyunsaturates are almost certainly essential in their own right. The long-chain ones are normal components of brain and retinal membranes, and seem to be crucial for normal brain development.

- Long-chain ω-3 polyunsaturates are prevalent in fish oil and they can be made from shorter chain varieties that are prevalent in some vegetable oils such as rapeseed oil and flaxseed oil, but in practice there is limited conversion to EPA and very little conversion to DHA in humans.

- Humans cannot inter-convert ω-6 and ω-3 fatty acids.

- Arachidonic acid ($20:4_{\omega-6}$) is the precursor of many potent eicosanoids which regulate a multitude of physiological processes including

the inflammatory response, blood coagulation, platelet aggregation, blood vessel tone, etc.

- Eicosanoids made from eicosapentaenoic acid ($20:5_{\omega-3}$) and dihomo γ-linolenic acid (DGLA; $20:3_{\omega-3}$) are generally less potent than those made from arachidonic acid.

- Oil of evening primrose and starflower oil contain large amounts of γ-linolenic acid.

- Many omnivorous diets contain relatively large amounts of arachidonic acid which inhibits the Δ6 desaturase which converts linoleic acid to γ-linolenic acid and thus to DGLA.

BLOOD LIPOPROTEINS

Fats are, by definition, insoluble in water, and so to transport them around the body in aqueous plasma they have to be associated with protein carriers and transported as lipid/protein aggregates, the **lipoproteins**. There are several subdivisions of lipoproteins in blood plasma which can be conveniently separated according to their density – the higher the proportion of fat in a lipoprotein, the lower its density because fat has low density. The protein components of lipoproteins are known as **apoproteins**. The subdivisions of the plasma lipoproteins and their approximate compositions are given in Table 11.6.

Chylomicrons are the form in which ingested fat is transported to the liver and tissues after its absorption from the intestine. They are normally absent from fasting blood. Levels of very-low-density lipoproteins (VLDL) should also be low in fasting blood because it is rapidly converted to low-density lipoprotein (LDL) (see below). This means that blood lipid determinations should be measured in fasting blood samples to avoid any distortion due to variable

amounts of postprandial chylomicrons and large amounts of VLDL. Intermediate-density lipoprotein (IDL) is a transitory intermediate that normally represents only a very small fraction of total lipoproteins. The principal lipoproteins in normal fasting blood are LDL, high-density lipoprotein (HDL) and relatively small amounts of VLDL.

Very-low-density lipoproteins are rich in triacylglycerol and thus measures of blood triacylglycerols are taken to indicate the amount of VLDL. Low-density lipoproteins are the major cholesterol-containing fraction and thus measures of total plasma cholesterol are often taken to indicate the LDL concentration. The normal function of VLDL is to transport triacylglycerol produced endogenously in the liver (largely from dietary fat) to the adipose tissue or the muscles where it acts as an energy source; LDL acts as an external source of cholesterol for cells unable to synthesize sufficient for use in membranes or as a precursor for steroid hormone synthesis. The main function of HDL is to transport excess cholesterol from tissues and other blood lipoproteins back to the liver.

Table 11.6 Subdivisions of the plasma lipoproteins and their approximate compositions (per cent)

	Triacylglycerol	Cholesterol	Phospholipid	Apoprotein
Chylomicrons	82	9	7	2
Very-low-density lipoproteins	52	22	18	8
Low-density lipoproteins	9	47	23	21
Intermediate-density lipoproteins	20	35	20	15
High-density lipoproteins	3	19	28	50

Epidemiological evidence and evidence from people with familial hyperlipidaemias suggests that high plasma LDL-cholesterol concentrations are causally associated with increased atherosclerosis and increased risk of coronary heart disease. High-density lipoprotein (HDL) on the other hand inhibits atherosclerosis and high HDL-cholesterol concentrations are protective against coronary heart disease. The LDL to HDL ratio is a better predictor of coronary heart disease risk than LDL concentration alone. Simple plasma cholesterol measurements do not indicate the distribution of the cholesterol between LDL and HDL but total cholesterol concentration is used as an indicator of LDL-cholesterol concentration. Raised VLDL is associated with obesity, glucose intolerance and high alcohol consumption. High VLDL is certainly an indicator of high risk of coronary heart disease but whether it is a significant independent risk factor for coronary heart disease is still a matter of debate (Grundy, 1998).

Key points

- Fats are insoluble in water and are transported in blood as lipoprotein complexes.

- Chylomicrons are the lipoproteins that carry absorbed fat from the intestine to the tissues and they are absent from fasting blood.

- Very-low-density lipoprotein (VLDL) is a triacylglycerol-rich fraction that transports fat produced in the liver to the muscles and adipose tissue.

- Low-density lipoprotein (LDL) is rich in cholesterol and acts as an external source of cholesterol for cells.

- LDL is atherogenic.

- High-density lipoprotein (HDL) is anti-atherogenic; it removes excess cholesterol to the liver.

- High plasma LDL is associated with increased risk of coronary heart disease but high HDL is associated with reduced risk.

DIGESTION, ABSORPTION AND TRANSPORT OF DIETARY LIPIDS

Figure 11.4 shows a summary scheme for the digestion and absorption of dietary fats. Dietary fat is emulsified by the action of bile salts and phospholipids in

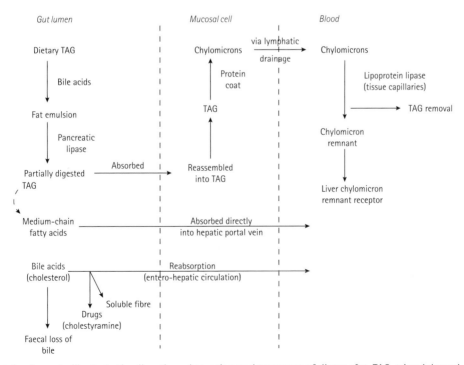

Figure 11.4 *A scheme to illustrate the digestion, absorption and transport of dietary fat. TAG, triacylglycerol.*

the intestine. This emulsified fat is then partially digested by the enzyme **lipase**, which is secreted into the gut in the pancreatic juice. Note that lipase is a water-soluble enzyme and so can normally digest water-insoluble fat only if it has first been emulsified. Lipase splits off (hydrolyses) fatty acids from the glycerol component of triacylglycerol. *In vivo*, this process does not result in total breakdown of triacylglycerol, the major end products in the gut are monoacylglycerols and free fatty acids. Lipase does not act on the fatty acid attached to the second (middle) carbon atom of the glycerol component.

Glands at the base of the tongue produce a lingual lipase, an enzyme that works at low pH and can readily digest the fat in milk globules before emulsification by bile salts. Lingual lipase is normally a minor contributor to fat digestion although it is important in suckling babies whose pancreatic function is not fully developed at birth. Churning of fat in the stomach with phospholipids and other digestion products has some emulsifying effect on dietary fat. The products of lipase action together with bile salts, phospholipids and fat-soluble vitamins form minute molecular aggregates known as **micelles**, and this effectively solubilizes them. Fat digestion products and fat-soluble vitamins diffuse from the micelles into the mucosal cells that line the small intestine and once inside they are reassembled into triacylglycerol and coated with protein to form the chylomicrons. Chylomicrons can be envisaged as droplets or packets of triacylglycerol surrounded by a thin protein coat. These chylomicrons enter the lymphatic vessels that drain the small intestine and pass into venous blood via the thoracic duct, which drains into the right subclavian vein. Most fat is absorbed in the duodenum and jejunum.

In the liver and adipose tissue, the triacylglycerol is removed from the chylomicrons by an enzyme called **lipoprotein lipase** that is located on the inner surface of the capillary. The products of this second digestion are absorbed into the cells and most is again reassembled into triacylglycerol for storage in adipose tissue or for transport in the liver. Liver cells clear the fat-depleted chylomicron remnants from the plasma via a specific chylomicron remnant receptor. These chylomicron remnants contain fat-soluble vitamins, and these are taken up and stored by the liver along with the chylomicron remnants. Some short- and medium-chain fatty acids are relatively more water soluble and they bypass this process. They are absorbed directly from the gut into the hepatic portal vein and transported to the liver bound to plasma albumin.

Large amounts of cholesterol-derived bile salts are secreted into the intestine each day in the bile. Most of this bile salt (cholesterol) is reabsorbed in the intestine and recycled to the liver – the **entero-hepatic circulation**. Some substances are thought to exert a lowering effect on plasma cholesterol by interfering with this entero-hepatic recycling leading to increased faecal losses of cholesterol derivatives. Soluble fibre and some plant sterols exert such an effect and the cholesterol-lowering drug cholestyramine is a resin that binds or chelates bile acids in the intestine preventing their reabsorption.

Key points

- Dietary fat is partly digested by pancreatic lipase in the small intestine; the products of this digestion are absorbed into the mucosal cells and most are re-esterified into triacylglycerol.

- Bile salts emulsify dietary fat so that it can be digested and solubilize fat digestion products so that they can be absorbed.

- Bile salts are reabsorbed in the ileum and returned to the liver (the entero-hepatic circulation).

- Chylomicrons carry the absorbed fat into the circulation via the lymphatic system.

- Lipoprotein lipase in tissue capillaries digests the triacylglycerol in chylomicrons so that it can be absorbed into the fat or liver cells and most is again reassembled into triacylglycerol.

- The chylomicron remnants are removed from the circulation by the liver along with the fat-soluble vitamins that they contain.

- Short- and medium-chain fatty acids can be absorbed directly into the hepatic portal vein and transported bound to plasma albumen.

TRANSPORT OF ENDOGENOUSLY PRODUCED LIPIDS

Figure 11.5 gives a summary of the origins and interrelationship of the non-chylomicron lipoproteins. Triacylglycerol-rich VLDL is produced in the liver by reassembling dietary fats and by endogenous

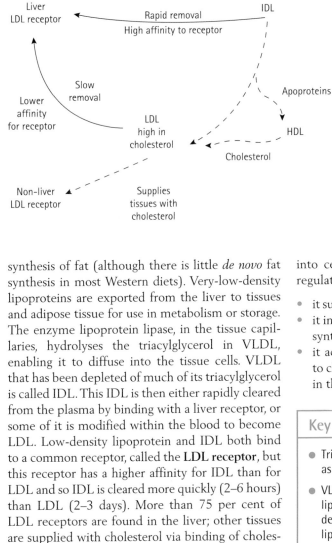

Figure 11.5 *The relationship between the various lipoproteins involved in endogenous lipid transport. After Brown and Goldstein (1984). VLDL, very-low-density lipoproteins; LDL, low-density lipoprotein; IDL, intermediate-density lipoprotein; HDL, high-density lipoprotein.*

synthesis of fat (although there is little *de novo* fat synthesis in most Western diets). Very-low-density lipoproteins are exported from the liver to tissues and adipose tissue for use in metabolism or storage. The enzyme lipoprotein lipase, in the tissue capillaries, hydrolyses the triacylglycerol in VLDL, enabling it to diffuse into the tissue cells. VLDL that has been depleted of much of its triacylglycerol is called IDL. This IDL is then either rapidly cleared from the plasma by binding with a liver receptor, or some of it is modified within the blood to become LDL. Low-density lipoprotein and IDL both bind to a common receptor, called the **LDL receptor**, but this receptor has a higher affinity for IDL than for LDL and so IDL is cleared more quickly (2–6 hours) than LDL (2–3 days). More than 75 per cent of LDL receptors are found in the liver; other tissues are supplied with cholesterol via binding of cholesterol-rich LDL to their LDL receptors (Brown and Goldstein, 1984). Around 80 per cent of LDL leaving the circulation is normally taken up by the liver and just 20 per cent by all other tissues. The perceived importance of the LDL receptor may be judged by the fact that its discoverers Brown and Goldstein were awarded the Nobel Prize for physiology and medicine in 1985. Once LDL is absorbed

into cells it releases its cholesterol, causing three regulatory responses in the cell:

- it suppresses synthesis of LDL receptors in the cell
- it inhibits the rate-limiting enzyme in cholesterol synthesis (**HMG CoA reductase**)
- it activates an enzyme that converts cholesterol to cholesterol esters that can be stored as droplets in the cell.

Key points

- Triacylglycerol produced in the liver is exported as very-low-density lipoprotein (VLDL).

- VLDL is depleted of triacylglycerol by lipoprotein lipase in tissue capillaries; this depleted VLDL is called intermediate density lipoprotein (IDL).

- Some IDL is cleared rapidly by the liver and some is converted within the circulation to LDL.

- Both IDL and LDL are cleared by LDL receptors although LDL is cleared much more slowly.

- Three-quarters of LDL receptors are in the liver; the other quarter is spread between the other tissues.

● When cells have surplus cholesterol, they produce less, convert some to cholesterol esters and suppress their synthesis of LDL receptors.

THE DIET–HEART HYPOTHESIS

According to Brown and Goldstein (1984), most people living in the Western industrialized countries have elevated plasma cholesterol concentrations making them prone to atherosclerosis and coronary heart disease. They concluded that this was due to reduced LDL receptor synthesis. This reduced receptor synthesis is one of the mechanisms that protect cells from cholesterol overload but it also leads to raised levels of circulating cholesterol. They suggested that dietary and other environmental factors that tend to raise the plasma LDL (e.g. high saturated fat and cholesterol intake) induce their effect by suppressing LDL receptor synthesis. Reduced LDL receptor synthesis would be expected not only to increase the lifespan of LDL but also lead to an increased rate of production because less IDL would be cleared and more would be converted within the blood to LDL. The raised level of LDL-cholesterol in the blood increases the tendency for it to be deposited in artery walls where it may trigger fibrotic changes, i.e. atherosclerosis or 'hardening of the arteries'.

When LDL-cholesterol levels in blood rise beyond a certain level then it is taken up by macrophages in the blood vessel walls and circulating monocytes. These LDL-laden macrophages are termed foam cells because they have a foamy appearance. Foam cells accumulate in the blood vessel wall giving rise to so-called fatty streaks, which are an early and relatively benign stage in the process of atherosclerosis. At this 'fatty streak' stage the process is clearly reversible; some fatty streaks disappear but others undergo hardening and fibrosis and become atherosclerotic plaques. High-density lipoprotein is involved in the process of removal of cholesterol from fatty streaks and plaques and returning it to the liver. Thus, as noted earlier, high HDL levels are known to be associated with reduced risk of coronary heart disease (CHD). It is not really clear why some fatty streaks regress and others develop into plaques but one suggested mechanism is that oxidation of the LDL can make it much more damaging to the artery wall. This theory has also led to suggestions that antioxidants, particularly in fruits and vegetables,

inhibit the progress of atherosclerosis (see Chapter 12 for further discussion of the oxidant theory of disease).

Reduced LDL receptor synthesis is seen as initiating a chain of events that can lead to increased atherosclerosis and ultimately increased risk of coronary heart disease and other atherosclerosis-linked diseases – the **diet–heart hypothesis** (Figure 11.6).

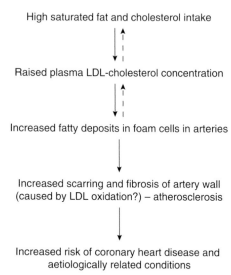

Figure 11.6 *The diet–heart hypothesis. LDL, low-density lipoprotein.*

There is overwhelming evidence that a raised plasma cholesterol concentration (which indicates a raised LDL-cholesterol) is linked to increased risk of coronary heart disease. Not least of this evidence, are studies on people with **familial hypercholesteraemia**, an inherited condition in which there is a defect in the LDL receptor gene. Even people who are heterozygous for this condition (i.e. one normal and one abnormal gene) become hypercholesteraemic and they have a markedly increased probability of dying prematurely from coronary heart disease, particularly if they are male. Those few people (one in a million) who are homozygous for this condition fail to produce any functional LDL receptors. They have to rely entirely upon other inefficient methods to clear LDL-cholesterol from blood and their plasma cholesterol concentrations may be up to six times normal. These individuals usually die from coronary heart disease in childhood. Injections of radioactively labelled LDL into such individuals confirms that it remains in the circulation about

2.5 times as long as in unaffected people and that the rate of endogenous LDL production is about doubled (Brown and Goldstein, 1984).

This diet–heart hypothesis could reasonably be described as a dominant theme of many nutrition-education campaigns in the UK and elsewhere. Dietary measures that would lead to lowered average plasma cholesterol concentrations are widely seen as central to nutrition education for health promotion. A figure of 5.2 mmol/L has been widely suggested as a desirable maximum for individual plasma cholesterol levels and yet the majority of the UK population exceed this level. Some frequently used cut-off points for plasma cholesterol concentration are given in Table 11.7. In Chapter 1, it was seen that in men the individual risk of coronary heart disease increases exponentially as the plasma

cholesterol concentration rises above this target value. However, most of the apparent excess population risk from high blood cholesterol seems to be concentrated in those men whose blood cholesterol levels are only slightly to moderately elevated. There are vast numbers of men (the majority of the population) who are apparently at some relatively small increased individual risk due to slight to moderate cholesterol elevation but only a small proportion at greatly increased risk due to very high cholesterol concentrations (see Table 11.8). The thrust of nutrition education has been to direct cholesterol-lowering dietary advice at the whole population with the aim of shifting the whole distribution downwards. In addition, intensive dietary counselling and perhaps cholesterol-lowering drugs may be used on those individuals identified as having substantially elevated cholesterol levels or existing coronary heart disease.

The distribution of plasma cholesterol concentrations in the UK adult population is shown in Table 11.8. Two-thirds of adults have values that are above the optimal range (i.e. above 5.2 mmol/L). There is a very pronounced trend in both sexes for plasma cholesterol to increase with age; in 19–24-year-olds only 16 per cent of men and 17 per cent of women have values that are above the optimal range and less than 1 per cent have values in the moderately or

Table 11.7 Some cut-off points for plasma cholesterol concentration

Plasma cholesterol concentration (mmol/L)	Classification
Below 5.2	Optimal range
5.2–6.5	Mildly elevated
6.5–7.8	Moderately elevated
Over 7.8	Severely elevated

Table 11.8 Distribution (per cent) of plasma cholesterol concentrations in UK adults by age and sex group[*]

Age group (years)	Serum cholesterol concentrations (mmol/L)			
	Below 5.2	5.2–6.5	6.5–7.8	7.8+
Men				
19–24	84	16	–	–
35–49	44	41	14	2
50–64	41	37	20	2
65–74[†]	29	51	18	4
75–84[†]	39	43	15	3
Women				
19–24	83	17	–	–
35–49	52	41	6	1
50–64	25	42	24	9
65–74[†]	24	32	29	15
75–84[†]	23	27	36	14

[*] Data from the NDNS survey of adults aged 19–64 years (Hoare et al., 2004) and the NDNS survey of adults aged over 65 years (Finch et al., 1998).
[†] Free living, excludes those living in care homes for the elderly.

severely elevated ranges. This distribution shifts sharply towards the higher values with each increase in age band so that, for example, in 65–74-year-old men 73 per cent are above the optimum and 22 per cent are over 6.5 mmol/L (76 per cent and 44 per cent, respectively, in women of this age).

In pre-menopausal women average values for plasma cholesterol level are lower than those of men, and the proportion in the higher categories of cholesterol level are also lower. However, this sex difference reverses at the menopause and so, for example, in the 65–74 years category 29 per cent of women have moderately and 15 per cent severely elevated cholesterol levels compared with corresponding values for men of 18 per cent and 4 per cent, respectively. When the plasma cholesterol levels recorded in the 2000–01 NDNS survey (Hoare *et al.*, 2004) are compared with those recorded in the earlier 1986–87 survey (Gregory *et al.*, 1990) there does seem to have been some improvement over the intervening years; average values for the whole sample were 5.8 mmol/L in 1986/7 and 5.2 mmol/L in 2000–01 and the percentage of the sample above the optimal values was around 66 per cent in 1986–87 but only 48 per cent in 2000–01.

Key points

- A high saturated fat intake leads to reduced LDL receptor synthesis and to raised levels of circulating LDL-cholesterol.

- LDL is taken up by foam cells in artery walls and forms fatty streaks which may trigger atherosclerosis, e.g. if the LDL becomes oxidized.

- Atherosclerosis predisposes to coronary heart disease (CHD).

- High saturated fat intake (and other environmental influences) triggers a chain of events that can ultimately lead to increased risk of coronary heart disease – the diet–heart hypothesis.

- Risk of CHD rises exponentially with plasma total cholesterol (an indicator of LDL-cholesterol concentration).

- People who are genetically prone to have markedly raised plasma LDL-cholesterol concentrations are at greatly increased risk of CHD.

- 5.2 mmol/L is the ideal upper limit for plasma total cholesterol concentration but two-thirds of the UK population exceed this level.

- People with markedly raised cholesterol levels are at greatest individual risk from CHD but much of the population risk is concentrated in the large numbers of people with mild to moderate cholesterol elevation.

- The health promotion priority has thus generally been to reduce average plasma cholesterol concentrations rather than solely seeking to identify and treat those with severely elevated cholesterol concentrations.

- Both average cholesterol level and the number in the elevated categories increase with age.

- Pre-menopausal women have lower average cholesterol levels than men and fewer are in the raised cholesterol categories but this situation reverses after the menopause.

- The NDNS surveys of 1986–87 and 2000–01 suggest that both average blood cholesterol levels and the percentage of people with raised levels have declined significantly in the 14 years between the two surveys.

CURRENT 'HEALTH IMAGES' OF DIFFERENT DIETARY FATS

Around 50 years ago, Keys *et al.* (1959) showed that, in short-term experiments with young men, total plasma cholesterol levels were significantly affected by the degree of saturation of the fat in the diet even when the diets were matched for total fat content. As a result of such experiments, saturated fat has acquired a negative health image. Saturated fat was found to raise plasma cholesterol concentration in such experiments and this is associated with increased atherosclerosis and increased risk of coronary heart disease. Polyunsaturated fats on the other hand were found to lower plasma cholesterol concentration when they replaced saturated fat. Results from these early experiments suggested that monounsaturated fatty acids were neutral in their effects on blood cholesterol level. Keys and his group concluded that saturated fatty acids were about twice as potent in raising serum cholesterol as polyunsaturated fatty acids were in lowering it. Keys *et al.*

(1965) produced an equation (the **Keys equation**) which enabled the change in plasma cholesterol of a group to be fairly well predicted in response to specified changes in its dietary fats.

Keys equation

$$\Delta C = (2.7 \times \Delta S) - (1.3 \times \Delta P) + 1.5Z^{1/2}$$

where:

- ΔC = change in plasma cholesterol concentration

- ΔS = change in per cent of energy from saturated fat

- ΔP = change in per cent of energy from polyunsaturated fat

- Z = dietary cholesterol (mg) per 1000 kcal (4.2 MJ).

As a result of such observations, some vegetable oils and soft margarine because of their high P:S ratios acquired a very positive health image and were for a time almost regarded as 'health foods'. In Keys and colleagues' experiments (1959), switching from a diet very high in saturates (P:S 0.16) to one very high in polyunsaturated fat (P:S 2.8) resulted in a rapid, but variable, reduction in an individual's plasma cholesterol concentration even though the total fat intake was kept constant (see Figure 3.10 in Chapter 3, p. 116). Since the 1960s, several attempts have been made to produce other such predictive equations that are better or more detailed than those of Keys *et al.*, (e.g. Yu *et al.*, 1995). Current dietary guidelines relating to dietary fats are detailed and discussed in Chapter 4.

Effects on LDL- and HDL-cholesterol

It is now known that the total plasma cholesterol consists of both LDL and HDL fractions. The LDL fraction is atherogenic, and regarded as 'the bad cholesterol' whereas the HDL fraction is anti-atherogenic and seen as 'the good cholesterol'. It would thus seem desirable to lower the LDL-cholesterol and raise the HDL-cholesterol. The LDL-cholesterol is generally considered to be readily responsive to dietary manipulation but the HDL

rather less so. High-density lipoprotein levels do rise in response to regular exercise and seem to be increased by moderate alcohol consumption. Current views on the ways in which the different dietary fat fractions affect these plasma cholesterol fractions and their current 'health image' are summarized below.

Total fat

In an assessment of current evidence, Mangiapane and Salter (1999) concluded that moderate reductions in total fat consumption without any change in fatty acid composition would not produce any favourable change in blood lipoprotein profiles. There are, of course, several other reasons for reducing our reliance on dietary fats such as improved weight control, better glucose tolerance and perhaps reduced susceptibility to some cancers (see Chapter 4). Better weight control and improved glucose tolerance would be expected to reduce risk of heart disease independently of any effects on plasma lipoprotein profiles.

The saturates

These generally raise the LDL-cholesterol concentration and so they have been and continue to be viewed very negatively by health educators. Saturated fats also cause a small compensatory rise in HDL-cholesterol but this is considerably outweighed by the effect on the LDL fraction. It does now seem that saturated fatty acids vary in their effects on plasma cholesterol. Palmitic acid (16:0) is by far the most common saturated fatty acid in the diet and, together with myristic acid (14:0), the most potent at raising LDL-cholesterol. Shorter chain, saturated fatty acids of 12 carbons or less (e.g. found in high amounts in coconut oil) have a smaller cholesterol raising effect. Stearic acid (18:0) is not atherogenic and may be closer to the monounsaturated fatty acid (oleic acid $18:1_{\omega-9}$) in its effects on plasma cholesterol levels (Yu *et al.*,1995). Stearic acid is found in large amounts in cocoa butter, which has been found to cause less increase in plasma cholesterol than other saturated fats. In general, if saturated fatty acids in the diet are replaced with either unsaturated fatty acids or with carbohydrate then this leads to a reduction in LDL-cholesterol concentration in plasma.

The monounsaturates

As a result of the early experiments of Keys *et al.* (1959) and other early workers, monounsaturates were regarded as neutral in their effects on plasma cholesterol concentration. More recent work suggests that when they replace saturated fatty acids, they have almost as great a lowering effect on the LDL fraction as polyunsaturated fats and are neutral in their effects on the HDL fraction (e.g. Mattson and Grundy, 1985; Yu *et al.*, 1995). At very high intakes they may actually increase HDL concentrations. Some Mediterranean men consume high-fat diets (40 per cent of energy from fat) and yet have very low incidence of CHD. Such Mediterranean diets are rich in olive oil and monounsaturated oleic acid. These monounsaturated fats are very much 'in fashion' at present, accounting for the current positive image of olive oil and, in the USA, of canola (rapeseed) oil.

The polyunsaturates

Polyunsaturated fatty acids of the ω-6 or n-6 series (the bulk of those in most vegetable oils) are still thought to lower the plasma LDL-cholesterol concentration – a beneficial effect. However, some studies have suggested that they may also lower HDL-cholesterol – a potentially harmful effect (Grundy, 1987). Such studies have been widely reported and helped to increase concern about the overall benefits of diets very high in polyunsaturated fat. Results from some of the early intervention trials using diets very high in polyunsaturated fats also suggested that very high intakes of these acids might have other detrimental effects including an increased cancer risk. Often such studies reported a non-significant decrease in cardiovascular mortality and a non-significant increase in mortality from other causes including cancer (see Oliver, 1981). Their high susceptibility to oxidation (see Chapter 12) is one possible mechanism by which high intakes might produce detrimental effects (COMA, 1991). Populations that consume high-fat diets and have a high proportion of their fat as ω-6 polyunsaturated acids have been historically rare because widespread use of large amounts of most extracted vegetable oils is a relatively recent phenomenon. Diets that are high in olive oil, palm oil or coconut oil have long been used but none of these contains high levels of ω-6 polyunsaturated fatty acids.

Safety concerns, together with this lack of historical precedent, have led many expert committees (e.g. COMA, 1991) to recommend that it would be prudent not to further raise current average intakes of polyunsaturated fatty acids in the UK and USA. It has also been recommended that individual consumption of polyunsaturated fatty acids should be limited to no more than 10 per cent of total energy. There is little hard evidence of deleterious effects of high polyunsaturated fat intake but nonetheless it would be fair to say that during the early 1990s some health educators viewed them less positively than they did in the 1960s and 1970s. More recent evidence suggests that polyunsaturated fatty acids are probably neutral in their effect on HDL and that any lowering effect on HDL only occurs at high intakes that are unlikely to be consumed in normal diets (Mangiapane and Salter, 1999).

The ω-3 series of acids are found in large amounts in marine oils and in variable amounts in different vegetable oils. For example:

- 11.4 per cent of total fatty acids in walnut oil
- 7 per cent in soya oil
- 10 per cent in rapeseed oil
- 0.29 per cent in sunflower seed oil.

ω-3 Fatty acids lower blood triacylglycerol concentrations and are generally thought to raise the HDL-cholesterol. They are also thought to have other apparently beneficial effects such as reducing inflammation and the tendency of blood to clot and therefore reducing the risk of thrombosis. They are very much 'in fashion' at present. Fish oils, the richest dietary source of the long-chain members of this series, are discussed more fully at the end of this chapter. According to Harris (1989) the overall effect of fish oil on LDL-cholesterol is minimal at practical levels of consumption.

Trans fatty acids

Diets containing only naturally occurring fatty acids would normally be low in *trans* fatty acids but certain types of margarine and vegetable shortening may contain quite large amounts of *trans* fatty acids, particularly the cheaper, hard margarines that have been phased out. *Trans* fatty acids are also generated when vegetable oils are heated, so frying adds some *trans* fatty acids to foods especially if the oil is re-heated several times. There has naturally been concern about whether there are any health implications in consuming relatively large amounts of these *trans* fatty acids because of their low levels in unprocessed foods. In particular, it has been suggested that they may have similar unfavourable effects on blood lipoproteins to saturated fatty acids.

The precise health implications of consuming large amounts of *trans* fatty acids is still unclear but they are generally classified as equivalent to saturated fatty acids in their effects on blood lipids. In short-term experiments, using both men and women, Mensink and Katan (1990) compared the effects of diets that were matched except for their *trans* fatty acid content. They concluded that *trans* fatty acids are at least as unfavourable as saturated fatty acids in their effects on blood lipids, tending not only to raise the LDL levels but also to lower HDL levels. Willett *et al.* (1993) in a large cohort study of American nurses reported a highly significant positive association between risk of coronary heart disease and dietary intake of *trans* fatty acids. These results achieved widespread publicity and led some margarine manufacturers to change their production methods and produce products that were free of *trans* fatty acids. Other workers have disputed the notion that high consumption of *trans* fatty acids is a major determinant of current risk of coronary heart disease. In 1989 average intakes of *trans* fatty acids in the UK were estimated at around 5 g/day (2 per cent of calories) but with very wide variation; some individuals consuming as much as five times this average value (COMA, 1991). COMA (1991) recommended that levels should not rise, and, as discussed and as quantified earlier in the chapter (see Table 11.3), they have been declining in recent years as consumption of hard margarine has declined, having been replaced by soft margarine containing much less and in some cases practically no *trans* fatty acids.

Dietary cholesterol

In short term experiments, dietary cholesterol does tend to raise the LDL-cholesterol level but, at usual intakes, this effect is small compared with the effects caused by altering the proportions of the various fatty acid fractions in the diet. Some animals such as rabbits are particularly susceptible to the hypercholesteraemic effects of dietary cholesterol. In these animals, dietary cholesterol suppresses LDL receptor production in liver cells and this reduces LDL clearance. Usual intakes of cholesterol are relatively small when compared with the normal rate of endogenous synthesis (around 10–20 per cent). Keys *et al.* (1965) calculated that a change in cholesterol intake from the top to the bottom of the range in 1960s American diets (i.e. from 1050 mg/day to 450 mg/day) would lower plasma cholesterol by only around 0.23 mmol/L. They concluded that dietary cholesterol should not be ignored in cholesterol lowering but that changing it alone would achieve very little.

Dietary cholesterol is usually given low priority in most sets of nutrition education guidelines (see Chapter 4). Note, however, that lowering saturated fat intake will probably result in some consequential fall in cholesterol intake because cholesterol is found only in animal products. Cholesterol intakes in the UK have fallen in line with the fall in fat and saturated fatty acid consumption (see Table 11.3). Some individuals are genetically susceptible to the hypercholesteraemic effects of dietary cholesterol and control of dietary cholesterol is more significant for such individuals (Brown and Goldstein, 1984). Note that eggs are the single most important source of cholesterol in most Western diets. Average daily cholesterol intake will be greatly affected by changes in egg consumption and those who are particularly sensitive to dietary cholesterol are advised to restrict their egg consumption.

Forty years ago dietary cholesterol was widely believed to be of predominant importance in the genesis of high blood cholesterol and atherosclerosis (e.g. Frantz and Moore, 1969). The contribution of experiments with herbivorous rabbits to this belief was critically discussed in Chapter 3. Since the 1960s, the evidence linking high plasma cholesterol levels with increased risk of atherosclerosis has strengthened but the view of dietary cholesterol as the major influence on plasma cholesterol concentration has faded.

Much of the apparent atherogenic effect of cholesterol seen in some rabbit experiments may have been due to the presence of highly atherogenic cholesterol oxides in the cholesterol used in these studies. Some old bottles of chemical cholesterol contain very large amounts of oxidized cholesterol. Oxidized cholesterol is many times more toxic to vascular endothelial cells than purified cholesterol. In fresh foods, cholesterol oxides concentrations are low but such oxides would be generated if these foods were subjected to prolonged heating and/or exposure to air, e.g. powdered egg, powdered whole milk and some cheeses. Jacobsen (1987) reported that *ghee* (clarified butter used in Indian cooking) has high levels of cholesterol oxides whereas fresh butter does not. Damage induced by oxidation of lipids in LDL is now considered to be an important factor in the aetiology of heart disease and oxidative damage has been implicated in the aetiology of cancer and other chronic diseases (see Chapter 12).

Plant sterols

Plants do not produce cholesterol but they do produce other sterols such as stigmasterol, ergosterol and β-sitosterol. It has been known for decades that these plant sterols although poorly absorbed in the gut do tend to inhibit the absorption of cholesterol. β-Sitosterol and other plant sterols were identified as possible cholesterol-lowering agents more than 30 years ago but their practical effect was small. More recently, β-**sitostanol**, a substance produced chemically from β-sitosterol has been reported to be a more effective cholesterol-lowering agent than other plant sterols. In a 1-year double blind trial, intake of 1.8–2.6 g/day of β-sitostanol ester incorporated into margarine was reported to reduce average cholesterol concentrations by 10 per cent in mildly hypercholesteraemic men (Miettinen *et al.*, 1995). The effectiveness of sitostanol is probably greater in those with higher dietary cholesterol intakes even though it may also have some effect on the reabsorption of biliary cholesterol. Several margarines and other dairy-type foods containing sitostanol-esters are now available in the UK and are marketed as functional foods that may help lower blood cholesterol (this is discussed further in Chapter 18).

Key points

- It has been known since 1960 that replacing dietary saturated fat with unsaturated fat lowers the total plasma cholesterol concentration.

- It is desirable to lower the plasma LDL-cholesterol and to raise the HDL-cholesterol.

- A moderate reduction in total fat intake does not produce significant improvement in blood lipoprotein profiles although it may be desirable on other grounds.

- Saturated fats and *trans* fatty acids raise the LDL-cholesterol concentration.

- Of the saturates, myristic acid (14:0) and palmitic acid (16:0) have the biggest cholesterol-raising effect, shorter chain acids (e.g. from coconut oil) have a smaller effect and stearic acid (18:0), found in cocoa butter, has no LDL raising effect.

- Monounsaturates are now thought to lower LDL-cholesterol when they replace saturated fat and to have a neutral effect on HDL. At very high intakes they may even raise the HDL.

- ω-6 polyunsaturates lower plasma LDL and are probably neutral in their effects on HDL although at very high intakes they may lower HDL.

- Some speculative safety concerns coupled with a lack of historical precedent of populations with very high intakes of ω-6 polyunsaturates has persuaded several expert committees to recommend that intakes of these fatty acids should not rise any further and they should not make up more than 10 per cent of food energy in any individual.

- The ω-3 series of polyunsaturated fatty acids lower blood triacylglycerol concentrations and raise HDL levels. At practical levels of consumption, they have little effect on LDL levels.

- Dietary cholesterol is now thought to be a relatively minor influence upon plasma cholesterol and lipoprotein profiles.

- Rabbits are very sensitive to the hypercholesteraemic effects of dietary cholesterol and some people may also be more sensitive to it.

- A reduction in saturated fat consumption will probably produce a consequent fall in cholesterol intake although eggs are the biggest single source of cholesterol in most diets.

- Oxidized cholesterol is much more atherogenic than cholesterol *per se* and would be present in increased amounts in foods subject to prolonged heating in air, e.g. powdered egg and whole milk, some cheeses and *ghee* (the clarified butter used in Indian cooking).

● Plant sterols inhibit the absorption of cholesterol from the gut and sitostanol-ester, a derivative of sitosterol may have a useful cholesterol-lowering effect when incorporated into margarine and other foods.

THE KEY TENETS OF THE DIET–HEART HYPOTHESIS

The diet–heart hypothesis (see Figure 11.6) can be broken up into two key tenets.

* *High total plasma cholesterol concentration causes an increased risk of coronary heart disease.* When the individual lipoprotein fractions in blood are considered then high LDL-cholesterol increases atherosclerosis and the risk of coronary heart disease, whereas HDL is thought to be protective against atherosclerosis. High VLDL is associated with increased CHD risk but it is difficult to say whether this is a direct harmful effect of high VLDL or a result of the link between high VLDL and obesity and diabetes, both of which are strong risk factors for CHD.
* *The amount and type of dietary fat is an important determinant of the plasma cholesterol concentration.* Current views on the effects of the various dietary fatty acids on blood lipoproteins were summarized earlier in the chapter.

There is substantial – many would say overwhelming – evidence in favour of both of these propositions. However there are several apparent weak links in the chain of evidence supporting the diet–heart hypothesis and the dietary guidelines that have evolved from it, e.g.:

* some populations appear to deviate from the usual trend of increasing saturated fat consumption associated with increasing average plasma cholesterol concentrations and increasing mortality from CHD
* there is a lack of correlation between plasma cholesterol concentration and the level of saturated fat in the diet when they are measured in individuals from within a population.
* many large-scale cholesterol-lowering intervention trials have failed to produce any measurable reduction in overall mortality in the test group.

In the next section, the evidence that underpins the diet–heart hypothesis is briefly discussed and explanations offered for these apparent anomalies.

Key points

According to the diet–heart hypothesis:

● An elevated plasma cholesterol concentration causes increased risk of atherosclerosis and coronary heart disease. The LDL fraction of plasma cholesterol is atherogenic whereas the HDL fraction is anti-atherogenic.

● The composition of dietary fats is a key determinant of total plasma cholesterol concentration and its distribution between the different lipoprotein fractions in plasma.

REVIEW OF THE EVIDENCE FOR THE DIET–HEART HYPOTHESIS

Descriptive epidemiology

Cross-cultural comparisons reveal a general tendency for plasma cholesterol concentration and CHD mortality to rise with increasing saturated fat and cholesterol consumption (e.g. Artaud-Wild *et al.*, 1993). In general, cross-cultural studies tend to support the diet–heart hypothesis but there are many exceptions to these general trends such as those listed below.

* The Masai of east Africa eat a diet based on milk, meat and blood which is high in saturated fat and cholesterol. Yet they are free of advanced atherosclerosis and their rates of coronary heart disease are very low. The traditional Masai are a fit and lean population and this could explain their protection from the effects of their apparently atherogenic diet. It has also been suggested that the presence of large amounts of fermented milk (yoghurt) may be significant (McGill (1979) contains a referenced summary of early studies on the Masai). Some fermented milk products are now marketed as **functional foods** (see Chapter 18).
* Some studies have reported that farmers have lower levels of CHD than non-farmers living in the same locality despite having similar fat intakes and higher plasma cholesterol concentrations. These studies also find farmers to be more

active, fitter and smoke and drink less than non-farmers (e.g. Pomrehn *et al.*, 1982).

- Recorded rates of coronary heart disease in France are low in comparison to other European countries with similar plasma cholesterol levels and despite saturated fat intake being relatively high in France. This is known as the 'French paradox'. One popular explanation is that high intakes of antioxidants in red wine might prevent oxidation of lipid infiltrates into artery walls and thus reduce the development of atherosclerotic lesions (Renaud and de Lorgeril, 1992). Low intakes of vegetables, which are more mundane sources of antioxidants, are also found in some of the countries that have unexpectedly high rates of CHD (Artaud-Wild *et al.*, 1993). It is also possible that this paradox is a measurement artefact caused by under-recording of CHD mortality in France.
- McKeigue *et al.* (1985) noted high rates of coronary heart disease among British Asians despite their having lower saturated fat and cholesterol intakes and lower blood cholesterol concentrations than the white population – these observations have since been confirmed several times. British Asians also have much higher prevalence of abdominal obesity, insulin resistance and **type 2 diabetes** than white Britons and this probably explains their high rates of CHD.

Dietary saturated fat intake is clearly only one of several factors that affect plasma cholesterol concentration, and plasma cholesterol is only one factor that governs the progression of atherosclerosis and the risk of coronary heart disease. Morris *et al.* (1980) illustrate this point. In an 8-year cohort study of male British civil servants, they found very low levels of fatal first coronaries in men who did not smoke and who participated in vigorous leisure-time activity. The rates were more than six times higher in cigarette smokers who did not participate in vigorous leisure-time activity. This study took no account of diet or plasma cholesterol and the data were collected before the current nutrition education campaigns aimed at lowering dietary fat intakes had gained much momentum in the UK.

Many factors that are not part of the diet–heart hypothesis in Figure 11.6 can influence plasma cholesterol concentration, the development of atherosclerotic lesions and the risk of CHD. These factors could obscure the relationship between dietary fats, plasma cholesterol and CHD risk. Some of these factors have been mentioned earlier and selected examples are listed below.

- Plasma total cholesterol is a crude indicator of CHD risk. It is the relative amounts of LDL (causative) and HDL (protective) that are important.
- Being overweight or obese increases the risk of CHD, particularly if much of the excess fat is stored in the abdominal cavity. It is also associated with increased plasma cholesterol levels.
- Insulin resistance and type 2 diabetes (both linked to abdominal obesity) also increase the risk of CHD.
- High levels of physical activity and fitness protect against CHD, perhaps partly mediated by a rise in HDL concentration.
- High blood pressure accelerates atherosclerosis and increases the risk of CHD. The effect of high blood pressure on atherosclerosis is independent of plasma cholesterol level.
- Some substances increase the oxidative damage to LDL in artery walls and so accelerate the process of atherosclerosis, e.g. some constituents of cigarette smoke. According to Steinberg *et al.* (1989) high levels of LDL only produce atherosclerosis if they are oxidized; this oxidation leads to infiltration and activation of macrophages in the artery wall. Some substance act as antioxidants and may inhibit the oxidation of LDL in arteries and so inhibit the process of atherosclerosis, e.g. **carotenoids** found in coloured fruits and vegetables and flavonoids in red wine (see Chapter 12).
- Soluble fibre (non-starch polysaccharide) may have a plasma cholesterol-lowering effect.
- Moderate intakes of alcohol may afford some protection against CHD, perhaps partly mediated by a rise in plasma HDL.
- Long-chain ω-3 polyunsaturated fatty acids may afford some protection against CHD.

From a health promotion viewpoint, undue emphasis placed on the P:S ratio of dietary fats and plasma cholesterol may deflect attention away from other, perhaps even more beneficial, changes in lifestyle. How significant is a moderately high-saturated-fat diet or perhaps even moderately elevated plasma cholesterol concentration in lean, active, non-smoking, moderate-drinking men who eat good amounts of fruit and vegetables? This question may be even more pertinent for women. How significant are reductions in saturated fat intakes for men who remain overweight, inactive, eat little fruit or vegetables and who smoke and drink heavily? Replacing butter with margarine or frying in oil rather than lard are relatively painless changes that may offer reassurance or salve the conscience but are unlikely to compensate for failure to alter any of these other risk factors. Some other descriptive epidemiological evidence that has been used to support the diet–heart hypothesis is:

- migrants and their descendants who move to areas where saturated fat intake is higher than in their country of origin have increased rates of CHD, e.g. Japanese migrants to the USA and British Asians
- white vegetarians and Seventh Day Adventists in the USA and UK have lower rates of CHD than the whole population; they also tend to have lower intakes of saturated fat
- marked changes in a population's consumption of saturated fat are often associated with corresponding changes in CHD incidence. In Britain, wartime rationing led to decreased saturated fat consumption and decreased rates of CHD. In Japan, marked increases in milk and meat consumption since the 1950s have been associated with marked increases in the prevalence of CHD (note also that Japanese life expectancy has also increased markedly since the 1950s).

In addition, the observation that atherosclerotic lesions of both animals and humans contain high concentrations of cholesterol adds weight to the belief that high plasma cholesterol helps to precipitate atherosclerosis.

Experimental studies

Numerous short-term experimental studies have shown that plasma cholesterol concentration, primarily the LDL fraction, is alterable by manipulating intake of dietary lipids (e.g. Keys *et al.*, 1959; Mattson and Grundy, 1985; Mensink and Katan, 1990; Yu *et al.*, 1995). Mangiapane and Salter (1999) give a concise referenced review of studies between 1959 and 1999 that have investigated the relationship between dietary fats and plasma lipoproteins. There is general agreement that increased intake of saturated fat tends to increase the plasma cholesterol whereas replacement of saturated with polyunsaturated fat tends to lower the cholesterol concentration. The probable effects of dietary cholesterol, monounsaturated fatty acids and *trans* fatty acids were discussed earlier in the chapter. Susceptibility to dietary manipulation of plasma cholesterol concentration varies between individuals and there is a general trend for those with the higher baseline levels to be more responsive to dietary change (Keys *et al.*, 1959). Despite the absence of any demonstrable effect on total mortality, most of the early cholesterol-lowering, dietary intervention studies did nonetheless produce significant reductions in plasma cholesterol in the test group (Oliver, 1981). However, according to Oliver (1981), plasma cholesterol was usually reduced by less than 10 per cent in free-living subjects despite some very major dietary modification and even drug use in many of these early studies.

'Experiments of nature'

People with several inherited hyperlipidaemias have a high propensity to premature CHD (see Mangiapane and Salter, 1999 for a useful summary). In **familial hypercholesteraemia** (Fredrickson type IIa) the primary genetic defect is in the LDL receptor gene. This genetic defect leads to reduce levels of functional LDL receptors and a marked rise in plasma LDL-cholesterol concentration. This condition is associated with marked atherosclerosis and greatly increased risk of premature CHD. This provides persuasive evidence of a direct causal link between high plasma LDL, atherosclerosis and CHD.

Cohort studies

Cohort studies whether within or between population generally indicate that, at least for young and middle-aged men, high serum cholesterol concentration is predictive of subsequent risk of death from coronary heart disease over the succeeding 5–20 years. In the Framingham study (Massachusetts, USA) there was a clear progressive increase in CHD mortality in all age groups of men with increasing plasma cholesterol level (see Figure 1.2, p. 20 and see Chapter 3 for a summary of the Framingham study).

The famous Seven Countries cross-cultural cohort study found a high correlation between dietary saturated fat intake and both plasma cholesterol concentration and incidence of coronary heart disease (summarized in Oliver, 1981).

In general, the relation between total plasma cholesterol and CHD is most convincing in middle-aged men and is much weaker in pre-menopausal women (e.g. Crouse, 1989) and elderly men (Shipley et al., 1991). This has caused some writers to question whether universal cholesterol-lowering was justified, particularly for women (e.g. in influential editorials in The Lancet and Circulation – see Hulley et al., 1992; Dunnigan, 1993). The lack of demonstrated holistic benefit in most cholesterol-lowering intervention trials prior to this time was an important reason why these authors recommended such caution. As will be seen below, some more recent intervention trials have provided much stronger evidence that lowering LDL-cholesterol can bring substantial net benefits. There are now good theoretical reasons to expect that total plasma cholesterol will be a relatively crude indicator of CHD risk. Measurement of individual lipoprotein fraction in blood should give a more sensitive indication of CHD risk. In the Framingham study, total plasma cholesterol was only a weak indicator of CHD risk in pre-menopausal women and older men but there was a very strong negative association (i.e. protective effect) between HDL concentration and CHD risk in these groups.

One of the gaps in the chain of evidence supporting the diet–heart hypothesis has been the failure to find any significant association between measures of dietary fat or saturated fat intake and plasma cholesterol concentration in most within-population studies. Oliver (1981) uses data from the Tecumseh study to illustrate this general finding; dietary intakes of fat, saturated fat, cholesterol and dietary P:S ratio were not significantly different when those in the highest, middle and lowest **tertiles** (thirds) for serum cholesterol concentrations were compared. In The Dietary and Nutritional Survey of British Adults, Gregory et al. (1990) found no significant correlation between any measures of dietary fat and serum LDL-cholesterol concentration in men except for a very weak (r = 0.08) one with dietary cholesterol; all correlation coefficients were less than 0.1. In women they found a weak but significant correlation with per cent of energy from

saturated fat and serum LDL-cholesterol concentration but only 2 per cent (r^2) of the difference in women's serum cholesterol could be explained by variation in their per cent of dietary energy from saturated fat.

Dietary differences in individual fat consumption do not appear to be an important factor in determining the position of any individual within the population distribution of plasma cholesterol concentrations. As already stated in Chapter 3, this may be because a host of other factors affect an individual's serum cholesterol concentration, e.g.:

- genetic variability in plasma cholesterol concentration, including variation in genetic susceptibility to dietary fats
- other dietary influences on plasma cholesterol
- other lifestyle influences on plasma cholesterol, such as exercise, age, smoking, alcohol, body mass index.

This lack of significant association is thus not incompatible with the proposal that dietary fat composition is a major determinant of a population's average plasma cholesterol concentration. It is still expected that widespread use of a diet with a higher P:S ratio and less cholesterol will lower the plasma cholesterol concentrations of adherents and lead to a downward shift in the distribution for plasma cholesterol of the population and thus to a reduction in average plasma cholesterol concentration. This general concept was discussed more fully in Chapter 3, using data in Figure 3.10 (p. 116) to illustrate it.

Intervention trials and clinical trials

Numerous trials of a variety of cholesterol-lowering interventions were carried out between 1960 and 1990. None of these produced a significant reduction in total mortality in the test group. Many did not even produced significant reductions in cardiovascular mortality although most succeeded in reducing plasma cholesterol to some extent. Some reported a non-significant fall in cardiovascular mortality that was offset by a non-significant rise in mortality from 'other causes'. In several of these early trials, the overall incidence of CHD was reduced largely as a result of a fall in the number of non-fatal myocardial infarctions (Oliver, 1981, 1991; McCormick and Skrabanek, 1988). Some early intervention trials that involved the use of cholesterol-lowering drugs actually reported increased mortality in the test group. One of the most spectacular of these 'failed' intervention trials was the Multiple Risk Factor Intervention Trial (MRFIT, 1982) which was discussed in Chapter 3.

Smith *et al.* (1993) conducted a combined (meta) analysis of 35 randomized controlled trials of cholesterol-lowering interventions published prior to 1993. They concluded that net benefit (i.e. reduced total mortality) from cholesterol-lowering intervention was confined to those at very high risk of coronary heart disease. Only those at greater risk than even asymptomatic patients under 65 years with hypercholesteraemia were reported to derive demonstrable net benefit from cholesterol-lowering interventions that had been used prior to 1993. Cholesterol-lowering drugs were used in more than two-thirds of the trials surveyed by these authors. They concluded that these drugs should be reserved for the small proportion of people at very high risk of death from CHD, perhaps only those with both existing coronary heart disease and hypercholesteraemia.

The apparent failure of these early intervention trials was explained by suggesting that the sample sizes in these trials were too small to get statistically significant reductions in overall mortality. Dunnigan (1993) estimated that a trial including 80 000 people over a 5-year period would be necessary to show whether there was any beneficial effect of cholesterol lowering on all-cause mortality even in patients with asymptomatic hypercholesteraemia under the age of 65 years. This is, of course, another way of saying that, at least within the time scale of an intervention trial, the difference in risk of dying is only minutely affected by being in the intervention or control group. As a result of such findings many scientists questioned the benefits of interventions and health promotion campaigns that were aimed at lowering average plasma cholesterol concentrations (e.g. Oliver, 1981, 1991; McCormick and Skrabanek, 1988).

Some more recent intervention trials using a new type of cholesterol-lowering drugs called **statins** has given strong evidence that lowering plasma cholesterol can have net beneficial effects both in patients with existing heart disease and those with asymptomatic hypercholesteraemia. These drugs inhibit the key enzyme in cholesterol biosynthesis (HMG CoA reductase) and produce a substantial and sustained reduction in LDL-cholesterol with few side effects.

In a 5-year study of over 4000 Scandinavians with existing CHD, the drug simvastatin reduced plasma LDL-cholesterol by 35 per cent and reduced total mortality by 30 per cent as a result of reduced cardiovascular mortality (SSSS Group, 1994). In a study of 6500 Scottish men with asymptomatic hypercholesteraemia, the drug pravastatin reduced LDL-cholesterol by 26 per cent, heart attacks by a third and total mortality by 22 per cent (Shepherd *et al.*, 1995). These latter authors estimated that treating 1000 healthy but hypercholesteraemic middle-aged men with pravastatin for 5 years would result in 20 fewer non-fatal myocardial infarctions and nine fewer deaths as well as less heart surgery and fewer investigative procedures. These two studies involve the use of drugs but nevertheless they do support the belief that dietary measures that lower average population plasma cholesterol concentration over the whole lifespan will shift the age distribution of deaths and disability from coronary heart disease upwards and lead to increased healthy life expectancy.

In more recent years it has become clear that lowering the plasma LDL-cholesterol concentration by the use of statin drugs lowers the risk of cardiovascular disease across the whole range of LDL levels found in industrialized countries and almost irrespective of the initial cholesterol concentration. This has led to the belief that cholesterol-lowering by statins is beneficial for anyone at increased risk of CHD or stroke irrespective of whether or not they have an elevated LDL-cholesterol concentration, e.g. if they have diabetes or hypertension. Group (2002) found that adding 40 mg of simvastatin to the existing treatments of high-risk patients with coronary disease, other occlusive arterial disease or diabetes reduced rates of strokes and heart attacks by around a third in those fully complying with the medication regimen. The size of the benefit depended on a patient's initial overall risk rather than their initial cholesterol level. Similarly, Sever *et al.* (2003) found that 10 mg/day of atorvastatin reduced rates of strokes and CHD in hypertensive patients who had total plasma cholesterol levels lower than 6.5 mmol/L.

These observations on the wide benefits of cholesterol lowering even to those without serious plasma cholesterol elevation together with low recorded levels of serious side-effects from these statins resulted in a decision in 2004 by the UK authorities to make low doses of simvastatin (10 mg) available without prescription in the UK. The possible side effects of statins are headaches, insomnia and digestive problems such as abdominal pain, wind and diarrhoea. Less commonly they can cause liver problems and so need to be used with caution in those with a history of liver disease or perhaps by heavy drinkers. They may rarely cause a serious myopathy (muscle wasting) and so any unexplained muscular pain or weakness needs to be reported to the doctor and investigated.

Key points

- The evidence supporting the diet–heart hypothesis is both impressive and varied.

- Populations with high saturated fat and cholesterol intakes tend to have higher plasma cholesterol concentrations and higher death rates from coronary heart disease (CHD) than those with low saturated fat intakes.

- Some vegetarian groups in the UK and USA with low intakes of saturated fat and cholesterol have lower rates of CHD than the rest of the population.

- Marked changes in a population's consumption of saturated fat have been accompanied by changes in CHD rates that are consistent with the diet–heart hypothesis.

- People who migrate from regions of low saturated fat consumption to regions of high consumption tend also to show increased rates of CHD.

- Experimental or therapeutic manipulations of dietary fat composition produce changes in plasma lipoprotein profiles that are consistent with the diet–heart hypothesis.

- People with genetic disorders that raise their plasma low-density lipoprotein (LDL)-cholesterol are at greatly increased risk of CHD.

- In cohort studies using single or several populations, a high plasma cholesterol concentration is associated with increased risk of CHD.

- Many cholesterol-lowering trials using drugs or diet have resulted in significant reductions in the combined number of fatal and non-fatal coronary events.

- Recent intervention trials using the statin drugs, which have a very potent cholesterol-lowering effect, have produced significant reductions in both deaths from CHD and total mortality.

- These statin trials suggest that population wide reductions in plasma cholesterol concentration over the whole lifespan would increase healthy life expectancy.

- Lowering cholesterol with statins has beneficial effects across the whole range of LDL-cholesterol concentrations normally found in industrialized countries almost irrespective of the initial cholesterol level.

- Statins reduce heart attack and stroke risk in high-risk patients such as people with diabetes and hypertension even where they do not have initial raised cholesterol levels.

- The wide benefits and infrequent incidence of serious side effects led to a low-dose statin being made available in the UK without prescription.

- A few anomalous observations are superficially inconsistent with the diet–heart hypothesis:
  - within populations there is little correlation between plasma cholesterol and saturated fat intakes
  - some populations with high saturated fat intakes or high plasma cholesterol concentrations seem to have lower rates of CHD than might be anticipated
  - until 1994, cholesterol-lowering intervention trials with diet and/or drugs failed to produce significant reductions in total mortality.

- There are plausible explanations for each of these anomalies:
  - many factors influence plasma cholesterol and any individual's saturated fat intake is only a minor determinant of where they lie in the population distribution of plasma cholesterol concentrations
  - high levels of fitness and activity, high intakes of antioxidants or consumption of fermented milk products are some of the factors that have been suggested might protect some populations from CHD.

- Clinical trials with statins have lowered both plasma cholesterol and total mortality and they work even in those without serious initial elevation of cholesterol levels.

FISH OILS

A series of papers published in the 1970s by Bang, Dyerberg and their colleagues reported that the Greenland Inuit had lower rates of CHD and lower rates of inflammatory joint disease than the Danes. The Inuit ate a traditional diet high in seal meat, whale meat and fish (e.g. Dyerberg and Bang, 1979). This low rate of CHD was despite a diet with similar total fat content to the Danes and despite the fact that most of the fat came from the animal kingdom. The lipid of the Inuit diet differs from the Danish diet in two major respects: first it is much lower in saturated fatty acids and second it has higher levels of ω-3 polyunsaturated fatty acids (reviewed by Kromhout, 1990).

Fish oils and other marine oils (e.g. from seals and whales) contain large amounts of long-chain ω-3 polyunsaturated fatty acids. The three longest chain members of this series, EPA ($20:5_{\omega-3}$), docosapentaenoic acid (DPA; $22:5_{\omega-3}$) and docosahexaenoic acid (DHA; $22:6_{\omega-3}$) account for around 20 per cent of the fatty acids in many oils from marine fish. As noted earlier in the chapter, the ω-3 fatty acids, because of their extra double bond, have a lower melting point and have greater fluidity at low environmental temperatures than the corresponding ω-6 fatty acid – this may explain their prominence in the fat of coldwater mammals and fish. These acids enter the marine food chain via their synthesis by marine plants and plankton, which then serve as food for higher marine organisms. These long-chain ω-3 polyunsaturates are widely believed to be the active agents that reduce risk of CHD and inflammatory joint diseases.

The reports on the health and mortality of the Inuit served to focus scientific attention on the protective and therapeutic potential of fish oils and the ω-3 polyunsaturates. The increased scientific interest in fish oils may be gauged by the output of research papers on fish oils; less than 10 per year in the 1970s but rising sharply during the 1980s to a level of several hundred per year in the early 1990s (see Simopoulos, 1991). Fish oils can be made available on prescription in the UK for the treatment of certain hyperlipidaemias and for patients with a history of CHD. The public perception of fish oils as health promoting is illustrated by the massive amount of shelf space occupied by fish oil products in health food shops, pharmacies and even supermarkets. In 2001, fish oils accounted for over a quarter of the UK market for natural food supplements.

Fish oil or fish liver oil

Fish liver oil, usually cod liver oil, has traditionally been taken as a good source of vitamins A and D; it is still widely used for this purpose and given the high prevalence of vitamin D inadequacy in most age groups in Britain there may well be a case for its wider use (see Chapters 12 and 13). A 10 mL dose of cod liver oil contains up to 1.5 times the reference nutrient intake (RNI) for vitamin A and up to 10 μg of vitamin D (the RNI for adults not regularly exposed to sunlight). Halibut and shark liver oil have even higher concentrations of these vitamins. Cod liver oil was traditionally taken in liquid form but because of the unpleasant taste many fish oil products are now taken as oil-filled capsules. Vitamins A and D are the most toxic of the vitamins when consumed in excess and so the recommended dose of fish liver oil should not be exceeded and they should not be taken by pregnant women because of the teratogenic effects of vitamin A.

The high concentrations of vitamins A and D in fish liver oil are now sometimes paradoxically seen as a handicap because they reduce the dose of the long-chain ω-3 fatty acids that they can safely provide. Fish body oil can be safely taken in much higher doses than fish liver oil and the US Food and Drug Administration (FDA) suggests that doses equivalent to 10–20 capsules per day should be generally regarded as safe although they may exacerbate clotting disorders or enhance the effect of anticoagulant drugs. A single capsule of fish (liver) oil should contain at least 100 mg of EPA and DHA and may contain up to 400 mg (the exact dose of any preparation should be shown on the label). This means that one capsule per day should provide between 1 g and 3 g of EPA/DHA per week. This compares with:

- 25 mg in a 100 g serving of cod
- 1.9 g in 100 g of mackerel
- 1.3 g in 100 g of herring
- 1.7 g in 100 g of sardines canned in tomato sauce
- 1.5–3 g in a 10 mL dose of cod liver oil.

COMA (1994a) recommended that average population intakes of long-chain ω-3 polyunsaturates should rise from 100 mg/day (0.7 g/week) to 200 mg/day (1.4 g/week). To achieve this aim COMA recommended that people should eat two portions of fish per week, one of which should be oily fish. People taking one capsule of fish oil each day should achieve this target dose of ω-3 polyunsaturates.

Possible protective mechanisms

There are a number of mechanisms by which long-chain ω-3 fatty acids have been suggested to reduce the risk of CHD and inflammatory joint diseases and some of these are discussed below.

Effects on the production of eicosanoids

Taking large doses of long-chain ω-3 fatty acids, especially large doses of EPA, leads to an increase in the production of eicosanoids from EPA and their partial replacement of those produced from arachidonic acid. Looking back at Figure 11.3 (p. 277) this means a decrease in production of the following eicosanoids produced from arachidonic acid:

- LTB_4 – a leukotriene that promotes inflammation
- TXA_2 – a thromboxane that promotes platelet aggregation
- PGI_2 – a prostaglandin with anti-aggregating effects on platelets.

These would be partly replaced by eicosanoids produced from EPA:

- LTB_5 – a leukotriene with low activity
- TXA_3 – a thromboxane with low activity
- PGI_3 – a prostaglandin with anti-aggregating effects on platelets.

The overall effect of these changes (see Figure 11.7) is predicted to reduce the risk of thromboses forming in blood vessels. This will reduce the risk of occlusive strokes (due to blockage of cerebral vessels with a clot) and myocardial infarction (heart attacks due to clots lodging in the coronary vessels). Inuits have extended bleeding times and are prone to frequent and longlasting nosebleeds and have high stroke mortality (most likely due to increased levels of cerebral haemorrhage). In short-term human and animal experiments, high consumption of fish oils has been found to reduce the tendency of blood to clot and to extend the bleeding time (Anon, 1984; Sanders, 1985).

These changes in eicosanoid production should also lead to a dampening of the inflammatory response

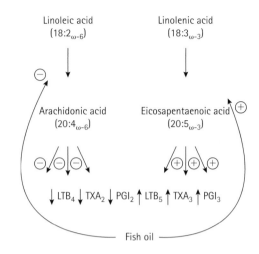

Figure 11.7 *Effects of fish oil consumption on the production of eicosanoids that affect platelet aggregation and inflammation.*

and so, for example, may reduce the damage caused by the inflammatory response after a myocardial infarction and may also explain the suggested benefits on inflammatory diseases such as arthritis and eczema. In a controlled, secondary intervention trial of fish oils in patients who had previously experienced a myocardial infarction, fish oils significantly reduced both cardiovascular and total mortality whereas the other treatments (low-fat diets or increased cereal fibre) did not (Burr *et al.*, 1989). In this trial, the patients taking fish oil did not have significantly less re-infarcts but these new infarcts were less likely to be fatal (consistent with reduced post-infarct inflammatory damage). A more recent intervention trial in Italy found reductions in both total mortality and non-fatal infarction in men receiving large supplements of ω-3 fatty acids (GISSI, 1999).

Kremer *et al.* (1985) reported that high intakes of EPA appeared to improve the clinical features of rheumatoid arthritis and the levels of LTB_4 were reduced by the treatment.

Effects on blood lipoprotein profiles

Fish oils reduce both fasting and postprandial blood triacylglycerol levels. They also raise the HDL-cholesterol concentration and the Greenland Inuit have been reported to have higher HDL levels than those living in Denmark and consuming less marine oils. At normal levels of consumption their effect on LDL-cholesterol is negligible.

Effects on plasminogen activation

Clots are broken down by plasmin, which is formed when the inactive blood protein plasminogen is activated. Experiments using fish oil supplements in patients with coronary artery disease indicate that they lead to reduced formation of a substance that inhibits the conversion of plasminogen to active plasmin. Clot-dissolving drugs such as streptokinase are often administered to patients in the immediate period after a myocardial infarction to reduce the damage done to the heart. It has been suggested that fish oils have a similar effect.

Effects upon heart rhythm

Irregular electrical activity (arrhythmia) in diseased or damaged heart muscle can have fatal consequences. There is evidence that changes in the balance of ω-3 and ω-6 fatty acids in the heart resulting from increased intakes of ω-3 fatty acids may reduce heart rate variability and arrhythmia and so reduce the risk of death following a heart attack (Buttriss, 1999).

Review of the evidence on the possible therapeutic and protective effects of fish oils

There is compelling evidence that in short-term, controlled experiments, fish oils affect the blood lipoprotein profile in ways that are currently considered to be beneficial. They also reduce the tendency of blood to clot in such trials and thus would presumably reduce the risk of thromboses forming within the circulation. There is also convincing evidence that in persons with established CHD, regular consumption of fatty fish or fish oil supplements produces overall benefits as measured by total mortality in the few years immediately after first infarction (Burr et al., 1989; GISSI, 1999). The Inuit and other populations consuming very large amounts of fish have a reduced tendency for blood to clot, prolonged bleeding times and a low incidence of CHD.

The epidemiological evidence for fatty fish consumption reducing the risk of CHD or still further, improving overall life expectancy is rather less convincing. The work on the Inuit and other populations consuming large amounts of fish has been some of the most positive of the epidemiological evidence in favour of fish oils having protective effects against the development of CHD (see Kromhout, 1990;

Buttriss, 1999). There is little evidence of an independent relation between fatty fish consumption and reduced risk of CHD in cross-population studies. Those comparisons that have been made have generally used total fish consumption as the independent variable (a crude predictor of total ω-3 fatty acid consumption) and the weak negative association with CHD mortality was dependent on the inclusion of the Japanese. In the famous Seven Countries Study there was no significant association between fish consumption and CHD mortality; some of those populations with negligible fish consumption in inland Yugoslavia had among the lowest rates of CHD whereas some of those with the highest fish consumption in Finland had among the highest rates of CHD. Fish consumption was related to subsequent mortality in a 20-year cohort study of 850 men in Zutphen, the Netherlands. In this cohort, death from CHD was inversely related to fish consumption; it was 50 per cent lower in men who ate 30 g of fatty fish per day (equivalent to about two servings per week) compared with those who ate no fish at all. Buttriss (1999) reviewed several other prospective cohort studies published prior to 1999 and concluded that most of these studies report a decrease in the risk of heart disease as fish consumption increases. She further adds that the effects of fish eating are most pronounced in populations that have low habitual fish consumption.

In general, the epidemiological evidence relating fatty fish consumption to reduced CHD risk is sporadic but this might not be unexpected even if regular consumption of long-chain ω-3 fatty acids is protective because:

* total fish consumption is a crude indicator of ω-3 fatty acid intake
* the relation between saturated fat intake and CHD might well obscure any lesser relation between fish consumption and CHD.

A major review on the effects of ω-3 fatty acids on cardiovascular diseases was recently commissioned by the Agency for Healthcare Research and Quality, AHRQ (Wang et al., 2004). This review generally confirmed the conclusions that ω-3 fatty acids from fish or fish oil supplements reduce all-cause mortality and various cardiovascular outcomes. Almost all of the randomized controlled trials included in this review had used subjects who already had diagnosed cardiovascular disease, i.e. secondary trials.

These consistently suggested that fish oil reduced all-cause mortality and other cardiovascular events in this type of subject, although it did not reduce the risk of stroke. With one exception, the studies that had addressed the possible primary preventative role of fish oil, i.e. in subjects with no previous clinical history of cardiovascular disease, were epidemiological cohort or case–control studies. Those three cohort studies that had specifically estimated fish oil intake (rather than just fish consumption) all reported a significant reduction in all-cause mortality, cardiovascular deaths and myocardial infarction associated with high fish oil consumption (average follow-up duration of 10 years).

The overall evidence at present seems consistent with the recommendation that fatty fish be included in healthful and diverse diets. A quantitative recommendation of two portions of fatty fish per week has been suggested. A few years ago, fish oil would have been regarded as just another source of fat in our already excessively fatty diets; it now has a much more positive image. There does also seem to be a case for specifically recommending increases in fatty fish consumption or even the use of fish oil supplements in those with established CHD or some types of hyperlipidaemia. Whether the current evidence is sufficient to warrant taking fish oil supplements is a matter of personal choice although the old fashioned daily dose of cod liver oil would reduce the high levels of vitamin D inadequacy reported in many sections of the UK population.

There have been several reports in the British press in 2006 of studies where schoolchildren have been given fish oil supplements and there are claims that it improves behaviour, especially in children with attention deficit hyperactivity disorder, and improves examination results. These claims are based upon a small number of small-scale single school studies, often without proper controls. In July of 2006 the Food Standards Agency concluded that insufficient evidence exists to warrant giving a daily dose of fish oil to all children and that there were 'too many inconsistencies' in the recent studies. The evidence was worthy of further study but not yet sufficient to make policy or support the use of supplement. However, one health authority in Britain (Bradford) has decided to offer free supplements of vitamin D to all children under 2 years of age because of high levels of vitamin D deficiency and rickets in the children especially those of south Asian origin.

Perhaps the traditional cod liver oil as a source of vitamin D might also offer some ω-3 fatty acids.

Some potential dangers of consuming large amounts of fish oil or omega-3 fatty acids are listed below although it must be emphasized that these are theoretical or speculative risks.

- High fish oil intakes reduce blood clotting and increase bleeding time. This should reduce the risk of thrombosis but may not be universally beneficial, e.g. those at risk of cerebral haemorrhage, those with clotting disorders or taking anticoagulant drugs.
- Fish oils seem to have some immunosuppressive effect because of their effects on eicosanoid production.
- ω-3 Fatty acids are highly susceptible to oxidation. Foods high in these acids are prone to go rancid and oxidative damage to them after absorption may have adverse consequences. Note that fish (liver) oil preparations contain vitamin E and normally more is added to them to reduce their rate of oxidative deterioration.
- Fish liver oil may have too much vitamin A and D especially for pregnant women, and the recommended dose should not be exceeded.
- There are preliminary reports of benefits in children's behaviour and performance when given fish oil supplements but these are as yet insufficient to justify providing supplements.

> ## Key points
>
> - Fish oils are the major dietary source of long-chain ω-3 fatty acids.
> - British consumers are advised to eat two portions of oily fish per week and to double their intake of long-chain ω-3 polyunsaturates.
> - Low rates of CHD and inflammatory joint disease among the Greenland Inuit focused scientific attention on the potential health benefits of eating oily fish and the ω-3 polyunsaturates.
> - Long-chain ω-3 fatty acids alter the balance of eicosanoid production in ways that should reduce platelet aggregation, blood clotting and inflammation.

- Fish oils reduce blood triacylglycerol concentrations and increase HDL levels.

- Increased consumption of ω-3 fatty acids may reduce the risk of potentially fatal cardiac arrhythmia.

- The Inuit and other populations consuming large amounts of fish have reduced blood clotting, extended bleeding times and low risk of CHD.

- Several within-population cohort studies indicate that high fish consumption is associated with reduced risk of CHD.

- Cohort studies that have specifically estimated fish oil consumption reported that high consumption was associated with reduced all-cause mortality, cardiovascular deaths and myocardial infarction in subjects without previous history of cardiovascular disease.

- Several secondary intervention trials have reported that fish oil consumption reduces total mortality of patients with existing coronary disease.

- Widespread consumption of large doses of fish oils as supplements may have potentially adverse effects for some people, e.g. impaired blood clotting, immunosuppression and increased susceptibility to oxidative damage by free radicals.

OTHER NATURAL OILS USED AS SUPPLEMENTS

Evening primrose oil supplements contain large amounts (8–11 per cent) of γ-linolenic acid (GLA) $(18:3_{\omega-6})$ and several other plant oils such as blackcurrant oil (15–25 per cent) and starflower oil (20–25 per cent) are also marketed as rich sources of γ-linolenic acid. There have been claims that products rich in γ-linolenic acid may reduce some of the symptoms of premenstrual syndrome especially breast pain (mastalgia) and may have some benefits for patients with atopic eczema. It is argued that in current diets the production of γ-linolenic acid and thus of DGLA $(20:3_{\omega-6})$ and its associated eicosanoids is low because large intakes of arachidonic acid from meat inhibit the desaturase that converts linoleic acid to γ-linolenic acid (see

Figures 11.2 and 11.3). Up until 2002 two evening primrose oil preparations were permitted to be sold as licensed medicines but their product licences were withdrawn in 2002 because it was considered that evidence of their efficacy was not sufficient to meet the standards for a medicine. Several placebo controlled trials have failed to show any beneficial effects of evening primrose oil supplements and there have been doubts cast upon the quality of some of the earlier positive research and even upon the integrity of some of those involved in testing and marketing this substance (see Webb, 2006).

Flaxseed oil or linseed oil is extracted from the flax plant and contains very high levels of α-linolenic acid $18:3_{\omega-3}$, the parent compound of the ω-3 series of fatty acids. It has been marketed as a vegetarian alternative to fish oils. However, Burdge (2004) has found that there is limited conversion of γ-linolenic acid to EPA and very little conversion to DHA. Wang et al. (2004) in their AHRQ review of ω-3 fatty acids found insufficient evidence to make any judgements about supplements containing γ-linolenic acid. Note that an algal extract containing large amounts of DHA is marketed as a source of DHA that is acceptable to vegetarians.

Key points

- Evening primrose oil, blackcurrant oil and starflower oil are rich in γ-linolenic acid.

- γ-Linolenic acid production may be limited on current diets because of large intakes of arachidonic acid and this might limit production of eicosanoids from dihomo-γ-linoleic acid.

- Claims about the benefits of evening primrose oil for mastalgia or atopic eczema are not currently substantiated by good-quality trials.

- Flaxseed oil contains large amounts of α-linolenic acid $(18:3_{\omega-3})$ and is sold as a vegetarian source of ω-3 fatty acids but there is only limited conversion to long-chain derivatives in humans.

- DHA is found in some algal extracts, which may be an acceptable source for vegetarians.

12

The micronutrients

SCOPE OF THIS CHAPTER

The previous three chapters have dealt with fats, carbohydrates and proteins, which are the energy yielding nutrients in food. They are present in relatively large amounts in the average diet and so are termed collectively the macronutrients. The substances covered in this section do not contribute to the body energy supply and are present in small amounts, milligrams or even microgram quantities, and so are collectively termed the micronutrients. The term micronutrient should strictly be reserved for those substances that are an essential component of the diet, the organic vitamins and the inorganic essential minerals and trace elements. The vitamins and minerals are specifically covered in Chapters 13 and 14. This chapter presents an overview of the general micronutrient adequacy of British adults' diets and the use of micronutrient supplements is discussed in the light of these observations about micronutrient adequacy (note that the micronutrient adequacy of other lifecycle groups is discussed in Chapter 15). Also discussed in this chapter are several groups of organic substances that are present in micro-quantities in the diet, and although they are not classified as essential nutrients may nevertheless have nutritional significance and are widely taken as dietary supplements. Those listed below are discussed in this chapter.

- *The antioxidants.* These substances either have inherent antioxidant activity or are part of antioxidant enzymes systems involved in the disposal of damaging oxygen free radicals. These free radicals are produced as a normal by-product of the oxidative processes in cells and can cause damage to cellular components unless quenched by antioxidant systems. It is widely believed that many chronic diseases and perhaps even ageing itself may be partly the result of cumulative damage by free radicals, the oxidant theory of disease. Some antioxidants are essential vitamins or minerals but others are substances that are not recognized as essential nutrients but which may nevertheless have useful antioxidant activity. The oxidant theory of disease and the role of antioxidants are, for convenience, discussed in this chapter irrespective of which category of substance the antioxidant belongs to.

- *The conditionally essential nutrients.* Several organic substances are not normally classified as essential micronutrients but may become essential in certain individuals or in particular circumstances. These are thus termed conditionally essential nutrients.

- *Other organic substances with vitamin-like cellular functions.* There are other organic compounds that are not usually considered to be even conditionally essential nutrients but also have vitamin-like functions in the body. Some of these substances are promoted as dietary supplements on the basis that extra supplies can have some physiologically beneficial effects, i.e. that the endogenously produced supply is insufficient for optimal health or that extra exogenous supplies can ameliorate certain disease states.

- *Secondary plant metabolites.* Plants produce many thousands of so-called secondary metabolites in addition to those produced in the primary cellular processes of respiration, photosynthesis, growth and development. Clearly, a diet rich in fruits and vegetables is associated with reduced risk of chronic diseases such as cancer and heart disease. Although conventional nutritional factors in plants, such as essential micronutrients and antioxidants, may explain all or much of this effect there is also a wide belief that secondary metabolites may confer particular health benefits. Indeed many substances in this category are used as conventional drugs or herbal remedies for the treatment or prevention of disease. This chapter includes a brief classification of these factors and considers the possible ways in which they may influence the development of chronic diseases.

Key points

- This chapter overviews the micronutrients – the essential vitamins and minerals that are required only in small amounts and do not act as sources of energy.

- The micronutrient adequacy of adult British diets will be overviewed and the case for the use of micronutrient supplements will be discussed and evaluated.

- The antioxidant theory of disease and the role of antioxidants (both essential nutrients and other plant chemicals) will be discussed in this chapter.

- This chapter also overviews several nutrients that are considered to be conditionally essential, i.e. normally synthesized in sufficient quantities to meet physiological needs but which may be essential under certain circumstances.

- Also discussed are other organic substances which, although having vitamin-like roles in the body, are not classified even as conditionally essential because they are synthesized endogenously. Many of these are used as dietary supplements in the belief that extra supplies can confer specific benefits.

- Plants produce many thousands of so-called secondary metabolites. This chapter presents a brief classification of these substances and discussed possible ways in which they may influence risk of developing chronic age-related diseases.

OVERVIEW OF DIETARY SUPPLEMENTS

Additional information and references may be found in recent book by the author (Webb, 2006) and concise overview can be found in a recent review (Webb, 2007). More than a third of UK adults take some form of dietary supplement. Almost anything that is taken in tablet or potion form that is not licensed as a medicine is by default legally classified as a dietary supplement, and these are subject to food law rather than the much more stringent rules governing medicines. There are several long and all-embracing definitions of dietary supplements, but almost all supplements fall in one of the following five categories.

- Preparations of vitamins or minerals – either singly or in combinations.
- Organic substances that have vitamin-like roles but are synthesized endogenously and so not classified as essential. They may act as coenzymes or as precursors in synthetic pathways. The distinction between essential and non-essential nutrients is not always clear cut; as mentioned earlier some nutrients are classified as conditionally essential and even some established vitamins only become essential under particular circumstances. Vitamin D is not essential in the diet if the skin is adequately exposed to sunlight; niacin is considered essential only if there is not sufficient tryptophan in the diet for endogenous synthesis (see Chapter 13). Some examples of these organic substances are briefly discussed later in the chapter.
- Natural fats and oils such as fish (liver) oil, evening primrose oil and flaxseed oil (see Chapter 11).
- Natural plant extracts or occasionally animal extracts that contain secondary metabolites that may be bioactive.
- The antioxidants, which span the other categories but are separated out for discussion as a single category in this chapter.

People take supplements for a range of individual reasons but most of these fall under the following four broad headings:

- to ensure micronutrient adequacy
- to compensate for some (perceived) extra need or defective metabolic handling of a nutrient, e.g.

poor absorption, increased need in pregnancy, increased loss in renal dialysis, an inborn error of metabolism
- to prevent or treat disease
- to improve athletic performance.

There are many potential hazards associated with taking dietary supplements. Some of these are listed below.

- They may be directly toxic. Many of the substances taken would not be found in any normal British diet, e.g. they may be herbal or ethnic medicines sold as dietary supplements for commercial convenience or they may contain much greater amounts of dietary constituents than would ordinarily be found in food. The larger the dose used and the longer the duration of use, the greater the risk of toxic effects. Even many essential nutrients are very toxic in excess, e.g. vitamins A and D and iron. If a micronutrient supplement is taken to ensure adequacy, the dose will probably be based on the reference nutrient intake (RNI)/recommended dietary allowance (RDA), but if it is taken for other purposes the dose may be many multiples of this.
- Supplements are not always subject to the strict regulation of good manufacturing process that governs the production of medicines. There may be problems with their purity, identity, dosage and bioavailability. They may be inadvertently contaminated (e.g. with heavy metals). There have been cases of medicinal drugs, even withdrawn drugs, having even been deliberately added to some products sold as dietary supplements. They may contain more or less than is stated on the label and sometimes with natural extracts the 'active' ingredient is uncertain. Some products may not disperse properly when swallowed and so may not be properly absorbed.
- They may divert attention away from more useful dietary and lifestyle changes and used as an easy alternative to such changes. An antioxidant supplement may be taken as an alternative to stopping smoking, milk thistle extracts may be taken to protect the liver from alcohol misuse and plant extracts taken as an alternative to eating five portions of fruit and vegetables.
- Some people may take supplements rather than their prescribed medication.

- Some supplements may interfere with prescribed drugs, e.g. they may increase their metabolic destruction by inducing enzymes in the liver that metabolize 'foreign' substances.

Several of these supplement issues and examples are addressed in this chapter. Some are dealt with in other chapters, e.g. oil supplements are discussed in Chapter 11, and vitamins and minerals (including their toxicity at high doses) are individually discussed in Chapter 13 and 14. Some substances discussed as functional foods in Chapter 18 are also taken as dietary supplements.

Key points

- Almost anything taken in medicinal form that is not a licensed medicine is legally classified as a dietary supplement.

- Most dietary supplements are covered by five categories: essential micronutrients, endogenously produced organic substances with vitamin-like roles, natural fats and oils, plant and animal extracts and the antioxidants.

- Supplements are taken to ensure adequacy, to compensate for some (perceived) increase in need, to prevent or treat disease or to enhance athletic performance.

- Some potential problems of supplement use:
  - direct toxicity
  - uncertain purity, identity, dosage and bioavailability
  - they may be used as an easy alternative to more useful dietary or lifestyle changes
  - they may affect the activity of prescription drugs or be taken as an alternative to prescribed medicines.

GENERAL MICRONUTRIENT ADEQUACY OF BRITISH ADULTS

Vitamins

The latest National Diet and Nutrition Survey (NDNS) of adults aged 19–64 years was conducted in Britain in 2000–01 (summary report by Hoare *et al.*, 2004). This found that for all vitamins, the mean intakes from food were above or very close to the RNI with the one exception of the vitamin A intakes of men and women in the 19–24-year-age group, the average intake for this was 80 per cent or less of the RNI. For several vitamins, the mean intake was well above the RNI with the mean being at least double the RNI in men and women for niacin, vitamin B_{12} and vitamin C and also for men only for thiamin and vitamin B_6. In general the average intakes of men were a higher proportion of the RNI than those for women although this was totally due to the higher total food intake of men; the nutrient density (amount of nutrient per calorie) of men's diets was actually lower than that of the women. The intakes of the youngest 19–24-year age groups were less than those of the total sample for every vitamin and in both sexes.

With the exception of the vitamin A intakes of the youngest adults the above mentioned results therefore tend to give reassurance about the vitamin adequacy of the diets of British adults. However, when one considers the distribution of individual intakes, the picture is not quite so reassuring. The averages do tend to conceal a substantial number of individuals whose intakes are unsatisfactory, i.e. below the lower RNI (LRNI).

- 7 per cent of men and 9 per cent of women have unsatisfactory vitamin A intakes and this rises to 16 per cent and 19 per cent respectively in the 19–24-year-olds.
- 3 per cent of men and 8 per cent of women have unsatisfactory intakes of riboflavin which again rises in the 19–24-year-olds to 8 per cent and 15 per cent, respectively
- For all of the vitamins except vitamin C between 1 and 2 per cent of women have unsatisfactory intakes and 5 per cent of 19–24 year old women have unsatisfactory vitamin B_6 intakes.

Note that these figures apply only to food intake of vitamins but around 35 per cent of those taking part in the survey were taking dietary supplements. When vitamins from supplements were included, the average vitamin A intake of young women in the 19–24-year age group was almost up to the RNI but the intake of young men in this age group remained well short of the RNI. Dietary supplements had little effect on the numbers of people with low vitamin intakes – they tend to be taken by those with the highest intake from food and who need them least.

All women who could become pregnant are advised to take a supplement of 400 μg/day of folic acid to minimize the risk of neural tube defects if they become pregnant (see Chapter 15), but the survey showed that well over 85 per cent of women of childbearing age took in less than this value from food and supplements combined. Around 2 per cent of women had dietary folate intakes below the LRNI of 100 μg/day (3 per cent in the 19–24 year age group).

The nutritional status for vitamins was also assessed biochemically in this survey by analysing blood samples. Significant findings from these blood analyses were as follows.

- 5 per cent of men and 3 per cent of women showed biochemical evidence of vitamin C depletion even though almost none had recorded unsatisfactory intakes of vitamin C and average recorded intakes were more than twice the RNI. This observation is difficult to explain although it is possible that the use of food tables overestimated the amount of vitamin C in food as it was eaten. Supplements would have raised average vitamin C intakes substantially but are less likely to have been taken by those with low intakes from food.
- 4 per cent of men and 5 per cent of women showed biochemical evidence of marginal folate status with higher prevalence in the youngest age groups
- 2 per cent of men and 4 per cent of women had biochemical evidence of vitamin B_{12} depletion even though average recorded intakes were three to four times the RNI and the number of individuals with unsatisfactory intakes was very low. Vitamin B_{12} deficiency is most often due to poor absorption, including pernicious anaemia.
- Two-thirds of the total sample showed biochemical evidence of riboflavin although the report noted that this assay is very sensitive to mild depletion of riboflavin in the tissues.
- Over 10 per cent of the total sample had biochemical evidence of vitamin B_6 deficiency.
- 14 per cent of the men and 15 per cent of the women showed biochemical evidence of vitamin D deficiency with almost double these proportions in the youngest age groups. There is no RNI for vitamin D for adults because it is assumed that the endogenous production in the skin when it is exposed to summer sunlight is the primary source of this vitamin for most people. Average dietary intakes of vitamin D were only 3–4 μg/day, which is far less than the 10–15 μg/day

Table 12.1 The vitamin adequacy of adult British diets aged 19–64*

Vitamin	Average intake (% RNI)				% Below LRNI				% Below biochemical threshold			
	Men (aged)		Women (aged)		Men (aged)		Women (aged)		Men (aged)		Women (aged)	
	19–64	19–24	19–64	19–24	19–64	19–24	19–64	19–24	19–64	19–24	19–64	19–24
A (retinol equivalents)	130	80	112	78	7	16	9	19	0	0	0	0
Thiamin	214	160	193	181	1	2	1	0	3	0	1	0
Riboflavin	162	129	146	126	3	8	8	15	66	82	66	77
Niacin equivalents	268	232	257	246	0	0	1	2				
B_6	204	189	169	165	1	0	2	5	10	4	11	12
B_{12}	431	296	319	266	0	1	1	1	2	0	4	5
Folate[†]	172	151	125	114	0	2	2	3	4	13	5	8
C	209	162	202	170	0	0	0	1	5	7	3	4
D[‡]	3.7 (μg)	2.9 (μg)	2.8 (μg)	2.3 (μg)	–	–	–	–	14	24	15	28

*Data from Hoare et al. (2004)
[†] Biochemical value is red cell folate indicating marginal status.
[‡] No adult RNI or LRNI for vitamin D – absolute values given.

recommended for those who do not get regular sunlight exposure. To emphasize this pre-eminence of sunlight as the main source of vitamin D, around 23 per cent of those sampled in the winter had low biochemical status for vitamin D compared with around 3 per cent of those sampled in the summer.

Table 12.1 summarizes average vitamin intakes as a percentage of the RNI, the percentage of people recording dietary intakes below the RNI and the percentage of those whose blood analysis fell below the value taken to indicate depleted status of the vitamin. It should be borne in mind that when viewing Table 12.1, and Table 12.2 later in the chapter, even where these tables indicate apparently low percentages of people with inadequate intakes of vitamins or mineral this will still translate into many thousands or even hundreds of thousands of affected individuals if these recorded intakes are truly representative of the usual intakes of British adults.

Minerals

As with vitamin intakes, the NDNS survey of adults showed a general tendency for average intakes of essential minerals to be lowest in the youngest 19–24-year age group. Male values were also substantially higher than female values reflecting the higher average food intakes of men. For older men the average intakes of all minerals were at or above the RNI but for magnesium, potassium, zinc and copper the intakes of men aged 19–24 were significantly below the RNI, as were the potassium intakes of men aged 25–34 years.

The average iron intakes of all age groups of women were substantially below the iron RNI except for the oldest group which was assumed to be post-menopausal and thus had the same lower RNI as men. In the youngest age group the recorded intake was only 60 per cent of the RNI. Average magnesium, potassium and copper intakes were significantly or substantially below the RNI for all age groups of women and the average iodine intake of the youngest age group of women was also below the RNI.

Around 25 per cent of women had unsatisfactory recorded iron intakes (below the LRNI) and this figure rose to 42 per cent in the youngest age group of women. Blood analysis indicated that 3 per cent of men and 8 per cent of women were anaemic (haemoglobin concentrations below 13 g/100 mL and 12 g/100 mL, respectively). Serum ferritin concentrations are regarded as a more sensitive

Table 12.2 The mineral adequacy of diets of British adults aged 19–64 years*

Mineral	Average intake (% RNI)				% Below LRNI				% Below biochemical threshold			
	Men (aged)		Women (aged)		Men (aged)		Women (aged)		Men (aged)		Women (aged)	
	19–64	19–24	19–64	19–24	19–64	19–24	19–64	19–24	19–64	19–24	19–64	19–24
Iron[†]	151	131	82	60	1	3	25	42	3 (4)	0 (4)	8 (11)	7 (16)
Calcium	144	123	111	99	2	5	5	8				
Magnesium	103	86	85	76	9	17	13	22				
Potassium	96	81	76	67	6	18	19	30				
Zinc	107	95	105	98	4	7	4	5				
Iodine	154	119	114	93	2	2	4	12				
Copper	119	95	86	76	–	–	–	–				

*Data from Hoare et al. (2004).
[†] The two biochemical values are the value for haemoglobin indicative of anaemia and in parentheses the value for serum ferritin indicative of iron store depletion.

indicator of iron status and 4 per cent of men and 11 per cent of women had values for serum ferritin indicative of depleted iron stores. The analysis of the distribution of individual intakes of minerals indicates that substantial proportions of men and women, particularly in the youngest age group, have unsatisfactory intakes of some minerals.

A summary of average mineral intakes expressed as a percentage of the RNI, the percentage individuals with recorded intakes below the LRNI and, for iron only, the percentage with blood values below the threshold value indicating depletion are shown in Table 12.2.

Summing up the vitamin and mineral adequacy of adult British diets

With a few exceptions this survey found that the average intake of most vitamins and minerals was above the RNI. However, it did highlight some problem areas as discussed earlier. When the distribution of individual intakes was assessed it was found that for many nutrients, significant numbers of individuals, particularly in the younger age groups, were recording intakes indicative of inadequacy. Even where the percentage of affected individuals is apparently low it should be noted that a 2 per cent frequency across all of the age and sex groups covered by this survey would translate into half a million affected people in the British population. The errors and uncertainties in measuring habitual

food intake and in translating this into nutrient intakes were discussed in Chapter 3 and must be borne in mind when interpreting the results of any survey of food and nutrient intakes. Another point is that the interpretation of measured values as indicating deficiency or adequacy is dependent on the validity of the standards against which they are compared, e.g.:

• according to the blood analysis around 66 per cent of adults are classified as having low riboflavin status whereas only 5–6 per cent recorded inadequate riboflavin intakes. Is this an indication that perhaps the biochemical assessment exaggerated the extent of deficiency or perhaps that the LRNI is set too low?

• less than 0.5 per cent of adults recorded vitamin C intakes below the LRNI whereas around 5 per cent had plasma vitamin C levels below the threshold value indicating vitamin depletion. Does this reflect a problem with the standards used or perhaps with the values used for the vitamin C content of some foods as eaten?

If the American RDA had been used to interpret the values obtained from this survey then the average values for zinc, folate and vitamin E would be below these for both sexes as would the calcium intakes for women. In general the interpretation would be substantially worse if the generally higher American dietary standards were used rather than the British ones.

Is there a case for more widespread use of vitamin and mineral supplements?

Around 35 per cent of British adults aged 19–64 years take a dietary supplement; 29 per cent of men and 40 per cent of women (Hoare *et al.*, 2004). The most commonly used supplements are vitamins, minerals, fish and fish liver oil. This is almost three times the rate of supplement usage reported in a similar survey conducted 14 years earlier. The percentage of supplement users rises with age, with no less than 55 per cent of women in the highest age category (55–64 years) taking supplements. In this and other similar surveys, there is a marked trend for supplement use to be highest in those individuals with the highest nutrient intake from food or to be concentrated in those age and social groups with the highest nutrient intakes from food. This means that those most likely to benefit from supplement use are the least likely to take them.

All nutritionists and dieticians would probably agree that the ideal way to ensure micronutrient adequacy is to eat a varied and prudent diet that uses all of the major food groups, has five daily portions of fruit and vegetables and provides sufficient energy to meet current needs. However, it may well take some time to persuade and facilitate those who do not already do it, to consume such a diet. There seem to be substantial numbers of British adults who are not currently eating this ideal diet and that, despite the absence of overt symptoms of micronutrient deficiency, are eating diets that are deemed to be deficient in one or more of the essential micronutrients. In the immediate short term some of the possible adverse physiological consequences of these vitamin and mineral deficiencies might be ameliorated by the targeted use of supplements containing moderate doses of the essential micronutrients. Current supplement usage, despite its very high prevalence, seems to do little to reduce these inadequacies because supplements are most often taken by those who do not need them. The use of such supplements, even when properly targeted and in moderate doses, must be seen as a short-term, pragmatic second best alternative to dietary improvement that would ameliorate only some of the consequences of a poor diet.

The Food Standards Agency (FSA, 2003) made recommendations about maximum supplemental doses of all vitamins and minerals. However, in the UK there is only legal regulation of maximum doses for general sale for those vitamins that are also licensed medicines, i.e. vitamin A (retinol), vitamin D, vitamin B_{12} and folic acid. Different regulations apply in different countries – even within the European Union (EU) – ranging from the liberal rules in countries such as the UK and Sweden where it is possible to legally buy large multiples of the RDA for most vitamins to more restrictive countries such as France where only doses up to the RDA or a low multiple of it can be sold as food supplements and higher doses must be sold as medicines. High multiples of the RNI of vitamins and minerals are taken in the belief that they may have additional benefits in preventing or alleviating disease or 'optimizing' health in some other way. In countries where only single or low multiples of the dietary standard are permitted, it is clearly implied that supplements should be taken to ensure adequacy. When high doses of vitamins and minerals are used for some other purpose, this becomes pharmacology rather than nutrition, i.e. they are being used as drugs not foods. There are plans to eventually harmonize regulations governing maximum permitted doses of vitamins and minerals across the EU. As part of the general harmonization of EU dietary supplement regulation, the Food Supplements Directive came into force across the EU in August 2005. This legislation contains two positive lists.

- A list of the vitamins and minerals which can be used in the manufacture of food supplements.
- A list of the chemical forms of these vitamins and minerals that can be used.

These lists can be viewed online in the Food Supplements (England) Regulations (HMSO, 2003).

The aim is that only substances on the above lists will be permitted and thus that anything not on these lists is by default forbidden. Transitional arrangements apply to substances on sale in the EU in July 2002 and for which an appeal dossier has been submitted. These regulations have attracted considerable hostility from certain individuals and pressure groups (see the website of the Alliance for Natural Health, www.alliance-natural-health.org). Some specific points of dispute are:

- omission of boron from the list of permitted minerals; it has been widely used in dietary supplements

- the only permitted form of folate in supplements is folic acid itself rather than the polyglutamates (i.e. folic acid conjugated to several glutamic acid residues) normally found in food.

Key points

- Average intakes of all vitamins of British adults are at or above the RNI with the exception of the vitamin A intakes of 19–24-year-olds.

- Average intakes of a few minerals are below the RNI and this is most pronounced in women and in the lowest age groups (19–24-year-olds).

- Analysis of the distribution of individual intakes of micronutrients indicates that large numbers of people have inadequate intakes of one or more vitamins or minerals, i.e. below the LRNI.

- Many individuals have intakes below the LRNI even where average intakes appear to be satisfactory.

- The frequency of inadequate intakes is generally higher in women than men and is generally highest in the youngest adults.

- Biochemical assessment of nutritional status for vitamins and for iron also indicates that relatively large numbers of individuals have values that lie on the wrong side of the normal threshold values for adequacy.

- Details of the intakes and measured biochemical status of individual vitamins and minerals are given in Tables 12.1 and 12.2.

- 35 per cent of adults take dietary supplements but they are taken by those with the highest intakes from food and thus by those who need them least.

- Supplements make a significant difference to average intakes of particular vitamins or minerals but make little difference to the number of people recording unsatisfactory intakes.

- Supplements could offset some of the adverse effects of low vitamin and mineral intakes but this must be seen as a short-term pragmatic alternative to the long-term goal of dietary improvement.

- The Food Supplements Directive came into force across the EU in August 2005 and this gives a list of permitted vitamins and minerals that can

be used in supplements and a list of the permissible chemical forms which can be used.

- British regulations are liberal by international standards and for many vitamins and minerals it is legal to sell supplements containing many multiples of the RNI.

- In some European countries, only single or low multiples of the RNI may be sold as supplements and higher doses are classed as medicines.

- There are long-term plans to harmonize permitted maximum doses across the EU.

- The use of high doses of vitamins and minerals could be regarded as a pharmacological (i.e. drug) use rather than a nutritional one.

ANTIOXIDANTS AND THE OXIDANT THEORY OF DISEASE

Nature and effects of free radicals

Free radicals are highly reactive species that have an unpaired electron, e.g. the **hydroxyl** and **superoxide** radicals. The electrons in an atom or molecule orbit the nucleus in shells or layers and the most stable configuration is when these electrons are in pairs that orbit in opposite directions. If an atom or molecule within the body loses or gains an electron then the resulting product is highly reactive and can react with and damage DNA, proteins, lipids or carbohydrates. Cellular damage caused by oxygen-derived free radical species has been implicated in the aetiology of a range of diseases including cancer, atherosclerosis, cataract and age-related macular degeneration (ARMD). It has also been suggested that many of the degenerative changes associated with ageing may be due to the cumulative effects of free radical damage. The reactions of free radicals involve the loss or gain of an electron and this can create another free radical that can initiate a damaging chain reaction unless the free radical is quenched by antioxidant systems and the chain reaction halted. This chain reaction has been likened to a line of dominoes: when one is knocked over it falls and knocks over the next one and so on along the line.

- Oxygen free radicals can react with DNA to cause breaks in the DNA chain and alteration of bases (mutation) – this could initiate carcinogenesis. The measurement of concentrations of unusual bases such as thymine glycol and 8-hydroxy guanine in urine is used as an experimental measure of the oxidative damage to DNA.

- Free radicals can peroxidize polyunsaturated fatty acid residues in **low density lipoprotein (LDL)** and this altered LDL is taken up by macrophages and generates foam cells and this ultimately leads to the scarring and fibrosis of artery walls seen in atherosclerosis. Unoxidized LDL is considered relatively benign in its effects on artery walls.
- Free radicals can peroxidize polyunsaturated fatty acid residues in membranes and this can alter membrane function. In this case, peroxidation of a polyunsaturated fatty acid will generate another unstable compound (the **lipid peroxyl radical**) and this reacts with another fatty acid to produce a stable lipid peroxide and another peroxyl radical and so on (see Figure 12.1). This chain reaction is stopped by vitamin E scavenging the peroxyl residue or by two peroxyl residues interacting to form the stable compound malondialdehyde. The concentration of malondialdehyde in plasma is used as a measure of 'oxidative stress'. Their supposed susceptibility to free radical damage is one of the concerns about diets with very high levels of polyunsaturated fat (Committee on the Medical Aspects of Food (COMA), 1991).
- Free radicals can cause fragmentation of proteins, oxidize sulphhydryl groups on sulphur-containing amino acids or disrupt sites where metal cofactors bind to proteins.
- Free radicals can degrade the complex polysaccharide hyaluronic acid found in synovial fluid and connective tissue and which acts as a viscous lubricant in joints. Neutrophils may generate free radicals in inflamed joints, and this inflammation may lead to osteoarthritic damage in the joint.

Oxygen free radicals are a normal by-product of the oxidative processes of the cell. Some of the processes that generate free radicals are listed below.

- Free radicals are a by-product of the electron transport chain.
- Dissociation of oxygen from haemoglobin generates superoxide radicals.
- Certain environmental factors increase the generation of free radicals, e.g. cigarette smoke, exposure to high oxygen tension, exposure to

ionizing radiation including sunlight, some chemicals including excesses of certain antioxidant nutrients such as iron and perhaps β-carotene.
- Phagocytic white cells generate oxygen free radicals to kill ingested bacteria and destroy other 'foreign bodies'. They can also secrete these reactive species into surrounding tissues (e.g. to kill large parasites) and this can cause significant damage to surrounding tissues. Injured and diseased tissue thus has high levels of free radicals. This notion that free radicals generated by neutrophils are responsible for killing tough bacteria and parasites has been used to emphasize their destructive potential and thus their capacity to produce the cellular damage that eventually leads to chronic disease. However, in a paper in the influential journal *Nature*, Ahluwalia *et al.* (2004) presented evidence that it is not the oxidative pulse of free radicals produced by neutrophils that kills ingested bacteria; rather it is due to protease enzymes that they produce. These authors imply that their results undermine the oxidant theory of disease because if free radicals are not as toxic as is generally believed then they may not have such a prominent role in the aetiology of chronic disease.

Physiological mechanisms to limit free radical damage

Free radicals are normal by-products of the oxidative processes in cells and there are thus necessarily several physiological mechanisms whose specific role is to neutralize these free radicals and limit their tissue-damaging effects. There are other mechanisms for the repair of the cellular damage induced by free radicals such as enzymes that repair damaged segments of DNA and selenium-containing enzymes that remove lipid peroxides.

Many metal-containing enzymes scavenge and dispose of free radicals. Several essential nutrients are components of, or cofactors for, enzymes that are involved in free radical disposal. Some examples are listed below.

- Zinc, copper and manganese are components of the enzyme **superoxide dismutase (SOD)**, which disposes of the superoxide radical by converting two superoxide radicals to hydrogen peroxide and oxygen. The SOD in the cytoplasm is a copper- and zinc-containing enzyme whereas that found in mitochondria requires manganese.

- Selenium is a component of the enzyme **glutathione peroxidase**, which neutralizes hydrogen peroxide (a powerful oxidizing agent) and converts it to water and oxygen. It also converts peroxidized lipids into stable and harmless products.
- Iron is a component of haem which is a prosthetic group within the enzyme **catalase**; this enzyme converts hydrogen peroxide to water and oxygen.
- The enzyme **glutathione reductase** regenerates the reduced form of glutathione, which is oxidized by the glutathione peroxidase reaction mentioned above. This enzyme is a flavoprotein and uses a riboflavin derivative as a prosthetic group.

In addition to these enzyme systems, some vitamins and other plant pigments have innate antioxidant properties and so have the capacity to scavenge free radicals, e.g. vitamin E in the lipid phase and vitamin C in the aqueous phase. Vitamins E is used as an antioxidant food additives by food manufacturers to prevent fatty foods becoming rancid and vitamin C is similarly used as a water-soluble antioxidant food additive. Some of the substances in food that are known to have, or probably have, an antioxidant effect are:

- the essential minerals selenium, zinc, copper and iron
- vitamins C and E
- β-carotene and the other carotenoids including lycopene (abundant in tomatoes), lutein (found in green vegetables), α-carotene, zeathanthin and cryptoxanthin
- other plant pigments such as the flavonoids found in some fruits, tea and red wine and the polyphenols found in many herbs and spices, some fruits, tea, chocolate and olive oil
- synthetic antioxidants like butylated hydroxytoluene (BHT) and butylated hydroxyanisole (BHA) used as food additives to prevent rancidity of fats
- other substances with vitamin-like roles but where endogenous synthesis is thought to be normally sufficient to meet physiological need and so they are not normally classified as essential nutrients, e.g. ubiquinone (coenzyme Q_{10}) from organ meats and yeast extract, lipoic acid from green leafy vegetables, glutathione from yeast extract and glutamine, an amino acid that acts as a glutathione precursor.

Figure 12.1 summarizes some of the mechanisms involved in the disposal of free radicals.

(1)   Superoxide dismutase converts superoxide radicals to hydrogen peroxide

$$O_2^{\bullet-} + O_2^{\bullet-} + 2H^+ \xrightarrow{\text{superoxide dismutase}} H_2O_2 + O_2$$

(2)   Glutathione peroxidase converts hydrogen peroxide to water

$$H_2O_2 + \text{reduced glutathione} \xrightarrow{\text{glutathione reductase}} H_2O + \text{oxidized glutathione}$$

(3)   Glutathione reductase regenerates reduced glutathione

$$\text{Oxidized glutathione} \xrightarrow{\text{glutathione reductase}} \text{reduced glutathione}$$

(4)   The enzyme catalase (iron-containing) converts hydrogen peroxide to water and oxygen

$$2H_2O_2 \xrightarrow{\text{catalase}} 2H_2O + O_2$$

(5)   Vitamin E can quench free radicals when it is oxidized

$$\text{Free radical} + \text{vitamin E} \longrightarrow \text{water} + \text{oxidized E}$$

$$\text{Lipid peroxyl radical} + \text{vitamin E} \longrightarrow \text{stable hydroperoxide} + \text{oxidized E}$$

(6)   Vitamin E can be regenerated by a mechanism that involves vitamin C

$$\text{Oxidized E} \xrightarrow{\text{regeneration (vitamin C)}} \text{vitamin E}$$

Figure 12.1 *Some of the mechanisms for the disposal of free radicals.*

Situations that might increase damage by free radicals

The following circumstances may increase the risk of disease due to free radical damage of cellular components.

- Increased generation of free radicals beyond the capacity of the mechanisms for their safe disposal and repair of the damage that they induce. This might be due to exposure to noxious environmental stimuli such as ionizing radiation (including sunlight), cigarette smoke, high oxygen concentration, certain toxic chemicals. It might also be caused by any infection or injury that leads to inflammation and the generation of excess free radicals by neutrophils that infiltrate the diseased or injured area.
- Impaired capacity of the disposal mechanisms to handle any free radicals that are generated, for example due to dietary deficiency of a key antioxidant nutrient. Thus it seems highly probably that deficiency of vitamin E, vitamin C or selenium, for example, would slow down the rate of free radical disposal and increase the cellular damage that they cause.

If premature babies are exposed to elevated oxygen concentration in their incubators, it can cause damage to the retina and lead to blindness – **retinopathy of prematurity**. This is one of the relatively few examples of a disease process being fairly strongly and causally linked to excess free radical production. High oxygen concentration is thought to lead to excessive generation of oxygen free radicals, which are responsible for the retinal damage. There is evidence that vitamin E, a free radical scavenger, protects these babies from the damaging effects of oxygen. High oxygen concentration of inspired air also produces lung damage in adults. When water is exposed to ionizing radiations then this generates hydroxyl radicals and they are responsible for much of the damage to living cells caused by ionizing radiations. There is also evidence that the toxic effects of excess iron may be due to free radical effects; *in vitro*, excess iron in serum stimulates lipid peroxidation and the formation of damaging hydroxyl radicals from hydrogen peroxide. Cigarette smoke and other air pollutants may exert some of their harmful effects by generating free radicals.

In most diseases there is increased formation of oxygen free radicals as a consequence of the disease process. Infiltration of white cells into damaged or diseased tissue will result in excess oxidant load because it has been generally thought that superoxide generation is used by these cells to kill pathogenic bacteria. However, note the earlier discussion of the study of Ahluwalia *et al.* (2004) which questioned the role of oxygen free radicals in killing bacteria ingested by neutrophils. Mechanical injury to tissue also results in increased free radical reactions. This means that injured or diseased tissue generates free radicals much faster than healthy tissue, and so reports that biochemical indices of free radical damage are raised in disease states should be treated with caution. These raised free radical indices may be a reflection of the disease process rather than an indication that free radical 'attack' is a key factor in initiating the disease and they do not necessarily indicate that free radical scavengers such as vitamin E will prevent or ameliorate the condition. For example, in experimental deficiency of vitamin E in rats there is a muscular atrophy that resembles that seen in the fatal, inherited human disease, muscular dystrophy. Indices of free radical damage are indeed also raised in the wasting muscles of boys afflicted with muscular dystrophy, but vitamin E does not alter the progress of the disease. In this instance, the free radical damage is almost certainly a result of the disease rather than its primary cause.

The antioxidant minerals, together with riboflavin, are essential components of enzyme systems involved in the safe disposal of free radicals. Deficiencies of these micronutrients might be expected to reduce the activity of these disposal mechanisms and thus increase tissue damage by free radicals. However, given this mode of action, it seems unlikely that high intakes would exert any extra protective effects. Selenium or zinc deficiency might be expected to increase free radical damage but it seems improbable that supplements of these minerals, in well-nourished people, would supply any extra protection against free radicals by increasing synthesis of their dependant enzymes. **Keshan disease** may be an example of a deficiency disease due to lack of one of these antioxidant minerals. In this condition there is a potentially fatal degeneration of the heart muscle (cardiomyopathy). This disease has been reported in certain areas of China where the soil is very low in selenium. Activity of the selenium-dependent enzyme, glutathione peroxidase, is low and the condition responds to selenium supplements and so the disease has been attributed to lack of dietary selenium with consequent failure of the free radical disposal mechanism.

The other antioxidant vitamins (E and C) together with the carotenoids and other non-nutrient antioxidants have the capacity to react with and quench free radicals without themselves becoming highly reactive. They thus have a free-standing antioxidant effect, independent of the enzyme mechanisms. There has, therefore, been considerable speculation whether high intakes of these micronutrients and plant pigments might protect against free radical damage and, in particular, reduce the long-term risk of cardiovascular disease and cancer. Epidemiological studies consistently report a negative association between high intakes of fruits and vegetables and risk of cancer and cardiovascular disease and these foods are the principal dietary sources of carotene, vitamin C and other plant pigments with antioxidant activity.

Figure 12.2 shows a theoretical scheme that seeks to explain how a free radical mechanism might be involved in the development of atherosclerosis. Such a scheme could explain the apparent interaction between several risk factors in the development of cardiovascular disease and it might also help to explain why plasma LDL-cholesterol concentration is such an imperfect predictor of cardiovascular risk. A high-saturated-fat diet tends to raise the low-density lipoprotein (LDL) cholesterol concentration; cigarette smoking increases free radical production, and lack of dietary antioxidants limits the capacity to scavenge free radicals and thus to minimize the damage that they can induce. Any unquenched free radicals can react with LDL to convert it to much more atherogenic oxidized forms. Oxidized LDL is taken up very readily by macrophages and these LDL-loaded macrophages become foam cells, which are characteristically found in atheromatous arterial lesions.

Figure 12.3 shows a summary scheme for the oxidant theory of disease and how various factors can interact to increase or decrease the cellular damage done by free radicals. Various environmental stimuli, inflammation or disease states can increase free radical generation above its normal level. Deficiencies of antioxidant nutrients or defective disposal mechanisms can impair their disposal whereas some drugs and non-nutrient antioxidants may facilitate their removal. Any surplus free radicals can cause damage to cellular components. If this damage exceeds the capacity of repair mechanisms, it may result in cumulative damage that ultimately leads to degenerative change and chronic disease.

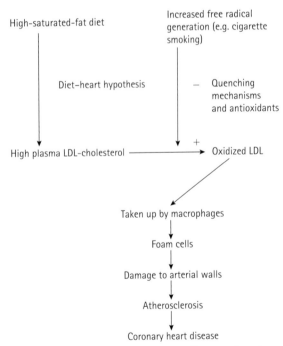

Figure 12.2 *A hypothetical scheme to illustrate how free radicals might contribute to the risk of cardiovascular disease. LDL, low-density lipoprotein.*

Key points

- Free radicals are highly reactive species that are normal by-products of metabolic processes and immune defence mechanisms.

- Free radicals can react with DNA, membrane phospholipids, proteins and other cellular components.

- Oxidative damage caused by reaction of free radicals with cellular components has been implicated in the aetiology of several chronic diseases and perhaps even in ageing.

- Free radical reactions generate further free radicals and this can set up a damaging chain reaction leading to extensive cellular damage.

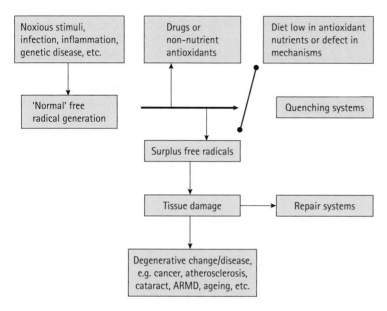

Figure 12.3 *The 'free radical theory of disease'. ARMD, age-related macular degeneration. Redrawn from Webb (2006) by kind permission of Blackwell Publishing.*

- Several cellular enzymes quench free radicals and these enzymes have riboflavin or a dietary mineral as essential cofactors.

- Vitamins E and C and some plant pigments such as the carotenoids have inherent antioxidant and free radical quenching activity.

- Increased free radical damage occurs when there is excess free radical production or impaired free radical disposal.

- Free radical production is increased in injured or diseased tissue and by certain environmental exposures such as radiation, sunlight, smoke or high oxygen pressure.

- Deficiencies of some antioxidant nutrients will impair the functioning of free radical quenching enzymes.

- There is much speculation that high intakes of those vitamins and plant pigments with inherent antioxidant activity may afford extra protection from free radicals and thus reduce the risk of chronic diseases like cancer and atherosclerosis.

DO HIGH ANTIOXIDANT INTAKES PREVENT HEART DISEASE, CANCER AND OTHER CHRONIC DISEASES?

Hundreds of compounds in the diet have been claimed to have antioxidant activity. Anyone reading through a catalogue of dietary supplements will likely find the term antioxidant mentioned for many of the products being promoted. However, relatively few of these potential antioxidants have been tested in high-quality clinical trials of substantial size and duration. In some cases, all that has been shown is that some food or supplement contains a chemical that has the potential to act as an antioxidant. In most cases the claims about the likely long-term health benefits of an 'antioxidant-rich' food or supplement are based on extrapolation from observational data or from short-term reductionist studies, e.g.:

- their effect on some marker of antioxidant stress in short-term studies with experimental animals or human volunteers
- their ability to inhibit chemically induced cancers in experimental animals
- their ability to inhibit growth of cultured tumour cells *in vitro*
- their ability to inhibit mutagenesis in bacteria which is used as an indicator of anti-cancer potential
- the epidemiological association between high estimated antioxidant intake and lowered risk of heart diseases or cancer.

Many of the trials that have been carried out with human subjects have had one or more of the following limitations:

- they have used small numbers of subjects
- they have been of short duration

- they have used reductionist outcome measures (e.g. a biochemical marker, a single symptom/disease)
- they have been poorly designed (e.g. not properly randomized and/or placebo controlled).

This following discussion therefore focuses on some of the antioxidants which have been subjected to more holistic testing of their long-term effects, namely:

- β-carotene and the other carotenoids
- vitamin E
- vitamin C
- coenzyme Q_{10}

The carotenoids

In an influential paper published in 1981, Peto *et al.* suggested that high intakes of β-carotene and other carotenoids might reduce the risk of human cancer. This effect was thought to be independent of their provitamin A activity. In the succeeding 25 years, hundreds of research papers have addressed the role of carotenoids in the prevention of cancer and other chronic, degenerative diseases.

The carotenoids are a group of over 600 naturally occurring plant pigments and about 10 per cent of these have provitamin A activity. β-Carotene, α-carotene and cryptoxanthin act as provitamin A but others found in significant amounts in human blood and tissues do not, e.g. lutein and lycopene. All of the carotenoids have antioxidant activity and are able to quench oxygen free radicals. Lycopene has the most potent antioxidant effect. Coloured fruits and vegetables are the richest sources of carotenoids, e.g. carrots, green vegetables, tomatoes, cantaloupe melon:

- carrots are rich in β-carotene
- tomatoes and watermelon in lycopene
- green leafy vegetables and red peppers are rich in lutein
- mangoes and sweetcorn are rich in cryptoxanthin.

Details of the chemical mechanisms by which carotenoids are thought to exert an antioxidant effect may be found in Ball (2004).

High fruit and vegetable intake is associated with reduced risk of chronic disease

There is an overwhelming body of evidence suggesting that diets high in fruits and vegetables are associated with low risk of cancers and other chronic diseases. This fruit and vegetable group is a major source of the antioxidant nutrients and also of the many other non-nutrients in the diet with antioxidant potential. This therefore means that diets high in carotenoids, vitamin C and other antioxidants have been associated with reduced cancer risk and heart disease in many case–control and in more reliable cohort studies. It is generally assumed that this association between fruit and vegetable intake is causal hence the numerous campaigns in different countries to promote a large and varied intake of fruit and vegetables (like the 5-a-day campaign in the UK). It is widely believed that the high antioxidant content of fruit and vegetables is responsible for much of this reduction in chronic disease risk associated with diets rich in fruits and vegetables. If this is correct then some of these benefits might also be gained by taking antioxidants in the form of dietary supplements, hence the prominence given to antioxidant effects of supplements in manufacturers' sales catalogues. There are of course several potential explanations for this association between high fruit and vegetable intake and lower risk of chronic disease, e.g.:

- the antioxidants in fruits and vegetables are directly protective against cancer and degenerative disease because of their antioxidant effects
- other components of fruits and vegetables might be exerting a protective effect and the raised antioxidant intake is merely coincidental
- high fruit and vegetable consumption is not directly protective but is merely a marker for a generally healthy diet, e.g. lower in fat, saturated fat or meat protein
- high fruit and vegetable consumption is a marker for a generally healthy lifestyle; people who eat the most fruits and vegetables are the most affluent, physically active and health conscious.

Other largely observational evidence also supports the notion that antioxidants protect against the development of chronic disease. Examples are listed below.

- Low blood levels of β-carotene and other carotenoids (especially lycopene) are also associated with increased risk of some cancers (Ziegler, 1991).
- In some studies, carotenoids have also been reported to protect against experimentally induced

cancers in laboratory animals despite very poor absorption of β-carotene by experimental animals.

- In a case–control study of 100 men with previously undiagnosed angina and 400 angina-free controls, Riemersma *et al.* (1991) found that blood levels of antioxidant vitamins were inversely related to risk of angina and that for vitamin E was significant even after correcting for confounding variables.
- Gey *et al.* (1991) reported an inverse correlation between blood levels of vitamin E and mortality from coronary heart disease in a cross-sectional study of men from 16 European countries, i.e. an apparent protective effect of vitamin E.
- In both of the previous studies it was assumed that the variation in blood vitamin E levels was due to variation in dietary intake rather than the use of supplements. Two large cohort studies have reported that in both women (Stampfer *et al.*, 1993) and men (Rimm *et al.*, 1993) consumption of high levels of vitamin E was associated with reduced risk of coronary heart disease. In both of these studies, the apparent benefit was only observed at doses of vitamin E beyond those consumed in typical US diets and was thus only observed in those taking supplements. Supplements were not associated with any significant reduction in overall mortality. These were not randomized controlled trials but epidemiological cohort studies and so the subjects using supplements were self-selecting. This means that the supplement users were probably not representative of the total study population in many respects and despite their best efforts the authors may not have been able to adequately correct for all of these confounding variables.

There is therefore a mass of observational and short-term experimental evidence to suggest a number of antioxidant substances may protect against chronic disease when taken in food or supplements. However, despite all of these hundreds of studies spread over more than 30 years there is still little direct holistic evidence that antioxidants, when take as supplements, afford any significant long-term protection against any major chronic disease or increase life expectancy in affluent well-nourished populations. COMA (1994a) in a major report on dietary aspects of cardiovascular disease concluded that the

evidence of a protective effect of the antioxidant vitamins E and C against cardiovascular disease was persuasive but not conclusive and that it would be premature to make specific recommendations about increased intakes of these vitamins until several of the large controlled trials then underway (and now completed) were known; they did warn that the use of pharmaceutical preparations containing high levels of vitamins cannot be assumed to be safe. They did, however, feel confident of recommending a diet rich in antioxidants, i.e. rich in fruits and vegetables and containing nuts and seeds. Four years later, when some of the ongoing intervention trials referred to by COMA (1994a) had been completed or terminated, the COMA (1998) report *Nutritional aspects of the development of cancer* concluded that even though there is epidemiological evidence indicating that high intakes of the antioxidant vitamins (β-carotene, vitamin C and vitamin E) are associated with reduced cancer risk, most of the intervention trials conducted have not confirmed a protective effect of these vitamins against cancer. The report also recommends caution in the use of purified micronutrient supplements and specifically counsels against the use of β-carotene supplements. The COMA panel concluded that there was insufficient evidence to reach any conclusions about the relationship between dietary selenium or zinc and cancer risk.

The Agency for Healthcare Research and Quality (AHRQ) commissioned an extensive report into the efficacy and safety of supplemental antioxidants (vitamins C, E and coenzyme Q_{10}) for the prevention and treatment of cardiovascular disease (Shekelle *et al.*, 2003). The authors of this report sifted through well over a thousand articles that had addressed this topic and identified 144 clinical trials. Their conclusions after reviewing and re-analysing this information are summarized below.

- The evidence available in the literature does not support there being any benefit for supplements of vitamin E (either alone or in combination) on either cardiovascular or all-cause mortality.
- Likewise there was no evidence of any harm caused by vitamin E supplements.
- There was no consistent evidence to suggest a beneficial effect of vitamin E on the incidence of fatal or non-fatal myocardial infarction.
- Vitamin E supplements do not appear to have any significant effects on plasma lipids.

- Their conclusions for vitamin C were similar to those for vitamin E.
- For coenzyme Q_{10} they found insufficient evidence to convincingly support or refute suggestions that supplements had any beneficial or harmful effects on cardiovascular outcomes.

The AHRQ also commissioned a similar report to investigate the effectiveness of these three antioxidants in the prevention and treatment of cancer (Coulter *et al.*, 2003). These authors also found no evidence to support beneficial effects of vitamin E and/or vitamin C in the prevention of new tumours, the development of colonic polyps or in the treatment of patient with advanced cancer.

One often cited intervention (experimental) study that did have an apparently positive outcome was conducted in the Linxian province of China. Using 30 000 middle-aged Chinese subjects, Blot *et al.* (1993) found that supplements containing β-carotene, selenium and vitamin E produced a substantial reduction in cancer incidence. However, people living in this area had low baseline intakes of micronutrients and indeed micronutrient insufficiency was a suspected cause of the very high incidence of certain cancers in this region. Any beneficial effect of β-carotene in this study was perhaps more likely to be related to its pro-vitamin A activity than its antioxidant effects.

Over the past decade or so there have been several, large controlled trials that have found no indication of benefit afforded by various antioxidant supplements and even some indication that β-carotene supplements may be harmful under some circumstances. Several examples are briefly described below.

- In an Italian study of vitamin E and ω-3 polyunsaturated fatty acid supplements in 11 000 men who had had a previous myocardial infarction, there was no indication of any benefit from the vitamin E supplements after 3.5 years (GISSI, 1999). (Note that this study did indicate beneficial effects of the fatty acid (fish oil) supplements as discussed in Chapter 11.)
- A 12-year trial of β-carotene supplements in 22 000 American doctors found no benefits of these supplements on either cancer or heart disease incidence (Hennekens *et al.*, 1996).
- A study of male Finnish smokers found no evidence of benefit for either β-carotene or vitamin E. On the contrary, it reported significantly

increased deaths from lung cancer, heart disease and strokes and increased total mortality (by 8 per cent) in those taking β-carotene supplements (Group, 1994). Smokers were originally chosen as subjects for this study because it was perceived that they might have most to gain from antioxidant supplements.

- The CARET trial tested the effects of combined retinol and β-carotene supplements using 18 000 American men identified as being at high risk of lung cancer because of smoking or work exposure to asbestos. This study was terminated prematurely because rates of lung cancer were higher in the supplemented group than in the placebo group (Omenn *et al.*, 1996).
- Rapala *et al.* (1997) reported increased death rates from coronary heart disease in those subjects (smokers) given β-carotene supplements compared with those receiving either the placebo or vitamin E supplements.
- In a trial of vitamin E supplements in 2000 with English men assessed from angiograms as being at high risk of having a heart attack, Stephens *et al.* (1996) reported that those taking the supplements had significantly fewer cardiac episodes but cardiovascular death was not significantly reduced – it was non-significantly higher.
- A recent placebo-controlled trial of vitamin C and E supplements in 2400 women at high risk of pre-eclampsia suggested no benefit from these antioxidant vitamins and perhaps a slight increase in risk with the pre-eclampsia onset occurring slightly earlier in those receiving the vitamin supplement (Poston *et al.*, 2006).

Vivekanathan *et al.* (2003) conducted a meta-analysis of seven large randomized trials of vitamin E supplements and eight trials of β-carotene supplements on long-term mortality and morbidity from cardiovascular disease. The vitamin E trials involved over 80 000 subjects and produced no evidence that these supplements reduced all-cause mortality, death from heart disease or from stroke. There was not even a non-significant trend supporting the use of vitamin E; the absolute death rate was very slightly, non-significantly higher in those receiving vitamin E supplements. There was also no evidence that vitamin E supplements conferred any benefits to patients who had already experienced a cardiovascular event. The analysis of the β-carotene trials suggested a small but statistically significant increase in all-cause mortality and cardiovascular deaths in those receiving supplements (doses were between 15 mg/day and 50 mg/day). The authors concluded that these data provide no support for the routine use of vitamin E supplements and that they contraindicate the use of supplements containing β-carotene. A major randomized controlled trial of vitamin E supplements (Lee *et al.*, 2005) has been published since the meta-analysis was conducted. It used 40 000 healthy women over 45 years and compared supplements of natural vitamin E or aspirin against a placebo. The average follow-up time was over 10 years, and the study found no overall benefit for vitamin E on major cardiovascular events, cancer, total mortality or either cardiovascular or cancer mortality. The authors concluded that their results did not support recommending supplements of vitamin E for prevention of cancer in healthy women.

In their major report on maximum safe levels of supplemental vitamin and mineral intakes, FSA (2003) suggested a safe upper level for β-carotene supplements of only 7 mg/day compared to the 15–50 mg/day used in these studies and compared with the 15 mg/day present in many supplements still on sale in March 2006. There seems to be no evidence that high intakes of vitamin E are harmful *per se*, and FSA (2003) suggested that prolonged intakes of 500 mg/day should be generally safe (*cf.* 'safe intakes' of 3–4 mg/day) and prolonged intakes of double this level gave no indication of any ill effects. Vitamin E is found in leafy vegetables, whole-grain cereals, liver and egg yolks but the richest sources are vegetable oils and the fat fractions of nuts and seeds. Recommending diets specifically aimed at raising vitamin E concentrations could thus conflict with the general advice to reduce total fat intakes although increased intakes of vegetables and whole-grain cereals is consistent with other recommendations. The requirement for vitamin E is increased by high intakes of polyunsaturated fatty acids because of their susceptibility to peroxidation by oxygen free radicals.

β-Carotene has generally been regarded as non-toxic even in very high doses of 300 mg/day (used to treat a condition called erythropoietic protoporphyria). However, data from intervention trials suggest that chronic use of doses of supplements as low as 15 mg/day leads to an increase in total mortality, heart disease mortality and, in particular, to an increased risk of lung cancer in those at high risk of

this disease because of cigarette smoking or workplace exposure to asbestos. It is ironic that smokers and asbestos workers were initially chosen as subjects for these trials because it was thought that beneficial effects of antioxidants in general and β-carotene in particular might be more readily shown in these high-risk subjects. Several theories have been put forward to explain why β-carotene might increase the risk of lung cancer under some circumstances. Paolini *et al.* (1999) suggested that β-carotene might exert a co-carcinogenic effect by inducing enzymes that activate certain environmental carcinogens. This was based on short-term experiments with rats. This theory could reconcile the paradox that epidemiological studies are consistent with a protective effect of high β-carotene diets on cancer risk whereas large supplements appear to increase lung cancer risk in those considered to be high risk of developing this disease. Good intakes of antioxidants, including β-carotene, might prevent initial oxidative damage to DNA in the initiation of cancer but high doses might activate carcinogens including those from cigarette smoke in those with high exposure to them.

Wang *et al.* (1999) used ferrets for some studies on the interaction between β-carotene and cigarette smoke because they are thought to be a good animal model for humans in the way they absorb and metabolize β-carotene. They exposed groups of ferrets to β-carotene supplements or cigarette smoke or both of these or neither of them. After 6 months of exposure the lungs of those receiving β-carotene supplements showed evidence of cell proliferation resembling the early stages of carcinogenesis. These changes were greater in those exposed to cigarette smoke and β-carotene but were not seen in the control group or the group just exposed to cigarette smoke.

Key points

- The carotenoids are a group of over 600 plant pigments that are found in green and other brightly coloured fruits and vegetables.

- A few carotenoids, such as β-carotene, have pro-vitamin A activity and all of them are antioxidants that can quench free radicals.

- Diets high in fruits and vegetables (thus also high in carotenoids and other antioxidants) are associated with reduced risk of cancer and chronic disease in both case–control and cohort studies.

- Low blood levels of carotenoids are also associated with increased cancer risk.

- High blood levels and dietary intakes of vitamin E and other antioxidants have been associated with reduced risk of cancer and/or coronary heart disease.

- Two large cohort studies have reported that the voluntary taking of vitamin E supplements is associated with reduced risk of coronary disease in men and women.

- It has been proposed that high intakes of β-carotene and other antioxidant carotenoids protect against cancer and chronic disease and this is independent of their pro-vitamin A activity.

- There are several other possible explanations for the epidemiological association between high carotenoid intake and low cancer risk, e.g. other components of fruits and vegetables may be protective or a high intake of fruit and vegetables may simply be a marker for a generally healthy diet or lifestyle.

- Large-scale intervention trials of β-carotene containing supplements in industrialized countries have failed to show any beneficial effects and have suggested that they increase lung cancer risk in high-risk groups such as smokers and asbestos workers.

- Large supplements of β-carotene may do more harm than good and this suggests more generally that one should exercise caution in the use of purified micronutrient supplements unless habitual dietary intakes are inadequate.

- Increased consumption of fruits and vegetables is recommended and would increase carotenoid intakes.

- Experiments with rats suggest that large doses of β-carotene may induce certain enzymes that activate environmental carcinogens and thus act as a co-carcinogen.

- A co-carcinogenic action of β-carotene might explain the increased cancer risk in those exposed to high levels of environmental carcinogens and given β-carotene supplements.

- Experiments with ferrets suggest that β-carotene supplements induce proliferative changes in the lung and this is increased by concurrent exposure to cigarette smoke.

- Vitamin E is a potent antioxidant.

- Intervention trials of vitamin E supplements suggest that supplements have no effect on risk of cancer or cardiovascular disease although there is no evidence that these supplements are harmful.

- Current evidence does not justify widespread use of vitamin E supplements.

- Leafy vegetables and wholegrain cereals contain vitamin E but the richest sources are vegetable oils and increased consumption of these is not consistent with general nutrition education guidelines.

- Increased consumption of polyunsaturated fatty acids increases vitamin E requirements.

- Vitamin C is also found in fruits and vegetables but there is no persuasive evidence that vitamin C supplements confer any benefit in terms of long-term risk of developing cancer or cardiovascular disease.

- There is insufficient evidence to make any firm judgements about the risks or benefits of taking coenzyme Q_{10} supplements.

- At the time of writing there are no large and convincing clinical trials that suggest a long-term, holistic benefit from taking supplements of any antioxidant.

USE OF SUBSTANCES OTHER THAN ESSENTIAL NUTRIENTS AS DIETARY SUPPLEMENTS

Dietary supplements or 'natural medicines'

A medicine is a substance that is used to cure, treat or prevent a disease. Clearly, many substances marketed as dietary supplements are being taken in the belief that they will offer medicinal benefits, such as:

- glucosamine and chondroitin sulphate to treat arthritis
- evening primrose oil to treat breast pain (mastalgia) and other symptoms of the pre-menstrual syndrome
- extracts of saw palmetto to treat benign prostatic hyperplasia (enlargement of the prostate gland)

- extracts of St John's wort (*Hypericum perforatum*) to treat clinical depression
- extracts of *Ginkgo biloba* leaves to treat age-related cognitive deficiency and perhaps to slow the progression of Alzheimer disease and other forms of dementia.

Despite these medicinal motives, there are considerable commercial advantages for companies to market their preparations as dietary supplements rather than medicines. In the UK, the control and licensing of medicines is the responsibility of the Medicines and Healthcare products Regulatory Authority (MHRA). Before the MHRA will grant a product licence for a medicine it must receive substantial evidence that the product is both safe and effective. To provide the evidence necessary to achieve licensing may take many years and cost many millions of pounds. However, products marketed as dietary supplements are covered by the less stringent food safety laws. There is no requirement to prove efficacy and safety prior to sale, although of course it is illegal to sell food that is injurious to health or to dishonestly advertize or describe a food. Enforcement of food safety laws is at the point of sale by local environmental health officers and trading standards officers, and the onus is on the enforcement authorities to 'prove' that a product is ineffective rather than on the provider to prove efficacy prior to sale. The major marketing limitation of selling a substance as a dietary supplement is that medicinal claims cannot be made for the product unless it has a medicinal licence. Thus one cannot claim that a dietary supplement cures or treats a disease but one can make more general health claims. The following claims would be legally acceptable:

- helps to maintain healthy joints
- helps to mop up damaging free radicals (these may contribute to many of the diseases of old age)
- helps to maintain a healthy skin
- helps to maintain an effective immune system
- helps to maintain normal blood cholesterol levels.

The following disease-orientated claims would not be permitted:

- helps to prevent or treat cancer
- helps to treat or prevent arthritis
- treats eczema
- prevents colds and flu.

The loose restrictions on health claims of dietary supplements seems like a relatively small price to pay for being free to market a substance that is intended in all but name to be used as a drug without having to go through the expensive and time-consuming process of getting it approved as a medicine. Other avenues can be used to make the supplement-buying public aware of the health claims that producers are legally prevented from making. Another point to bear in mind is that even these limited restrictions can easily be circumvented for products that are sold on the internet from outside British jurisdiction. British (and EU) food and supplement labelling laws do not, for example, apply in the Channel Islands, and several major supplement suppliers to the UK by post are based in these islands. This means that these suppliers can make claims that would not be permitted under British law and supplements that are not permitted to be sold in the UK can easily be obtained by post. Regulations similar to those in the UK apply in many other countries including the USA. Note that in the USA there is a list of permitted specific health claims relating to the cure or prevention of disease which can be made on qualifying foods and there are also some so-called 'qualified health claims'. These are discussed in Chapter 18 in the section dealing with food labelling.

Key points

- Many dietary supplements are taken in the belief that they will treat or prevent specific diseases, i.e. they are used as medicines.

- There are considerable commercial advantages to marketing a substance as a dietary supplement rather than seeking to licence it as a medicine.

- Medicines must be proved to be safe and effective prior to marketing whereas the onus is on the authorities to show that claims for a supplement are false or that it is unsafe.

- In theory, it is not permitted to claim that supplements or foods alleviate or prevent a specific disease.

- It is permissible to make a number of more general health claims for dietary supplements.

- British and EU regulations on labelling and sale of supplements can be circumvented by selling them by post from outside British legal jurisdiction.
- Whilst US regulations relating to health claims are broadly similar to British regulations there are some permitted health claims relating to prevention or cure of disease that are permitted on foods in the USA (see Chapter 18).

Conditionally essential nutrients?

In addition to the accepted essential nutrients, some other substances may be required under particular circumstances or by particular groups of people, e.g. only required in premature infants, in people with certain genetic defects or in people with certain pathological conditions. Harper (1999) terms these substances as conditionally essential and suggests that a conditionally essential nutrient is one that 'is not ordinarily required in the diet but which must be supplied exogenously to specific groups that do not synthesize them in adequate amounts'. Using this definition, one could classify vitamin D as conditionally essential because a dietary supply is only necessary if there is inadequate exposure of the skin to sunlight for the endogenous synthesis of the vitamin.

- Carnitine is a cellular component that is synthesized from the amino acid lysine. It is essential for fatty acid metabolism; fatty acids with 16 or more carbon atoms can only enter the mito-chondrion as carnitine esters. Healthy people normally synthesize enough carnitine to satisfy their physiological needs, even those who are strict vegetarians and get almost none from their diet. There are several rare inherited disorders of fatty acid metabolism in which carnitine becomes an essential nutrient. It is also widely regarded as essential for infants, especially if they are premature.
- The amino acid glutamine may be essential in people with serious illness or injury because their utilization exceeds synthesis and plasma glutamine concentrations drop. Some clinical trials have shown that supplemental glutamine may have beneficial effects in these circumstances.
- The amino acids cysteine and tyrosine are conditionally essential for premature infants because the enzymes for their synthesis do not develop until the end of gestation.

Harper (1999) list three conditions that must be met before a nutrient can be classified as conditionally essential:

- the level of the substance in plasma must decrease to below the normal physiological range
- this decline must be associated with some biochemical, structural or functional abnormality
- supplements of the nutrient must raise the plasma level and correct the abnormalities.

Many substances that are normally present in the body but are not classified as essential nutrients or even as conditionally essential nutrients are widely promoted and taken as dietary supplements. These substances usually have clear biochemical functions akin to those of vitamins but are not classified as essential because endogenous synthesis is regarded as normally sufficient to meet physiological needs, e.g. creatine, glucosamine and s-adenosyl methionine. The implication behind their use as supplements is that endogenous synthesis is not always sufficient to ensure optimal health or becomes insufficient in certain pathological states, i.e. that these should be considered as potential conditionally essential nutrients. Often it is implicit in their promotion that they may be beneficial in the treatment or prevention of particular diseases. Several of these substances are briefly discussed below but no attempt is made to give a reasoned assessment of their effectiveness in preventing or treating disease; fuller referenced accounts may be found in Webb (2006).

L-Carnitine

A typical adult man synthesizes 11–34 mg/day of carnitine from the essential amino acid lysine. The diet of an omnivore would contain 20–200 mg/day of L-carnitine whereas that of a vegan would contain almost none. Vegans do have slightly lower levels than other adults and this difference is larger in vegan children. Only the L-isomer of carnitine is synthesized in the body, so supplements containing mixture of D- and L-isomers should not be taken.

Fatty acids of 16 carbon atoms or more can only enter the mitochondrion for oxidation when they are in the form of carnitine esters. In the cytoplasm of the cell, coenzyme A derivatives of fatty acids are converted to carnitine esters and the reduced coenzyme A released for re-use. Also when there is high rate of coenzyme A production from β-oxidation of fatty acids then the acetyl moiety can be transferred to carnitine so that coenzyme A availability for carbohydrate metabolism is maintained.

Certain rare genetic disorders of fatty acid metabolism (e.g. deficiency of the enzyme propionyl CoA carboxylase) can lead to deficiency of carnitine as can a genetic deficiency in the enzyme that transports carnitine across the plasma membrane. Haemodialysis can increase carnitine requirements as can certain anticonvulsant drugs and certain antibiotics. Carnitine is added to infant formula especially soy-based formula (essentially carnitine free) to bring its level up to that found in breast milk. There is no evidence that growth is impaired in normal babies fed on unsupplemented soya formula, although their blood levels of carnitine fall and their blood levels of free fatty acids rise. Premature babies have around 10 times less carnitine in their muscles than adults; it is thus widely regarded as a conditionally essential nutrient for babies and especially for premature babies.

Carnitine has been claimed to boost athletic performance and to be beneficial for people with chronic fatigue syndrome and Alzheimer disease. There is little evidence to support these claims (see Webb, 2006).

Glucosamine and chondroitin sulphate

Polysaccharides known as glycosaminoglycans are major structural components of cartilage and chondroitin sulphate is one of these glycosaminoglycans. Chondroitin sulphate is obtained commercially from either the cartilage of fish-like sharks or from the trachea of farm animals. All of these glycosaminoglycans contain repeating disaccharide units in which glucosamine or galactosamine is combined with glucuronic acid. Glucosamine is synthesized endogenously by substitution of an amino group onto carbon 2 of glucose and it is produced commercially by the acid hydrolysis of the shells of shellfish such as prawns, shrimps and crabs.

Both glucosamine and chondroitin are claimed to be of benefit in the prevention and treatment of osteoarthritis. It is suggested that endogenous glucosamine production is insufficient for optimal repair and remodelling of cartilage in joints and so a supplemental exogenous supply will boost cartilage production and promote the efficient maintenance of healthy joints and encourage repair of eroded arthritic joints. Chondroitin may also have anti-inflammatory effects within the joint. Chondroitin is a large polymer and so might not necessarily be expected to pass across the intestinal wall in its polymeric form. However, there is evidence that some chondroitin is absorbed as large molecular weight moieties and some absorbed as low molecular weight breakdown products.

In vitro studies suggest that in high concentrations glucosamine can increase the rate of cartilage synthesis in cultured chondrocytes although whether the concentrations used are of relevance to the *in vivo* situation is a matter for debate. Evidence from meta-analyses of clinical trials suggests that both glucosamine and chondroitin may confer some positive measurable effects on both symptoms of osteoarthritis and more objective measures of disease progression. This evidence of benefit is by no means conclusive and there is considerable debate about the clinical significance of any benefits (see Manson and Rahman, 2004; Webb, 2006 for more details).

Coenzyme Q_{10} or ubiquinone

Coenzyme Q_{10} or ubiquinone is a key component of the electron transport system in mitochondria which generates ATP from the re-oxidation of reduced $NADH_2$ and $FADH_2$ (oxidative phosphorylation). It is a lipid-soluble substance which has a quinone moiety within its structure: an aromatic ring with two carbonyl (C=O) groups which can be reversibly reduced by the addition of two hydrogen atoms to hydroxyl (C–O–H) to give the quinol form ubiquinol:

$$\text{Ubiquinone (CoQ}_{10}) + H_2 \leftrightarrow \text{ubiquinol}$$

The reduced quinol form of coenzyme Q_{10} is found in the lipid phase of most membranes where it is believed to have an important role as an antioxidant that protects membrane components from oxidative damage by free radicals. Coenzyme Q_{10} is synthesized in most tissues and as the name ubiquinone (ubiquitous quinone) suggests it is widely distributed in many foods, being especially prevalent in meat, fish, nuts and certain vegetable oils.

Although supplements of coenzyme Q_{10} are absorbed there is little evidence that they increase tissue levels in young people or animals. It has been suggested that it might be useful as an antioxidant that helps prevents chronic disease but, as was discussed earlier, two major reviews (Coulter *et al.*,

2003; Shekelle *et al.*, 2003) found no evidence that supplements of coenzyme Q_{10} conferred any protective benefits against cardiovascular disease or cancer.

It has been speculated that because of its pivotal role in cellular energy production, large supplements of coenzyme Q_{10} might improve athletic performance, but there is no significant evidence to support this or even to suggest that supplements increase levels of coenzyme Q_{10} in muscles. Levels of coenzyme Q_{10} decline in some tissues in old age and so once again it has been speculated that it might reduce the effects of ageing but with no significant evidential support.

Creatine

The adult human body typically contains 120–160 g of the amino acid creatine which is largely concentrated in muscle. It can be synthesized in the body from other amino acids and so is not considered to be an essential nutrient. The amount synthesized is enough to maintain the normal body pool size and depends on the amount present in the diet; vegetarian diets contain almost no creatine whereas omnivores typically take in around 2 g/day, which is largely derived from meat and fish.

Creatine acts as a short-term energy store in muscle where ATP is used to phosphorylate creatine to phosphocreatine and this phosphocreatine can then be used to regenerate ATP during periods of intense activity. It is normally taken as a supplement by athletes involved in explosive events requiring short periods of intense maximal activity or those whose sport involves repeated short bursts of intense activity. Its usefulness as a supplement is discussed further in Chapter 16 in the section dealing with diet and athletic performance.

α-Lipoic acid

α-Lipoic acid is a sulphur-containing compound that is synthesized by both animals and plants and so is widely distributed in foods. It is not considered an essential nutrient because of this endogenous synthesis. The α-lipoic acid in food is covalently bound to lysine residues of the enzymes for which it acts as a cofactor. Human gut enzymes do not break the bonds between lipoic acid and lysine and so dietary lipoic acid from food is absorbed as lipolysine. Free lipoic acid is only present in blood if supplements of pure lipoic acid are being taken. The amount in supplements is probably at least 10 times

that found in normal diets. Only one optical isomer of lipoic acid is normally synthesized in cells whereas chemically synthesized supplements often contain a racaemic mixture of both isomers and the other isomer would not normally be present in the body. α-Lipoic acid is a cofactor for several important enzymes including pyruvate dehydrogenase (converts pyruvate to acetyl CoA), succinyl CoA dehydrogenase in the Krebs cycle and some of the enzymes in the metabolism of amino acids. α-Lipoic acid can be reduced to α-dihydrolipoic acid and this has the potential to act as an antioxidant via its oxidation back to α-lipoic acid.

α-Lipoic acid is marketed as a supplement with claims that it can act as an antioxidant, and that it can improve memory and energy levels in the elderly although there is very little evidence to support any of these claims. It is also used in large pharmacological doses, especially in Germany, to treat peripheral nerve damage in people with diabetes (peripheral diabetic neuropathy) but such pharmacological use is beyond the scope of this book (see Ziegler *et al.*, 1999).

Lecithin and choline

Lecithin is the term used by scientists to describe the phospholipid, phosphatidylcholine. Dietary supplements of lecithin are usually extracted from soybean oil and also contain lesser amounts of two other phospholipids, phosphatidylinositol and phosphatidylethanolamine. Choline is a component of the important neurotransmitter acetylcholine. Choline can also act as a methyl donor in cellular reactions and it is an important component of the phospholipids in membranes and in plasma phospholipids.

In the UK, COMA (1991) specifically excluded choline and lecithin from its list of essential nutrients. However, in the USA, the Food and Nutrition Board added choline to its list of essential nutrients in 1998 because it could not guarantee that the synthetic pathway was capable of producing adequate amounts of choline at all stages of the lifecycle. Note that choline is found in many foods, especially in soya beans, nuts, eggs, liver, meat, cauliflower and lettuce, so even if there is a dietary requirement deficiency would be very unlikely.

On the basis of its presence in acetylcholine and the low levels of synthesis of this transmitter in the brains of patients with Alzheimer's disease, supplements of choline and lecithin have been tested in patients with dementia but even in large doses they did not confer any measurable benefit (Higgins and Flicker, 2003). Large doses of lecithin have also been found not to have any cholesterol-lowering effect despite earlier reports to the contrary (Oosthuizen *et al.*, 1998).

s-Adenosylmethionine

s-Adenosylmethionine is synthesized in the body from the sulphur-containing amino acid methionine. It is the most important source of methyl groups for a host of methyl transfer reactions in biochemical pathways including synthesis of nerve transmitters, synthesis of creatine, glutathione, carnitine, phospholipids, DNA and RNA. A healthy adult synthesizes several grams of *s*-adenosylmethionine each day.

It was not until the late 1990s that a preparation of *s*-adenosylmethionine that could be administered orally was first produced and supplements first went on sale in the USA in 1999. It has become a big-selling supplement in just a few years. Many potential benefits have been suggested for *s*-adenosylmethionine supplements and these implicitly suggest that despite the high rate of endogenous synthesis there may be occasions when the supply of *s*-adenosylmethionine is rate limiting in one or more of the pathways noted earlier. Thus additional supplemental *s*-adenosylmethionine may confer benefits under these circumstances. In a very detailed and thorough evaluation of clinical trials of supplemental *s*-adenosylmethionine, Hardy *et al.* (2002) concluded that it may:

- have clinically useful effects in the treatment of depression
- have some effect in reducing osteoarthritic pain
- reduce some of the symptoms of liver disease such as severe itching.

Key points

- Conditionally essential nutrients are normally synthesized in adequate amounts but may become essential under particular circumstances, e.g. in certain pathological conditions or in certain lifecycle groups.

- If a nutrient is conditionally essential, the plasma level must be abnormally low, this must give rise to adverse consequences and supplements must raise the blood level and correct the consequences.

- Examples of conditionally essential nutrients are:
  - vitamin D becomes essential in the diet when there is inadequate exposure to sunlight
  - L-carnitine is essential for those with some rare, inherited disorders of fatty acid metabolism and probably for premature babies
  - glutamine may become essential during severe illness or injury.

- Some supplements that are frequently taken as dietary supplements fulfil vitamin-like biochemical roles but are not normally classified as essential or conditionally essential.

- The above section briefly outlined the biochemical roles of and the rationale for the use as dietary supplements of: L-carnitine, glucosamine, chondroitin sulphate, coenzyme Q_{10}, creatine, α-lipoic acid, lecithin, choline and *s*-adenosylmethionine.

Secondary metabolites in plant extracts

Secondary metabolites are substances that are produced by plants in addition to those involved in the primary processes of photosynthesis, respiration, growth and development. Although the 'primary metabolites' will be widely distributed and common to most or even all plants, plants are much more individual in their profiles of secondary metabolites. Some secondary metabolites may only be found in one plant or a group of related plants whereas others may be widely distributed in plants. These secondary metabolites serve roles such as:

- acting as attractants for pollination and seed dispersal
- imparting an unpleasant taste to a plant or producing unpleasant symptoms when eaten so as to discourage consumption of the key parts of the plant
- protecting the plant from bacterial and fungal damage
- protecting the plant against damage by ultraviolet light.

The total number of these secondary metabolites runs into many tens of thousands but they can be broken down into a small number of categories as listed below (classification based on Crozier, 2003).

- *The terpenoids.* This is a diverse group of over 25 000 substances composed of varying numbers of five carbon (C5) isoprene units and are derived from the precursor substance isopentyl diphosphate:

$$CH_2 = C - CH_2 - CH_2 - O - P - P$$
$$|$$
$$CH_3 \quad \text{(isopentyldiphosphate)}$$

  where P is a phosphate moiety.

  The different categories of terpenoids are classified according to the number of isoprene units. These are the hemiterpenes (C5), the monoterpenes (C10), the sesquiterpenes (C15), the diterpenes (C20), the triterpenoids (C30), the tetraterpenoids (C40) and the higher terpenoids (C40). Several volatile oils that give plants their characteristic odour are monoterpenes such as geraniol in lemon oil, linalool in coriander oil and menthol in peppermint oil. Ginkgolide A, found in *Ginkgo biloba*, is derived from a diterpene. Two of the compounds that help give ginger its characteristic smell are sesquiterpenes. The important plant sterols sitosterol and stigmasterol are triterpenoids as are the saponins which have surfactant properties and which form a stable foam when shaken in aqueous solution. The large group of carotenoid pigments are all tetraterpenoids and ubiquinone (CoQ_{10}) is a higher terpenoid derivative.

- *The phenols and polyphenols.* These are a group of more than 8000 compounds which have at least one aromatic ring and at least one hydroxyl (-OH) group attached to it. They vary from simple compounds with a single aromatic ring like the phenolic acids and hydroxycinnamates through the stilbenes and flavonoids with two aromatic rings and up to complex polymeric forms and complexes of phenols conjugated with other substances. Flavonol glycosides that have an attached sugar residue make up a quarter of the weight of *Ginkgo biloba* leaf extract. Examples of substances in this large grouping include:
  - flavonols such as quercetin and kaempferol found in tea, red wine, green vegetables, onions and berries
  - simple monomeric flavanols such as the catechins found in green tea and apricots and more complex polymeric forms found in chocolate and red wines. Tannins from tea are complex flavanols

  - isoflavones found particularly in soya beans some of which, e.g. genistein and daidzein, are termed phytoestrogens because they have weak oestrogenic activity in humans (see the section on phytoestrogens in Chapter 16).

- *The alkaloids.* These are a group of around 12 000 nitrogen-containing compounds that are mainly synthesized from amino acids but a few like theobromine in chocolate and caffeine in tea and coffee are synthesized from purine bases like adenine. Many substances from within this category have pharmacological activity; some are potent poisons and some are used as medicinal drugs. Examples include:
  - atropine from deadly nightshade which blocks acetylcholine receptors at parasympathetic nerve endings
  - nicotine from the tobacco plant which stimulates acetylcholine receptors except those at parasympathetic endings
  - curare from a vine which grows in South American rain forests blocks acetylcholine receptors on skeletal muscle and so causes paralysis include respiratory arrest
  - the anti-cancer drug vincristine extracted from the blue periwinkle
  - cocaine from the coca plant is used as an illegal recreational drug and was formerly used as a local anaesthetic
  - codeine and morphine from the opium poppy are important narcotic analgesics
  - quinine from the bark of the *Cinchona* tree was the first effective treatment for malaria.

- *Sulphur-containing secondary metabolites.* These consist of the glucosinolates from members of the cabbage or *Brassica* group of vegetables and the s-alkyl sulphoxides from the onion or *Allium* genus.

  All of the cruciferous vegetables contain substances called glucosinolates which further contain both nitrogen and sulphur. These are synthesized from the amino acids tyrosine, methionine or tryptophan. The Cruciferae include not only the cabbage family (e.g. sprouts, broccoli and cauliflower) but also rape, horseradish, mustard, turnip, swede, watercress and rocket. The breakdown products of the glucosinolates produced when the vegetable is cut or chewed are responsible for the hot or bitter tastes of some of these vegetables (e.g. horseradish and mustard). Rape seeds normally have a bitter taste due to their glucosinolate content and this makes them unpalatable for use as animal feed but a genetically modified version has been produced that tastes better because it does not synthesize this glucosinolate.

Members of the *Allium* or onion family produce sulphur-containing compounds called *s*-alkylcysteine sulphoxides from the sulphur containing amino acid cysteine. The side chain of cysteine is oxidized and alkylated (addition of a hydrocarbon group) to give compounds that have side chains with the following general formula:

$$-CH_2 - \overset{\displaystyle \overset{O}{\|}}{S} - R$$

where R is an alkyl or hydrocarbon group.

Some examples of these compounds are *s*-methylcysteine sulphoxide found in most *Allium* species, *s*-propylcysteine sulphoxide found in chives and *s*-propenylcysteine sulphoxide found in onions (it is metabolites of this compound that irritate the eyes when onions are cut). The compounds found in garlic are of particular interest because of the many claims for medicinal properties that have been made for garlic, attributed to its *s*-alkylcysteine sulphoxide content. The predominant compound in garlic is *s*-allylcysteine sulphoxide or alliin. This compound has little smell and whole undamaged garlic cloves also have little smell but when they are cut or crushed, an enzyme called allinase cleaves off the side chain of alliin and two of these side chains condense to produce allicin which is regarded as the 'active ingredient' in garlic:

$$CH_2 = CH - CH_2 - S - S - CH_2 - CH = CH_2$$
(allicin)

Although one clove of garlic can produce around 4 mg of allicin, it is degraded to other sulphur compounds during cooking and is relatively unstable even if crushed garlic is not cooked.

Role of secondary plant metabolites in preventing chronic disease

Many plant extracts are sold as dietary supplements and are implied to be of benefit in the treatment of particular health problems or to produce specific short-term health benefits. It is the secondary plant metabolites that are usually believed to afford these therapeutic effects; a number of conventional drugs are derived from plant secondary metabolites (some examples were listed earlier in the section on alkaloids). Detailed discussion of these issues is beyond the scope of a general nutrition text and is an area that is at the fringes of nutrition *per se* and there is considerable overlap here with both herbal and allopathic medicine (the use of some of the more popular herbal extracts is discussed more fully in Webb, 2006).

It has already been noted and discussed several times in this book that people with a high fruit and vegetable intake are less prone to chronic diseases such as cancer and cardiovascular disease. The exact reasons for this association is still not clear but it is generally believed that the association is cause and effect, i.e. that high fruit and vegetable intake protects against chronic disease hence the campaigns in many countries to encourage higher fruit and vegetable intake (5-a-day in the UK). If this association is causal, there are several ways in which fruit and vegetables might be protective, such as:

- they contain relatively large amounts of potassium
- they contain relatively large amounts of antioxidant vitamins and minerals
- they are rich in (soluble) dietary fibre.

It is also possible that the high and varied intake of secondary plant metabolites in those eating lots of fruit and vegetables may be responsible for some of this apparent protective effect. Listed below are some of the potential ways in which plant secondary metabolites might afford some protection against chronic disease (after Jackson, 2003).

- A number of plant secondary metabolites have antioxidant potential, e.g. the carotenoids and many flavonoids. These antioxidants might act to prevent DNA damage by carcinogens that add hydroxyl or alkyl groups to bases in DNA and thus induce mutations that may initiate carcinogenesis. LDL-cholesterol is much more damaging to arterial walls when it is oxidized and so antioxidants might help to reduce the risk of cardiovascular disease by inhibiting this LDL-oxidation.
- Potential carcinogens and other foreign chemicals are detoxified in the body by so-called phase I

and phase II enzymes. Phase I enzymes convert the foreign substance into a water-soluble metabolite to facilitate its excretion and phase II enzymes convert foreign chemicals to harmless metabolites. In some cases the action of phase I enzymes may convert some environmental carcinogens into a more damaging and more mutagenic form. It has been suggested that certain plant secondary metabolites, including the glucosinolates from *Brassica* vegetables, might act to prevent this metabolic activation of potential carcinogens. The sulphur-containing compounds found in garlic and other members of the onion family might activate phase II enzymes and thus speed up the detoxification of foreign and potentially harmful chemicals. High intakes of some plant secondary metabolites, especially if concentrated supplements are used, might therefore affect the metabolism of prescribed drugs (also foreign chemicals) and thus influence their effectiveness; extracts of St John's wort, for example, are thought to accelerate the breakdown of several prescription drugs, and in 2000 the UK Department of Health (DH) issued a warning that St John's wort should not be used with certain prescription drugs and that anyone taking this 'supplement' should advise their doctor or pharmacist if they were taking this with any prescription drug (DH, 2000).

- Once cancerous change has been initiated in a tissue then substances called promoters may stimulate the abnormal cells to develop into tumours and spread to other sites. A number of chemicals in food may have such cancer-promoting activity. The female hormone oestrogen promotes many breast cancers and the phytoestrogens found particularly in soya foods might inhibit this promotion. The phytoestrogens are only weakly oestrogenic and so in women who are producing oestrogen their net effect may be to reduce the oestrogen stimulus by competing with the more potent human oestrogen for binding sites on the cancer and other cells (see Chapter 18 for further discussion of phytoestrogens).

- A high plasma LDL-cholesterol level is known to be a risk factor for atherosclerosis and cardiovascular disease. Some plant secondary metabolites might reduce plasma LDL-cholesterol. According to Mulrow *et al.* (2000), an analysis of 37 trials of garlic supplements on plasma total cholesterol found that these supplements produced a small fall in cholesterol levels that was statistically but not clinically significant. Further analysis suggested that perhaps even this small fall was only transitory and did not persist if the supplements were taken for 6 months or more.

- Heart attacks, strokes and pulmonary embolisms are the result of a blood clot or thrombus lodging in and blocking arteries that supply the heart muscle, brain or lungs. Some plant secondary metabolites may reduce blood platelet aggregation and/or the clotting process *per se* and thus lessen the chance of thrombosis. Certain polyphenols and the salicylates (aspirin-type compounds) inhibit platelet aggregation *in vitro* and phytoestrogens may also have an anti-clotting effect.

- Some carotenoids are found in the human retina, and they may protect it from damage by ultraviolet light and thus inhibit the degenerative changes seen in age-related macular degeneration.

In his discussion of this list, Jackson (2003) warns that most of the studies on which these theoretical mechanisms are based are short-term experiments with purified chemicals using laboratory animals or *in vitro* systems. Such studies can only be a first step in providing reliable evidence of the protective effect of crude plant extracts or even whole foods in free-living people. They do not justify the use of supplemental extracts or even the consumption of a particular food on purely health grounds; they are interesting observations worthy of further study!

Key points

- Plants produce many thousands of so-called secondary metabolites.

- The complement of secondary metabolites may be unique to a plant or group of plants.

- These secondary metabolites are classified as follows:
  - the terpenoids – based on multiple isoprene units
  - the phenols and polyphenols – which have at least one aromatic ring and one hydroxyl group attached to it
  - the alkaloids from which many potent drugs and poisons originate and which are nitrogen-containing compounds derived from either amino acids or purine bases
  - sulphur-containing compounds: the glucosinolates from members of the cabbage or *Brassica* group and *s*-alkyl sulphoxides from the *Allium* or onion family.

- Plant secondary metabolites may contribute to prevention of chronic degenerative diseases by:
  - acting as antioxidants
  - affecting the phase I and phase II enzymes involved in detoxification of potential carcinogens and other xenobiotics
  - preventing cancer 'promotion'
  - favourably affecting the blood lipoprotein profile
  - reducing platelet aggregation or reducing blood coagulability
  - plant pigments may reduce damage by ultraviolet radiation.

- The evidence that underpins these mechanisms is largely derived from reductionist experiments with isolated cells, animals or cell-free systems and can thus only be regarded as preliminary.

13

The vitamins

SOME GENERAL CONCEPTS AND PRINCIPLES

What is a vitamin?

Vitamins are a group of organic compounds that are indispensable to body function. Some vitamins cannot be synthesized in the body and others cannot be synthesized in sufficient quantity to meet the metabolic needs or can only be synthesized from specific dietary precursors. Vitamins or their precursors must therefore be provided in the human diet. Vitamins are only required in small amounts and they do not serve as sources of dietary energy. Vitamins or their derivatives now have clearly defined roles in particular biochemical pathways or physiological processes, e.g.:

- the active principle of **rhodopsin**, the light-sensing pigment in the rods of the retina, is a derivative of vitamin A. One of the early consequences of vitamin A deficiency is night blindness.
- **Thiamin pyrophosphate** is an essential cofactor for several key enzymes in metabolism including pyruvic oxidase, the enzyme responsible for the conversion of pyruvic acid to acetyl coenzyme A in carbohydrate metabolism (see Chapter 5). In thiamin deficiency, the metabolism of carbohydrates is progressively blocked at this step and the function of other thiamin pyrophosphate-dependent enzymes is similarly impaired.
- Niacin (nicotinic acid) is a component of the important coenzymes **nicotinamide adenine dinucleotide** (**NAD**) and the phosphorylated derivative (**NADP**). Both NAD and NADP serve as hydrogen acceptors and donators in numerous oxidation and reduction reactions. They are essential in many human biochemical pathways.
- Vitamin D (**cholecalciferol**) is the precursor of a hormone produced in the kidney, **1,25-dihydroxy cholecalciferol** (**1,25-DHCC**) or **calcitriol**. This hormone stimulates the synthesis of proteins essential for calcium absorption in the gut. In vitamin D deficiency (**rickets**) children absorb insufficient calcium for normal skeletal development.

Key points

- Vitamins are organic compounds that are only required in small amounts in the diet and do not serve as sources of energy.
- Many of the precise biochemical functions of vitamins are now known.
- Most vitamins cannot be synthesized at all by the body or can only be synthesized form specific dietary precursors.

Classification

Vitamins are divided into two broad categories according to their solubility characteristics. Vitamins A, D, E and K are insoluble in water but soluble in lipid or lipid solvents and they are thus classified as the **fat-soluble vitamins**. The B group of vitamins and vitamin C are the **water-soluble vitamins**. The term B vitamins describes a group of eight different vitamins which were originally grouped together as the B complex because they were found together in, for example, yeast extract. The B vitamins are:

- thiamin (B_1)
- riboflavin (B_2)
- niacin (B_3)
- vitamin B_6 (pyridoxine and related compounds)
- vitamin B_{12} (cobalamin)
- folic acid (folate, folacin)
- pantothenic acid
- biotin.

In general, the fat-soluble vitamins are stored in the liver and thus daily consumption is not required provided that average consumption over a period of time is adequate. Excesses of these vitamins are not readily excreted and so if intakes are very high, toxic overload is possible (vitamins A and D are the most toxic of the vitamins but vitamins E and K have low toxicity). Concentrated supplements are the most likely cause of toxic overload, but some very rich food sources can also produce symptoms of toxicity. For example, the livers of marine mammals and fish may contain toxic amounts of vitamins A or D and even liver from farm animals may contain enough vitamin A to cause birth defects if eaten by pregnant women. Fat-soluble vitamins are normally absorbed from the gut and transported along with the fat. Thus malabsorption of fat or disorders of fat transport can increase the risk of fat-soluble vitamin deficiency. For example, in cystic fibrosis, the lack of pancreatic fat-digesting enzymes may precipitate fat-soluble vitamin deficiencies (see Chapter 16).

The water-soluble vitamins leech into cooking water and this can result in very substantial losses during food preparation. Stores of these vitamins tend to be smaller than for the fat-soluble vitamins and excesses tend to be excreted in the urine. A more regular supply is required than for the fat-soluble vitamins and symptoms of deficiency tend to occur much sooner (vitamin B_{12} is a clear exception to this generalization). Toxicity is much less likely because of their water solubility and urinary excretion and is all but impossible from natural foodstuffs.

Key points

- Vitamins are subdivided into those that are fat soluble (A, D, E and K) and those that are water soluble (B group and C).

- Fat-soluble vitamins are stored in the liver so clinical deficiency states usually manifest only after chronic deprivation.
- Fat-soluble vitamins are not readily excreted and so toxic overload is possible even from rich food sources.
- Fat malabsorption can precipitate fat-soluble deficiency diseases.
- Substantial losses of water-soluble vitamins can occur by leeching into cooking water.
- Stores of most water-soluble vitamins are relatively low and so deficiency states manifest after relatively short periods of deprivation.
- Water-soluble vitamins are excreted in urine and so toxic overload is unlikely.

Vitamin deficiency diseases

Dietary deficiencies of vitamins give rise to clinically recognizable deficiency diseases that are cured by administering the missing vitamin. Vitamin discoveries in the first half of the twentieth century greatly increased the perception of good nutrition as a vital prerequisite for good health. Common and frequently fatal diseases could be cured by the administration of small amounts of vitamins or vitamin-containing foods. These cures probably unreasonably raised the expectation of the ability of nutrition to cure or prevent other non-deficiency diseases. In many cases, the symptoms of these deficiency diseases, or at least some of them, are readily explicable from knowledge of the cellular functions of the vitamin as illustrated by the examples below.

- The impaired night division seen in vitamin A deficiency is explained by its role as a component of visual pigments.
- The inadequate bone mineralization seen in rickets is because vitamin D is required to produce the hormone calcitriol that is required for calcium absorption and normal bone mineralization.
- The breakdown of connective tissue seen in **scurvy** can be explained by the role of vitamin C in the production of the structural protein **collagen**.
- The **megaloblastic anaemia** seen in vitamin B_{12} and folic acid deficiency is because these two vitamins are required for DNA synthesis and thus for cell division and red cell production in bone marrow.

- The haemorrhagic disease seen in vitamin K deficiency in newborn babies is because this vitamin plays an essential role in the synthesis of active **prothrombin** and several other blood clotting factors.

Several of these deficiency diseases have in the past represented major causes of human suffering:

- *beriberi* in Japan, China and several other rice-eating parts of the Far East
- *pellagra* in southern Europe, north Africa, south Africa and even some southern states of the USA where maize was the dominant staple
- *rickets* was rife among poor children living in industrial cities of Britain and northern Europe
- *scurvy* was a major hazard for sailors and others undertaking long sea voyages by sail.

These deficiency diseases are now rare in industrialized countries and are generally confined to those with predisposing medical or social problems, e.g. alcoholics and frail elderly people. Although average intakes of most vitamins appear to be satisfactory, this may obscure the fact that the individual intakes of large numbers of British adults may be unsatisfactory and substantial numbers may have biochemical indications of unsatisfactory status for some vitamins (discussed in Chapter 12). Even in developing countries, most of the historically important deficiency diseases are now relatively uncommon. However, a few vitamin deficiencies still represent important public health problems in parts of the world, e.g.:

- vitamin A deficiency is still widespread among children in many parts of the developing world where it causes blindness and is associated with high child mortality
- vitamin D deficiency is an important precipitating factor for osteoporosis and bone fractures among elderly housebound people in Britain and some other industrialized countries
- lack of folic acid is an important cause of anaemia in several developing countries
- pellagra is still endemic in parts of southern Africa
- subclinical thiamin deficiency may still be prevalent in some rice-eating populations.

- Often the symptoms of deficiency diseases are explained by their known functions.
- Some deficiency diseases still represent important public health problems in some areas although in the industrialized countries they are usually confined to those with predisposing social and medical problems.
- Average vitamin intakes of UK adults are almost always above the current reference nutrient intake (RNI) although many individuals may have less than satisfactory intakes of one or more vitamins.

Precursors and endogenous synthesis of vitamins

Vitamins may be present in food in several different forms and some substances may act as precursors from which vitamins can be manufactured. In a few cases, external supply of the pre-formed vitamin may make a relatively minor contribution to the body supply of the vitamin. Some examples of these 'alternative' sources of vitamins are given below.

- The plant pigment **beta (β)-carotene** and several other carotenoids can be converted to vitamin A (**retinol**) by enzymes in the intestinal mucosa, liver and other human tissues.
- The amino acid tryptophan can be converted to the vitamin niacin. Niacin can obtained either directly from the vitamin present in food or indirectly by the conversion of tryptophan in dietary protein to niacin.
- The principal source of vitamin D for most people is endogenous synthesis in the skin. Ultraviolet radiation, from sunlight, acts on the substance 7-dehydrocholesterol, which is produced in the skin and initiates its conversion to cholecalciferol or vitamin D_3.
- Most mammals can convert glucose to ascorbic acid (vitamin C) but primates, guinea pigs and a few exotic species lack a key enzyme on this pathway and thus they require a dietary supply of this vitamin.

Key points

- Vitamin deficiencies cause clinically recognizable deficiency diseases that can be cured by vitamin therapy.

Key point

Some vitamins are present in several forms in the diet and some can be manufactured from other dietary precursors.

Circumstances that precipitate deficiency

People meeting their energy needs and eating a variety of different types of foods seldom show clinical signs of vitamin deficiency. Dietary deficiencies arise when either the total food supply is poor or the variety or nutritional quality of the food eaten is low, or a combination of these factors. Vitamin deficiencies may occur as an added problem of general food shortage and starvation. They may also be associated with diets that are heavily dependent upon a single staple food that is deficient in the vitamin or associated with some other very particular circumstance or dietary restriction. Some examples of circumstances associated with deficiency states are listed below.

- Beriberi (thiamin deficiency) has historically been associated with diets based on white rice. Rice is inherently low in thiamin and most of it is located in the outer layers of the rice grains, which are removed by milling.
- Pellagra (niacin deficiency) epidemics have usually been associated with diets based on maize (or sometimes sorghum). Maize protein (zein) is low in the amino acid tryptophan which can serve as a niacin precursor, and most of the niacin present in maize is present in a bound form (**niacytin**) that is unavailable to humans. Sorghum and maize contain large amounts of the amino acid leucine, which inhibits the conversion of tryptophan to niacin.
- Scurvy (vitamin C deficiency) is not a disease of famines; it occurred principally among people living for extended periods on preserved foods, e.g. those undertaking long sea voyages or taking part in expeditions to places where the fruits and vegetables that normally provide our vitamin C were unavailable.
- Vitamin B_{12} is naturally confined to foods of animal origin and micro-organisms and so strict vegetarians (**vegans**) are theoretically at risk of dietary deficiency of the vitamin unless they obtain supplementary B_{12}. The usual cause of B_{12} deficiency is poor absorption of the vitamin. An autoimmune disease, **pernicious anaemia**, results in damage to the parietal cells of the stomach that produce an **intrinsic factor** that is necessary for the absorption of B_{12} from the gut.
- Inadequate exposure of the skin to sunlight is regarded as the primary cause of vitamin D deficiency, e.g. in elderly people who are immobile and unable to go outside.

- Primary dietary deficiency of vitamin K is almost never seen but some anticoagulant drugs (e.g. warfarin) exert their effect by blocking the effects of vitamin K and lead to reduced levels of clotting factors in blood and risk of bleeding and haemorrhage. Therapeutic overdose of these drugs or accidental consumption of warfarin-based rodent poisons leads to excessive bleeding and vitamin K acts as an antidote in these circumstances.
- In affluent countries, alcoholics are at particular risk of vitamin deficiencies – most obviously because high alcohol consumption is likely to be associated with low food and nutrient intake. Poor alcoholics spend their limited money on alcohol rather than food. High alcohol consumption may also increase the requirement for some nutrients and reduce the efficiency of absorption of others. Several of the deficiency diseases listed earlier do occur in alcoholics in affluent countries, and in many cases there are multiple deficiencies. Some of the harmful effects of very high alcohol intakes may be attributable to dietary deficiency rather than harmful effects of alcohol *per se*. Alcoholics are particularly prone to thiamin deficiency and some neurological manifestations of thiamin deficiency – **Wernicke–Korsakoff syndrome**.
- Very-low-fat diets may precipitate fat-soluble vitamin deficiencies. These diets contain low amounts of fat-soluble vitamins and the absorption of the vitamins may also be impaired by the lack of fat. Poor fat absorption (e.g. in cystic fibrosis and coeliac disease) may also be associated with fat-soluble vitamin deficiencies.

> **Key points**
>
> - Vitamin deficiency diseases can be a secondary consequence of general food shortage.
> - Vitamin deficiencies are usually associated with very specific dietary or other lifestyle circumstances such as consumption of a restricted range of foods, high alcohol consumption, lack of exposure to sunlight or low absorption of fat from the diet.

THE INDIVIDUAL VITAMINS

Readers with limited biochemical background are urged to refer back to Chapter 5 to facilitate their understanding of the significance of particular biochemical lesions that result from vitamin deficiency. In Chapter 3 there is some discussion of the methods used to determine vitamin requirements and assess vitamin status. Table 3.6 (p. 92) contains a summary of some of the biochemical tests of vitamin status. The relevant chapters in Gropper *et al.* (2004), Geissler and Powers (2005) and Shils *et al.* (2006) are recommended as a reference source for factual information about the vitamins and the pathological consequences of deficiency; Ball (2004) has written a substantial monograph on the vitamins and their functions. Chapters in these texts dealing with individual vitamins will not be specifically referenced. Figures related to high UK intakes and recommendations for maximum safe intakes are taken from Food Standards Agency (FSA, 2003). Figures for average UK adult intakes and numbers with low intakes or low biochemical status for vitamins are taken from Hoare *et al.* (2004).

The sections that follow contain brief reviews of the individual vitamins.

Vitamin A – retinol

Key facts

- *Names and dietary forms* – **retinol**; β-carotene and other carotenoids; vitamin A activity is expressed as retinol equivalents.
- *Dietary standards.* UK RNI M/F 700/600 μg/day of retinol equivalents; lower RNI (LRNI) 300/250 μg/day; American recommended dietary allowance (RDA) 900/700 μg/day.
- *Dietary sources.* Retinol in dairy fat, eggs, liver, fatty fish and supplemented foods like margarine; carotene in many dark green, red or yellow fruits and vegetables:
  - 1 cup whole milk – 110 μg retinol equivalents
  - 40 g cheddar cheese – 150 μg
  - 1 portion (90 g) fried lamb liver – 18 500 μg
  - 1 egg – 110 μg
  - 1 tomato – 75 μg
  - 1 serving (95g) broccoli – 400 μg
  - 1 serving (65 g) carrots – 1300 μg
  - 1 banana – 27 μg
  - half cantaloupe melon – 700 μg.
- *Biochemical functions.* Precursor of 11-*cis* retinal, a component of visual pigments;

maintains integrity of epithelial tissues and immune system; synthesis of glycoproteins. Retinoic acid has an important role in the regulation of gene expression.

- *Effects of deficiency.* Night blindness; xerophthalmia leading to permanent blindness; poor growth; thickening and hardening of epithelial tissue; reduced immunocompetence.
- *Risk factors for deficiency.* Poor diet, based on starchy staple and not supplemented with dairy fat, fatty fish or fruits and vegetables; very-low-fat diet or fat malabsorption.
- *Biochemical measure of nutritional status.* At normal levels of dietary intake plasma retinol concentration is homeostatically regulated and only correlates well with dietary intake when it is very low or very high. For adults, plasma retinol concentrations below 0.35 μmol/L are considered severely deficient and concentrations of 0.35–0.7 μmol/L indicate marginal status.
- *Prevalence of deficiency.* Common in some developing countries and a major factor in child mortality and blindness in these areas. Average UK intakes from food of men and women aged 19–24 years < 80 per cent of the RNI; 7 per cent of UK men and 9 per cent UK women below LRNI rising to 16 per cent and 19 per cent, respectively, in those aged 19–24 years.
- *Toxicity.* Retinol is teratogenic in high doses. Acute vitamin A poisoning occurs with doses of around a hundred times the RNI and produces abdominal symptoms, blurred vision, anorexia, headaches. Chronic toxicity leads to cracked lips, dry hard skin, conjunctivitis, liver damage, headaches, bone mineral loss and joint pain.
- *Recommendations on high intakes.* Supplements may not contain more than 2400 μg/day in the UK. Pregnant women should not take vitamin A containing supplements without medical supervision. A maximum daily retinol intake of 1500 μg/day is recommended. β-Carotene has low acute toxicity with doses of 300 mg/day well tolerated but it is recommended that supplements should not exceed 7 mg/day because of adverse outcomes noted in long-term trials.
- *Typical highest UK intakes.* These are estimated at 6000 μg/day of retinol per day from food for top 2.5 per cent of consumers and this is usually associated with regularly eating liver. The highest consumers take in around 7 mg/day of β-carotene from food and supplements may contain up to 20 mg/day.

Nature and sources of vitamin A

The chemical structure of vitamin A or retinol is shown in Figure 13.1. If the alcohol (CH_2OH) group at carbon 15 is oxidized to an aldehyde group (CHO) then this is retinal and if it is oxidized to a carboxyl group (COOH) then this is retinoic acid. All of the double bonds in the side chain of retinol are in the *trans* configuration. Retinol is fat soluble and only found in the fat fraction of some foods of animal origin, e.g. butter and milk fat, liver, egg yolk, oily fish or fish liver oil. There is very little retinol in muscle meat or white fish but margarine, some breakfast cereals, some processed milks and infant foods are fortified with the vitamin.

Humans can also make retinol from β-carotene and several other members of the carotenoid group of pigments although 90 per cent of the 600 carotenoids do not have vitamin A activity. β-Carotene can be cleaved by humans to yield two units of vitamin A (retinol). Absorption of carotene is less efficient than that of retinol and so 6 μg of carotene (12 μg of other carotenoids with vitamin A activity) is by convention taken to be equivalent to 1 μg of retinol. Note that in practice the absorption of carotene varies from food to food (e.g. less than 10 per cent from raw carrots but over 50 per cent when dissolved in palm oil). The vitamin A content of the diet is expressed in **retinol equivalents (RE)**:

$$1 \, \mu g \, RE = 1 \, \mu g \text{ of retinol} = 6 \, \mu g \text{ of }$$
$$\beta\text{-carotene} = 12 \, \mu g \text{ of other provitamin A}$$
$$\text{carotenoids}$$

β-Carotene, and any other similar plant pigments with vitamin A activity, must all be converted to retinol equivalents to give the total vitamin A activity of foods or diets. Dark green vegetables, orange and yellow fruits and vegetables and palm oil are rich plant sources of vitamin A.

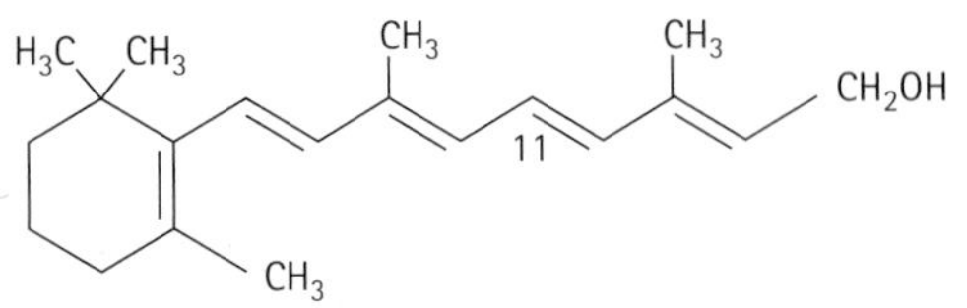

Functions

Rhodopsin is the light-sensitive pigment in the rod cells of the retina. It is comprised of 11-*cis* retinal (the chromophore) and a protein called opsin. Within the eye, all *trans* retinol (vitamin A) is converted by enzymes to 11-*cis* retinal and this binds spontaneously with opsin to form rhodopsin. Light induces isomerization of the 11-*cis* retinal in rhodopsin to all *trans* retinal and this causes the opsin and retinal to dissociate and the pigment to become bleached. It is this light-induced *cis* to *trans* isomerization that generates the nervous impulses that we perceive as vision. Enzymes in the eye then regenerate 11-*cis* retinal and thus rhodopsin (summarized in Figure 13.2). Rhodopsin is the most light sensitive of the human visual pigments and is responsible for our night vision. In bright light rhodopsin is completely bleached and other less sensitive pigments in the cones of the eye are responsible for day vision. During dark adaptation, rhodopsin is being regenerated. Note that 11-*cis* retinal is the chromophore in all known visual pigments including those in the cones of the eye. The light-absorbing characteristics of the chromophore are modified by binding to different proteins but the essentials of the light response are as described for rhodopsin.

Vitamin A maintains the integrity of epithelial tissues in the eye, respiratory tract, gut and elsewhere.

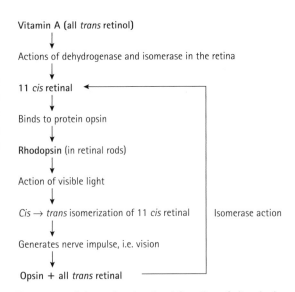

Figure 13.2 *Scheme for the visual function of vitamin A in the rods of the retina*

Figure 13.1 *The structure of vitamin A (all* trans *retinol).*

In vitamin A deficiency there are pathological changes in the integrity of epithelial tissues. Normal epithelial tissue has columnar or cuboidal cells and goblet cells produce mucus, which moistens the epithelial surface. In vitamin A deficiency there is overgrowth of undifferentiated flat cells, which are dry and keratinized (hard). Retinoic acid acts as a hormone, which binds to specific receptors within epithelial cells and controls the expression of numerous genes; these receptors are similar to those that mediate the actions of steroid and thyroid hormones. This control of gene expression and protein synthesis regulates the proliferation and differentiation of epithelial cells. Retinol also has a role in the synthesis of cell surface glycoproteins, which contain the sugar mannose.

Vitamin A is essential for proper functioning of the immune system. It is well established that vitamin A deficiency is associated with reduced resistance to infection and increased child mortality. In experimental vitamin A deficiency in rats, both antibody and cell-mediated immune responses are impaired and they improve when vitamin A is administered. In vitamin A deficiency there is reduced antibody production, reduced numbers of natural killer cells in the circulation and neutrophils show a reduced ability to ingest and kill pathogens and tumour cells. Loss of integrity of epithelial surfaces, which normally act as a primary barrier to infection, also increases vulnerability to infection.

Vitamin A is necessary for normal fetal development. Fetal abnormalities occur both in vitamin A deficiency and vitamin A overload and this has been confirmed by experimental studies with animals. These effects on development are mediated by the effects of retinoic acid on gene expression in the fetus.

Requirements and assessment of vitamin A status

The estimated adult requirements for vitamin A are given in the key facts section and the origin of these values was discussed in Chapter 3. In practice, the biochemical assessment of individual vitamin A status using plasma retinol concentration is insensitive because plasma levels only change after prolonged deprivation or oversupply. Healthy adults have large stores of vitamin A in their livers, which take many months to deplete. Poor dark adaptation and lack of goblet cells and other histological changes

in smears of corneal epithelium are often used as clinical indicators of inadequate vitamin A status.

Deficiency states

The most obvious effects of vitamin A deficiency are on the eye. Night blindness due to reduced production of rhodopsin is an early indication of vitamin A deficiency. The corneal epithelium is also affected by vitamin A deficiency. There is drying and hardening of the cornea and the appearance of **Bitot spots** (white clumps of keratinized epithelial cells on the surface of the cornea). In the early stages, these changes in the eye can be reversed by vitamin A but as they progress they become irreversible and permanent blindness results. Infection and necrosis of the cornea may eventually result in the extrusion of the lens. The clinical terminology used to describe the various levels of ocular pathology in vitamin A deficiency is complex but the term **xerophthalmia** is used to cover all of the ocular manifestations of vitamin A deficiency. Other consequences of vitamin A deficiency are:

- impaired growth
- depressed immune function and increased susceptibility to infection
- overgrowth and keratinization of other epithelial tissues, e.g. in the trachea.

Vitamin A deficiency is very prevalent in southeast Asia, the Indian subcontinent and several developing countries in Africa and South America. It is the major cause of child blindness in these regions and also causes high child mortality from infections. The World Health Organization (WHO) has estimated that there may be 6–7 million new cases of xerophthalmia each year with about 10 per cent of these being severe enough to cause corneal damage. More than half of this 10 per cent with ocular damage die within a year and three-quarters of the survivors are totally or partially blind. As many as 20–40 million children have mild vitamin A deficiency that leads to reduced resistance to infection and increased child mortality. Eradication of vitamin A deficiency is a major aim of the WHO.

Risk factors for deficiency

A diet that is almost entirely composed of starchy roots or cereals (e.g. rice or cassava) has no significant source of either retinol or the provitamin A carotenoids. Such a diet is also very low in fat and this reduces the absorption of any carotene that is present in the diet. Vitamin A deficiency can also be a secondary consequence of poor fat absorption in cystic fibrosis, coeliac disease, obstructive jaundice or of cirrhosis of the liver because of inability to store the vitamin. Deficiency does not usually manifest while children are being breastfed even if it is only partial breastfeeding.

Benefits and risks of high intakes

It has been claimed that the carotenoids may have protective effects against cancer and other chronic diseases because of their antioxidant properties and independent of their pro-vitamin A functions. This is discussed in Chapter 12.

Retinol is relatively toxic when taken in excess but carotene is not. Chronic consumption of 10 times the RNI (RDA) of retinol causes:

* loss of hair
* dry itchy skin
* swollen liver and spleen with permanent liver damage possible.

Very large single doses can also be toxic. Excess retinol in pregnancy is teratogenic (causes birth defects).

The epithelial changes seen in vitamin A deficiency resemble some of those seen in the early stages of epithelial carcinogenesis. Some prospective case–control studies published in the 1970s and early 1980s (e.g. Wald *et al.*, 1980) reported that low plasma retinol concentrations were associated with increased risk of cancer. There are many reasons why the results from such studies might not necessarily indicate a protective effect of dietary vitamin A on cancer risk (see Chapter 3 for fuller discussion of this example). Two very obvious criticisms of such studies are:

* changes in plasma retinol concentration may be an early consequence of cancer rather than a cause
* plasma retinol concentration is not a sensitive indicator of individual vitamin A intake and is affected by hormonal and other non-dietary factors.

Many epidemiological studies have found that a low intake of vitamin A is associated with an increased risk of cancers of epithelial origin and experimental vitamin A deficiency is associated with increased cancer incidence. There are overwhelming grounds,

unrelated to cancer risk, for measures to ensure adequacy of vitamin A intake in areas of the world where deficiency exists. There is, however, no convincing evidence that supplemental intakes of retinol, well in excess of the RNI/RDA, are likely to be beneficial; given the known toxicity and teratogenicity of vitamin A, they are undesirable.

Natural and synthetic retinoids have been widely and successfully used in the treatment of skin diseases including acne, psoriasis and skin cancer. They have been used both for topical application and oral administration. When given orally these retinoids have toxic effects like those described for vitamin A and this limits the doses that may be used. Pregnancy is a contraindication for the use of these retinoids because of their teratogenic effects.

Vitamin D – cholecalciferol

Key facts

* *Names and dietary forms.* **Cholecalciferol** (D_3) is the normal form found in animal foods; **calciferol** (D_2) is used in supplements and supplemented foods only.
* *Dietary standards.* None for adults in UK if they are regularly exposed to sunlight; USA RDA 5 μg/day.
* *Dietary sources.* Dairy fat, eggs, liver, fatty fish and supplemented foods such as margarine and some breakfast cereals:
  - 1 cup whole milk (UK unsupplemented) – 0.03–0.06 μg
  - 1 egg – 1.2 μg
  - 40 g cheddar cheese – 0.1 μg
  - 5 g cod liver oil – 10.5 μg
  - 1 portion (90 g) fried lamb liver – 0.5 μg
  - 100 g fatty fish: herrings (most), salmon, tuna, pilchards, sardines (least) – 6–22 μg
  - 5 g pat of butter/margarine – 0.04/0.4 μg.
* *Biochemical functions.* Precursor of 1,25 dihydroxycholecalciferol (calcitriol), a hormone produced in the kidney which increases the capacity of gut and kidney tubule to transport calcium; it regulates deposition of bone mineral. It may have a role in regulating immune responses.
* *Effects of deficiency.* Rickets/osteomalacia with skeletal abnormalities; increased risk of osteoporosis in the elderly; low plasma calcium;

muscle weakness, possibly tetany; growth failure; increased risk of infection.

- *Risk factors for deficiency.* Inadequate exposure to sunlight for a variety of reasons such as dress customs, being housebound, working indoors for long hours. Lack of back-up from the limited range of vitamin D-rich animal foods or supplemented foods exacerbates the problem. Risk increased in people with pigmented skin.

- *Biochemical assessment of nutritional status.* Plasma concentration of 25-hydroxycholecalciferol (25-OHD), a metabolite of vitamin D which is the main circulating form. A plasma 25-OHD concentration of less than 25 nmol/L has traditionally been taken as an indicator of poor vitamin status.

- *Prevalence of deficiency.* 15 per cent of UK adults (19–64 years) have plasma 25-OHD levels below the threshold with values worst in the younger age groups. Evidence of widespread poor vitamin D status has also been reported in UK children and elderly people (see Chapter 15).

- *Toxicity.* The most acutely toxic of the vitamins. Overdose leads to elevated calcium concentrations in blood and urine with calcification of soft tissues and high risk of kidney stones.

- *Recommendations on high intakes.* Long-term intakes of up to a maximum of 25 μg/day from all sources should be generally safe and higher doses should only be used under medical supervision.

- *Typical highest UK intakes.* Those with highest intakes may get 9 μg/day from food. The maximum permitted dose in supplements in the UK is 10 μg/day; note fish liver oil supplements contain substantial amounts of vitamin D.

Nature, sources and requirements for vitamin D

Vitamin D_3 or cholecalciferol is formed in the skin of animals by the action of UV light (sunlight) on 7-dehydrocholesterol. This latter compound is made by inserting an extra double bond into cholesterol (in the B ring of the steroid nucleus). The chemical structures of 7-dehydrocholesterol and cholecalciferol are shown in Figure 13.3. Almost all of the vitamin D found naturally in food is vitamin D_3 and it is, like retinol, obtained only from foods of animal

origin like eggs, butter, liver, oily fish and fish liver oil. Irradiation of the plant sterol ergosterol (e.g. from yeast) yields vitamin D_2, which has similar activity to cholecalciferol in mammals. This form of vitamin D is often used in the production of vitamin tablets and to supplement foods such as margarine, milk in the USA, baby foods and breakfast cereals.

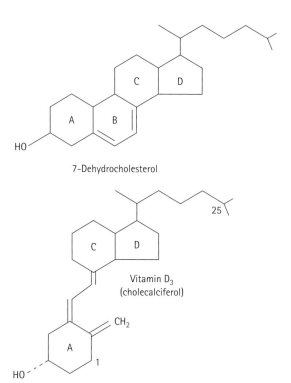

Figure 13.3 *The structures of 7-dehydrocholesterol and cholecalciferol (vitamin D_3).*

For most people, endogenous synthesis of cholecalciferol in the skin is the primary source of the vitamin and a dietary supply is not necessary. Dietary supply of the vitamin becomes much more important in people who do not get adequate exposure to sunlight, e.g. housebound elderly people. Vitamin D does not strictly classify the criteria for an essential nutrient if the skin is adequately exposed to sunlight, but it could be classified as conditionally essential in people without adequate exposure to summer sunlight. In the UK, winter sunlight does not contain the correct UV wavelengths for vitamin D production but production and storage during the summer months should be adequate to last through the winter. In British adults the proportion recording low biochemical status for vitamin D was around five times higher in those sampled in the period January to March than those samples in July to September. In white-skinned people, short periods of exposure of the hands and face to summer sunlight is sufficient to maintain adequate vitamin D status but much longer exposure is required if the skin is black or brown. One theory suggests that the evolution of white races in northern latitudes and those with darker skins near the equator might have been due to differences in ability to produce vitamin D.

Functions of vitamin D

Vitamin D (cholecalciferol) is required for the synthesis of the hormone 1,25 dihydroxycholecalciferol or calcitriol. Cholecalciferol is hydroxylated to 25-hydroxycholecalciferol in the liver and this is the main circulating form of the vitamin in plasma. This compound is further hydroxylated to calcitriol in the kidney by an hydroxylase whose activity is regulated by the parathyroid hormone.

Calcitriol acts like a steroid hormone. It binds to receptors within the nucleus of its target tissues and affects gene expression, i.e. the synthesis of particular proteins. Overall, the best documented effect of vitamin D is in the maintenance of calcium homoeostasis. In the intestine, it increases the synthesis of several proteins that are involved in the absorption of calcium. In vitamin D deficiency the gut absorbs calcium very inefficiently. In the bone, calcitriol has several effects. It induces undifferentiated bone cells to become osteoclasts and these cells release calcium and phosphorus from bone when plasma calcium is low and they are activated by parathyroid hormone. It also stimulates bone resorption by osteoclasts. Calcitriol also induces the synthesis of some of the proteins that are prominent in the bone matrix (e.g. osteocalcin) and it is necessary for normal bone development, mineralization and remodelling. Calcitriol is also necessary for the efficient reabsorption of filtered calcium in the renal tubule.

Several tissues that are not associated with maintenance of calcium homoeostasis have cellular receptors for calcitriol including lymphocytes and skin cells. Calcitriol has a role in the regulation of cell proliferation and differentiation in several tissues. It has been used in the treatment of psoriasis, a condition in which there is excessive proliferation and keratinization of epidermal cells in the skin. In experimental animals, calcitriol has immunosuppressive effects and in pharmacological doses reduces several autoimmune conditions. This suggests that it has a role in the normal regulation of immune responses.

Deficiency states

Rickets in children and **osteomalacia** in adults are due to lack of vitamin D. During the late nineteenth century and early twentieth century, rickets was extremely prevalent among poor children living in the industrial cities of Britain. The symptoms arise from a failure to absorb calcium from the gut, which leads to reduced plasma calcium concentration, and reduced calcification of bones. Muscle weakness, gastrointestinal and respiratory infections are general symptoms of rickets. There is a series of skeletal abnormalities characteristic of the disease, such as:

- bowing of the legs or knock knees
- swelling of the wrist
- beading of the ribs at the normal junction of cartilage and bone (rickety rosary)
- pelvic deformities which may cause problems in childbirth in later years.

In severe rickets, plasma calcium concentration may fall low enough to induce uncontrolled convulsive muscle contractions (tetany). Chronic vitamin D deficiency is now regarded as a major cause of osteoporosis (brittle bones) in very elderly housebound people (see Chapter 14 for further discussion of osteoporosis). Inadequate exposure of the skin to sunlight is regarded as the primary cause of vitamin D deficiency. Poor dietary supply of the vitamin is usually regarded as an exacerbating factor. Average intakes of vitamin D in UK adults are 2–3 µg/day which is considerably less than the RNI of 10 µg/day that is given for those adults who do not get out in the sun. The risk of vitamin D deficiency is increased by any factor that reduces exposure of the skin to the correct ultraviolet wavelengths such as:

- living in northern latitudes
- atmospheric pollution
- skin pigmentation
- some traditional costumes
- being housebound because of illness or immobility
- working indoors for very long hours and other cultural or social factors that prevent people getting out of doors during the daytime.

As was noted in Chapter 12 around 15 per cent of adults in the UK have low biochemical status for vitamin D with a much higher proportion in those sampled in the winter months compared to those sampled in the summer. The number of adults with low status is higher in the younger age groups. Many children and elderly people also show biochemical evidence of poor vitamin D status (see Chapter 15). Relatively high levels of rickets and osteomalacia have been a problem among Asian women and children who have recently migrated to Britain from the Indian subcontinent.

Toxicity

Vitamin D is the most toxic of the vitamins and as little as five times the dietary standard (50 μg/day) may be enough to cause hypercalcaemia when taken for 6 months, thus FSA (2003) recommended that the usual safe maximum should be regarded as 25 μg/day. Vitamin D poisoning does not occur if the skin is overexposed to the sun because of natural regulation. Poisoning is due to over-fortification of foods or excessive use of supplements. Excess vitamin D causes hypercalcaemia and this leads to anorexia, nausea, vomiting, hypertension, kidney stones, renal failure and possible calcification of soft tissues. It may have fatal consequences if severe and prolonged. In the 1950s some British babies developed a vitamin D-induced hypercalcaemia because of excessive fortification of milk and other foods. Ordinary UK milk is no longer fortified with vitamin D although it is in the USA.

Vitamin E – a-tocopherol

Key facts

- *Names and chemical forms.* α-Tocopherol; other tocopherols have vitamin activity; vitamin E activity expressed as α-tocopherol equivalents.
- *Dietary standards.* UK 'safe intake' M/F 4/3 mg/day; American RDA 15 mg/day.
- *Dietary sources.* Vegetable oils, wheat germ and whole grain cereals, dark green leaves of vegetables, seeds and nuts:
  - 1 egg – 1 mg
  - 5 g pat of butter/polyunsaturated margarine – 0.1/1.25 mg
  - 1 slice wholemeal bread – 0.05 mg
  - 5 g sunflower/olive/rapeseed oil – 2.5/0.26/1.2 mg.
- *Biochemical functions.* Antioxidant in the lipid phase; scavenges free radicals and prevents lipid peroxidation.
- *Effects of deficiency.* Progressive degeneration of nerves, muscle atrophy and retinopathy. In rats deficiency produces infertility and reabsorption of fetuses in pregnant animals.
- *Risk factors for deficiency.* Overt deficiency almost never seen and is usually confined to persons with medical disorder that impairs fat and/or fat-soluble vitamin absorption.
- *Biochemical measure of nutritional status.* Plasma tocopherol, often expressed as the ratio of α-tocopherol to total cholesterol in plasma. The lower limit of normality is deemed to be a tocopherol to cholesterol ratio of at least 2.25 μmol/mmol.
- *Prevalence of deficiency.* Overt deficiency rare. Only 1 per cent of UK men aged 19–64 years had plasma tocopherol to cholesterol ratios below the satisfactory level (2 per cent of women).
- *Toxicity.* Little evidence of toxicity even at very high intakes.
- *Recommendations on high intakes.* Prolonged intakes of as much as 500 mg/day generally regarded as safe and little indication of ill effects at double this value.
- *Typical highest UK intakes.* Estimated that the highest 2.5 per cent of UK adults take in around 18 mg/day from food; supplements (which are widely used) may contain up to 670 mg/day.

Overview

There are several compounds synthesized by plants that have vitamin E activity and the most active and important is α-tocopherol (structure shown in Figure 13.4). Vitamin E is widely distributed in plant foods and is particularly concentrated in plant oils that typically contain 10–50 mg of vitamin E per 100 g. Animal fats contain small amounts of vitamin E. The estimated requirements for vitamin E are given in the key facts section.

Vitamin E is readily oxidized and so acts as an antioxidant. Its primary function is to prevent oxidative damage by **free radicals** to polyunsaturated fatty acids in membrane phospholipids. Free radicals and antioxidants are discussed more fully in Chapter 12.

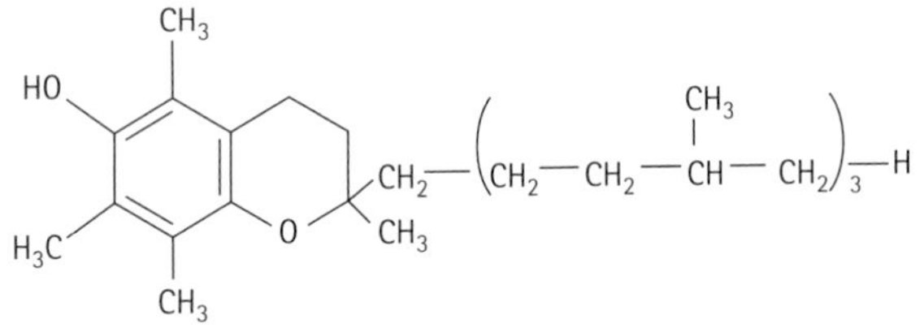

Figure 13.4 *The structure of vitamin E (α-tocopherol).*

Overt deficiency of vitamin E is rare and is usually associated with some disorder of fat absorption or fat transport. As discussed in the previous chapter, there is considerable debate about whether low intakes of vitamin E may allow increased oxidative damage to membranes and thus increase the risk of chronic disease. Nerve degeneration, muscle atrophy and retinopathy are seen in both animals and people with prolonged vitamin E deficiency. Early studies of experimental vitamin E deficiency in rats found that it produced sterility and this is the origin of its ineffective use in preparations that are claimed to increase sexual potency or act as aphrodisiacs. Many people take very large supplements of vitamin E, and doses up to 800 mg/day seem to produce no acute toxic effects.

Vitamin K – phylloquinone

Key facts

- *Names and chemical forms.* **Phylloquinone (K_1)** from plants; menaquinone (K_2) produced by intestinal bacteria. The synthetic water-soluble forms menadione (K_3) and menadiol (K_4) are no longer permitted to be used in supplements under EU regulations.
- *Dietary standards.* UK 'safe intake' 1 µg/kg body weight/day; American RDA M/F 120/90 µg/day.
- *Dietary sources.* Liver, green leafy vegetables, some vegetable oils, milk.
- *Biochemical functions.* A cofactor for the enzyme γ-glutamyl carboxylase which

carboxylates glutamic acid residues in the synthesis of several clotting factors including prothrombin. May have a role in bone metabolism; there are several proteins with carboxylated glutamic acid residues found in bone.

- *Effects of deficiency.* Excessive bleeding, especially brain haemorrhage in the newborn.
- *Risk factors for deficiency.* Normally confined to newborn, especially premature infants; in adults usually a secondary result of poor fat absorption. Overdoses of warfarin and other coumarin-type drugs may precipitate symptoms of vitamin K deficiency.
- *Toxicity.* Few reports of any toxic effects although it will interfere with anticoagulant treatment because coumarin-type drugs act as anti-metabolites to vitamin K.
- *Recommendations on high intakes.* Intakes of 1 mg/day of natural vitamin K should be safe.
- *Typical highest UK intakes.* Little data, supplements may contain up to 200 µg/day.

Overview

Phylloquinone (vitamin K_1) is found largely in plant foods particularly green leafy vegetables although it is found in smaller amounts in many foods. An alternative form of the vitamin menaquinone is produced by bacteria. Human gut bacteria produce significant amounts of vitamin K, which probably contribute to vitamin K intakes. The structure of phylloquinone is shown in Figure 13.5.

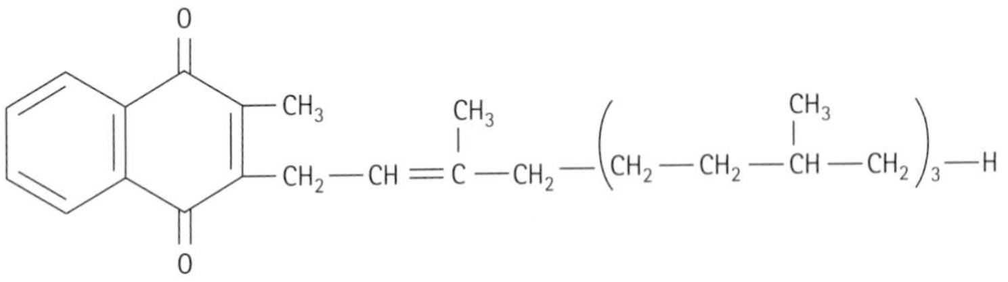

Figure 13.5 *The structure of vitamin K (phylloquinone).*

Several clotting factors, including prothrombin, only become functional when several residues of the amino acid glutamic acid within their structures are carboxylated (addition of COOH group); this carboxylation occurs after translation. The enzyme responsible for this carboxylation (γ-glutamyl carboxylase) requires vitamin K as a coenzyme. These proteins with carboxylated glutamic acid residues are know as Gla proteins and they bind calcium much more readily than the non-carboxylated form. This binding of calcium to clotting factor proteins produces the conformational changes that make them biologically active.

Vitamin K deficiency leads to a reduced efficiency of the blood clotting system and thus to a tendency to bleed. Primary dietary deficiency of vitamin K is almost never seen but malabsorption, for example in coeliac disease, can precipitate deficiency and lead to bleeding. The coumarin group of anticoagulant drugs (e.g. warfarin) exert their effect by blocking the effects of vitamin K and lead to reduced levels of clotting factors in blood. Therapeutic overdosage of these drugs or accidental overdosage due to warfarin-based rodent poisons leads to bleeding and vitamin K acts as an antidote to warfarin. Some newborn babies, especially premature babies, may develop intracranial haemorrhages shortly after birth; this tendency to haemorrhage can be prevented by prophylactic administration of vitamin K and the routine administration of vitamin K is common in maternity units. In 1992, Golding et al. reported that vitamin K injections in the newborn were associated with an increased risk of childhood cancer. This report naturally raised concerns about the safety of this prophylactic use of vitamin K but subsequent studies (e.g. Eklund et al., 1993) have suggested that these concerns were probably unwarranted.

Similar carboxylated Gla proteins are found in other tissues although the significance of these proteins is not clear. There are, for example, three Gla proteins in bone; osteocalcin, matrix Gla protein and protein S. The presence of these proteins in bone has led to suggestions that vitamin K may have an important role in bone metabolism and thus that vitamin K insufficiency may be a contributory factor in the cause of osteoporosis. Ball (2004) has summarized evidence that provides some preliminary support for an association between vitamin K insufficiency and osteoporosis risk and this is summarized below although it would be extremely premature to assume that there is a cause and effect relationship.

- On a normal diet with normal blood clotting, the osteocalcin that circulates in the blood is not fully carboxylated and substantial supplements are needed to achieve full carboxylation.
- In very elderly women there is reduced carboxylation of circulating osteocalcin.
- High levels of under-carboxylated osteocalcin in elderly women is associated with reduced bone density at the hip and increased risk of fracture.
- Low intakes of vitamin K have been associated with increased hip fracture risk.
- Women in the lowest quartile of vitamin K intakes have been reported to have lower bone density than those in the highest quartile.

Thiamin – vitamin B$_1$

Key facts

- *Names and chemical forms.* Thiamin (vitamin B$_1$).
- *Dietary standards.* UK adult RNI M/F 1.0/0.8 mg/day; UK LRNI 0.6/0.45 mg/day; American RDA M/F 1.2/1.1 mg/day.
- *Dietary sources.* Found in all plant and animal tissues but only whole cereals, nuts, seeds and pulses are rich sources:
  - 1 slice wholemeal bread (UK) – 0.12 mg
  - 1 egg – 0.04 mg
  - 1 pork chop – 0.7 mg
  - 1 cup whole/skimmed milk – 0.06 mg
  - 30 g peanuts – 0.27 mg
  - 1 serving (165 g) brown/white rice – 0.23/0.02 mg
  - 1 serving (75 g) frozen peas – 0.18 mg
  - 1 serving (200 g) baked beans – 0.14 mg
  - 1 teaspoon (5 g) yeast extract – 0.16 mg.
- *Biochemical functions.* Gives rise to thiamin pyrophosphate, a coenzyme for pyruvic oxidase (carbohydrate metabolism), transketolase (pentose phosphate pathway) and α-oxyglutarate oxidase (Krebs cycle).
- *Effects of deficiency.* Beriberi and the neurological disorder Wernicke–Korsakoff syndrome.

- *Risk factors for deficiency.* Diet very heavily dependent on polished rice; alcoholism.
- *Biochemical measure of nutrient status.* Erythrocyte transketolase activation coefficient (ETKAC) with values greater than 1.25 indicative of deficiency.
- *Prevalence of deficiency.* Average UK intakes around double the RNI with around 1 per cent recording intakes below the LRNI; 3 per cent of men and 1 per cent of women had ETKAC above the threshold value for thiamin deficiency.
- *Toxicity.* Few reports of any toxic effects.
- *Recommendations on high intakes.* Daily doses of 100 mg/day regarded as safe but doses well in excess of this may well be safe.
- *Typical highest UK intakes.* Thiamin-only supplements may contain as much as 300 mg/day but normal multinutrient supplements contain 1–5 mg/day.

Nature and sources

The chemical structure of thiamin is shown in Figure 13.6. Thiamin is water soluble and so can leach into cooking water. It is oxidized when heated in alkaline solution. It is found in wholegrain cereals where it is concentrated in the bran and germ layers. Much of the thiamin is removed from cereals when they are refined, e.g. when milled to produce white flour or white rice. White rice is particularly low in thiamin but white flour is fortified with thiamin in the UK and USA. Thiamin is present or added to many breakfast cereals and is found in pulses, vegetables, milk, organ meat and pork.

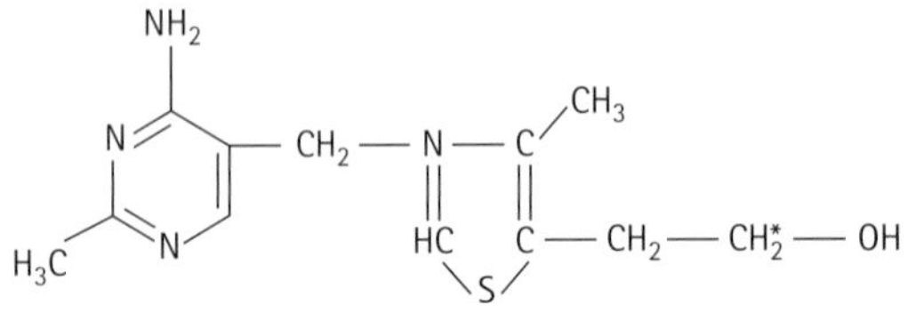

Figure 13.6 *The structure of thiamin.*

Functions

Thiamin is the precursor of the important coenzyme thiamin pyrophosphate. Thiamin pyrophosphate is formed by addition of pyrophosphate (two phosphate groups) at the position marked by the asterisk in Figure 13.6. It is an essential coenzyme in several key reactions in metabolism (see Chapter 5), including:

- conversion of pyruvate to acetyl CoA in carbohydrate metabolism
- conversion of α-ketoglutarate to succinyl CoA in the Krebs cycle
- reactions catalysed by transketolase in the pentose phosphate pathway.

In thiamin deficiency there is a progressive block at these steps in metabolism. The pyruvate dehydrogenase enzyme that converts pyruvate to acetyl CoA seems to be particularly sensitive to thiamin deficiency. Thiamin deficiency leads to an inability to metabolize carbohydrate aerobically and pyruvate and lactate accumulate in the blood and tissues. The block in the pentose phosphate pathway restricts the production of reduced NADP which is essential for lipid biosynthesis including the synthesis of **myelin** (the fatty sheath that surrounds many nerves).

Requirements and assessment of status

The estimated adult requirements for thiamin are given in the key facts section. The requirement for thiamin increases as energy expenditure increases and the UK RNI is set at 0.4 mg per 1000 kcal (4.2 MJ) and the LRNI set 0.23 mg per 1000 kcal. The **ETKAC** is used to assess thiamin status with values of greater than 1.25 taken as an indication of thiamin deficiency. The theoretical basis of these enzyme activation tests is discussed in Chapter 3.

Deficiency states

Beriberi and **Wernicke–Korsakoff syndrome** are caused by thiamin deficiency. The major symptoms of beriberi are:

- lactic acidosis
- peripheral neuropathy – degeneration of peripheral nerves with tingling and loss of sensation at the extremities followed by gradual loss of motor function, muscle wasting and paralysis (dry beriberi)
- heart failure and oedema (wet beriberi).

Wernicke–Korsakoff syndrome is the neurological and psychiatric manifestation of thiamin deficiency that is often associated with alcoholism. This syndrome is characterized by paralysis of eye movements or rapid jerky eye movements (nystagmus), unsteadiness when walking or standing and mental derangements including loss of memory and the ability to learn. Post-mortems on such patients show lesions in various parts of the brain ranging from loss of myelin to complete necrosis.

The clinical manifestations of beriberi can be largely explained by the known biochemical functions of thiamin pyrophosphate. Under conditions of normal eating, nervous tissue relies on carbohydrate metabolism for its energy generation and the metabolism of heart muscle also relies heavily on the aerobic metabolism of glucose. As thiamin deficiency impairs carbohydrate metabolism it is thus not surprising that many of the symptoms of beriberi are associated with changes in nerve and cardiac function. Production of the fatty sheath (myelin) covering nerve fibres is dependent on the enzyme transketolase in the pentose phosphate pathway; this enzyme requires thiamin pyrophosphate as a coenzyme and demyelination of nerves is a feature of beriberi and Wernicke–Korsakoff syndrome. The accumulation of lactic acid in blood and tissues that results from impaired pyruvic oxidase functioning may exacerbate the oedema of wet beriberi.

Beriberi has been known in China and the Far East for several thousand years but large-scale epidemics occurred in the late nineteenth and early twentieth centuries and were probably precipitated by the introduction of machine milling for rice. Epidemics of beriberi are associated with diets that are based on white (polished) rice. Rice is low in thiamin and if rice is efficiently milled then most of this thiamin is removed with the bran. The high carbohydrate content of rice may also increase requirements. The poorest members of these eastern societies often escaped beriberi because they ate the cheaper brown rice with its thiamin still present. Only those who could afford the more expensive and higher prestige white rice were vulnerable to this condition including the armed forces of Japan and China.

In the late nineteenth century, a Japanese naval surgeon noted that many supplementary foods were effective in curing and preventing beriberi and he proposed that it might be caused by protein deficiency. In 1890, Eijkmann noted that beriberi in patients at a military hospital in Java seemed to be associated with eating polished rice but not brown rice. He induced symptoms similar to human beriberi in chickens by feeding them with boiled polished rice. These symptoms could be prevented by feeding them rice bran. In 1926, Jansen and Donath working in Eijkmann's lab in Java purified thiamin from rice bran. Most parts of India have escaped epidemics of beriberi because of different milling practices. The rice is soaked and then steamed or boiled prior to milling (parboiled), and this greatly increases the retention of B vitamins within the rice grain after milling. Introduction of less harsh milling practices, fortification of white rice with thiamin and diversification of the diet have all contributed to the decline in beriberi. Intakes of thiamin are, however, still low in many rice-eating countries and offer little margin of safety.

It is very common for alcoholics to be thiamin deficient, and Wernicke–Korsakoff syndrome is largely confined to alcoholics. There are several reasons for this:

- the diet of alcoholics is poor and thiamin intake is low
- high alcohol intake impairs the absorption of thiamin
- alcohol may increase the requirement for thiamin
- high alcohol intake may impair the activity of the enzyme that converts thiamin to the active coenzyme thiamin pyrophosphate.

Thiamin deficiency may also contribute to **fetal alcohol syndrome**, a syndrome seen in some babies born to alcoholic mothers and described more fully in Chapter 15. Given the frequent association of manifestations of thiamin deficiency in those with excessive alcohol consumptions, there may be some grounds for suggesting high alcohol consumers who cannot be persuaded to reduce their alcohol intakes might gain some benefit from additional thiamin intakes in the form of supplements.

Riboflavin – vitamin B$_2$

Key facts

- *Names and chemical forms.* **Riboflavin** (vitamin B$_2$).
- *Dietary standards.* UK adult RNI M/F 1.3/1.1 mg/day; LRNI 0.8 mg/day in both sexes; American RDA M/F 1.3/1.1 mg/day.

- *Dietary sources.* Small amounts in many foods; rich sources are liver, milk, cheese and egg:
  - 1 slice wholemeal bread (UK) – 0.03 mg
  - 1 egg – 0.21 mg
  - 1 cup whole milk – 0.33 mg
  - 40 g cheddar cheese – 0.16 mg
  - 1 portion (90 g) fried lamb liver – 4 mg
  - 1 teaspoon (5 g) yeast extract – 0.55 mg
  - 1 serving (95 g) broccoli – 0.19 mg.
- *Biochemical functions.* Component of flavin nucleotides which are cofactors for several enzymes involved in oxidation-reduction reactions.
- *Effects of deficiency.* Cracking at the corners of the mouth; raw red lips; enlarged nasal follicles plugged with sebaceous material.
- *Risk factors for deficiency.* Absence of milk from the diet.
- *Biochemical measure of nutrient status.* The **erythrocyte glutathione reductase activation coefficient** (EGRAC) and a value of 1.3 is taken as the upper limit of normality.
- *Prevalence of deficiency.* Mild to moderate deficiency regarded as common. Around 3 per cent of UK men and 8 per cent of women have measured intakes below the LRNI with much higher numbers in the youngest age group. Two-thirds of UK adults have an EGRAC above the threshold level.
- *Toxicity.* Little evidence of toxicity in humans; its low solubility may prevent absorption of sufficient amounts to cause toxicity.
- *Recommendations on high intakes.* Regular intakes of 40 mg/day should be safe but no evidence that values well in excess of this produce any adverse effects.
- *Typical highest UK intakes.* Maximum from food sources around 4 mg/day and supplements may contain up to 100 mg/day.

Nature and sources

The structure of riboflavin is shown in Figure 13.7. Dairy products, meat, fish, eggs, liver and some green vegetables are rich sources, although it is widely distributed in many foods. Milk is an important contributor to total riboflavin intakes in the UK. Cereals are generally a poor source unless they are fortified.

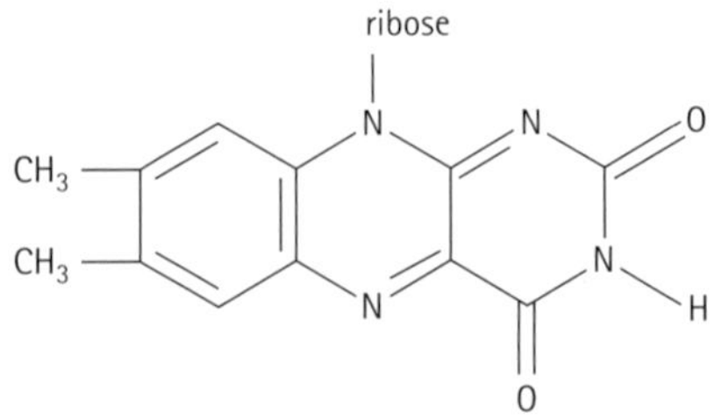

Figure 13.7 *The structure of riboflavin.*

Functions

Riboflavin gives rise to **flavin mononucleotide (FMN)** and **flavin adenine dinucleotide (FAD)**. These flavin nucleotides are essential components (prosthetic groups) of several key **flavoprotein** enzymes involved in oxidation–reduction reactions. These flavin nucleotides are used in both the Krebs cycle and oxidative phosphorylation, and so riboflavin deficiency leads to a general depression of oxidative metabolism. Glutathione reductase, an enzyme involved in disposal of free radicals, also has a flavin prosthetic group.

Requirements and assessments of status

The adult requirements for riboflavin are given in the key facts section. Riboflavin status may be assessed by the EGRAC and a value in excess of 1.3 taken to indicate poor riboflavin status. Around two-thirds of British adults have EGRAC values in excess of 1.3 with the frequency rising to around 80 per cent of those aged 19–24 years. The theoretical basis for these enzyme activation tests is discussed in Chapter 3. The high proportion of adults recording values in excess of the threshold value for the EGRAC may indicate the need to re-evaluate the suitability of this threshold value.

Riboflavin deficiency

Mild riboflavin deficiency has long been considered to be relatively common even in industrialized countries but no severe and characteristic deficiency disease has been described for this vitamin. This may be because the wide distribution of small amounts of the vitamin in food prevents mild deficiency progressing to major life-threatening illness. Also, riboflavin deficiency is usually associated with concurrent beriberi and the severe symptoms of beriberi mask the symptoms of riboflavin deficiency. In volunteers deliberately made riboflavin deficient, the following symptoms have been observed:

- chapping at the corners of the mouth (angular stomatitis)
- raw red lips (cheilosis)
- enlarged follicles around the sides of the nose which become plugged with yellow sebaceous material (nasolabial seborrhoea).

Niacin – vitamin B3

Key facts

- *Names and chemical forms.* **Niacin/nicotinic acid**, vitamin B_3; it may also be synthesized from the amino acid tryptophan. The amount in food is expressed as **niacin equivalents**.

- *Dietary standards.* UK RNI M/F 17/13 mg niacin equivalents/day; LRNI M/F 11/9; American RDA M/F 16/14.

- *Dietary sources.* Widely distributed in small amounts in many foods but good amounts in meat, offal, fish, wholemeal cereals and pulses; in some cereals, especially maize, much of the niacin may be as unavailable niacytin; the tryptophan in many food proteins is also a potential source of niacin:
  - 1 slice wholemeal bread (UK) –
    1.4 mg + 0.6 mg from tryptophan
  - 1 portion (90 g) lamb liver – 13.7 mg + 4.4 mg
  - 1 pork chop – 6.1 mg + 4.9 mg
  - 1 serving (95 g) canned tuna – 12.3 mg + 4.1 mg
  - 1 egg – 0.04 mg + 2.2 mg
  - 1 cup whole milk – 0.16 mg + 1.5 mg
  - 1 portion (75 g) frozen peas – 1.1 mg + 0.7 mg

- *Biochemical functions.* Component of NAD and NADP, which are coenzymes involved in many oxidation–reduction reactions.

- *Effects of deficiency.* Pellagra.

- *Risk factors for deficiency.* A diet that is heavily dependent on maize (or sorghum) and not supplemented by high-protein foods.

- *Biochemical measure of nutrient status.* Urinary N' methyl nicotinamide excretion mg/nicotinamide/g creatinine. Values above 1.6 mg/g indicate normality and values less than 0.5 indicate frank deficiency.

- *Prevalence of deficiency.* Given the high protein content of current diets, then deficiency is unlikely in industrialized countries.

- *Toxicity.* High doses of nicotinic acid have been used to lower plasma cholesterol and this led to reports of adverse symptoms associated with these high pharmacological doses such as flushing, itching, nausea and vomiting.

- *Recommendations on high intakes.* Doses of nicotinamide of up to 500 mg/day should not have any adverse effects.

- *Typical highest UK intakes.* The highest consumers will take in around 60 mg/day from food (as tryptophan and niacin). Multivitamins may contain up to 150 mg/day and single niacin preparations up to 250 mg/day.

Nature and sources

Niacin is also called nicotinic acid and is designated vitamin B_3. Its chemical structure is shown in Figure 13.8. Pre-formed niacin is found in red meat, liver, pulses, milk, wholegrain cereals, fish and it is added to white flour and many breakfast cereals. Much of the niacin present in cereals may be in a bound form that is not readily available to humans.

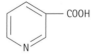

Figure 13.8 *The structure of niacin (nicotinic acid).*

The amino acid tryptophan can also act as a source of niacin. Niacin can therefore be obtained from the diet either directly as vitamin present in the food or indirectly by the conversion of tryptophan in dietary protein to niacin. This means that early suggestions that pellagra was due to protein deficiency were partly correct because high-protein foods, by providing tryptophan, could permit endogenous niacin synthesis and cure or prevent deficiency. The niacin content of foods and diets is expressed in milligrams of **niacin equivalents**.

In calculating the niacin equivalents in a food then 60 mg of tryptophan is usually taken to be equivalent to 1 mg of niacin. In the typical British or American diet, tryptophan makes up just over 1 per cent of the total dietary protein.

1 mg niacin equivalent = 1 mg niacin or 60 mg tryptophan

Functions

Niacin is a component of the important coenzymes NAD and the phosphorylated derivative NADP. NAD and NADP serve as hydrogen acceptors and donators in numerous oxidation and reduction reactions in all human biochemical pathways. It is during the re-oxidation of the reduced NAD, produced during the oxidation of foodstuffs, that most of the ATP yielded by aerobic metabolism is produced in the mitochondria of human cells (see Chapter 5).

Dietary requirements and assessment of status

The adult dietary standards for niacin are given in the key facts section. The requirement for niacin varies with energy expenditure and the UK RNI is set at 6.6 mg of niacin equivalents per 1000 kcal (4.2 MJ). There is no ideal method for assessing niacin status, but the urinary excretion of N' methyl nicotinamide is one method that can be used. This is usually expressed as milligrams nicotinamide per gram of creatine in the urine because this value is more meaningful than simple urinary concentration, which obviously fluctuates according to fluid intake.

Niacin deficiency

Niacin deficiency causes the disease **pellagra**. The symptoms of the disease are often referred to as the 3Ds – dermatitis, diarrhoea and dementia – and if it prolonged and severe then the fourth D is death. An early sign of pellagra is itching and burning of the skin which becomes roughened and thickened; skin exposed to sunlight is most liable to show dermatitis and a ring of affected skin around the neck (Casal's collar) is a common manifestation. Gastrointestinal symptoms, including diarrhoea, are a characteristic manifestation of pellagra. Early neurological symptoms are weakness, tremor, anxiety, depression and irritability and, if there is severe prolonged deficiency, eventually dementia. The disease has high mortality and at its peak in the late 1920s and early 1930s caused thousands deaths in the southern USA. It is still endemic in parts of southern Africa.

Pellagra has usually been associated with diets based on maize. Maize protein is low in tryptophan and the pre-formed niacin present in maize is present in a bound form (**niacytin**) that is unavailable to humans. Introduction of maize from the Americas has been associated with major epidemics in those parts of the

world where it became established as the dominant staple, e.g. in southern Europe, north Africa and south Africa. In the early decades of this century it was so prevalent in some southern states of the USA that it was thought to be an infectious disease.

Davies (1964) gave an analysis of the factors that led to the rise and fall of pellagra in the southern USA. At the turn of the twentieth century the diets of poor Southerners were based on corn (maize), pork fat and molasses. The first recorded outbreak of pellagra in the southern USA was in 1907 and Davies attributes this to changes in the way that the corn was milled. At the turn of the century, large-scale machine milling replaced the old inefficient water driven mills and this harsher milling produced a finer and more palatable corn meal. However, it also removed the germ of the corn grain and reduced its vitamin content. Paradoxically the disease started to decline at the height of the Great Depression. Davies suggests that this was because demand for cotton, the principal agricultural product of the region, declined sharply leading many farmers to cultivate gardens and smallholdings to produce food crops. He thus attributes the decline in pellagra, at a time of great economic deprivation, to departure from the cash-crop monoculture rather than to increased knowledge of the causes of the disease and methods of prevention. Note that introduction of machine milling may have been an important factor in precipitating epidemics of both beriberi and pellagra. Harsh machine milling is very efficient at removing the nutrient-rich outer layers of the cereal grain. Traditional hand milling methods were less efficient in removing these outer layers and left more of the vitamins in the final product.

Among the people of Central America, where maize originated, its consumption was not associated with pellagra. The traditional method of tortilla preparation resulted in the release of niacin from its bound state; the maize grains were mixed with slaked lime (calcium hydroxide) and subject to prolonged heating prior to grinding and cooking.

Sorghum consumption is associated with pellagra in some parts of India and China despite the fact that sorghum contains reasonable amounts of tryptophan (almost as much as rice, which is not pellagragenic). Bender (1983) concluded that this is because of the high content of another amino acid, leucine, in sorghum, which inhibits key enzymes in the conversion of tryptophan to niacin. The high leucine content of maize may also increase its potential to cause pellagra.

Vitamin B₆ – pyridoxine

Vitamin B$_6$ – pyridoxine

> ### Key facts
>
> - *Names and dietary forms.* **Pyridoxine** and related compounds are collectively termed vitamin B$_6$.
> - *Dietary standards.* UK RNI M/F 1.4/1.2 mg/day; UK LRNI M/F 1.0/0.9 mg/day; American RDA 1.3 mg/day for both sexes.
> - *Dietary sources.* Liver is a rich source, cereals, meats, fruits and vegetables all contain moderate amounts.
> - *Biochemical functions.* Precursor of pyridoxal phosphate, a coenzyme involved in amino acid metabolism.
> - *Effects of deficiency.* Overt deficiency rare, convulsions reported in infants fed on B$_6$-depleted formula.
> - *Risk factors for deficiency.* Overt deficiency is rare.
> - *Biochemical measure of nutrient status.* The **erythrocyte aspartate aminotransferase activation coefficient (EAATAC)** with values of greater than 2.0 indicative of vitamin B$_6$ deficiency.
> - *Prevalence of deficiency.* 5 per cent of young women (19–24 years) in the UK have recorded intakes that are below the LRNI and more than 10 per cent of adults have EAATAC values above 2.0, i.e. biochemical indication of B$_6$ deficiency.
> - *Toxicity.* In animal studies, high doses of vitamin B$_6$ have been shown to be neurotoxic with abnormalities in gait and balance and histological evidence of peripheral nerve damage. There have been some reports of sensory neuropathy in people taking large supplemental doses with early symptoms being tingling sensations in the hands and feet.
> - *Recommendations on high intakes.* A lifetime dose of 10 mg/day should pose no risk but there are insufficient data to judge whether doses well in excess of this are safe.
> - *Typical highest UK intakes.* Food may contain up to 4 mg/day and although most supplements contain up to 10 mg/day a few provide as much as 100 mg/day.

Nature and sources

Vitamin B$_6$ is present in food as pyridoxine, pyridoxal or pyridoxamine, which are all biologically active and inter-convertible. The structures of these are given in Figure 13.9.

The different forms of vitamin B$_6$ are widely distributed in both plant and animal foods. Liver, eggs, meat, fish, green leafy vegetables, pulses, fruits and wholegrain cereals all contain significant amounts of B$_6$.

Functions

Vitamin B$_6$ is a precursor of the important coenzyme pyridoxal phosphate. This coenzyme is essential in many biochemical reactions particularly those involving the metabolism of amino acids. Some of the reactions/pathways where pyridoxal phosphate acts as a coenzyme are:

- **transamination** reactions – transfer of amino groups to produce non essential amino acids (see Chapter 5)
- decarboxylation of amino acids, e.g. to produce the nerve transmitters γ-aminobutyric acid (GABA), histamine, dopamine and 5-hydroxytryptamine (5-HT; serotonin)
- synthesis of niacin from tryptophan

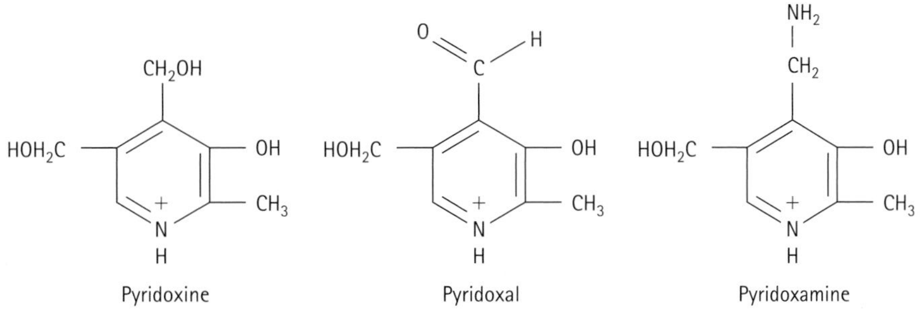

Figure 13.9 *The structure of the three forms of vitamin B$_6$.*

- breakdown of glycogen by the enzyme glycogen phosphorylase
- synthesis of the haem component of haemoglobin.

Requirements and assessment of status

The adult requirements for vitamin B_6 are given in the key facts section. A wide range of tests of vitamin B_6 status have been developed including the measurement of pyridoxal phosphate concentrations in blood or erythrocytes. Erythrocyte enzyme reactivation tests (see Chapter 3) using the EAATAC or alanine amino transferase are used as measures of long-term B_6 status and the critical value for the EAATAC is given in the key facts section.

Deficiency and toxicity

Overt primary dietary deficiency of vitamin B_6 is rare. In the 1950s B_6 deficiency was seen in some American babies who had been fed formula depleted of its vitamin B_6 by a fault in the processing. These babies had convulsions and abnormal findings on electroencephalography. Symptoms of deficiency in adults include anaemia, raw red lips, smooth inflamed tongue, lesions at the corners of the mouth, dermatitis and fatigue. Note that although overt symptomatic deficiency is rarely seen, many British adults have unsatisfactory status for this vitamin. Certain drugs used in the treatment of tuberculosis, rheumatoid arthritis and epilepsy increase the requirement for B_6 and supplements of the vitamin are usually given with these drugs.

There has been much speculation about whether vitamin B_6 alleviates the symptoms of pre-menstrual syndrome primarily because of its involvement in the synthesis of nerve transmitters. It has been widely used as a self-medication for this purpose. Some cases of B_6 toxicity have been reported in women who consume very large doses of this vitamin on a long-term basis. The symptoms are sensory neuropathy of the hands and feet. FSA (2003) suggested a safe lifetime dose of 10 mg/day largely on the basis of animal studies that have found that high doses of the vitamin can be neurotoxic. Although there are reports of sensory neuropathy in people taking higher doses (up to 200 mg/day) FSA felt that there were insufficient data to judge the risk posed by such doses.

Vitamin B_{12} – cobalamins

Key facts

- *Names and chemical forms.* **Cyanocobalamin** and related compounds are collectively termed vitamin B_{12}.
- *Dietary standards.* UK RNI 1.5 μg/day; UK LRNI 1 μg/day; American RDA 2.4 μg/day.
- *Dietary sources.* Meat (especially organ meat), fish, milk, eggs and fermented foods or foods contaminated with mould or other micro-organisms. Note that the algal product *Spirulina* is not a source of active vitamin B_{12} despite having been promoted as such, although another algal product *Chlorella* does contain the active vitamin.
- *Biochemical functions.* Interacts with folate in methylation reactions necessary for DNA synthesis and cell division; required for production of the myelin sheath around many nerves.
- *Effects of deficiency.* Megaloblastic anaemia; degeneration of the spinal cord leading to progressive paralysis.
- *Risk factors for deficiency.* Vegan diet; poor absorption as in pernicious anaemia due to inadequate production of intrinsic factor by the parietal cells of the stomach.
- *Biochemical measure of nutrient status.* Serum B_{12} concentration with a value of 118 pmol/L taken as the lower limit of normality in adults.
- *Prevalence of deficiency.* Average intakes are three to four times the RNI. Less than 1 per cent of adults have unsatisfactory intakes; 2 per cent of men and 4 per cent of women have blood levels indicative of deficiency suggesting that inadequate absorption is the main factor causing deficiency. Note that 6 per cent of free-living elderly UK adults and 9 per cent of those living in institutions have blood levels below the threshold value.
- *Toxicity.* High oral intakes are poorly absorbed and excessive amounts in blood are excreted in urine so potential for toxicity is low.
- *Recommendations on high intakes.* Long-term consumption of 2 mg/day should not produce any adverse effects.
- *Typical highest UK intakes.* Some UK adults may get as much as 20 μg/day from food, and supplements may provide up to 3 mg/day.

Nature and sources

Vitamin B_{12} comprises a group of complex molecules, which contain the element cobalt. The structure of cyanocobalamin is given in Figure 13.10. All of the vitamin B_{12} ordinarily present in the diet is in foods of animal origin. The ultimate source of the cobalamins is their synthesis by micro-organisms and any foods contaminated by micro-organisms will contain B_{12}.

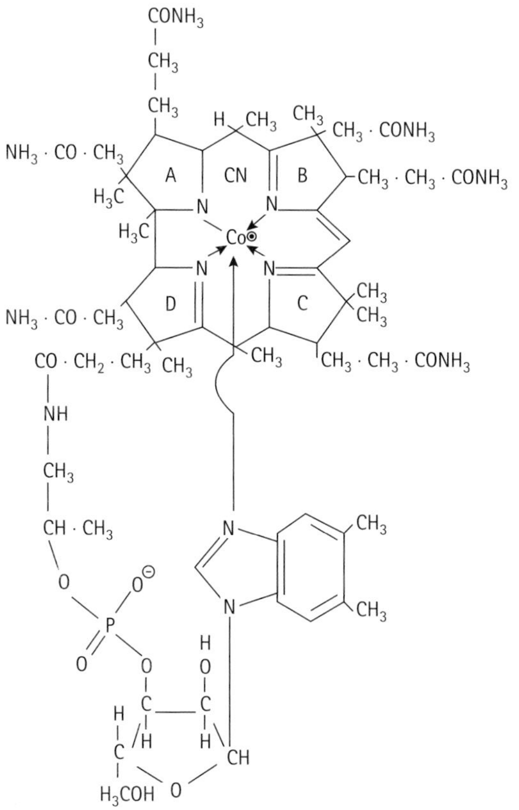

Figure 13.10 *The structure of cyanocobalamin (vitamin B_{12}).*

Functions

Together with folic acid, vitamin B_{12} is essential for the synthesis of the nucleotide thymidylate. This nucleotide is found exclusively in DNA and so its production is essential for DNA synthesis and cell division. This means that cell division including the production of red blood cells will be impaired by lack of B_{12} or folic acid. Vitamin B_{12} is also required as a coenzyme for a reaction that is essential for the metabolism of fatty acids with odd numbers of carbon atoms (methylmalonyl CoA conversion to succinyl CoA).

Requirements and assessment of status

Human requirements for vitamin B_{12} are only 1–2 µg/day and healthy omnivorous adults have several years' supply stored in their livers. Vitamin B_{12} status is assessed by measurement of serum B_{12} concentrations. Quantitative details are given in the key facts section.

Deficiency of B_{12}

Lack of vitamin B_{12} or folic acid causes a macrocytic (large cell) or **megaloblastic anaemia.** In this type of anaemia red blood cells are large, irregular and fragile. In severe cases, the blood haemoglobin concentration may fall to less than a third of the normal level. Dietetic lack of B_{12} is rare and usually associated with a strict vegetarian (**vegan**) diet. Folic acid deficiency is, on the other hand, common in some developing countries and high intakes of folic acid can compensate for lack of B_{12} and mask the haematological consequences of B_{12} deficiency. Prolonged B_{12} deficiency also leads to irreversible damage to the spinal cord – **combined subacute degeneration.** This nerve damage manifests initially as loss of sensation or tingling sensation in the fingers and toes which leads to progressive paralysis. These consequences of B_{12} deficiency on the nervous system are not corrected by folic acid and so misdiagnosis and treatment of B_{12} deficiency with folic acid may mask the haematological consequences but allow the insidious progression of the irreversible spinal cord damage; this is one potential danger if common foods are supplemented with folic acid.

Vitamin B_{12} is naturally confined to foods of animal origin and to micro-organisms, although meat substitutes must contain added B_{12} in the UK. This means that strict vegetarians (vegans) may avoid all foods that naturally contain B_{12} and thus be at risk of dietary deficiency of the vitamin unless they eat supplemented foods or take B_{12} supplements. In practice, even among those theoretically at risk, dietary deficiency is uncommon because requirements are very small and an omnivore has stores that represent several years' turnover of the vitamin. Contamination of food with micro-organisms, insects, faecal matter or perhaps synthesis by gut bacteria may contribute significant amounts of B_{12} to the diet of even the strictest vegetarian (e.g. mould on nuts, insects or insect droppings on fruit or vegetables). Algal preparations like *Spirulina* and *Chlorella* have been marketed as sources of vitamin B_{12} that are suitable for vegetarians but the form of the vitamin found in *Spirulina* is almost certainly not active in humans (Watanabe *et al.*, 1999) although that in *Chlorella* is bioavailable (Kittaka-Katsura *et al.*, 2002). Some lactovegetarian Asian women in the UK develop signs of deficiency despite the presence of B_{12} in milk – this is explained by suggesting that the traditional practice of boiling milk with tea may destroy the B_{12} in the milk. It may take many years of dietary deficiency of vitamin B_{12} before clinical symptoms of deficiency manifest in adults.

The usual cause of B_{12} deficiency is not dietary lack but inadequate absorption. An autoimmune disease, **pernicious anaemia**, results in damage to the parietal cells of the stomach that produce an **intrinsic factor** that is necessary for the absorption of B_{12} from the gut. Until the 1920s, pernicious anaemia was an inevitably fatal condition; nowadays the effects of the resulting B_{12} deficiency can be alleviated by monthly injections of the vitamin. The efficiency of absorption of vitamin B_{12} declines in elderly people.

Folate – folic acid, folacin

Key facts

- *Names and chemical forms.* **Folate/folic acid** (folacin). Note that folate is the generic name for all dietary forms but folic acid refers to the parent compound used in supplements but not normally present in food.
- *Dietary standards.* UK RNI 200 μg/day (note that women of childbearing age currently recommended to take supplements of 400 μg/day); UK LRNI 100 μg/day; American RDA 400 μg/day.
- *Dietary sources.* Liver, nuts, green vegetables, wholegrain cereals are good sources:
  - 1 portion (90 g) lamb liver – 220 μg
  - 1 slice wholemeal bread (UK)–14 μg
  - 30 g peanuts – 33 μg
  - portion (95 g) broccoli – 100 μg
  - 1 banana – 30 μg
  - 1 orange – 90 μg
  - 1 teaspoon (5 g) yeast extract – 50 μg.

- *Biochemical functions.* Involved with B_{12} in methylation reactions necessary for DNA synthesis and thus important in cell division.
- *Effects of deficiency.* Megaloblastic anaemia; see also neural tube defects (Chapter 15).
- *Risk factors for deficiency.* Poor diet – deficiency common in tropical countries; prolonged heating (e.g. of pulses) destroys folate; poor absorption, e.g. in coeliac disease; some drugs (e.g. anticonvulsants) may interfere with folate functioning.
- *Biochemical measure of nutritional status.* Red cell folate concentration with values below 230 nmol/L considered to indicate severe deficiency and values less than 345 nmol/L indicative of marginal deficiency.
- *Prevalence of deficiency.* 4–5 per cent of UK adults have red cell folate levels indicative of marginal status but less than 1 per cent have values indicating severe deficiency. In elderly people in the UK, 8 per cent of free-living subjects and 16 per cent of those living in institutions have red cell folate concentrations indicative of severe deficiency and another 20 per cent have marginal values.
- *Toxicity.* Direct toxicity is very low but high doses can mask the haematological effects of vitamin B_{12} deficiency. However, they do not prevent the damage to the spinal cord. It may also reduce the effectiveness of drugs that work by affecting folate metabolism.
- *Recommendations on high intakes.* Doses of up to 1.5 mg/day should not have any adverse effects but note previous section.
- *Typical highest UK intakes.* The highest consumers may get in excess of 500 μg/day from food and supplements aimed at women, may provide up to 800 μg/day.

Nature and sources

Folic acid or pteroylmonoglutamic acid is the parent compound for a group of substances known collectively as folate or folacin in the USA. Folic acid is made up of three components – pteridine, *para*-amino benzoic acid (PABA) and glutamic acid (see Figure 13.11). Within the body, metabolically active folates have multiple glutamic acid residues conjugated to them. Also the pteridine ring is usually reduced to dihydrofolate or tetrahydrofolate and there are various single carbon units that can be

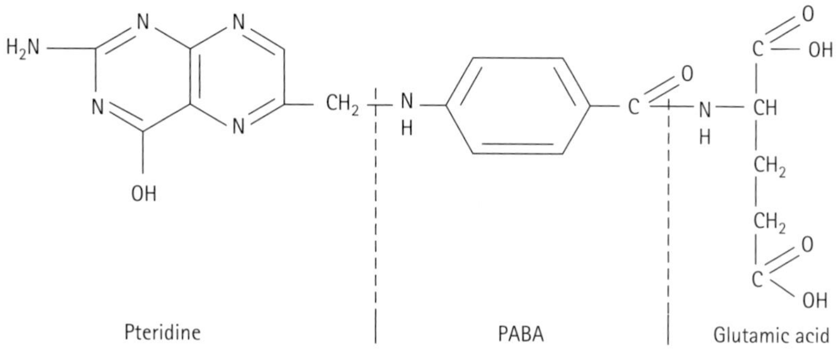

Figure 13.11 *The structure of folic acid. PABA, para-amino benzoic acid.*

attached to the nitrogen atoms in this ring (see Ball, 2004 for details of the structures of the different forms of folate). Folates are found in good amounts in green vegetables, liver, yeast extract, mushrooms, nuts and wholegrains. It has been a source of considerable controversy that the only permitted form of folate in the EU Food Supplements Directive is folic acid itself rather than the conjugated forms which are usually present in food.

Functions

Folate interacts with vitamin B_{12} in the transfer of methyl groups. The synthesis of thymidylate, the nucleotide necessary for DNA synthesis, involves methyl transfer and requires both folate and B_{12}. As with B_{12}, deficiency of folic acid limits DNA synthesis and thus cell division.

Requirements and assessment of folate status

The estimated adult requirements for folate are given in the key facts above. Long-term folate status can be assessed by measurements of red cell folate concentrations. The critical values are also given in the key facts above. Serum folate concentration is used as a measure of recent folate consumption.

Folate deficiency

Megaloblastic or macrocytic anaemia is a symptom of both folic acid and B_{12} deficiency. The bone marrow's ability to produce blood cells is affected by the reduced ability to synthesize thymidylate and thus DNA. Large, immature and unstable red cells are found circulating in the blood in megaloblastic anaemia as well as abnormal white cells and platelets. Other rapidly dividing tissues are also affected, such as the gut lining. High doses of folic acid will mask the haematological consequences of

B_{12} deficiency but will not prevent the neurological consequences so it is important that the cause of megaloblastic anaemia is determined before treatment is undertaken. Some degree of folate deficiency is relatively common in those living on a poor diet in developing countries, i.e. a diet lacking in green vegetables and pulses and made up largely of a low folate starchy staple. Several drugs, including some antiepileptics, increase folate requirements and alcoholics often have poor folate status. Folate deficiency may also be precipitated by diseases that affect absorption of folate, e.g. coeliac disease and tropical sprue.

There is now overwhelming evidence that folate supplements given preconceptually and in early pregnancy reduce the risk of the baby developing a **neural tube defect**. All women are now advised to take folic acid supplements in the first trimester of pregnancy and ideally all women at risk of becoming pregnant should take supplements. Some foods are now fortified with folic acid in an attempt to increase the folic acid status of women who have unplanned pregnancies and in a few countries there is mandatory or widespread fortification (see Chapter 15 for further discussion of this issue).

There is now preliminary evidence which suggests that increased intakes of folic acid may have more widespread benefits. Homocystinuria is an inherited condition in which there is increased concentration of the amino acid homocysteine in blood. This homocysteine is toxic to vascular endothelial cells, promotes LDL oxidation and increases the risk of thrombosis (COMA, 1994a). It has been suggested that perhaps more mildly elevated levels of homocysteine may also increase the risk of cardiovascular disease and that folic acid supplements may lower homocysteine levels and thus reduce the risk of cardiovascular disease (reviewed in Ball, 2004).

Biotin

Key facts

- *Names and chemical forms.* **Biotin.**
- *Dietary standards.* UK 'safe intake' 10–200 μg/day; USA 30 μg/day.
- *Dietary sources.* Widely distributed in many foods at low concentrations but good amounts in liver and organ meat, egg yolk, wholegrain cereals and yeast.
- *Biochemical functions.* A cofactor for several carboxylase enzymes that add carboxyl or —COOH groups.
- *Effects of deficiency.* Dermatitis and other symptoms.
- *Risk factors for deficiency.* Simple dietary deficiency is rare – can occur as a side effect of certain treatments like dialysis or **total parenteral nutrition** or in some rare genetic abnormalities.
- *Biochemical measure of nutritional status.* Plasma biotin with values below 1.02 nmol/L thought to indicate deficiency – rarely measured.
- *Prevalence of deficiency.* Nutritional deficiency is rare.
- *Toxicity.* Little evidence of toxicity associated with oral biotin consumption.
- *Recommendations on high intakes.* Doses of up to 0.9 mg/day should not have any adverse effects but doses 10 times higher than this have no reported adverse effects.
- *Typical highest UK intakes.* The highest UK consumers may get around 70 μg/day from food and over-the-counter supplements may contain up to 2 mg/day.

General overview

Biotin was originally known as the 'anti egg white injury factor' because it cured a dermatitis induced in rats by feeding them large amounts of raw egg white. A protein present in raw egg white inhibits the absorption of biotin but this is denatured when eggs are cooked. Biotin deficiency in humans is rare and usually associated with eating large amounts of raw egg or other bizarre diets. It has been reported in the past in patients being fed by total parenteral nutrition for long periods. Human milk is relatively low in biotin and some cases of biotin-responsive dermatitis have been reported in babies breastfed by poorly nourished mothers.

Biotin functions as a coenzyme for several important carboxylase enzymes, i.e. enzymes that add a carboxyl (COOH) group via fixation of carbon dioxide. The enzyme pyruvate carboxylase is important in gluconeogenesis (production of glucose from pyruvate and amino acids – see Chapter 5). Other carboxylase enzymes are important in fatty acid synthesis (acetyl CoA carboxylase) and the metabolism of branched chain amino acids.

Biotin requirements have not been clearly established partly because gut bacteria may make some indeterminate contribution to biotin supply but the current dietary standards are given in the key facts above. Biotin is present in good amounts in liver, cooked eggs, cereals and yeast.

Pantothenic acid

Key facts

- *Names and chemical forms.* Pantothenic acid; it is present as coenzyme A in food.
- *Dietary standards.* UK 'safe intake' 3–7 mg/day; USA 5 mg/day.
- *Dietary sources.* Present as CoA in most animal and plant cells so widely distributed in foods.
- *Biochemical functions.* It is the precursor of coenzyme A (CoA) and CoA-containing compounds are key intermediates in many biochemical pathways, e.g. acetyl CoA and succinyl CoA.
- *Effects of deficiency.* 'Burning feet syndrome', in which there are abnormal skin sensations induced by warmth, has been associated with deficiency of pantothenic acid.
- *Biochemical measure of nutritional status.* A plasma pantothenic acid concentration of less than 100 μg/L is indicative of low intake but it is rarely measured.
- *Prevalence of deficiency.* Overt dietary deficiency rarely seen.
- *Toxicity.* No reports of toxic effects.

- *Recommendations on high intakes.* Supplemental doses of 200 mg/day should not have any harmful effects although no harmful effects have been reported with doses over 10 times this amount.
- *Typical highest UK intakes.* Food may provide up to 12 mg/day and over-the-counter supplements may contain 550 mg/day.

Pantothenic acid is a precursor of coenzyme A which is essential for many metabolic processes – note the acetyl CoA in carbohydrate and fatty acid metabolism and the succinyl CoA of the Krebs cycle. The vitamin is widely distributed in food and clinical deficiency is rare. A 'burning feet' syndrome has been reported in severely malnourished prisoners of war and in experimental deficiency. Requirements for pantothenic acid are difficult to estimate accurately.

Vitamin C – ascorbic acid

Key facts

- *Nature and chemical forms.* **Ascorbic acid.**
- *Dietary standards.* UK RNI 40 mg/day; UK LRNI 10 mg/day; USA RDA M/F 90/75 mg/day.
- *Dietary sources.* Fruit, fruit juices, salad and leafy vegetables are good sources:
  - 1 serving (95 g) broccoli – 30 mg
  - 1 serving (75 g) frozen peas – 10 mg
  - 1 portion (150 g) boiled potatoes – 14 mg
  - 1 portion (45 g) sweet pepper – 45 mg
  - 1 tomato – 15 mg
  - 1 orange – 95 mg
  - 1 banana – 8 mg
  - 1 serving (100 g) strawberries – 60 mg
  - 1 apple – 2 mg
  - 1 glass (200 g) orange juice – 70 mg.
- *Biochemical functions.* Important in synthesis of collagen; promotes non-haem iron absorption; cofactor in synthesis of carnitine, synthesis of several nerve transmitters and peptide hormones. An important water-soluble antioxidant.
- *Effects of deficiency.* Scurvy.
- *Risk factors for deficiency.* Living on preserved foods, absence of fruit and vegetables from the diet.
- *Biochemical measure of nutritional status.* Plasma vitamin C concentrations of less than 11 μmol/L are indicative of biochemical depletion.
- *Prevalence of deficiency.* 5 per cent of UK adult men and 3 per cent of women had plasma concentrations below the threshold value. Around 14 per cent of free-living elderly UK adults had plasma levels below the threshold and this rose to around 40 per cent in those living in institutions.
- *Toxicity.* Several grams of vitamin C can cause diarrhoea due to unabsorbed vitamin entering the large bowel. There are claims that high doses can increase the risk of calcium oxalate kidney stones because oxalate is a metabolite of the vitamin but the data are conflicting.
- *Recommendations on high intakes.* Doses of 1 g/day are unlikely to have any significant adverse effects even in susceptible groups and doses well in excess of this are widely used without any apparent ill effects.
- *Typical highest UK intakes.* The highest consumers may get 200 mg/day from food and supplements may provide as much as 3 g/day.

Nature and sources

The structure of vitamin C or ascorbic acid is shown in Figure 13.12. Most species are able to make ascorbic acid from glucose but primates, guinea pigs, bats and some birds lack a key enzyme (gulonolactone oxidase) on this synthetic pathway. Details of this synthetic pathway may be found in Gropper *et al.* (2004). Ascorbic acid is water-soluble and in solution is readily oxidized to dehydroascorbic acid and thus it acts as an antioxidant. It is sometimes used in food processing as an antioxidant.

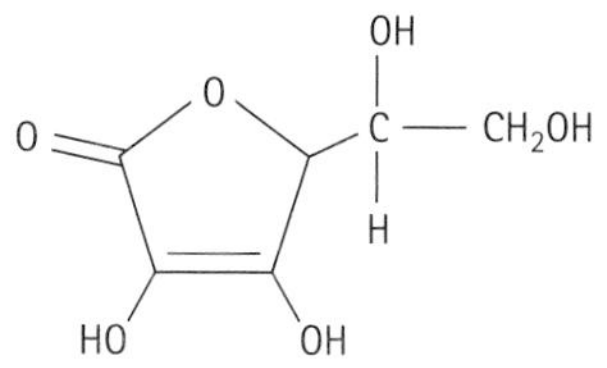

Figure 13.12 *The structure of vitamin C (ascorbic acid).*

Fruits and vegetables (including potatoes) are the classical sources of vitamin C. Significant amounts of vitamin C are also present in offal and fresh cow milk. There may even be traces in fresh raw meat and fish. Because of its use as an antioxidant additive, it may also be present in foods such as ham, sausages and pâté.

Functions

Vitamin C (ascorbic acid) is necessary for the functioning of the enzyme **proline hydroxylase**. This enzyme hydroxylates residues of the amino acid proline to hydroxyproline once it has been incorporated into the important structural protein **collagen**. Collagen is a major structural protein, it has the capacity to form strong insoluble fibres; it is the most abundant protein in mammals and serves to hold cells together. It is a structural component of bones, skin, cartilage, blood vessels and indeed fulfils a structural role in most organs. The hydroxylation of proline residues occurs after incorporation of the amino acid into procollagen (the precursor of collagen) and the hydroxylation is necessary for the structural properties of collagen; hydroxyproline is almost exclusively confined to collagen. A similar vitamin C dependent hydroxylation of lysine residues in procollagen also occurs. Some other functions of vitamin C are given below.

- It acts as an antioxidant in the aqueous phase (see Chapter 12).
- It is a cofactor in the synthesis of the important nerve transmitter noradrenaline (norepinephrine).
- It is a cofactor in the synthesis of carnitine, which is necessary for the transfer of long-chain fatty acids into the mitochondrion where β-oxidation occurs.
- Large doses of vitamin C increase the absorption of non-haem iron from the gut.
- It is involved in the synthesis of several peptide hormones and transmitters, e.g. oxytocin, gastrin, calcitonin and antidiuretic hormone. These hormones all have a glycine residue at their C-terminal that has to be converted to an amide to make the active hormone.

Requirements and assessment of status

The dietary standards for vitamin C are shown in the key facts above. Vitamin C status can be assessed by measurement of plasma vitamin C concentration and values below 11 µmol/L are taken as indicative of biochemical depletion.

Deficiency states

Scurvy is the disease caused by lack of vitamin C. Most of the symptoms of scurvy can be attributed to impaired synthesis of the structural protein collagen, i.e. bleeding gums, loose teeth, subdermal haemorrhages due to leaking blood vessels, impaired wound healing and breakdown of old scars. Large areas of spontaneous bruising occur in severe scurvy and haemorrhages in heart muscle or the brain may cause sudden death. Sudden death from haemorrhage or heart failure may occur even when the outward manifestations of scurvy do not appear particularly severe. Anaemia is usually associated with scurvy almost certainly because vitamin C is an important promoter of iron absorption from the gut. The organic bone matrix is largely collagen and so osteoporosis may also occur in scurvy.

Scurvy occurs in people deprived of fresh foods for extended periods, especially diets lacking in both fruits and vegetables. Outbreaks of scurvy commonly occurred among people living for extended periods on preserved foods, e.g. those undertaking long sea voyages or taking part in expeditions to places where fresh foods were unavailable. The curative and preventative effects of fresh vegetables, fruits and fruit juices were documented almost two centuries before the discovery of vitamin C. In 1795, the regular provision of lime juice (or some suitable alternative) to British naval personnel resulted in the 'limey' nickname for British sailors. This nickname is still sometimes used to describe the British.

Benefits and risks of high intakes

Around 10 mg/day of vitamin C is enough to prevent scurvy but some sources recommend intakes of several grams per day for 'optimal health'. This issue is covered in Chapter 12 where the role of vitamin C as an antioxidant is discussed with the conclusion that there is no convincing evidence to support the suggestion that high supplemental intakes of vitamin C (or any other antioxidant) reduce the long-term risk of developing cancer or cardiovascular disease. Many people take very large doses of vitamin C (1–5 g/day) without any obvious toxic effects. When the body pool of the vitamin exceeds 1500 mg, it starts to be excreted in the urine along with its metabolites because the reabsorption system for vitamin C in the kidney becomes saturated.

The UK panel on dietary reference values (COMA, 1991) listed at least eight benefits that have been suggested for intakes of vitamin C that are well in excess of those needed to prevent or to cure scurvy. The panel was nevertheless not persuaded to allow any of these suggested benefits to influence its decisions about the reference values for vitamin C. The size of the body pool of vitamin C is maximized at intakes of 100–150 mg/day. At higher intakes, the absorption of vitamin C from the intestine becomes saturated and there is increased renal excretion of vitamin C. It has been suggested at one time or another that high intakes might have the following beneficial effects:

- a serum cholesterol-lowering effect
- improved physical work capacity
- improved immune function
- reduced formation of carcinogenic substances called nitrosamines in the stomach and thus reduced risk of stomach cancer
- improved male fertility
- extended survival time in patients with terminal cancer when gram quantities are administered. There is no consistent or persuasive evidence to support this
- impaired wound healing and dental problems are symptoms of vitamin C deficiency and so supplements might have beneficial effects on wound healing and gum health for those with low baseline status.

Perhaps the most persistent of these claims is that intakes of more than 10 times the RNI/RDA for vitamin C might help prevent the development of the common cold. This view was popularized by a book published in the early 1970s written by the double Nobel prize winner Linus Pauling (1972). The original basis for advocating very high intakes of vitamin C was based largely on either cross-species extrapolations of the amounts synthesized by the rat or on the amounts consumed by other primates requiring vitamin C such as gorillas.

Since 1970 there have been dozens of controlled trials on the efficacy of vitamin C in preventing colds and/or reducing their duration. Despite this plethora of research effort there remains no convincing evidence that high vitamin C intakes affects the frequency of colds. In a meta-analysis of 29 clinical trials involving over 11 000 subjects, Douglas et al. (2004) found no evidence that vitamin C supplements reduced the risk of developing a cold. They concluded that 'routine mega-dose prophylaxis is not rationally justified for community use'. There was some suggestion that vitamin C prophylaxis may have a small but statistically significant effect in reducing the duration and severity of cold symptoms. Four trials using doses of up to 4 g/day of vitamin C found no evidence that it had any beneficial effects when taken at the onset of symptoms.

Many thousands of people (maybe a third of Americans) are unconvinced by arguments against the efficacy of vitamin C supplements and in such individuals the placebo effect may mean that they do in practice derive benefit from these preparations. Such widespread consumption of doses that are far in excess of those that can be obtained from normal human diets means that the potential toxicity of these preparations needs to be considered. Despite the widespread use of supplements, reports of adverse effects are few and the vitamin appears to be non-toxic even at doses many times the RNI/RDA, say 1 g/day, and much of the excess is excreted in the urine. Some concerns about intakes of gram quantities of the vitamin are:

- large excesses may lead to diarrhoea and gastrointestinal symptoms because the absorption system is saturated and vitamin C remains in the gut
- products of vitamin C metabolism may increase risk of gout and kidney stones in susceptible people; the risk for healthy people is probably small
- large doses of vitamin C may interfere with anticoagulant treatment
- large amounts of vitamin C excreted in the urine may make urinary tests for diabetes and faecal tests for occult blood unreliable.

Doses of up to 1 g/day can probably be tolerated for very long periods with no obvious ill effects in most people and doses several times higher than this are frequently taken without obvious ill effects. Use of gram quantities of vitamin C or any other vitamin is the province of the pharmacologist rather than the nutritionist.

14

The minerals

INTRODUCTION

In the UK, Dietary Reference Values are given for 11 minerals and safe intakes listed for another four (Committee on the Medical Aspects of Food (COMA), 1991). These same 15 minerals are also deemed to warrant a recommendation of some type in the USA. There is, therefore, international acceptance that at least 15 dietary minerals are essential. Several of these essential minerals are required only in trace amounts and in some cases requirements are difficult to establish with confidence. COMA (1991) considered the possible essentiality of another 19 minerals, most of these were classified as non-essential or of unproved essentiality, a few they regarded as probably essential in trace amounts. The new legislation in European countries based on the European Union (EU) Food Supplements Directive allows 15 minerals to be used in supplements. These are:

- calcium
- molybdenum
- chromium
- potassium
- copper
- selenium
- fluoride
- zinc
- iodine
- chloride
- iron
- phosphorus
- magnesium
- sodium
- manganese.

The incidence of clinically recognizable, acute dietary deficiency states is extremely rare for most essential minerals. Only two such deficiencies diseases have either historically or currently been seen as anything other than extremely rare or localized, i.e. **goitre**, a swelling of the thyroid gland caused by lack of dietary iodine, and iron deficiency anaemia. This has not prevented active debate about whether suboptimal intakes and subclinical deficiencies of other minerals are widespread particularly for calcium, selenium and zinc.

The first part of this chapter presents a series of brief reviews of 10 of the essential minerals starting with a key facts section. This is followed by a discussion of four mineral-related issues that have been singled out for more detailed discussion. These topics are:

- iodine and the iodine deficiency diseases
- iron and iron deficiency anaemia
- calcium, diet and osteoporosis
- salt (sodium chloride) and hypertension.

The role of dietary fluoride in dental health is discussed in Chapter 9 and so is only mentioned briefly in this chapter. Fluoride has not been proved to be an essential nutrient, and in both the UK and the USA only safe intakes are given. In the UK, even this safe intake is restricted to infants. The roles of zinc, selenium, iron and copper as prosthetic groups for antioxidant enzyme systems are discussed in Chapter 12 in the section dealing with free radicals and antioxidants. It is noted in Chapter 12 that the average intakes of several minerals are below the reference nutrient intake (RNI), especially in young women. Substantial numbers of individuals in both sexes and across the adult range (19–64 years) recorded intakes of one or more minerals that were below the lower RNI (LNRI) in the latest National Diet and Nutrition Survey (NDNS) conducted in Britain in 2000–01 (Hoare *et al.*, 2004). Further information on individual minerals can be found in Geissler and Powers (2005), Gropper *et al.* (2004) and particularly recommended is Shils *et al.* (2006); the individual chapters in these texts dealing with particular minerals are not individually referenced here.

Key points

- There are at least 15 essential minerals.
- Iodine and iron deficiency are two of the most prevalent micronutrient deficiencies in the world.
- Acute, clinical deficiency of most other minerals is rare or localized.
- Whether intakes of several other minerals are suboptimal has been a topic of active debate in nutrition.
- Data presented in Chapter 12 showed average intakes of several minerals were below the RNI in women and that many individuals of both sexes recorded unsatisfactory intakes of at least one mineral.

CHROMIUM

Key facts

- *Dietary standards.* UK 'safe' intake >25 μg/day; American recommended dietary allowance (RDA) males (M)/females (F) 35/25 μg/day.
- *Dietary sources.* Relatively large amounts in processed meats, wholegrain cereals and pulses. Only the trivalent form is present in food, and this is the only form permitted in supplements within the EU.

- *Biochemical functions.* It potentiates the actions of insulin and it is proposed that a chromium containing oligopeptide called chromomodulin stimulates the kinase activity of the insulin receptor.
- *Effects of deficiency.* Impaired glucose uptake, increased fat utilization and other signs of reduced insulin action seen in patients on total parenteral nutrition (TPN) who have not been given chromium in their solution.
- *Risk factors for deficiency.* Overt deficiency only seen in TPN patients.
- *Biochemical measure of nutritional status.* No reliable indicator available.
- *Prevalence of deficiency.* Overt deficiency almost never seen.
- *Toxicity.* Compounds permitted for use in supplements have very low toxicity.
- *Recommendations on high intakes.* Doses of 10 mg/day should not have any adverse effects.
- *Typical highest UK intakes.* The highest consumers may get 200 μg/day from food and supplements may provide a further 600 μg/day.

Overview

Chromium-responsive symptoms of reduced insulin response have been reported in isolated cases of patients on long-term TPN when their infusion solution was not supplemented with chromium. These symptoms included weight loss, peripheral neuropathy, reduced glucose utilization, hyperglycaemia and a low respiratory quotient (indicative of high fat utilization). Reduced insulin response has also been reported in experimental chromium deficiency in animals. It is suggested that chromium is a component of a factor that enhances the response to insulin and variously known as 'glucose tolerance factor' and chromomodulin. Early studies of chromium supplementation in patients with impaired glucose tolerance suggested that these supplements did have measurable beneficial effects but this has not been confirmed in a more recent analysis of randomized controlled trials. The results of chromium supplements in diabetic patients have also yielded conflicting results, and there seems to be no case for widespread use of chromium-containing supplements. High doses of permitted supplemental forms seem to have no harmful effects and this may be partly due to its poor absorption. High doses of chromium picolinate have been reported to cause DNA damage in mammalian cells and it has been linked to individual case reports of renal failure; this form is not permitted for use in dietary supplements in the EU.

COPPER

Key facts

- *Dietary standards.* Adult RNI in the UK is 1.2 mg/day, but there were insufficient data to set an LRNI; American RDA 0.9 mg/day.
- *Dietary sources.* Nuts, seeds, shellfish, offal and cocoa powder and chocolate are good sources of copper, but it is widely distributed in plant and animal foods.
- *Biochemical functions.* There are several copper-containing enzymes and other proteins in the body involved in transmitter synthesis, iron metabolism, electron transport and disposal of free radicals.
- *Effects of deficiency.* Experimental deficiency in animals results in anaemia, low white cell count and osteoporosis.
- *Risk factors for deficiency.* Overt deficiency rarely seen in humans but has been reported in patients receiving TPN and in premature babies fed on milk diets.
- *Prevalence of deficiency.* Only seen in special circumstances.
- *Toxicity.* Acute copper poisoning is rare because copper compounds have an unpleasant taste and an emetic effect, they cause abdominal pain and diarrhoea. The risk of chronic overload is reduced because of homoeostatic regulation of gut absorption.
- *Recommendations on high intakes.* An upper safe limit for lifetime consumption has been set at 10 mg/day.
- *Typical highest UK intakes.* The highest intakes from food in the UK are around 3 mg/day and over-the-counter supplements may contain up to 2 mg/day.

Overview

Copper has clearly been established as an essential nutrient but overt deficiency of the mineral is rarely seen. As was seen in the key facts section, copper requirements of adults are of the order of 1 mg/day and several rich food sources contain between 0.3 mg/100 g and over 2 mg/100 g including shellfish, nuts, seeds, cocoa powder, legumes, the bran and germ component of cereals, liver and other organ meats. Many other foods have intermediate amounts of copper (0.1–0.3 mg/100 g) including many fruits and vegetables (including potatoes), chocolate products, most meats, and most grain products. Drinking water may also contain significant amounts of copper. Although estimates of current copper intakes are below those recorded in the past this largely reflects improved analytical procedures and reduced use of Bordeaux mixture, a fungicide used in horticulture which contains copper sulphate. Its wide distribution in food and low requirement makes overt dietary deficiency of copper improbable. Note that cows' milk is particularly low in copper.

Experimental copper deficiency has been induced in animals and it results in anaemia, low neutrophil count, osteoporosis and skeletal abnormalities. In humans, there have been isolated reports of copper deficiency in patients receiving TPN which was not supplemented with copper and in premature babies fed on milk diets. The symptoms in humans are similar to those induced by experimental deficiency in animals. There is a rare hereditary disorder called Menkes disease which is associated with reduced copper uptake but this condition is not alleviated by copper administration and the sufferer dies in early childhood. It has been proposed, but not established, that marginal copper deficiency might lead to raised blood cholesterol, reduced skin pigmentation and impaired glucose tolerance.

There are a number of important copper-containing proteins in the body. These include:

- some types of superoxide dismutase which is involved in free radical disposal and is discussed in Chapter 12
- enzymes involved in the synthesis of the catecholamine group of nerve transmitters from tyrosine (e.g. adrenaline, noradrenaline and dopamine)
- enzymes involved in the synthesis of the pigment melanin responsible for, among other things, skin pigmentation
- cytochrome *c* oxidase involved in the electron transfer system in mitochondria

- ceruloplasmin, which is involved in the transport and oxidation of iron that is necessary for haemoglobin synthesis.

Acute copper poisoning is rare because copper compounds have an unpleasant taste and cause gastrointestinal symptoms when consumed in excess. There is homoeostatic regulation of copper absorption from the gut which reduces the risk of chronic poisoning. There are two rare inherited conditions called Wilson disease and Indian childhood cirrhosis that lead to excessive accumulation of copper in the body. In both cases the excess copper causes cirrhosis of the liver, and in Wilson's disease it accumulates in the brain and causes neurological damage. Both conditions can be treated with chelating agents that hasten copper excretion and by preventing the consumption of copper-rich diets.

FLUORIDE

It is generally agreed that fluoride is not strictly an essential nutrient but that it can be a beneficial dietary substance that reduces the risk of dental decay especially if consumed in optimal amounts by young children. A level of 1 mg/kg in drinking water is regarded as optimal for dental health. In the USA more than half of the population drink water that has been fluoridated up to this optimal level but fluoridation is much less widespread in the UK. In the UK a 'safe intake' of 0.05 mg/kg/day is given for fluoride but only for infants, whereas in the USA there are 'adequate intakes' for all age groups ranging from 0.5 mg/day for children aged 6–12 months up to 4 mg/day for adult men. Tea and seafood are the richest sources of fluoride in the British diet and tea may provide up to 70 per cent of the fluoride in the British diet.

In the UK fluoride supplements are sold as medicines rather than dietary supplements and the amount that is recommended to be taken varies with the concentration in the local water supply. The British Dental Association recommend that supplements should not be given before 6 months of age and not used at all if the water concentration exceeds 700 µg/L. They further recommend that if the water concentration is below 300 µg/L then supplement doses are as follows:

- 250 µg/day – 6 months to 3 years
- 500 µg/day – at 3–6 years
- 1 mg/day – from 6 years until puberty.

If the water concentration is between 300 µg/L and 700 µg/L then the following supplement doses should be used:

- 200 µg/day – 3–6-year-olds
- 500 µg/day – those over 6 years.

The role of fluoride in dental health has been discussed more fully in Chapter 9.

MAGNESIUM

Key facts

- *Dietary standards.* Adult UK RNI (M/F) 300/270 mg/day; UK LRNI 190/150 mg/day; American RDA 400/310 mg/day.
- *Dietary sources.* Leafy vegetables, wholegrains, nuts, seafood and legumes are good sources. Some drinking water may contain 50 mg/L in hard water areas.
- *Biochemical functions.* Many magnesium-dependent enzymes exist and most biochemical pathways have magnesium-dependent enzymes.
- *Effects of deficiency.* Induced magnesium deficiency leads to muscle weakness, spasms, personality changes, anorexia, nausea and vomiting.
- *Risk factors for deficiency.* Symptomatic, primary dietary deficiency is almost never seen but can be a secondary consequence of renal disease, uncontrolled diabetes, alcoholism and gut conditions. There is a rare hereditary condition in which there is defective absorption from the gut – primary idiopathic hypomagnesia.
- *Biochemical measure of nutritional status.* Assessment of magnesium status is difficult because only 1 per cent is extracellular. Normal serum magnesium concentration is 16–26 mg/L.
- *Prevalence of deficiency.* Primary symptomatic deficiency is rare but average adult intakes are below the RNI in UK and many adults, children and elderly Britons have recorded intakes below the LRNI.
- *Toxicity.* Oral toxicity is normally low although diarrhoea may result from excessive intake and many laxatives and antacids contain magnesium salts (e.g. Epsom salt).
- *Recommendations on high intakes.* Supplements of 400 mg/day should not have any adverse effects but there are insufficient data to set proper upper limits.

Overview

As seen in Chapter 12 many adults have recorded intakes if magnesium that are below the LRNI. This is also true for many older children and about a quarter of elderly people in the UK (see Chapter 15). Some enzymes like DNA and RNA polymerase contain magnesium which binds to the enzyme and makes it active. Magnesium can also affect enzyme activity by binding to the substrate and increasing its affinity for the enzyme, e.g. it complexes with ATP which increases its affinity for kinases. About 60–65 per cent of body magnesium is present in bone, 1 per cent is in extracellular fluids and the rest is found within soft tissues, especially muscle. There are over 300 enzyme reactions in which magnesium is important including many kinases and enzymes involved in glycolysis, Krebs cycle, the pentose phosphate pathway, β-oxidation of fatty acids, creatine phosphate formation in muscle and nucleic acid, and RNA and DNA synthesis.

As has been noted in the key facts section, many people in different age groups have intakes of magnesium that are regarded as suboptimal or even frankly inadequate and yet primary symptomatic deficiency of magnesium is rare although it may occur as a secondary consequence of several conditions (as also listed in the key facts section). Chronic low magnesium status has been linked to increased risk of coronary heart disease (CHD) and this has been used to explain the slightly lower incidence of CHD in hard water areas. There is, however, little substantial evidence to support this. There are claims that magnesium supplements may lower blood pressure in healthy people or those with moderate hypertension (e.g. Sacks *et al.*, 1998). There is also little evidence to support claims that supplements enhance athletic performance or help to prevent osteoporosis.

MANGANESE

Key facts

- *Dietary standards.* UK 'safe intake' 1.4mg/day (1.8 mg/day in the USA).
- *Dietary sources.* Manganese is present in reasonable amounts in most plant foods especially wholegrain cereals, nuts, dried fruits, leafy vegetables and tea.

- *Biochemical functions.* There are several important manganese-containing enzymes including pyruvate carboxylase in gluconeogenesis and mitochondrial superoxide dismutase.
- *Effects of deficiency.* Not seen in humans.
- *Biochemical measure of nutritional status.* Rarely measured.
- *Prevalence of deficiency.* Not seen, average UK intake is three times the 'safe intake'.
- *Toxicity.* Very low.
- *Recommendations on high intakes.* Intake of 12 mg/day unlikely to have any adverse effects but little evidence to judge.
- *Typical highest UK intakes.* Highest UK intakes from food around 8 mg/day and supplements may provide up to 10 mg/day. Tea drinkers have high intakes but bioavailability of this manganese may be low.

Overview

Although experimental manganese deficiency can be induced in animals and has been reported in individual cases of patients receiving TPN, it is almost never seen. Average intakes are high in relation to requirements. Most plant foods contain reasonable amounts but the concentrations in animal tissues are low and thus the amounts in meat, fish and milk are low. Two manganese-containing enzymes are listed in the key facts section and a number of other enzymes are activated by manganese, although many of these are also activated by magnesium.

MOLYBDENUM

Key facts

- *Dietary standards.* UK 'safe intake' 50–400 μg/day in the USA 45 μg/day.
- *Dietary sources.* Widespread in foods and the amount depends on soil content.
- *Biochemical functions.* At least three molybdenum requiring enzymes exist – xanthine oxidase, aldehyde oxidase and sulphite oxidase.
- *Effects of deficiency.* Reduced activity of the above enzymes.

- *Risk factors for deficiency.* TPN only.
- *Biochemical measure of nutritional status.* Not usually measured.
- *Toxicity.* Has low toxicity and symptoms may resemble copper deficiency.
- *Recommendations on high intakes.* Few data but may require 10+ mg/day to produce any ill effects
- *Typical highest UK intakes.* Highest UK intakes from food may be 250 µg/day and supplements may contain further 330 µg/day. Highest total intake is usually at least an order of magnitude below toxic effects.

Overview

Experimental molybdenum deficiency can be induced in animals but just one verified case of molybdenum deficiency has been reported in a single TPN patient. Molybdenum is a cofactor for:

- xanthine oxidase, an enzyme involved in purine breakdown
- aldehyde oxidase, an enzyme involved in nucleotide breakdown from nucleic acids
- sulphite oxidase involved in breakdown of sulphur-containing amino acids.

Note that reduced excretion of sulphate and uric acid was recorded in the one confirmed case of human molybdenum deficiency.

PHOSPHORUS

Around 80 per cent of the body calcium is in bone mineral as the calcium salt hydroxyapatite. Phosphorylation and dephosphorylation reactions are an important feature of biochemical reactions (note ATP and creatine phosphate). Phosphorus is a component of phospholipids which are important in membranes and is important in some buffering systems. In the UK the RNI for phosphorus is set at 550 mg/day, which is the molar equivalent of the calcium RNI, and in the USA the RDA is 700 mg/day. Phosphate is a major component of all plant and animal cells and so is found in all natural foods.

POTASSIUM

Key facts

- *Dietary standards.* Adult UK RNI 3500 mg/day; adult LRNI 2000 mg/day; American RDA 4700 mg/day.
- *Dietary sources.* Fruits and vegetables are the best sources although there is some in milk and flesh foods:
  - 1 orange – 490 mg
  - 1 banana – 470 mg
  - 1 apple – 145 mg
  - 1 portion (95 g) broccoli – 210 mg
  - 1 portion (75 g) frozen peas – 100 mg
  - 1 tomato – 220 g
  - 1 portion (265 g) chips (French fries) – 2700 mg
  - 1 glass (200 g) canned orange juice – 260 mg.
- *Biochemical functions.* It is the major cation in intracellular fluid; nerve impulse transmission; contraction of muscle and heart; acid–base balance.
- *Effects of deficiency.* Primary symptomatic deficiency is rarely seen but secondary hypokalaemia leads to muscle weakness, changes in cardiac function, reduced gut motility, alkalosis, depression and confusion.
- *Biochemical measure of nutritional status.* Normal serum concentrations of potassium are 3.6–5.0 mmol/L but variations are due to disease (e.g. renal disease) rather than dietary variation.
- *Prevalence of deficiency.* Recorded average adult intakes are below the RNI and 19 per cent of women have intakes below the LRNI (more in the younger age groups). Many children and a quarter of elderly Britons have intakes below the LRNI.
- *Toxicity.* Not reported.
- *Recommendations on high intakes.* Supplemental doses of 3700 mg/day have no adverse effects.
- *Typical highest UK intakes.* Total maximum UK intake around 5 g/day with most of this from food – supplements contain up to 200 mg/day.

Overview

The richest sources of potassium are fruits and vegetables but it is present in all animal and plant tissues and is present in milk. The body of an average man contains around 135 g of potassium and the actual amount in any person's body is a reflection of their lean tissue mass. All but 5 per cent of the body's potassium is found within cells and it is the principal cation in intracellular fluid. Measures of total body potassium are used to estimate lean tissue mass and thus body composition.

Potassium is the principal cation in intracellular fluid and sodium the principal cation in extracellular fluid. This differential distribution of these two ions on either side of the cell membrane is maintained by active cellular pumps that use energy to pump sodium out of the cell in exchange for pumping potassium in. This differential distribution of these two cations is crucial for many cellular processes including the generation and propagation of nerve impulses, active transport processes and the maintenance of acid–base balance.

Potassium is present in most foodstuffs and so overt dietary deficiency is improbable. However, as noted in the key facts section and noted in more detail in Chapters 12 and 15, many people of all age groups have intakes of potassium that are considered unsatisfactory. This low potassium intake is likely to be due to low consumption of fruits and vegetables and is yet another adverse consequence of low fruit and vegetable intake. The low recorded intake of potassium in many British people adds more weight to the campaign to increase fruit and vegetable intake up to five portions per day. Low blood potassium may be a secondary consequence of other conditions or situations, such as prolonged diarrhoea, vomiting, laxative abuse or excessive secretion of the hormone aldosterone by the adrenal cortex. This low blood potassium leads to a range of symptoms listed in the key facts section.

Later in this chapter there is an extended discussion of the influence of dietary factors, especially dietary salt intake, on blood pressure and the incidence of hypertension. Reduced sodium (salt) intake and reducing the prevalence of obesity are the primary focus of attempts to reduce average population blood pressure, the incidence of hypertension and thus reduce the adverse consequences of high blood pressure. Nevertheless, there is a substantial body of evidence to suggest that high potassium intake may have some effect in reducing blood pressure (Cappuccio and Macgregor 1991; COMA 1991, 1994a). COMA (1994a) recommended that average potassium intake should be increased to 3.5 g/day from current level of around 2.8 g/day by increasing consumption of fruit and vegetables.

SELENIUM

Key facts

- *Dietary standards.* UK RNI M/F 75/60 μg/day; UK LRNI 40 μg/day; American RDA 55 μg/day.
- *Dietary sources.* Meat (particularly organ meat), eggs, fish and cereals.
- *Biochemical functions.* Component of enzyme system glutathione peroxidase, involved in disposal of free radicals. There are also other selenium-containing enzymes, including one that is involved in converting the thyroid hormone thyroxine into its more active form triiodothyronine.
- *Effects of deficiency.* Keshan disease, a progressive cardiomyopathy.
- *Risk factors for deficiency.* Low levels of selenium in the soil.
- *Biochemical measure of nutritional status.* Plasma or serum selenium is regarded as a good short-term indicator of selenium intake and red cell selenium a more long-term measure of intake.
- *Prevalence of deficiency.* Estimates of selenium intake are not reliable because the food database is incomplete for this mineral. There are probably substantial numbers of people in the UK with values below the LRNI although symptomatic deficiency does not occur.
- *Toxicity.* Selenosis leads to skin lesions, changes to the hair and nails and is followed by a range of neurological symptoms; it occurs in areas of the world where soil levels of selenium are particularly high.
- *Recommendations on high intakes.* A safe intake for lifetime consumption is set at 450 μg/day.
- *Typical highest UK intakes.* It has been estimated that highest intakes from food in the UK are around 100 μg/day and supplements may provide up to a further 300 μg/day.

Overview

Selenium is present in the food sources listed in the key facts section largely as the selenium-containing amino acids selenomethionine and selenocysteine, where selenium replaces the sulphur present in the parent amino acids cysteine and methionine. The selenium content of the soil in any particular region will have a major effect on the selenium content of food grown in that area and thus on the dietary intakes of the people who live there. Affluent populations tend not to be so reliant on food grown locally and may eat selenium-rich seafood, and so are to some extent protected from these localized problems. Thomson and Robinson (1980) give figures for the blood selenium concentrations of people living in different regions, which vary from approximately 0.22 mg/L in people sampled in the USA where selenium soil content is reasonably high down to approximately 0.06 mg/L in some areas of New Zealand where the selenium content of the soil is low. Areas of China have low intakes of selenium in the soil and this is where a progressive cardiomyopathy (Keshan disease) attributed to selenium deficiency has been reported.

A number of selenoproteins are important enzymes and the best known of these are the enzymes, including glutathione peroxidase, that are involved in free radical disposal mechanisms and were discussed in Chapter 12. Note that despite its apparent role in protecting against free radical damage, COMA (1998) found no substantial evidence to support the suggestion that supplements of selenium might have cancer-preventing effects.

ZINC

Key facts

- *Dietary standards.* UK adult RNI M/F 9.5/7 mg/day; LRNI 5.5/4 mg/day; RDA in the USA 11/8 mg/day.
- *Dietary sources.* Meats, wholegrain cereals, pulses and shellfish:
  - 1 slice wholemeal bread – 0.7 mg
  - 1 pork chop – 2.8 mg
  - 1 portion (75 g) frozen peas – 0.5 mg
  - 1 portion fried lamb liver – 4 mg
  - 1 serving (70 mg) canned crabmeat – 3.5 mg.
- *Biochemical functions.* Numerous zinc-containing enzymes are involved in DNA synthesis (and so cell division) and in the synthesis and metabolism of fats, carbohydrates and proteins. Superoxide dismutase involved in disposal of free radicals is a zinc-containing enzyme. Insulin is stored as a complex with zinc in the pancreas.

- *Effects of deficiency.* Experimental zinc deficiency leads to anorexia and growth reduction, reduced immune function, slow healing, hypogonadism and delayed sexual maturation, skin lesions and hair loss.
- *Risk factors for deficiency.* Diets with lots of unleavened bread and thus high in phytate may reduce zinc absorption.
- *Biochemical measure of nutritional status.* Serum or plasma zinc concentration with a value of less than 700 µg/L are indicative of deficiency.
- *Prevalence of deficiency.* Average intakes in the UK are around the RNI but 4 per cent of adults have intakes below the LRNI with higher prevalence in older children and in the elderly (see Chapter 15).
- *Toxicity.* Excess zinc interferes with copper absorption and precipitates symptoms of copper deficiency and may also interfere with iron absorption. Excess zinc can also depress the activity of superoxide dismutase in red cells (an enzyme involved in free radical disposal). Zinc supplements can cause gastrointestinal symptoms.
- *Recommendations on high intakes.* The safe upper limit for lifetime supplemental zinc intake is 25 mg/day.
- *Typical highest UK intakes.* The highest UK consumers may get around 17 mg/day from their food and occasionally water may contain up to 10 mg/day. Supplements in the UK may contain as much as 50 mg/day.

Overview

Zinc was clearly established as an essential nutrient for experimental animals in the 1930s and in humans in 1961. Zinc is found in all living tissue where it is concentrated in the cell nuclei and good food sources are wholegrain cereals, pulses, meat and shellfish. Overt symptomatic dietary deficiency of zinc is uncommon although it may be a contributory factor to low growth rates in some children. Zinc deficiency can be precipitated by high intakes of phytate from unleavened bread which impairs zinc absorption. Some cases of zinc deficiency associated with high consumption of such bread were reported in Egypt and Iran in the 1960s. Note that the phytate in cereals is destroyed when bread dough is raised by yeast.

More than 200 zinc-containing enzymes have been recorded and these are involved in DNA synthesis and metabolism and synthesis of the three major macronutrients. Zinc is important in cell division. The role of the zinc-containing enzyme superoxide dismutase in free radical disposal was discussed in Chapter 12. When animals are fed on experimental zinc-deficient diets there is rapid onset of anorexia and growth retardation. Response to zinc deficiency is classified as a type II response where there is rapid reduction in growth and conservation of body zinc for essential metabolic functions (in the more common type I response there is depletion of body stores to maintain normal functions followed by reduction of the nutrient-dependent functions when stores become depleted). Studies conducted in the USA have suggested that marginal zinc deficiency may be a contributory factor in low growth rates of children. Healthy children selected because of their low weight for height showed increased growth when given small zinc supplements compared to those given a placebo. Zinc supplements given to random samples of children had no effect on growth rates. Zinc deficiency also occurs in a rare inherited condition acrodermatitis enteropathica as a result of impaired zinc absorption. The condition is controlled by zinc supplements. As detailed in Chapter 12 average adult intakes of zinc are just above the RNI and about 4 per cent of adults have unsatisfactory intakes with higher numbers in older adults and in older children.

As well as the effects on growth, zinc deficiency also causes reduced immune function, slow healing, delayed sexual maturation and hypogonadism, and skin lesions. Given the effects on the immune system and wound healing it might seem prudent to ensure that people with injuries, those at high risk of infection and those undergoing surgery have good zinc status and small zinc supplements might well be an appropriate way of ensuring this. Of course proper evaluation of the effectiveness of these supplements would require assessment of prior zinc status in those receiving them, i.e. does the zinc have an effect in those who are deficient and does it confer any additional benefits in those whose zinc status is normal? Zinc supplements have also been promoted as being of benefit in the treatment of anorexia nervosa and in treating male infertility but this is based on the symptoms of zinc deficiency and there is no evidence that they are effective.

Reference to the key facts section indicates that some people taking zinc supplements may have zinc intakes that are significantly above the safe upper limit for lifetime consumption.

IODINE AND IODINE DEFICIENCY DISEASES

Key facts

- *Dietary standards.* Adult UK RNI 140 μg/day; LRNI 70 μg/day; American RDA 150 μg/day.
- *Dietary sources.* The richest natural sources are seafood; amounts in fruits, vegetables and meat depend on soil content of iodine; modern farming and processing methods increase the amounts in milk and some bakery products; iodized salt.
- *Biochemical functions.* A component of the thyroid hormones thyroxine and triiodothyronine.
- *Effects of deficiency.* Goitre/iodine deficiency diseases, including cretinism and myxoedema.
- *Risk factors for deficiency.* Living in inland areas where soil iodine content is low and no seafood is eaten.
- *Biochemical measure of nutritional status.* Usually based on clinical assessment.
- *Prevalence of deficiency.* 1.6 billion people worldwide at risk of iodine deficiency; 4 per cent of UK adult women have estimated intakes below the LRNI but average intake is well above the RNI and symptomatic dietary deficiency is not seen in developed countries.
- *Toxicity.* High intakes can lead to disturbances of thyroid function which usually manifests as hyperthyroidism and toxic nodular goitre but occasionally it may manifest as hypothyroidism.
- *Recommendations on high intakes.* Supplements of up to 500 μg/day should cause no problems.
- *Typical highest UK intakes.* The highest consumers may get up to 450 μg/day from their food and drinking water may provide a further 30 μg/day and supplements may provide up to 490 μg/day.

Distribution and physiological function of body iodine

Iodine is a component of the thyroid hormones, **thyroxine** and **triiodothyronine**. The thyroid gland traps and concentrates absorbed iodine very efficiently;

if radioactively labelled iodine is taken in, then this radioactivity can be shown to be rapidly concentrated within the thyroid gland. The ability of the thyroid to concentrate 'labelled' iodine is used diagnostically as a measure of thyroid function. High doses of radioactive iodine may be used as an alternative to surgery to selectively destroy thyroid tissue in some cases of hyperthyroidism or thyroid carcinoma, especially in elderly people. Nuclear emissions released after accidents or explosions contain large amounts of relatively short-lived radioactive iodine and this accumulates in the thyroid where it can ultimately cause thyroid carcinoma. Administration of iodine-containing tablets can be used as a public health measure after nuclear accidents to compete with and competitively reduce the uptake of the radioactive iodine into the thyroid.

Iodine deficiency

In goitre, there is a swelling of the thyroid gland. This swelling ranges from that which is only detectable to the trained eye to massive and sometimes nodular overgrowth. The thyroid swells because of excessive stimulation by the pituitary hormone, **thyrotrop(h)in**. Thyrotropin output is normally inhibited by circulating thyroid hormones and so any reduced output of thyroid hormones caused by iodine deficiency leads to compensatory increases in thyrotropin output and consequent thyroid growth (see Figure 14.1). In some cases, the swelling of the thyroid is the only apparent symptom of iodine deficiency.

In severe iodine deficiency, there are symptoms of thyroid hormone deficiency. In children, iodine deficiency can lead to **cretinism**, a condition characterized by impaired mental and physical development. In adults, iodine deficiency causes not only goitre but can also lead to impaired mental functioning, low metabolic rate, hypotension, weight gain and other symptoms of thyroid hormone deficiency. In places where goitre is endemic it causes increased rates of spontaneous abortion and stillbirth and the birth of large numbers of children with congenital physical and neurological abnormalities, e.g. deaf-mutism, spasticity and mental deficiency. There is a general impairment of intellectual performance and psychomotor skills in children from iodine-deficient areas. If a goitre is very large it may lead to problems with breathing or swallowing that may require surgery and occasionally large nodular goitres may become malignant. Controlled studies

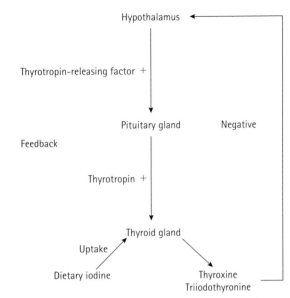

Lack of dietary iodine reduces negative feedback and leads to overproduction of thyrotropin, which causes over-stimulation and swelling of the thyroid – goitre.

Figure 14.1 *The regulation of thyroid hormone output and the origins of goitre.*

by David Marine in Ohio in the 1920s showed that iodine supplements were effective in the treatment and prevention of goitre in schoolchildren. Women and girls are more susceptible to goitre than males.

Causes and scale of the problem

The richest sources of dietary iodine are seafoods. The smaller amount of iodine in other foods varies according to the iodine level in the soil. The iodine content of drinking water gives a good indication of the general iodine level in the soil in an area. In many regions of the world, the soil iodine content is low, especially in mountainous regions and flooded river valleys where glaciation, and run off from melting snow and heavy rain, have leached much of the iodine from the soil. The area around the Great Lakes in America and in Derbyshire and the Cotswold areas of England were once goitre areas. The Himalayas, Andes, Alps and the mountains of China together with the Ganges valley and other river valleys in Asia are all areas where soil iodine content is inadequate. In areas where the soil iodine content is low and where seafood is not consumed, then the iodine deficiency diseases, manifesting most apparently as goitre, have been, and often still are, endemic. Iodine deficiency is one of the most common nutrient deficiencies in the world and is the most common cause of preventable mental deficiency in children. The World Health Organization (WHO) estimated that in 1993 there were over 1.6 billion people in the developing world at risk of iodine deficiency, with around 200 million suffering from goitre and around 20 million of these having some degree of resultant mental defect. More than 5 million people have gross cretinism and learning disabilities. Iodine deficiency is endemic in large parts of Central and South America, large parts of India, China and Southeast Asia, some regions of Africa and the Oceanic islands; around 85 per cent of those with overt cretinism are in Asia.

Nowadays, few affluent communities rely solely on food produced in their locality and this reduces the risk of goitre. In both the UK and USA, the iodine content of cow milk is high because of iodine supplementation of feed and the use of iodine disinfectants. In many goitre areas, including Switzerland and the USA, iodized salt has been effectively used as a prophylactic measure to prevent goitre. Kelp is a form of seaweed that is marketed as a dietary supplement partly on the basis of its high iodine content and the recommended dose typically contains one to two times the adult RNI/RDA. Note that persons with thyroid disorders should not take this supplement as it may interfere with the management of their condition. In some iodine-deficient areas, injections of iodized oil have been used and a single injection gives protection for 2–3 years. Iodized oil can be administered orally but the duration of effectiveness is reduced to about a year.

One problem with assessing iodine intakes and levels of dietary adequacy is that the food tables may not always be a totally reliable guide to the iodine content of food grown in a particular locality. Zimmerman and Delange (2004) have suggested that two-thirds of people in western Europe live in areas that are iodine deficient. They go on to suggest that most women in Europe are iodine deficient during pregnancy, and that all pregnant women in Europe should receive supplements containing 150 µg/day.

Requirements and intake of iodine

The adult RNI (RDA) for iodine is 140 (150 µg/day and intakes are typically double this in the UK and more than double this in the USA. The very high intakes in the US, which reached a peak of 800 µg/day in 1974, have been a cause for concern. Very high intakes can cause toxic nodular goitre and hyperthyroidism. The Food Standards Agency (FSA, 2003) suggested a safe upper limit of 500 µg/day from supplements which equates to a total maximum intake of around 1000 µg/day. Some Japanese populations who habitually consume seaweed have intakes many times this suggested maximum with no apparent ill effects and Hetzel and Clugston (1999) suggest that populations that have been iodine deficient may be much more sensitive to the toxic effects of excess iodine.

Certain foods of the cabbage (*Brassica*) family and cassava contain goitrogenic substances that either block the uptake of iodine by the thyroid gland or block the synthesis of thyroid hormones. The presence of such goitrogens may precipitate deficiency where intakes of iodine are at the borders of adequacy. Cassava, in particular, may be a significant factor in precipitating iodine deficiency in some tropical areas where it is the principal energy source for around 200 million people. Intakes of iodine should be doubled to 200–300 µg/day where there is high intake of these goitrogens.

> ## Key points
>
> - Iodine is essential as a component of the hormones thyroxine and triiodothyronine.
> - In iodine deficiency, reduced thyroid hormone output causes increased thyrotropin output from the pituitary, which stimulates the thyroid and causes it to swell (goitre).
> - Severe iodine deficiency in children causes impaired mental and physical development (cretinism) and leads to symptoms of thyroid insufficiency in adults.
> - In goitre areas there is general impairment of mental performance and increased numbers of abortions, stillbirths and birth of children with mental and physical defects.
> - Iodine deficiency occurs in mountainous areas and frequently flooded river valleys where melting snow and floodwater have leached the iodine from the soil.
> - One to two billion people in the world are at risk of iodine deficiency and 20 million have some degree of mental defect as a result of iodine deficiency.

- Iodine deficiency is the most common cause of preventable mental deficiency in children.
- Access to seafood and food from various geographical regions reduces the risk of iodine deficiency.
- Iodized salt and injections of iodized oil have been used to prevent and treat iodine deficiency.
- Very high intakes of iodine may cause toxic goitre and hyperthyroidism but those people with chronically low iodine intakes may be particularly susceptible.
- Certain foods such as cabbage and cassava contain goitrogens that increase the requirement for iodine.

IRON AND IRON DEFICIENCY ANAEMIA

Iron nutrition

Key facts

- *Dietary standards.* UK adult RNI M/F 8.7/14.8 mg/day; LRNI 4.7/8 mg/day; American RDA 8/18 mg/day.
- *Dietary sources.* Meat (particularly offal); fish; cereals; green vegetables; the biological availability of iron is much higher from meat and fish than from vegetable sources:
  - 1 pork chop – 1 mg
  - 1 portion (90 g) fried lamb liver – 9 mg
  - 1 egg – 1.1 mg
  - 1 serving (80 g) peeled prawns – 0.9 mg
  - 1 serving (85 g) canned sardines – 3.9 mg
  - 1 portion (75 g) frozen peas – 1.1 mg
  - 1 portion (95 g) broccoli – 1 mg
  - 1 50 g bar of dark (plain) chocolate – 1.2 mg
  - 1 serving (130 mg) spinach – 5.2 mg
  - 1 slice wholemeal bread – 1 mg.
- *Biochemical functions.* Component of haemoglobin, myoglobin and cytochromes; there are several iron-containing enzymes such as catalase.
- *Effects of deficiency.* Iron deficiency anaemia.
- *Risk factors for deficiency.* Chronic blood loss due to, e.g. heavy menstrual bleeding, malignancy, intestinal parasites or repeated pregnancies; a vegetarian diet that is low iron, has low bioavailability and lacks promoters of absorption such as vitamin C.

- *Biochemical measure of nutrient status.* Low haemoglobin concentration in blood is indicative of anaemia and WHO lower limits are 130 g/L for men and 120 g/L for women. Serum ferritin concentration is used to indicate level of iron stores and the normal range is 20–300 μg/L for men and 15–150 μg/L for women.
- *Prevalence of deficiency.* The most common micronutrient deficiency in the world with 700 million suffering from iron deficiency anaemia and many more with depleted iron stores. Even in the UK 9 per cent of pre-menopausal women are anaemic and 12 per cent have depleted iron stores.
- *Toxicity.* Acute effects of high iron intakes are due to its irritant effects on the gastrointestinal system, i.e. constipation or diarrhoea, nausea and vomiting. Severe and/or chronic iron overload will cause tissue damage, especially cirrhosis of the liver.
- *Recommendations on high intakes.* Supplements of 17 mg/day should cause no serious problems unless genetically susceptible to iron overload (this figure has been based on a safety factor of three, i.e. a third of the dose that might be expected to cause some problems).
- *Typical highest UK intakes.* Highest intakes from food in the UK are around 25 mg/day and supplements may provide a further 20 mg/day.

Distribution of body iron

An average well-nourished male body will contain about 4 g of iron. Around 70 per cent of this total will be present in the respiratory pigments **haemoglobin** in blood (67 per cent) and **myoglobin** in muscles (3–4 per cent). Most of the body's non-haem iron will be stored as the iron–protein complex, **ferritin**. Small amounts of iron will also be found in a variety of important iron-containing enzymes and proteins and bound to the protein **transferrin** in plasma that is responsible for the transport of iron around the body. The first effect of iron deficiency is depletion of iron stores and this is followed by reduced levels of the iron-containing respiratory pigments haemoglobin and myoglobin, i.e. iron deficiency anaemia.

Requirement for dietary iron

Iron is very efficiently conserved by the human body with daily losses of body iron in a typical healthy male amounting to only around 1 mg/day (i.e. only 0.025

per cent of normal body iron content). This tiny net loss of iron compares with around 20 mg of iron in the ageing red blood cells that are removed from the circulation and destroyed each day. The iron released from broken down red cells is recycled and the small amount of iron lost from the body is that present in lost skin, nails, hair, body fluids and sloughed cells from the alimentary and genito-urinary tracts. In pre-menopausal women, losses of menstrual blood and the losses of iron at parturition and during lactation also contribute to body iron loss. Average menstrual blood loss represents an additional increment of around 80 per cent to the general iron losses of women but in some women (say 10 per cent) these extra menstrual losses may represent an addition of 150 per cent or more to the general iron loss. Any condition which results in chronic blood loss will deplete body iron stores and increase the risk of anaemia, e.g. ulcers, intestinal parasites, intestinal cancer.

Average intakes of iron in the UK are around 13.2 mg/day in men and 10.0 mg/day in women, i.e. around 13 times average daily losses in men and, even in those women with particularly high menstrual losses, still around four times estimated losses. The iron RNI is 8.7 mg/day for men and 14.8 mg/day for pre-menopausal women. According to COMA (1991) even this RNI may be insufficient for those women with particularly high menstrual losses. The very large differences in estimated requirements for iron and estimated losses are because only a small and variable proportion of dietary iron is absorbed. The proportion of dietary iron that is absorbed varies with several factors. These are listed below.

- The iron status of the individual; inorganic iron absorption is two to three times higher in subjects who are iron deficient compared to those with good iron stores. There is also a substantial increase in the efficiency of iron absorption during pregnancy.
- The form in which the dietary iron is present, haem iron from meat and fish and organic iron in milk is much better absorbed than inorganic iron from vegetable foods. Most of the inorganic iron in food is in the trivalent or ferric state whereas that in most supplements is in the divalent ferrous state, which is better absorbed.
- The presence of promoters of inorganic iron absorption such as vitamin C, alcohol and meat protein.

- The presence of inhibitors of inorganic iron absorption in the diet such as phytate (e.g. from unleavened bread), tannin (e.g. from tea) and perhaps even large amounts of dietary fibre.

Haem iron from meat and fish is far better absorbed (10–30 per cent) than the iron in vegetable foods (2–10 per cent). Absorption of haem iron is also unaffected by the presence of inhibitors and promoters. Vitamin C, stomach acid and the presence of meat and fish all promote iron absorption. Vitamin C is a major factor in promoting the absorption of iron from vegetable foods. Fibre, phytate (from unleavened bread) and tannin in tea all tend to hinder iron absorption. Alcohol increases gastric acid secretion and facilitates iron absorption.

COMA (1991) assumed an average efficiency of absorption of iron of about 15 per cent when making their calculations of dietary reference values.

Regulation of iron balance and iron overload

The principal physiological mechanism for regulating body iron balance is by controlling the efficiency of absorption. When iron stores are low, iron is absorbed more efficiently than when body iron stores are full. The efficiency of iron absorption may more than double when iron stores are depleted. This regulatory system is usually sufficient to prevent iron toxicity from dietary sources even when moderate doses of therapeutic iron are consumed chronically by people who do not need them. Chronic iron overload can lead to cirrhosis of the liver. Single very high doses of iron can cause diarrhoea, vomiting, gastrointestinal bleeding, circulatory collapse and liver necrosis. Iron poisoning resulting from children consuming pharmaceutical preparations of iron is one of the most common causes of accidental poisoning. Consumption of alcoholic drinks containing large amounts of iron can precipitate iron overload and contribute to liver cirrhosis. Some wines and Normandy cider contain large amounts of iron and cirrhosis due to iron overload has been common among Bantu people of South Africa who consumed large amounts of beer brewed in iron pots. White et al. (1993) found a positive association between alcohol consumption and level of iron stores in both men and women. As there is no physiological mechanism for excreting excess iron, iron overload and toxicity is a major problem for those with certain conditions that require repeated blood transfusions, e.g. the inherited blood disorder, thalassaemia. Drugs that bind or chelate iron and facilitate its excretion can be used to treat or prevent iron overload. Hereditary haemochromatosis is an inherited condition in which there is chronic over-absorption of iron, which can lead to liver and other tissue damage unless it is treated by regular therapeutic bleeding.

Determination of iron status

Iron deficiency will eventually impair the ability to synthesize haemoglobin. Iron status has traditionally been diagnosed by measurement of blood haemoglobin concentration. Iron deficiency anaemia is characterized by reduced blood haemoglobin concentration and reduced red blood cell size – a **microcytic anaemia** (small cell) as compared with the **macrocytic anaemia** (large cell) of vitamin B_{12} or folic acid deficiency. A blood haemoglobin concentration of less than 12 g/100 mL (120 g/L) of blood has traditionally been taken as 'the level below which anaemia is likely to be present' and the prevalence of anaemia has usually been established by use of a cut-off value like this. Currently the WHO suggests a value of less than 13 g/100 mL for men and 12 g/100 mL for women at sea level (because living at altitude increases red cell count and haemoglobin concentration).

Other measures of iron status have been increasingly used in recent years. The plasma ferritin level indicates the state of body iron stores and these stores may become depleted without any fall in blood haemoglobin concentration. Plasma ferritin is a more sensitive measure of iron status than blood haemoglobin concentration. Normal ranges for plasma ferritin are given in the key facts section and a value of less than 15 μg/L is indicative of iron depletion in women. In iron deficiency, the concentration of the iron transport protein, transferrin, in the plasma rises but the amount of iron in plasma drops and so low ratio of iron to transferrin in plasma, the **transferrin saturation**, indicates low iron status. When the percentage saturation of transferrin with iron is below 15 per cent, the ability to synthesize haemoglobin is impaired.

The symptoms of anaemia result from the low haemoglobin content of blood leading to impaired ability to transport oxygen and they include general fatigue, breathlessness on exertion, pallor, headache and insomnia.

Key points

- An adult male body contains about 4 g of iron with 70 per cent in haemoglobin and myoglobin, small amounts in iron-containing enzymes and the rest stored as the iron–protein complex ferritin.
- A healthy male loses less than 1 mg of iron per day but menstrual losses, pregnancy and lactation increase the average losses of younger women.
- Iron requirements greatly exceed iron losses because only a proportion of dietary iron (approximately 15 per cent) is absorbed.
- The efficiency of iron absorption increases in iron deficiency and decreases when iron stores are full. The gut is the main site of regulation of body iron balance.
- Haem iron is absorbed more efficiently than inorganic iron from vegetable sources.
- Substances such as phytate and tannin inhibit inorganic iron absorption whereas alcohol, gastric acid and vitamin C promote its absorption.
- There is no route for excreting body iron.
- Chronic high consumption of iron can lead to cirrhosis of the liver and other tissue damage due to iron overload.
- Single high doses of iron can cause acute poisoning, typically in children accidentally consuming iron tablets.
- Iron deficiency eventually impairs haemoglobin synthesis and the capacity of blood to transport oxygen – iron deficiency anaemia.
- Iron deficiency anaemia is a microcytic (small red cells) anaemia and leads to pallor, fatigue, breathlessness on exertion and headache.
- Iron status may be assessed by measuring blood haemoglobin concentration, plasma ferritin concentration or plasma transferrin saturation.
- Plasma ferritin is a more sensitive indicator of iron status than blood haemoglobin concentration because iron stores become depleted before anaemia occurs.

Iron deficiency

Prevalence of iron deficiency and anaemia

A major problem in determining the prevalence of iron deficiency is to decide on the criteria that are to be used to define it. In a series of studies, Elwood and colleagues found that women with haemoglobin concentrations that would indicate mild to moderate anaemia showed little or no evidence of clinical impairment, even cardiopulmonary function under exercise appeared to be little affected by this degree of apparent anaemia (reviewed by Lock, 1977). More recently it has been suggested by several groups that functional impairment due to iron deficiency (as measured by plasma ferritin) may occur in the absence of anaemia (COMA, 1991). Reduced work capacity and changes in certain brain functions that adversely affect attention span, memory and learning in children are some of these suggested adverse consequences of iron deficiency.

Iron deficiency is considered to be the most common nutrient deficiency in the world. WHO estimates put the worldwide incidence of iron deficiency at around 40 per cent with perhaps a third of these having frank iron deficiency anaemia. There may be something like 700 million people with iron deficiency anaemia in the world. The incidence is higher in women than in men because of the extra demands of menstruation, pregnancy and lactation on body iron stores. In the developed countries, the condition is considered to be uncommon in young men. The low iron intakes and poor iron status of many British women is discussed in some detail in Chapters 1 and 12. Evidence is presented suggesting that many British children and elderly people also have intakes of iron that are below the LRNI and many have biochemical evidence of iron depletion or iron deficiency anaemia.

Preventing iron deficiency

In people consuming the same type of diet, then iron intake is likely to be directly related to total energy intake. On a good mixed European or American diet iron intake will be around 5–7 mg per 1000 kcal (4.2 MJ). This means that if the diet provides enough iron for women to meet their dietary standard then men consuming the same type of diet are likely to take in around double theirs. Young vegetarian women who restrict their food intake to control their weight are clearly at increased risk of iron deficiency. Any food fortification programme that seeks to eliminate iron deficiency anaemia in those women with particularly high needs will increase still further the surplus intake of men.

Some risk factors for iron deficiency are listed below.

- A diet that is low in absorbable iron, i.e. a diet that is low in haem iron, has low amounts of vitamin C or relatively high amounts of tannins or phytate that inhibit iron absorption. Vegetarians (10 per cent of adolescent girls) are therefore an obvious high-risk group but high intakes of vitamin C may make the inorganic iron in such diets more bioavailable.
- High menstrual blood losses, repeated pregnancies or prolonged lactation. Any other condition that leads to chronic blood loss will increase iron losses and so increase the risk of iron depletion. Infestation of the gut with parasites that cause blood loss; hookworm infestation is a major precipitating factor in many tropical countries.
- Any condition that reduces production of stomach acid reduces iron absorption from surgical gastrectomy through to simple age-related decrease in gastric acid production (achlorhydria).
- Athletes have been said to be at increased risk because of suggestions that endurance training increases iron losses. This perception of increased iron deficiency in athletes has been increased because endurance training has a haemodilution effect; it leads to increases in plasma volume that are greater than the increase in circulating haemoglobin, thus causing a fall in the measured concentration of haemoglobin in blood even though the total circulating mass of haemoglobin is increased. True anaemia in athletes is usually due to low iron intake due to dietary restriction (Maughan, 1994).

There are essentially three strategies that can be used to try to prevent and treat iron deficiency:

- provision of iron supplements to those with or at high risk of deficiency
- fortification of a core food(s) with iron
- education aimed at general improvement in the dietary iron content or increasing its bioavailability.

Of course, where chronic blood loss is identified as a precipitating factor, this problem should also be appropriately dealt with.

In Sweden, the prevalence of iron deficiency was reduced by three-quarters over a 10-year period from the mid-1960s (Anon, 1980). Increased fortification of flour with iron, widespread use of prophylactic iron preparations and increased intakes of vitamin C were considered to be some of the factors that contributed to this decline in anaemia. In 1974 sales of pharmaceutical iron preparations in Sweden amounted to almost 6 mg per head per day. Indiscriminate use of pharmaceutical preparations leads to risk of minor side effects, accidental poisoning, and chronic iron overload in susceptible people. In the UK, all flour other than wholemeal must be fortified with iron and there is also iron fortification in the USA. The iron added to British and American flour is in a form that is very poorly absorbed and so probably makes little contribution to preventing iron deficiency. Any fortification programme designed to eliminate anaemia in women with high iron needs inevitably results in men and even many women receiving iron intakes greatly in excess of their needs. This excess iron intake might cause harm, particularly to subjects inherently sensitive to iron overload. Another factor thought to have contributed to the decline in iron deficiency anaemia in Sweden was increased vitamin C intake; high intakes of vitamin C may account for the relatively low levels of anaemia found in vegetarians.

If pre-menopausal women and other groups at increased risk of anaemia are advised to eat a diet containing more available iron, such a diet would probably contain more meat (and/or fish). This could lead to increased intake of saturated fat and might not be

entirely consistent with other nutrition education guidelines. It might also be unacceptable or impractical for many women. Nevertheless, lean meat and fish are important sources of iron and other nutrients and moderate amounts should be promoted as important components of a healthy diet, especially for those at high risk of anaemia. Many young women mistakenly view red meat as particularly fattening and nutrition education should aim to correct this misconception. Current advice to increase consumption of fruits and vegetables would increase vitamin C intake and thus increase iron absorption. Several fruits and vegetables are also good sources of available iron, e.g. tomatoes, cabbage and broccoli. Large increases in consumption of cereal fibre might tend to reduce iron availability. In developed countries, iron supplements are clearly appropriate for those with poor iron status. The case for higher levels of intervention will clearly be much stronger in developing countries where the scale and severity of iron deficiency is much greater than in developed countries.

Key points

- Some past studies have reported little impairment of physiological functioning in women with mild anaemia but more recent studies suggest that symptoms of iron deficiency may occur in the absence of anaemia.

- Iron deficiency is the most common micronutrient deficiency in the world and 700 million people worldwide may have frank anaemia.

- Even in the UK a third of pre-menopausal women may have relatively low iron stores and half of these have frank depletion of their iron stores.

- Children, adolescents, pregnant women and the elderly may all be regarded as at increased risk of anaemia although it is generally uncommon in young men.

- Risk of anaemia is increased by chronic blood loss, lack of available iron in the diet, repeated pregnancies, prolonged lactation and lack of stomach acid.

- Strategies for tackling iron deficiency include increased use of iron supplements, food fortification and nutrition education aimed at improving iron availability in the diet.

- On a normal mixed diet, iron intake will be roughly proportional to energy intake.

- Any supplementation programme aimed at increasing iron intakes of high-risk women will lead to some men consuming large excesses of iron.

- Iron from fortified bread (UK and USA) is often poorly absorbed.

- Increased use of prophylactic iron preparations may result in some women taking supplements that they do not need.

- Excess iron from fortified food or supplements may cause harm, particularly to people who are inherently sensitive to iron overload.

- Increased consumption of meat is the most obvious way of improving iron availability.

- Modest amounts of lean meat are consistent with a healthy diet and nutrition education should counteract the view of many girls and young women that red meat is very fattening.

- Increased consumption of fruits and vegetables would increase vitamin C intake and thus increase inorganic iron uptake; several fruits and vegetables are also good sources of available iron.

CALCIUM, DIET AND OSTEOPOROSIS

Calcium homoeostasis

Key facts

- *Dietary standards.* Adult UK RNI 700 mg/day; LRNI 400 mg/day; USA 1000 mg/day with higher values for the elderly and adolescents.

- *Dietary sources.* Milk and milk products are rich sources with high biological availability; fish, especially if fish bones can be eaten as in tinned fish; green vegetables; pulses; nuts; wholegrain cereals (white flour is supplemented in the UK); the calcium in vegetables and in cereals may have relatively low biological availability:
  - 1 cup (195 g) milk – 225 mg
  - 40 g slice of cheddar cheese – 290 mg
  - 1 serving (20 g) almonds – 50 mg
  - 1 slice wholemeal bread – 19 mg
  - 1 serving (95 g) broccoli – 72 mg
  - 1 serving (75 g) cabbage – 40 mg
  - 1 portion (85 g) canned sardines – 390 mg
  - 1 serving (80 g) peeled prawns – 120 mg
  - 1 portion (130 g) grilled cod – 13 mg.

- *Biochemical functions.* 99 per cent of body calcium is in bone mineral but the other 1 per cent plays vital roles in nerve and muscle function, release of hormones and nerve transmitters, blood clotting and acts as an intracellular regulator of metabolism.

- *Effects of deficiency.* Overt, primary calcium deficiency is rare. Vitamin D deficiency leads to poor absorption of calcium and the disease, rickets/osteomalacia. Osteoporosis has been suggested as a long-term consequence of calcium insufficiency that is probably secondary to vitamin D deficiency and poor absorption.

- *Risk factors for deficiency.* Vitamin D deficiency and lack of sunlight exposure lead to secondary deficiency through poor absorption. Low intake is associated with lack of dairy products in the diet.

- *Biochemical measure of nutritional status.* No routine method available.

- *Prevalence of deficiency.* As noted in Chapter 12, 5 per cent of British women have unsatisfactory calcium intakes with higher prevalence in older children and older British adults living independently. Vitamin D deficiency is very prevalent and leads to inadequate calcium absorption.

- *Toxicity.* At high doses gastrointestinal symptoms may occur and in those taking medicinal calcium supplements a milk alkali syndrome sometimes occurs and results in hypercalcaemia, calcification of tissues, alkalosis, hypertension, neurological symptoms and renal impairment.

- *Recommendations on high intakes.* Supplemental doses of 1500 mg/day should have no adverse effects.

- *Typical highest UK intakes.* The highest UK consumers may get 1700 mg/day from food with up to a further 600 mg/day supplied by drinking water in some hard water areas. Over-the-counter supplements may provide up to 2400 mg/day.

Halliday and Ashwell (1991b) have written a general review of calcium nutrition and Prentice (1997) and Phillips (2003) have reviewed osteoporosis and the role of diet in its aetiology. The National Osteoporosis Society website (www.nos.org.uk) is also recommended as a good source of information about osteoporosis. This site also lists a range of inexpensive publications produced by the society that can be ordered online. Most of the uncited primary sources used for this section are listed in these reviews.

Distribution and functions of body calcium

A typical adult human body contains more than 1 kg of calcium and 99 per cent of this calcium is in the skeleton. The skeletal calcium is present as the calcium phosphate substance **hydroxyapatite**, which gives bone its mechanical strength. The small amount of body calcium that is outside the skeleton has a multitude of other vital functions such as those listed below.

- Calcium plays a major role in the release of hormones and neurotransmitters.
- Calcium is an important intracellular regulator.
- It is an essential cofactor for some enzymes and is necessary for blood clotting.
- It is involved in nerve and heart function.
- Electrical excitation of muscle cells leads to release of calcium from intracellular storage sites and this calcium release triggers muscle contraction.

Any variation in the calcium concentration of body fluids can thus have diverse effects on many systems of the body and the calcium concentration in extracellular fluids is under very fine hormonal control. The skeletal calcium not only strengthens bone, but also serves as a reservoir of calcium. The skeleton can donate or soak up excess calcium and thus enable the concentration in extracellular fluid to be regulated within narrow limits. A fall in blood calcium concentration, as seen after removal of the parathyroid glands or in extreme vitamin D deficiency, leads to muscle weakness and eventually to tetany and death due to asphyxiation when the muscles of the larynx go into spasm. A rise in plasma calcium is seen in vitamin D poisoning and in hyperparathyroidism. This hypercalcaemia can lead to gastrointestinal symptoms, neurological symptoms, formation of kidney stones and in some cases may lead to death from renal failure.

Hormonal regulation of calcium homoeostasis

The hormone **1,25 dihydroxycholecalciferol (1,25DHCC or calcitriol)** is produced in the kidney from vitamin D and is essential for the active absorption of dietary calcium in the intestine. Calcitriol promotes the synthesis of key proteins involved in active transport of calcium in both the gut and kidney. Some passive absorption of calcium occurs independently of vitamin D and this passive absorption increases with increasing dietary intake. Parathyroid hormone and calcitonin (from the thyroid gland) regulate deposition and release of calcium from bone and also the rate of excretion of calcium in the urine. Parathyroid hormone also indirectly regulates the intestinal absorption of calcium by activating the renal enzyme that produces calcitriol. Typical daily fluxes of calcium and the hormonal influences on these calcium fluxes are summarized in Figure 14.2.

Requirement and availability of calcium

The adult RNI for calcium in the UK is 700 mg/day for both males and females, this is significantly less

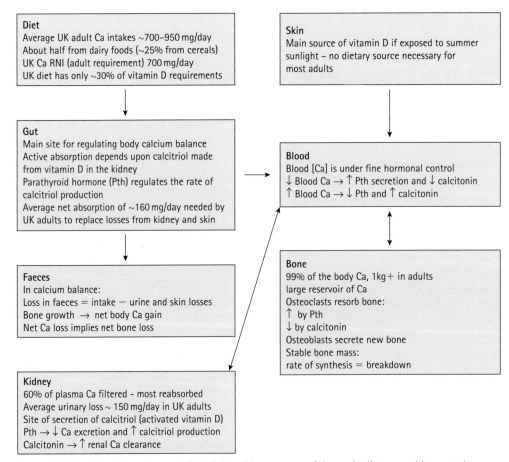

Figure 14.2 *Typical calcium fluxes in UK adults with summary of the main dietary and hormonal influences upon calcium homeostasis.*

than the American RDA of 1000 mg/day. The extra increments allowed for growth and pregnancy are also generally higher in the USA than the UK. Probably two thirds of non-pregnant women in the USA fail to meet the current RDA. A very substantial minority of British women also take in less than the RNI and 5 per cent take in less than the LRNI; many older children and independently living elderly people also take in less than their LRNI. In the UK, COMA arrived at the dietary standards by calculating the amount needed to replace typical urinary and skin losses (~160 mg/day), assuming that around 30 per cent of the dietary intake is absorbed. In Western countries, 50–70 per cent of dietary calcium is from dairy produce and the calcium in dairy produce tends to be well absorbed. This predominance of dairy produce as the major source of dietary calcium makes calcium intake vulnerable to changes in the image of dairy produce induced by health education messages. In the UK, daily calcium intake fell by 20 per cent over the period 1975–95 as a result of reduced total food intake and milk consumption. This trend was most pronounced in young women and teenage girls but according to the most recent NDNS survey (Hoare *et al.*, 2004) there has been a significant improvement in average adult calcium intake over the past decade. Note that lower-fat milks contain just as much calcium as whole milk and so reduced intake of dairy fat does not inevitably lead to reduced calcium intake. The calcium contents of typical portions of some common foods are listed in the key facts section.

The efficiency of absorption of calcium varies according to the phase of the lifecycle, the food source of calcium and the total intake (see examples below).

- The efficiency of calcium absorption increases markedly in pregnancy but is reduced in elderly people.
- Calcium from vegetable sources is generally less well absorbed than that from milk and cheese. Efficiency of absorption from breast milk is higher than from infant formula.
- At low calcium intakes the active, vitamin D-dependent absorption process predominates whereas at high intakes the less efficient passive process predominates so that the proportion of the oral load that is absorbed tends to decline with increasing intake.

Many populations who do not consume large amounts of dairy produce as adults have average calcium intakes that are less than half the current UK RNI and thus below even the current LRNI. Despite this, overt symptoms of acute dietary deficiency are not seen. For example, Prentice *et al.* (1993) reported calcium intakes in pregnant and lactating women in rural Gambia in 1979 of only around 400 mg/day. A follow-up report by Jarjou *et al.* (1994) suggested that this had fallen still further, to less than a quarter of the current UK RNI for lactating women. Despite this there is no overt evidence of acute calcium deficiency and rates of bone fractures in the Gambia are low. There is evidence that individuals who consume chronically low calcium amounts of calcium can adapt to these low intakes by increasing efficiency of absorption and by reducing their urinary losses of calcium.

Key points

- An adult body contains over 1 kg of calcium and 99 per cent of this is in the bone mineral.
- Calcium has numerous functions in addition to being a component of bone mineral.
- Large fluctuations in the calcium concentration of extracellular fluid have adverse effects on several systems and it is subject to fine hormonal control.
- Bone mineral acts as a large reservoir of calcium.
- Calcitriol is the hormone produced in the kidney from vitamin D.
- Calcitriol induces key proteins necessary for the active absorption of calcium.
- Parathyroid hormone and calcitonin control the flow of calcium into and out of bone and the rate of calcium excretion in the urine.
- Parathyroid hormone indirectly controls the intestinal absorption of calcium by regulating the renal enzyme that produces calcitriol.
- The UK RNI for calcium is 700 mg/day for men and women and substantial numbers of UK women do not take in this much and 5 per cent take in less than the LRNI.
- This RNI is calculated as the amount needed to replace daily losses assuming that 30 per cent of the dietary intake is absorbed.

- More than half of the calcium in Western diets is from milk and dairy products.
- UK intakes of calcium have fallen in recent decades as total food intake and milk consumption have dropped, although this trend seems to have been reversed in the past 10 years.
- Low-fat milk has just as much calcium as full-fat milk.
- Calcium from dairy products is much better absorbed than that from vegetable sources.
- The efficiency of calcium absorption increases in pregnancy but declines in the elderly.
- At low calcium intakes the active vitamin D-dependent process predominates but at high intakes this becomes saturated and passive absorption becomes increasingly prominent.
- Calcium intakes of many populations are much lower than in the UK and well below the current LRNI; however, these populations show no overt signs of calcium deficiency and often have very low rates of bone fractures.

CALCIUM AND BONE HEALTH

The nature of bone

The skeletal calcium is present as **hydroxyapatite**, a crystalline complex of calcium, phosphate and hydroxide ions. These crystals are laid down upon an organic matrix that is largely composed of the protein collagen. Hydroxyapatite makes up around half the weight of the bone and is responsible for conferring its mechanical strength. There are two types of mature bone, 80 per cent is cortical or compact bone and 20 per cent is trabecular bone. Cortical bone is on the outside whereas trabecular bone has a honeycomb structure with marrow filling the spaces. It is found in the centre of bones such as the pelvis, vertebrae and the ends of the long bones.

Effects of age and sex on bone density and fracture risk

Bones are not fixed and inert but living dynamic structures. The processes of bone deposition and bone breakdown continue throughout life. Bones are continually being remodelled by cells that synthesize new bone (osteoblasts) and cells that reabsorb bone and cartilage (osteoclasts). Thus if a bone's weight remains constant this is the result of a dynamic equilibrium, a balance between synthesis and breakdown. Bone mass increases throughout childhood as the skeleton grows and the rate of bone deposition exceeds the rate of breakdown. A newborn baby has 25–30 g of calcium in its skeleton and by the time the **peak bone mass** (**PBM**) is reached the skeletal calcium content has risen to well over 1 kg. People reach their PBM in their thirties and for a few years bone mass remains fairly constant because of a dynamic equilibrium between synthesis and breakdown. During middle and old age, the rate of breakdown exceeds the rate of bone formation and there is a steady decline in bone mass in these older adults (see Figure 14.3). This decrease in bone mass involves loss of both organic matrix and mineral matter. As people age, their bones become thinner, less strong and increasingly prone to fracture when subjected to trauma. Smith (1987) suggested that thinning of the bones may take them below a 'fracture threshold' when they become liable to fracture when subjected to relatively minor trauma such as a fall from a standing position. This thinning of the bones and consequent increase in fracture risk is termed **osteoporosis**.

In healthy men and pre-menopausal women, the age-related decline in bone mass is relatively slow, around 0.3–0.4 per cent of bone lost per year. In women, the decade immediately after the menopause is associated with a marked acceleration in the rate of bone loss. This post-menopausal acceleration in the rate of bone loss is due to the decline in oestrogen production and means that women usually reach the 'fracture threshold' bone density long before men (see Figure 14.3). Osteoporosis-related fractures are much more common in women than men, e.g. Spector *et al.* (1990) recorded a 4:1 female to male ratio in the age-specific incidence of hip fracture in the UK. The high female to male ratio in fracture rates is only seen in countries where rates of osteoporosis are high (Cummings *et al.*, 1985).

Bone density can be measured in living subjects by techniques such as dual-energy X-ray absorptiometry. These bone density measurements are regarded as reliable indicators of bone strength. Although a sub-threshold density is a necessary permissive factor for osteoporotic fracture, bone mineral density measurements are imperfect predictors of individual susceptibility to fracture especially for fractures of the hip (Cummings *et al.*, 1986; Smith, 1987). Leichter *et al.* (1982) measured bone density

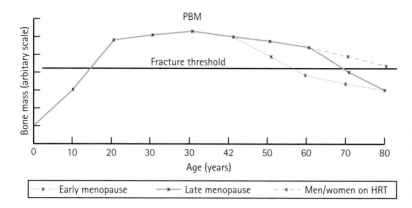

Figure 14.3 *Change in bone mass throughout life. PBM, peak bone mass; HRT, hormone replacement therapy. From Webb and Copeman (1996).*

and the shear stress required to fracture the femoral neck using isolated human bones obtained from cadavers. As expected, they found a high statistical correlation between shear stress at fracture and both bone density and bone mineral content. Breaking stress, bone density and bone mineral content all declined with the age of the subject. However, they found that breaking stress declined with age much faster than either bone density or bone mineral content. They concluded that changes in bone strength are apparently influenced by factors other than just bone density and mineral content, e.g. changes in the micro-architecture of the bone.

The imperfect association between fracture risk and measured bone density needs to be borne in mind when evaluating reports of weak associations between environmental/lifestyle variables and bone density. This also means that evidence that interventions can have acute effects on bone density need to be treated with caution. Will any short-term increase be maintained in the longer term? Will small measured increases in bone density significantly reduce fracture risk?

Key points

- Bone consists of crystals of the calcium phosphate salt, hydroxyapatite, deposited on an organic matrix consisting largely of the protein collagen.
- Hydroxyapatite makes up half of the bone weight and increases its mechanical strength.
- Bones are living dynamic structures that are continually being broken down and re-synthesized.

- Cells called osteoblasts synthesize new bone and osteoclasts cause bone breakdown.
- During childhood, rate of bone synthesis exceeds breakdown as the skeleton grows.
- In early adulthood the peak bone mass is reached and for a few years rate of synthesis and breakdown are matched.
- In middle and old age there is a net loss of bone and bones become thinner.
- Thinning of bones in old age weakens them and can take them below a 'fracture threshold' where they break in response to relatively minor trauma – this is called osteoporosis.
- There is a marked acceleration in bone loss in women around the menopause that is due to decreased oestrogen production.
- Women usually reach their 'fracture threshold' before men and so elderly women are more prone to bone fractures than elderly men.
- Non-invasive bone density measurements are indicators of bone strength.
- Bone strength decreases more rapidly with age than bone density, probably due to age-related changes in bone micro-architecture.
- Bone density is thus an imperfect measure of fracture risk and this should be borne in mind when assessing the results of studies where bone density has been used as the measured outcome.

Incidence of osteoporosis

The thinning of the bones in osteoporosis is responsible for increased rates of bone fracture in older people especially fractures of the vertebrae, wrist and the neck of the femur (hip fracture). Rates of osteoporotic fractures increased very substantially in many industrialized countries during the second half of the twentieth century. Adult bone mass declines with age so the increased prevalence of osteoporosis is partly accounted for by the increased numbers of people surviving into old age. Wickham *et al.* (1989) in a prospective study of 1400 elderly British people found that incidence of hip fracture was four times higher in women over 85 years than in women in the 65–74-year age band. Figure 14.4 shows the age and sex distribution of hip fractures in one region of England. The proportion of fractures rises exponentially with increasing age and the higher prevalence in females is also illustrated. The number of people aged over 85 years in the UK doubled in the last two decades of the twentieth century, and this group now represent 2 per cent of the UK population. There has, however, also been a real increase as demonstrated by the large increases in age-specific incidence of fractures seen in the UK (Spector *et al.*, 1990).

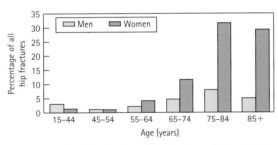

Figure 14.4 *Age distribution of hip fractures in the Trent region of England 1989/1990. Data source Kanis, 1993. Source: Webb and Copeman (1996).*

Up to 3 million people in the UK may be affected by osteoporosis, which results in around 70 000 hip fractures, 50 000 wrist fractures and more than 40 000 vertebral fractures each year. As many as 1 in 3 women and 1 in 12 men in the UK will develop osteoporosis during their lifetime (National Osteoporosis Society; www.nos.org.uk). Fractures of the hip are currently considered to be the major public health priority. A significant proportion of those affected die within a few months of the initial fracture and many more are permanently disabled or never regain full mobility after the fracture. Up to 20 000 deaths each year in the UK may be consequences of hip fracture or the associated surgery. Prentice (1997) suggested that a third of all orthopaedic beds in UK hospitals were occupied by patients with osteoporosis and this probably costs

the National Health Service in excess of a billion pounds each year. In the USA there are over 200 000 hip fractures each year that are attributable to osteoporosis. Cummings *et al.* (1985) and Johnell *et al.* (1992) give comparative rates of osteoporotic fracture in different countries.

Types of osteoporosis

There are two main types of osteoporosis.

- *Type I or menopausal osteoporosis.* This occurs in the 50–75-age group and results mainly in wrist and vertebral fractures. Loss of oestrogen is considered the major precipitating factor and it is six times more common in women than men.
- *Type II or senile osteoporosis.* This manifests mainly as fractures to the hip and vertebrae in those aged over 70 years. The incidence in women is only twice that of men; note that actual numbers of fractures in women will be much greater because women increasingly outnumber men in the older age groups. It is suggested that vitamin D deficiency and consequent increase in parathyroid hormone secretion are important causative factors.

General and lifestyle risk factors for osteoporosis

Box 14.1 lists some of the known or possible risk factors for osteoporosis. It is clear from the box that one should expect risk of osteoporosis and fractures to increase with age and elderly women to be at increased risk compared to elderly men. Projected increases in the elderly populations of many countries (see Chapter 15) makes it likely that the number of people affected by osteoporosis will rise over the coming decades unless prevention and treatment become more effective. The over-85 age group has been and will continue to increase more rapidly than the total elderly population. Women outnumber men by 3 to 1 in the over-85 age group.

The accelerated bone loss associated with menopausal oestrogen loss suggests that anything that diminishes sex hormone output might be likely to increase bone loss and fracture risk. Many conditions in which there is reduced sex hormone output are indeed associated with reduced bone density. For example:

- early menopause or surgical removal of the ovaries
- cessation of menstruation due to starvation or anorexia nervosa

- Old age; risk of osteoporosis increases with age and accelerates in women when they reach the menopause
- Being female; rates are higher in women than men in western Europe and North America
- Lack of sex hormones; factors that reduce sex hormone secretion, e.g. early menopause or ovarian removal, increase risk and hormone replacement therapy reduces risk
- Being white; there are distinct racial differences in bone density and considerable genetic variations within races
- Never having borne a child
- A sedentary lifestyle
- Smoking
- High alcohol consumption
- Being small or underweight
- Inadequate calcium intake in childhood?
- High consumption of carbonated, cola drinks?
- Being an omnivore; vegetarians have lower rates of osteoporosis

- amenorrhoea due to extremely high activity and low body fat content in women athletes
- hypogonadism in men.

Hormone replacement therapy (HRT) in post-menopausal women prevents or reduces the post-menopausal acceleration in rate of bone loss and reduces the risk of osteoporotic fracture. This treatment is widely accepted as being effective in the prevention of osteoporosis. The controversy about HRT is whether this and other benefits of the treatment are sufficient to outweigh any possible risks such as increased risk of uterine cancer or perhaps of breast cancer. Up until around 2002 many older women were being prescribed HRT for the long-term prevention of osteoporosis; many family doctors routinely encouraged their older female patients to use HRT. In 2002 a study by Nelson et al. suggested that HRT might increase the risk of heart disease in post-menopausal women whereas in the past it had been thought to be cardio-protective. This study has been criticized because most of the subjects were elderly and had existing heart disease and so were unlikely to benefit from any cardio-protective effects of HRT. These critics have suggested that if started in younger women when menopausal symptoms first appear it may still have

these benefits. Beral et al. (2003) looked at the relationship between breast cancer and HRT in a study that involved over a million women. They seemed to confirm what had long been suspected: that long-term HRT use is associated with a small increase in breast cancer risk. These studies have led to advice to family doctors that they should not routinely prescribe HRT to post-menopausal women to prevent osteoporosis although its use for alleviation of acute menopausal symptoms like 'hot flushes' is still recommended. Phytoestrogens from soya products have been marketed as an alternative to HRT for alleviation of menopausal symptoms and prevention of osteoporosis in older women (see Chapter 18).

There are clear racial differences in bone density; people of European and Asian origin have bones that are less dense than those of African origin. In the USA, white women are much more likely to have osteoporotic fractures than black women. Even within racial groups there is almost certainly a very large inherited variability in bone density and susceptibility to fracture. According to Prentice (1997) around 80 per cent of the variation in bone mineral status can be attributed to genetic factors.

The increasingly sedentary lifestyle of those living in the industrialized countries is widely believed to be a major factor in the increased age-specific incidence of osteoporotic fracture. There are numerous observations that suggest inactivity reduces bone density and that weight-bearing exercise increases it. Some examples are listed below.

- Immobilization or extreme inactivity, e.g. confinement to bed or the weightlessness experienced by astronauts results in loss of bone mass.
- When bones are repeatedly mechanically stressed they thicken and become stronger. Thus tennis players have much thicker bones in their racket arms than their other arm and runners have higher than average bone density in their vertebrae. Experimental studies have shown that jumping up and down using a small trampoline increases bone density in pre-menopausal women although not in post-menopausal women (Bassey *et al.*, 1998).
- Increased activity in the childhood and adolescence increases the PBM. Children who spent more than 2 hours daily in weight-bearing activity were reported to have greater bone mineral density than those who spent less than an hour daily in such activity (see Cooper and Eastell, 1993).

- Weight-bearing exercise in older people slows down the rate of age-related bone loss. In a cross-sectional study of 600 post-menopausal women, Coupland *et al.* (1999) were able to show that reported levels of stair climbing and brisk walking was positively associated with bone density at the hip and over the whole body. In 1400 elderly British people sampled by Wickham *et al.* (1989), risk of hip fracture was reduced in those people with higher levels of outdoor physical activity.
- Pocock *et al.* (1986) found a significant correlation between measured fitness level and bone mineral density in normal women. In the post-menopausal women in this sample, fitness was the only measured variable that correlated significantly with bone mineral density.

Being underweight is associated with a higher risk of osteoporotic fracture and in the elderly this is often as a result of low lean body mass caused by inactivity. More active and fitter elderly people may also be less prone to osteoporotic fracture because they are better co-ordinated and stronger and therefore less prone to falling or less liable to injury if they do fall.

Many studies have suggested that cigarette smoking is associated with reduced bone density and with increased fracture risk. In their sample of elderly British people, Wickham *et al.* (1989) reported a strong association between cigarette smoking and risk of hip fracture. Smoking is associated with:

- lower body weight
- reduced physical activity
- early menopause
- reduced blood oestrogen concentration (even in women receiving HRT).

These are all known associates of high fracture risk. High alcohol consumption has also been widely reported as a risk factor for osteoporosis. Heavy drinking is associated with extensive bone loss even in relatively young adults (Smith, 1987). High alcohol consumption might also be expected to increase risk of falling.

Dietary risk factors for osteoporosis

A vegetarian lifestyle is generally associated with higher bone density and reduced risk of osteoporosis (see Chapter 17). To what extent, if any, this as a result of meat avoidance *per se* is difficult to establish. There are numerous differences between Caucasian vegetarians and the general white population which would be confounding variables in this association between meat avoidance and osteoporosis. See Chapter 17 for discussion of the health aspects of vegetarianism.

The extent to which calcium nutrition affects the risk of osteoporosis has been widely investigated and the emerging consensus is that there is little evidence of any relationship between bone density and calcium intake in young and middle-aged adults but that calcium supplements may slow the rate of bone loss in post-menopausal women especially those whose habitual intakes from food are low (Phillips, 2003). Cross-cultural comparisons indicate that it is unlikely that low calcium intake is of itself a major causative factor for osteoporosis or a major determinant of bone density. Osteoporosis is uncommon in some populations with low calcium intakes but prevalence is high in many populations with relatively high calcium intakes, e.g. in the USA, UK and northern Europe. For example rural Bantu women have only one-tenth the fracture incidence of Western women despite taking in only half as much calcium (Rolls, 1992) and the similar findings of Prentice *et al.* (1993) in rural Gambia were discussed earlier. Gatehouse and Webb (unpublished observations) found a significant *positive* association between age-standardized hip fracture rates in women and *per capita* consumption of fresh milk products in eight western European countries; consumption of fresh milk products is a good predictor of calcium intakes in such countries. Hegsted (1986) also found a *positive* correlation between calcium intake and incidence of hip fracture in a genetically and culturally more diverse sample of nine countries in Europe, the Far East, Australasia and North America. International comparisons may be of limited usefulness in proving cause and effect relationships, especially when used rather anecdotally as above, but they are more persuasive when used to argue against such a relationship. If high calcium intake is associated internationally with high rates of osteoporosis this makes it improbable that calcium deficiency is an important causal factor. It is still possible, of course, that high calcium intakes or calcium supplements might have some role in offsetting an increase in osteoporosis risk even though it is primarily due to other causes. Double-blind placebo-controlled trials of calcium supplements in childhood suggest that for the first few months they do cause a small increase in measured bone density but this effect disappears once the supplements are stopped (reviewed by Prentice, 1997 and Phillips, 2003).

As was noted in Chapter 13, good vitamin D status is essential for the efficient absorption of calcium from the intestine and biochemical evidence of widespread vitamin D inadequacy has been found in children, adults and elderly people in Britain (see Chapters 12 and 15). Some of the beneficial effects of calcium supplements in slowing the rate of bone loss in older people may be because they compensate for poor vitamin D status; at high calcium intakes, more calcium is absorbed by non-vitamin D-dependent mechanisms.

Prevention and treatment of osteoporosis

Several strategies may be employed to try to reduce the number of fractures attributed to osteoporosis (see below).

- Promotion of changes in diet and lifestyle of children and young adults that increase the PBM. This increases the amount of bone that can be lost in later life before the fracture threshold is reached.
- Encourage dietary and lifestyle changes that slow down the rate of bone loss in older people, particularly in post-menopausal women. This means that it will take longer to reach the fracture threshold from any given PBM.
- Try to reverse the process of osteoporosis in older people. Promotion of dietary, behavioural and pharmacological measures that will increase bone density in those with low bone density or frank osteoporosis.
- Try to reduce the risk of bones being subjected to the traumas that cause them to fracture. Fractures of the hip usually occur after a fall. High risk of falling contributes towards the increased risk of all fractures in the elderly. In someone with advanced osteoporosis, measures that reducing the tendency to fall or to protect the faller from injury may offer the greatest potential for reducing the risk of fractures. Design and maintenance of accommodation for the elderly should pay particular attention to the risks associated with a fall for this group. Measures designed to

improve muscle strength in the elderly may reduce the risk of falling. In contrast with the enormous amount of work done looking at factors that affect bone density, relatively little work has been done on the causes of falls in the elderly.

It is often argued that a high intake of calcium in childhood together with ensuring good vitamin D status is likely to increase PBM and thus reduce the later risk of osteoporosis. Calcium intakes substantially below the dietary standard during childhood may limit PBM and poor vitamin D status certainly has adverse effects on skeletal development. However, in observational studies there is little or no correlation between calcium intake and bone density in children. According to Prentice (1997) and Phillips (2003) calcium supplementation studies in children suggest that supplements can have a small effect on bone density. This effect seems to be greatest in the first few months of supplementation and the effect disappears quickly once the supplements are stopped. In contrast, there is clear evidence that active children have denser bones than those who do little load-bearing exercise. Increasing the activity levels of children can be promoted on many grounds and would seem to be the most effective long-term strategy for improving bone health. Good intakes of milk and cheese in growing children will, in most cases, be necessary for children to achieve calcium intakes that reach dietary standard values. Vitamin D is produced by the action of sunlight on the skin and so outdoor activity should have a double effect on bone health.

As discussed earlier, there is little evidence that normal variation in dietary calcium intake has any major effect on bone density in adults. Supplemental calcium in women during the menopause is generally ineffective at preventing oestrogen-related bone loss but supplements in the elderly may reduce the rate of bone loss at the hip (Prentice, 1997; Phillips, 2003). There is compelling evidence that elderly people (and other age groups) in Britain often have poor vitamin D status and this is probably a major contributory factor to type II osteoporosis and to the high rates of hip fractures in the elderly. Inadequate exposure to sunlight during the summer months is the primary cause of this widespread vitamin D deficiency. The importance of vitamin D produced endogenously in the skin when it is exposed to summer sunlight is confirmed by the observation that only about 1 per cent of men sampled in the period July to September had unsatisfactory vitamin D status compared to 24 per cent of those sampled in January to March. Elderly housebound Britons like the rest of the population are very unlikely to obtain adequate amounts of vitamin D from their diet and as a result of this and poor sunlight exposure, up to 40 per cent of elderly British people living in residential homes have biochemical indications of poor vitamin status.

Chapuy *et al.* (1994) showed that calcium and vitamin D supplements given to institutionalized, elderly women in France substantially reduced risk of hip and other fractures over a 3-year period. Many of their sample had raised parathyroid levels and low serum 25-hydroxycholecalciferol concentrations, which are indicative of poor vitamin D status. The treatment lowered serum parathyroid hormone levels whereas levels rose in the placebo group. High parathyroid hormone levels were associated with lowered bone density measurements. However neither calcium supplements nor vitamin D supplements were effective in preventing fracture recurrence in elderly people with a history of established osteoporosis (Record Trial Group, 2005). So calcium and vitamin supplements may prevent or slow down the age-related loss of bone but they cannot reverse the process once the bones are seriously weakened.

An expert report in the UK (Caroline Walker Trust (CWT), 1995) recommended that architects designing residential accommodation for older people should take particular account of the need of residents for regular exposure to sunlight. They suggested the provision of sheltered alcoves on the south side of buildings and well-paved pathways with hand rails and no steps. There is a clear case for vitamin D supplements in elderly housebound people. The case for inactivity as a cause of osteoporosis was made earlier and so the case for encouraging increased amounts of load-bearing exercise in all age groups is overwhelming. There are many other reasons for encouraging increased activity and physical fitness (summarized in Chapter 17).

There is compelling evidence that the administration of oestrogen (HRT) to menopausal women prevents or reduces the post-menopausal acceleration in rate of bone loss and reduces fracture risk. Detailed discussion of this issue is beyond the scope of this book but there is further discussion of the effects of phytoestrogens on bone density and as possible 'natural' alternatives to HRT are discussed in Chapter 18. The treatments for osteoporosis include:

- administration of sex hormones or synthetic analogues – oestrogen replacement therapy in women and testosterone injections in men
- supplements of vitamin D and calcium
- use of calcitonin injections or the bisphosphonate group of drugs which both inhibit bone breakdown by osteoclasts
- a new drug called teriparatide has recently become available for those women most severely affected by osteoporosis. It is a synthetic analogue of part of the parathyroid hormone molecule. It can be administered only by injection and at the moment its use is restricted to 18 months but the benefits last beyond this period. It stimulates new bone formation, so unlike other treatments it does reverse the process of osteoporosis.

Conclusions

An active lifestyle, absence of cigarette smoking, moderate alcohol consumption and a diet that meets the standards for essential nutrients is both consistent with general health education guidelines and offers expectation of reducing the risk of osteoporosis and bone fractures. There seems to be no convincing evidence that calcium supplements *per se* will prevent osteoporosis or be effective in its treatment. Good intakes of calcium in childhood and early adulthood may contribute to increased peak bone mass but other lifestyle factors (e.g. activity level) are probably more significant and the case for calcium supplements seems unconvincing. Widespread vitamin D deficiency in the elderly is probably an important cause of increased fracture risk and so increased exposure to sunlight and/or supplements of vitamin D and calcium should be encouraged. Although much of the current health promotion focus is concerned with the undoubted dangers of overexposure to strong sunlight and avoidance of sunburn, it does seem that many British people in all age groups do not get enough regular sunlight exposure to maintain good vitamin D status.

Detailed discussion of the pros and cons of HRT is beyond the scope of this book but, on the narrow question of whether it reduces the risk of osteoporosis, the evidence is compelling. The development of a new class of drugs that reverse the process of osteoporosis rather than just slowing or arresting it is encouraging for those people with, or at risk of developing, this disabling disease.

Key points

- Osteoporotic fracture rates rose during the twentieth century not only because of the growth of the elderly population but also because the age-specific incidence increased.
- In the UK 150 000–200 000 fractures each year are attributed to osteoporosis.
- Many of the 70 000 people who annually suffer hip fractures die within a few months of the initial fracture or never regain full mobility.
- A third of all orthopaedic beds in the UK are occupied by people with osteoporosis.
- Menopausal oestrogen loss is thought to be a major precipitating factor for type I osteoporosis and vitamin D deficiency for the type II that occurs principally in very elderly people.
- The risk factors for osteoporosis are listed in Box 14.1.
- The projected growth of the very elderly population together with the 3:1 ratio of women to men in this age group indicates that fracture rates are likely to increase in the coming decades.
- Lack of sex hormones in men or women increases bone loss and oestrogen replacement therapy slows bone loss.
- There are inherent racial and individual differences in bone density, and perhaps 80 per cent of the variation in bone mineral status can be attributed to genetic factors.
- Bones thicken when exposed to repeated stress and they become thinner when immobilized.
- Experimental and epidemiological studies suggest that load-bearing exercise:
  - increases bone deposition in children and increases peak bone mass
  - slows the rate of bone loss in older adults
  - increases bone density in older adults.
- Cigarette smokers and alcoholics have reduced bone density but vegetarians usually have higher than average bone density.

- International comparisons suggest that osteoporosis is often most prevalent in those countries with the highest calcium intakes which makes it unlikely that low calcium intake is a primary cause of osteoporosis.
- Calcium intakes seem to have a small positive effect on bone density in children but only as long as the supplements continue to be taken.
- Calcium supplements slow the rate of bone loss in elderly women, especially in those whose intake from food is low. These supplements may be compensating for poor vitamin D status.
- Many elderly people have little exposure to sunlight and low vitamin D status.
- Combined supplements of vitamin D and calcium have been shown to reduce fracture risk in very elderly housebound women but not in those who already have established osteoporosis and have already experienced a fracture.
- Osteoporosis would be reduced by the following:
  - increased weight-bearing activity in children and ensuring they have good vitamin D and calcium status
  - increased participation in load-bearing activity in all adults
  - ensuring the vitamin D status of elderly people by increasing access to sunlight or the provision of supplements
  - measures to reduce the risk of falling in the elderly or to decrease the risk of injury in elderly fallers
  - increased use of hormone replacement therapy by post-menopausal women
  - less tobacco use and alcohol misuse.
- A new class of drugs, e.g. teriparatide, which are analogues of parathyroid hormone seem to reverse the process of osteoporosis and result in new bone synthesis.

SALT AND HYPERTENSION

Key facts

- *Dietary standards.* Sodium adult RNI 1.6 g, chloride 2.5 g (these are equivalent in molar terms and represent 4.1 g of salt); sodium LRNI 575 mg/day chloride 888 mg/day (c.1.5 g salt/day). US values: sodium 1.5 g/day and chloride 2.3 g/day.

- *Dietary recommendations.* Average population salt intake should be reduced to around 6 g/day.
- *Dietary sources.* Processed foods are the major source with small amounts in natural foods and some discretionary salt is added at the table and during home cooking. The salt content of some typical food portions:
  - 2 medium slices bread – 1 g
  - 60 g cheddar cheese – 1.1 g
  - 60 g Danish blue cheese – 2.1 g
  - 4 fish fingers – 0.9 g
  - 1 portion cornflakes (25 g) – 0.7 g
  - 1 portion all-bran (45 g) – 1 g
  - 90 g prawns – 3.7 g
  - 1 gammon steak (120 g) – 6.5 g
  - 2 slices (60 g) corned beef – 1.5 g
  - 2 large sausages – 1.5 g
  - 1 packet of crisps – 0.4 g
  - 1 bowl of canned tomato soup (200 g) – 2.3 g
  - 1 portion baked beans (200 g) – 2.4 g
  - sardines in tomato sauce (100 g) – 0.9 g
  - 1 takeaway cheeseburger – 2.2 g
  - lime pickle (15 g) – 0.2 g
  - takeaway vegetable curry – 2 g
  - beef chow mein – 5.5 g.
- *Biochemical functions.* Sodium is the major cation in extracellular fluid; it maintains fluid and electrolyte balance, is important in nerve transmission and in acid–base balance. Chloride is the major anion in the body and is important in maintaining fluid and electrolyte balance.
- *Effects of deficiency.* Dietary deficiencies do not usually occur.
- *Risk factors for deficiency.* Unaccustomed heavy physical activity in a warm environment can lead to substantial salt losses in sweat and this may cause short-term increases in salt requirement but adaptation occurs and results in the production of a much more dilute sweat.

Overview

Historical importance of salt

Salt has been prized throughout history for its ability to flavour and preserve foods. Roman soldiers used to be paid partly with salt (their *salarium*) which is the origin of the word salary and of the common expression 'to be worth one's salt'. Salt has been an important trading commodity with whole empires built on the revenues derived from the salt trade. Salt has also been attributed with mystical and purifying properties by many cultural groups and it certainly does have useful antiseptic properties. In their excellent monograph on salt, MacGregor and de Wardener (1999) devote a whole chapter to these non-culinary uses of salt – the image of Sumo wrestlers purifying the fighting arena with handfuls of salt is one example that is familiar to many of us. In past times in the USA, salt was left in the room of a dead person to purge their sins and it was common practice in parts of Britain to sprinkle salt on a corpse or place salt in the coffin. MacGregor and de Wardener even reproduce an ancient woodcut of French women sprinkling salt on their husbands' genitals to enhance their sexual performance! This monograph is entitled 'Salt, diet and health' and contains a good introduction to work concerning the health consequences of a high salt intake and lists and discusses many of the landmark studies in this field.

The problems with salt

High salt intake has long been suspected of being involved in the aetiology of essential hypertension. Note that essential hypertension is the most common type of high blood pressure where the cause is unknown and the hypertension is not a secondary consequence of some other known pathology. Salt (sodium chloride) is made up of the two mineral elements sodium and chlorine. It is the sodium component that has been generally regarded as significant in causing hypertension although this has been questioned; this discussion generally refers to salt rather than to sodium alone. Even in people with hypertension, salt (sodium) balance is very effectively hormonally regulated; if salt intake is raised or lowered then urinary excretion rapidly rises or falls so as to restore the balance between intake and output. This homoeostatic mechanism is so effective that salt excretion is generally regarded as the best way of measuring salt intake. Despite this homoeostatic mechanism, it has been argued that prolonged excess salt intake can lead to excess salt retention and therefore increased fluid retention and hypertension. Evidence from dialysis patients and those with endocrine disorders confirms that salt retention does indeed lead to increased blood pressure.

MacGregor and de Wardener (1999) suggest that the kidneys of patients with essential hypertension have an impaired ability to excrete salt. When large amounts of salt are consumed by susceptible people their kidney defect means that there is a tendency to retain excess salt which triggers several compensatory mechanisms that increase salt excretion and restore homoeostasis. A rise in blood pressure and consequent increase in renal filtration of salt is one of these compensatory mechanisms. They cite as evidence for this theory, cross-transplantation studies in rats. When the kidneys of genetically hypertensive and normal rats were surgically swapped, the blood pressure rose in the normal rats with hypertensive strain kidneys but remained normal in the hypertensive strain rats with normal kidneys. They claim that limited observations on patients receiving therapeutic kidney transplants show a similar trend.

High salt intake has also been implicated in the aetiology of gastric cancer. One theory suggests that salt acts as a gastric irritant and that continued irritation due to high salt intake leads to atrophy of the acid secreting glands in the stomach. Reduced acid secretion in the stomach then allows proliferation of bacteria, and they produce carcinogenic substances (nitrosamines) from some components of food. Again there is considerable support for the latter part of the hypothesis; patients with pernicious anaemia who produce less gastric acid have markedly increased rates of gastric cancer. In recent years it has become clear that infection with the bacterium *Helicobacter pylori* is the most important predisposing factor for gastric cancer. Chronic infection with this organism leads to atrophic gastritis and eventually to cancer. Most early studies on the relationship between diet and cancer have taken no account of the presence or absence of this organism. There is moderately consistent evidence that diets rich in salted meats and fish, and salted pickled vegetables are associated with increase risk of this cancer but these foods are not generally consumed in the UK (COMA, 1998).

MacGregor and de Wardener (1999) review evidence that high salt intake may be a factor in the aetiology of osteoporosis. In short-term studies, increases in salt intake and excretion also increase the renal excretion of calcium although one would expect homoeostatic mechanisms to compensate for this by increasing the intestinal absorption of calcium. One study has reported a positive correlation between rates of bone loss and urinary salt excretion in older women.

Affluent populations have generally been advised to substantially reduce their dietary salt intake. The WHO has suggested a move towards a population average salt intake of 5 g/day. In both Britain (COMA, 1991, 1994a and Scientific Advisory Committee on Nutrition (SACN), 2003) and the USA (National Research Council (NRC), 1989b) it is recommended that salt intake should be limited to 6 g/day. The principal aim of such recommendations is to reduce the 20–25 per cent incidence of essential hypertension in the adult populations of affluent countries and thus to reduce the morbidity and mortality from diseases precipitated by high blood pressure, namely strokes, myocardial infarction, renal failure and retinopathy. Adults can be classified into four categories when trying to assess the prevalence of high blood pressure:

- normotensive and untreated – systolic blood pressure <160 mmHg, diastolic <95 mmHg and not taking drugs to control their blood pressure
- normotensive treated – systolic blood pressure <160 mmHg, diastolic <95 mmHg and taking drugs to control their blood pressure
- hypertensive treated – systolic blood pressure >160 mmHg and/or diastolic >95 mmHg and taking drugs to control their blood pressure
- hypertensive untreated – systolic blood pressure >160 mmHg and/or diastolic >95 mmHg but not taking drugs.

All of the latter three categories are people who have developed high blood pressure and they represent about 22 per cent of all adults in Britain. The prevalence of hypertension rises steeply with age, as can be seen from the rates in different age groups:

- 1 per cent of those aged 16–24 years have high blood pressure
- 3 per cent of those aged 25–34
- 7 per cent of those aged 35–44
- 18 per cent aged 35–44 years
- 38 per cent aged 55–64 years
- 57 per cent aged 65–74 years
- 70 per cent aged over 75 years.

A wide variety of antihypertensive drugs are now available that are effective in lowering blood pressure, at least in the short term. These drugs also seem to be effective in reducing the renal and cerebrovascular complications of hypertension although some of them, particularly the older drugs, are less effective in reducing the coronary conditions associated with high blood pressure and may even be associated with increased coronary risk. As with any drug, there may be acute side effects and possible long-term problems are of particular concern because antihypertensives may need to be taken for the rest of the patient's life. There have been suggestions that use of some antihypertensives can be associated with increased overall mortality (e.g. Multiple Risk Factor Intervention Trial (MRFIT, 1982). Despite the availability of this wide range of antihypertensive drugs, the idea that moderation of dietary salt intake might prevent hypertension or be a useful alternative to drugs in the treatment of hypertension is still an attractive proposition. Salt restriction may also be used in conjunction with antihypertensive drugs to increase their effectiveness or reduce the doses needed. High intakes of potassium and possibly calcium have also been suggested as having possible protective effects against the development of hypertension.

Key points

- It is widely believed that high salt intake is an important cause of essential hypertension.
- High blood pressure increases the risk of strokes, myocardial infarctions, renal failure and retinopathy.
- One theory suggests that the kidneys of hypertensives have an impaired ability to excrete salt and that a rise in blood pressure is a compensatory mechanism that increases renal filtration and salt excretion.
- There is very effective renal regulation of daily salt balance even in hypertensives.
- Salt has also been implicated in the aetiology of gastric cancer and less convincingly in the aetiology of osteoporosis.
- In the UK (and USA) a maximum salt intake of 6 g/day has been recommended compared with the current average of around 10 g/day.
- Reduced salt intake is expected to reduce the prevalence of hypertension and thus ultimately the risk of the hypertension-linked diseases.
- Salt restriction may also be a useful adjunct to or alternative to antihypertensive drug treatment.
- 20–25 per cent of all UK adults may be hypertensive and the proportion rises steeply with age.

Requirement for salt

There is no doubt that the sodium and chloride that comprise salt are essential nutrients. Sodium is the principal cation in extracellular fluid and the standard 70 kg man has around 92 g of sodium in his body, equivalent to around 250 g of salt. Around half of total body sodium is in the extracellular fluid, 38 per cent in bone and the remaining 12 per cent in the intracellular fluid; potassium is the dominant cation in intracellular fluid. Despite its undoubted essentiality, the habitual intake of most affluent populations greatly exceeds minimum requirements. Almost all ingested salt is absorbed in the intestine and the homoeostatic control of salt excretion by the endocrine system enables individuals, even those with hypertension, to remain in salt balance over a huge range of intakes. Some populations, such as the Kalahari Bushmen and New Guinea Highlanders, manage on habitual salt intakes of around 1 g/day whereas other populations (e.g. some regions of Japan and Korea) habitually take in more than 25 g/day. Average urinary excretion of salt in a sample of adult Yanomamo Indians in Brazil was found to be only 50 mg per day, which is less than 1 per cent of that excreted by an average Briton (see MacGregor and de Wardener, 1999 for substantial detail on comparative salt intakes of different populations).

The American NRC (1989a) estimated that minimum requirements for sodium chloride were only around 1.25 g/day. This minimum figure did not provide for large prolonged losses from the skin through sweat. Individuals adapt to salt restriction during heavy exercise or in a hot environment by producing very dilute sweat. The UK RNIs for sodium and chloride amount to a salt intake of around 4 g/day; the panel felt that this value allowed for losses in sweat during exercise and high temperatures once adaptation had occurred but that in the short term, extra intake might be required under these circumstances (COMA 1991).

Amount and sources of dietary salt

It is generally accepted that **discretionary salt**, used in cooking and at table makes the traditional methods of dietary analysis using food tables an unreliable method of assessing salt intake. The best method of estimating salt intake is by measurement of sodium excreted over a 24-hour period. This method relies on the assumption that, whatever the intake, individuals are in approximate salt balance on a day-to-day basis and thus that sodium excretion is equal to sodium intake. The method usually involves collecting a 24-hour urine specimen from the subjects. Normally well over 90 per cent of total body sodium loss is via the urine and the figure can be corrected for losses via the skin and in faeces, which are small under most circumstances. If there is severe diarrhoea or unaccustomed heavy sweating due to physical activity, high ambient temperature or fever, then losses by these other routes may of course be very considerable. Ideally, a marker substance should be used to ensure that the 24-hour urine specimen is complete, i.e. a substance that is consumed by the subject and excreted in the urine; only where there is complete recovery of the marker is the sample considered to be complete.

In a large sample of British adults Gregory *et al.* (1990) found a very poor correlation (r = 0.25) between salt intake as measured by 24-hour urinary sodium excretion and that calculated from the average salt content of foods recorded during a 7-day weighed inventory. Several factors may contribute to this poor agreement between the two methods:

- the sodium excretion method used just 1 day, which was at a different time to the 7 days of the weighed inventory (the intake of many nutrients fluctuates widely from day to day)
- no allowance was made for salt added during cooking or at the table in the weighed inventory
- no marker was used to ensure completeness of the 24-hour urine specimen.

Nevertheless, the lack of agreement between these methods underlines the difficulty of estimating a subject's habitual salt intake in order to correlate this with, for example, blood pressure in epidemiological studies. Both methods have been used as the measure of habitual intake in epidemiological studies. Nutrient intakes fluctuate from day to day and several days intake needs to be recorded to get a useful estimate of average daily intake. The length of the necessary recording time varies from nutrient to nutrient depending on its distribution in food (see Chapter 3). This means that this disagreement between the two methods is in line with what is found with other nutrients. For example, potassium intake in food and 24-hour excretion of potassium were also both measured in this sample of people. In this case there is no discretionary intake from table and cooking use. Despite this the correlation between the two methods for potassium intake were almost as bad as for sodium. This strongly suggests that even though 24-hour sodium excretion may be an accurate reflection of sodium intake on that day, large day-to-day variations may make it a relatively poor predictor of the habitual salt intake of an individual.

Average 24-hour sodium excretion should be a much better reflection of the habitual intake of a population or group. Using this method, James *et al.* (1987) concluded that average salt intake in the UK was around 10.7 g/day for men and 8.0 g/day for women. More recently, Hoare *et al.* (2004) reported average intakes for British men of 11 g/day and 8.1 g/day for women using the 24-hour excretion method; only 15 per cent of men and 31 per cent of women were below the 6 g/day recommended maximum. The intakes recorded by James *et al.* (1987) were less than previous measurements (e.g. those assumed by National Advisory Committee on Nutrition Education (NACNE), 1983). These authors suggested that this was because those using more traditional methods had not recognized that as much as 75 per cent of cooking salt is not actually consumed and most is discarded with cooking water.

James *et al.* provided their subjects with pots of table and cooking salt that had been 'labelled' with lithium; recovery of lithium in urine enabled them to estimate what proportion of the total excreted was from these sources. By comparing the amount removed from the pot with recovery they were also able to make their estimate of the proportion of this salt that was not consumed, e.g. discarded in cooking water or in uneaten food. They concluded that discretionary salt made up only about 15 per cent of total intake, 9 per cent from table salt and 6 per cent from cooking salt. They estimated that another 10 per cent of total intake was from salt naturally present in foods but that the remaining 75 per cent was derived from salt added by food manufacturers during processing (the salt content of some common foods is shown in the key facts section). Such figures indicate that there is very limited scope for individuals to reduce their salt intake by restricting their discretionary use of salt. If salt intake is to be substantially reduced then either the salt content of manufactured foods must be reduced or the contribution of high salt manufactured foods to the total diet must be reduced. The most recent NDNS survey (Hoare *et al.*, 2004) estimated salt intake by 7-day weighed food intake at 8.3 g/day for men and 5.8 g/day for women – this excludes salt added during cooking or at the table and estimates of total salt intake using urinary sodium excretion give figures of 11 g/day in men and 8.1 g/day in women. (These latter values are slightly higher than those reported by Gregory *et al.* (1990) in the previous NDNS of British adults – 10.1 g/day for men and 7.7 g/day for women.) Hoare *et al.* (2004) also presented an analysis of the contribution of different foods to the total food intake from food:

- cereals and cereal products provided over 35 per cent of the salt in food with white bread alone contributing 14 per cent of the total
- meat, meat dishes and meat products provided 26 per cent of the total with bacon and ham contributing 8 per cent
- milk and milk products provided 8 per cent of the total
- vegetables and vegetable dishes (excluding potatoes) contributed 7 per cent
- fish and fish products contributed 4 per cent
- miscellaneous foods, which include soups, sauces and relishes, contributed 8 per cent
- all other categories of food provided substantially less than 5 per cent each.

Reduced salt versions of several salty foods are now widely available in Britain, e.g. cured meats and some canned foods. In late 1998, an announcement by a major British supermarket chain that they were going to reduce the salt content of their own brand of prepared foods by 25 per cent achieved much publicity. Many other supermarket chains and food producers claimed that they were already reducing the salt content of their manufactured food products. Since then there have been periodic announcements by various food manufacturers and retailers of reductions in salt content of their food. Encouraging food manufacturers to use less salt may not be entirely without problems; salt is used by manufacturers not only as a flavouring agent but also as a preservative and processing aid. Reduced salt content of processed foods may have effects other than on their palatability. In particular, shelf-life may be adversely affected thus increasing costs and the microbiological safety of the food may also be threatened. If salt is replaced by alternative preservatives then this increased intake

of alternative preservatives may itself be undesirable. In a chapter entitled 'The industrial conspiracy', MacGregor and de Wardener (1999) argue that salt producers and food processors have resisted pressure to reduce the salt content of manufactured foods for commercial reasons rather than out of any necessity to maintain food safety or quality.

> ## Key points
>
> - A normal man's body contains around 250 g of salt and sodium is the major cation in extracellular fluid.
> - Sodium and chlorine are essential minerals but current salt intakes are 10 times minimum requirements.
> - Individuals adapt to low salt intakes by reducing the sodium concentrations of sweat and urine.
> - The UK RNIs for sodium and chlorine are equivalent to about 4 g/day of salt.
> - 24-hour sodium excretion is regarded as the best measure of salt intake.
> - There is very poor correlation between salt intake as measured by conventional dietary analysis and 24-hour sodium excretion.
> - 24-hour sodium excretion is a good measure of any day's salt intake or the average intake of a population: it is a poor measure of an individual's habitual salt intake because of large day-to-day variations.
> - A 1987 estimate found that more than 75 per cent of UK dietary salt is from manufactured foods and only around 15 per cent is salt added at the table and during home cooking.
> - Substantial reductions in total salt intake require that either less is used by food processors or that consumption of high-salt processed foods is reduced.
> - The salt content of many processed foods has been reduced and low-salt versions of a number of processed foods are now available although this has not reduced average salt intakes.

A review of the evidence for a salt–hypertension link

In some populations that have very low salt intakes of approximately 1 g/day, hypertension is practically unknown and there is no general increase in blood pressure with age as is seen in the UK and USA (e.g. Kalahari Bushmen and the Yanomamo Indians of Brazil). In countries such as Japan and Korea average salt intake may be two to three times that seen in the UK and there is very high incidence of strokes and gastric cancer, which have both been causally linked to high salt intake. The low-salt populations often have diets and lifestyle that are very different from those of affluent Westerners. Any number of confounding variables could explain the apparent link between salt and hypertension, e.g. high physical activity, low levels of obesity, low alcohol and tobacco use and high potassium intake of those populations with low salt intake. There are, however, some examples of fit, active populations still leading a fairly traditional lifestyle who nonetheless have high salt intakes and who have blood pressure and hypertension profiles that are more typical of those seen in Western populations. For example, Solomon Islanders who cooked their food in seawater have eight times the incidence of hypertension compared with those living on nearby islands whose salt intake is low. Tobian (1979) and MacGregor and de Wardener (1999) both provide interesting summaries of the early work in this area.

The levels of salt in these low-salt populations, such as that in the Yanomamo Indians, is so low as to be a totally unrealistic goal for those living in affluent countries. However, more extensive cross-population studies, such as those of Gliebermann (1973), suggested that there was a near linear relationship between the average salt intake of a population and the average blood pressure in middle-aged and elderly people (see Figure 3.7, p. 103). This would mean that even modest reductions in population salt intake could be expected to lead to reduced average blood pressure, reduced incidence of hypertension and thus eventually to reduced morbidity and mortality from those conditions that are precipitated by hypertension. In Gliebermann's paper, the reliability and validity of many of the measures of salt intake were questionable. As in all such cross-cultural studies, there was the recurring problem of confounding variables. Gliebermann's data also included some black populations that are genetically salt sensitive and prone to hypertension and this could account for some of the most divergent points on her graphs.

In a more recent cross-population study, Law et al. (1991a) related blood pressure to salt intake from reported data on 24 populations around the world. They overcame some of the criticisms of Gliebermann's earlier work (see list below).

- They restricted their analysis to data in which salt intake was measured by 24-hour sodium excretion.
- They excluded African and other black populations from their study.
- They analysed data from developed and economically underdeveloped countries separately so as to reduce the problem of confounding lifestyle variables.
- Their study included people across a wide age range enabling them to look at the relationship between salt intake and blood pressure in different age groups.

Despite these improvements in methodology their conclusions were similar to those of Gliebermann. They found a highly significant relationship between average blood pressure and population salt intake in both developed and the economically underdeveloped populations. The effect of salt intake on blood pressure increased with age and with initial blood pressure level. They derived an equation that they suggested would predict the average change in blood pressure of a group that would result from a specified change in salt intake. The variables in this equation were: the group's age, current salt intake and initial blood pressure. They predicted, for example, that in a developed country such as the UK a 60 per cent reduction in salt intake in 60–69-year-olds with a systolic pressure of 183 mmHg might be expected to lead to a 14 mmHg reduction in systolic pressure.

Studies of migrant populations confirm that much of the international variation in blood pressure and incidence of hypertension-related diseases is due to environmental rather than genetic factors. People of Japanese origin in the USA, where salt intake is much lower than in Japan, have reduced incidence of strokes as compared with Japanese people living in Japan. Samburu tribesmen in Kenya have a traditional low-salt diet in their villages but if they join the Kenyan army the high-salt army rations are associated with a rise in their average blood pressure after 2–3 years (see Tobian, 1979).

Reduced reliance on salting as a means of food preservation during this century has been associated with falling mortality from strokes and gastric cancer in both the USA and UK, and indeed in most industrialized countries. On an international basis, there is a strong positive correlation between stroke and gastric cancer mortality in industrialized countries. This is consistent with there being a common causative factor for the two diseases. Joossens and Geboers (1981) regressed mean death rates for gastric cancer in 12 industrialized countries with those for stroke; they found a very strong linear correlation between 1955 and 1973 (see Figure 3.8, p. 105). In a more recent study, Joossens et al. (1996) reported a strong positive correlation between average salt intake and death rate from stomach cancer in a study of 24 populations from around the world.

The weak point in the evidential link between salt intake and hypertension has traditionally been the lack of association between salt intake and blood pressure in individuals from within the same community. This lack of association has been a fairly consistent finding in many within-population studies (Tobian, 1979; Law et al., 1991b) and may be because of the general tendency for the influence of other factors on blood pressure to obscure the relationship with salt intake (see Chapter 3). The difficulty of reliably measuring habitual salt intake would also be an important factor – many studies have used 24-hour sodium excretion as the measure of habitual salt intake but it is almost certainly a very poor measure of this. Others have argued that this lack of association is because only a relatively small proportion of the population is salt sensitive. There will inevitably be genetic variation in salt sensitivity, but if this variation is so great that effectively only a small subgroup of the population is salt sensitive, this would greatly weaken the case for population intervention to reduce salt intake.

Frost et al. (1991) in a complex re-analysis of 14 published within-population studies of the relationship between salt intake and blood pressure concluded that the results were consistent with the results predicted from their equation derived from between-population analysis (Law et al., 1991a). They argued that day-to-day variation in an individual's salt intake tends to obscure the true association between sodium intake and blood pressure in within-population studies. This is consistent with the poor correlation between 24-hour sodium excretion and salt content of food in weighed inventories reported by Gregory et al. (1990) that was discussed earlier in the chapter.

There have been several intervention trials that have aimed to reduce salt intake of a population as a means of reducing blood pressure and the incidence of hypertension. The results of trials conducted in Japan and Belgium are consistent with the belief that salt restriction will have beneficial effects on blood pressure but are less than conclusive (see MacGregor and de Wardener, 1999). Forte et al. (1989) report the effects of an intervention trial using two small, rural populations in Portugal. Over a 2-year period, the intervention succeeded in reducing average salt intake by at least 25 per cent in the test village whereas that in the control village did not change. By the end of the study period the average systolic blood pressure in the test village had fallen by 13 mmHg relative to the control village.

Denton et al. (1995) conducted a 2-year controlled study of the effects of salt on the blood pressure of chimpanzees. Salt was added to the normal vegetable and fruit diet of the experimental group and over the first 18 months of the study blood pressure rose substantially in 10 of the 13 animals in the experimental group. When the salt supplements were withdrawn, the blood pressure of these chimps returned to normal within 20 weeks.

The SACN (2003) report Salt and health concluded that the evidence for an association between salt intake and blood pressure had increased over the previous 10 years and that this effect was consistently found in a variety of different study populations and different ethnic groups. They discussed data from the Dietary Approaches to Stop Hypertension Trial (Appel et al., 1997) which showed that a diet rich in fruits, vegetables and low-fat dairy products and reduced saturated and total fat coupled with a low-salt diet was the most effective dietary strategy for reducing hypertension. A systematic review of the long-term effects of advice to reduced dietary salt consumption (Hooper et al., 2002) resulted in significant reductions in blood pressure at 6–12 months but that these were not sustained in the longer term and neither was the initial reduction in average sodium excretion. The authors concluded that these data illustrate the difficulties of sustaining a low-salt diet when most of the salt consumed originates in processed foods. This committee re-affirmed earlier recommendations that average daily salt intake should be reduced to 6 g/day and that this lowering posed no significant risks. They concluded that reduced salt intake would lower blood pressure for the whole population.

Is salt restriction an effective antihypertensive therapy?

Moderation of salt intake is widely promoted as a preventive measure, but it has also long been used as a method of treating hypertension. Before the advent of the antihypertensive drugs, extreme salt restriction was one of the few treatments available for severe hypertension. The Kempner rice and fruit diet aimed to restrict salt intake to 1 g/day. This diet was effective in some individuals but it was associated with poor compliance, anorexia and side effects that greatly limited its practical usefulness. These early therapeutic studies of patients with severe (malignant) hypertension generally suggested that although extreme salt restriction was effective in some hypertensives, more moderate salt restriction (say 2.5+ g/day) was not effective. The advent of antihypertensive drugs heralded a general loss of interest in this method of treating severe hypertension. There is now, however, renewed interest in the use of moderate salt restriction as a treatment for those people with asymptomatic mild to moderate hypertension where the principal aim is to reduce the long-term risk of hypertension-linked diseases. Drug therapy is effective in reducing hypertension in such subjects but lifelong consumption of antihypertensive drugs is clearly not an ideal solution and may be associated with a new range of hazards.

Several trials of the effectiveness of salt restriction in the treatment of hypertension have been conducted in recent decades, e.g. note the rigorous double-blind, random crossover study of MacGregor et al. (1982) discussed in Chapter 3. Law et al. (1991b) analysed the results of 78 controlled salt reduction trials. They concluded that in those trials where salt restriction was for 5 weeks or more, the results obtained closely matched those that they had predicted from the cross-population analysis of Law et al. (1991a). Effects of salt restriction were less than predicted when shorter periods of salt restriction were used. They concluded that in 50–59-year-olds in industrialized countries, a reduction in salt intake of 3 g/day could be expected to lead to an average reduction in systolic blood pressure of 5 mmHg with greater reductions in those who were hypertensive. They argue that such a level of salt reduction would, if universally adopted, lead to major reductions in stroke and heart disease mortality.

Other factors involved in the aetiology of hypertension

Much of the evidence implicating salt in the aetiology of hypertension could also be used to support the proposition that high potassium intake is protective against hypertension. In acute studies of sodium loading in both salt-sensitive rats and in people, high potassium intake seems to ameliorate the effects of high sodium loads. Some correlation between the sodium/potassium ratio and blood pressure may be found in within-population studies where no relationship can be shown between blood pressure and sodium intake alone. The SACN (2003) concluded that it is difficult to relate blood pressure to specific nutrients because of strong correlations between potassium, calcium, magnesium and fibre intakes. It did find consistent evidence that increased intake of fruit and vegetables did have a positive effect in lowering blood pressure (e.g. Appel et al., 1997).

There is some epidemiological evidence that low calcium intake may be associated with increased risk of hypertension. People with osteoporosis also have higher incidence of hypertension, a finding consistent with a common aetiology. Some have used this latter observation to suggest that high salt may cause osteoporosis whereas other have argued that low calcium intake might be a factor in hypertension. Several intervention trials have suggested that calcium supplements may reduce blood pressure, at least in a proportion of hypertensives.

Overweight and obesity are generally agreed to lead to increases in blood pressure and weight loss reduces blood pressure in the overweight hypertensive. White et al. (1993) reported that in their representative sample of English adults, blood pressure rose with increasing body mass index. Increased physical activity reduces the tendency to gain excessive weight and also contributes directly to a reduction in blood pressure. Excessive alcohol consumption also leads to a rise in blood pressure and increases the risk of stroke even in the absence of hypertension. White et al. (1993) found that blood pressure was positively associated with alcohol consumption in male drinkers but they also found that non-drinkers had higher blood pressures than low and moderate drinkers. The SACN

(2003) reviewed evidence accumulated since 1994 and concluded that this confirms that:

- blood pressure rises with increasing adiposity and that weight reduction in hypertensive patients is associated with a reduction in blood pressure
- alcohol is an independent risk factor associated with hypertension
- increased physical activity and especially aerobic exercise has been associated with reductions in blood pressure.

Box 14.2 lists several factors associated with an increase in blood pressure and an increased risk of hypertension.

Box 14.2 Factors associated with increased risk of hypertension

- Being black; prevalence is higher among black people in the USA and UK than in white people, there are almost certainly also large individual variations in susceptibility within races
- Overweight
- High alcohol consumption
- Sedentary lifestyle
- High population salt intake
- High dietary fat intake
- Low potassium or calcium intakes?

Conclusions

An active lifestyle, moderate alcohol consumption and good control of body weight are undoubtedly factors that will lessen the risk of hypertension and the hypertension-linked diseases. Increased intakes of fruits and vegetables will have a beneficial effect on blood pressure. Fruit and vegetables increase potassium intakes and lower the sodium/potassium ratio in the diet; processing of foods generally involves an increase in this ratio by some loss of potassium and addition of salt; this is one favoured mechanism by which fruits and vegetables may exert their effects on blood pressure. There are general grounds for assuring that calcium intakes meet dietary standard levels and this may have some beneficial effect on population blood pressure.

There is compelling evidence of some causal link between dietary salt intake and hypertension. The argument tends to be about how significant and widespread the benefits of salt restriction would be – would salt intake moderation lead a general fall in average population blood pressure or would effects be limited to a relatively small proportion of salt-sensitive people? Moderate salt restriction will almost certainly be of some value to some salt-sensitive people and the general consensus (see SACN, 2003) is that it would have wider benefits. Salt restriction may also be useful in the treatment of mild to moderate hypertension either as an alternative to drug use or as an adjunct to drug treatment. Processed foods contain most of the salt in Western diets, and so any substantial reduction in salt intake requires either less reliance on these high-salt foods or reduced use of salt by food manufacturers. It is difficult for populations to sustain a reduction in salt intake in the current environment because of the predominance of processed food as our main source of salt.

Key points

- Cross-population studies show that average blood pressure of adult populations is highly correlated to average salt intakes.

- This correlation remains strong even when developed and developing countries are analysed separately.

- When migration is accompanied by changes in salt intake then measured changes in blood pressure or stroke mortality are consistent with salt intake being a cause of hypertension.

- Falls in salt consumption over the past century have been associated with reductions in stroke mortality.

- Internationally, death rates from stroke and gastric cancer are highly correlated and this suggests a common aetiology.

- An international correlation between average salt intake and gastric cancer mortality has also been reported.

- In general, there is no correlation between salt intake and blood pressure in individuals from the same population. This is not unexpected and is partly because the usual measure of salt intake, 24-hour sodium excretion, is a poor measure of habitual salt intake.

- Limited evidence from population interventions is consistent with the salt–hypertension hypothesis.

- When salt is added to the fruit and vegetable diets of chimpanzees, their blood pressure rises relative to control animals and falls when the supplemental salt is withdrawn.

- Several clinical trials suggest that sustained moderate reductions in salt intake reduce the blood pressures of people with mild to moderate hypertension.

- Very severe salt restriction was the first partly effective treatment for severe hypertension although it fell into disuse with the advent of effective antihypertensive drugs.

- Other factors associated with increased risk of hypertension are listed in Box 14.2 and attention to these will contribute to a reduction in hypertension prevalence.

- Reduced salt consumption will almost certainly help to reduce the prevalence of hypertension; the debate is really about how widespread these benefits will be.

PART FOUR

VARIATION IN NUTRITIONAL REQUIREMENTS AND PRIORITIES

15

Nutrition and the human lifecycle

INTRODUCTION

When I show my students Table 15.1 and ask for their comments, they almost invariably consider it a very bad diet because it so far removed from the dietary guidelines for adults discussed in Chapter 4. Many of them doubt whether anyone could actually be eating such a diet because it is also very different from the average intakes recorded in dietary surveys and household budget surveys. Table 15.1 in fact shows the approximate composition of mature human milk, the ideal food for babies. This extreme example illustrates the general point that nutritional needs and priorities are likely to change during the human lifecycle; in this case it shows that what is nutritionally ideal for newborn babies is far from ideal for fully grown adults. One would also, for example, expect the relative nutritional needs of an active rapidly growing adolescent to be markedly different to those of an elderly housebound person or even of a sedentary middle-aged person. Such differences mean that the dietary reference values (DRVs) vary with age, sex and reproductive status,

Table 15.1 An unbelievably bad diet?

	% **Energy**
Fat	53
Saturated fat	23
Carbohydrate	39
Sugars	39
Starch	0
Protein	8
Fibre (g)	0

and they also mean that there should be differences in the priority and nature of the general dietary guidelines offered for different lifecycle groups. This chapter focuses on the differing requirements and nutritional priorities of different lifecycle groups.

Overt deficiency diseases are uncommon in industrialized countries but this is no guarantee that many people are not more subtly affected by suboptimal nutrition. Thus in Chapter 12 evidence was presented that many adults have intakes of essential vitamins and minerals that are considered inadequate or have biochemical indications of poor nutrient status even where average intakes of the nutrient are considered satisfactory; in a few cases even average intakes were less than ideal. Those people who are subject to particular nutritional stresses, such as pregnancy, lactation, or rapid growth are likely to be the most sensitive to any marginal deficiencies or suboptimal intakes of nutrients.

If essential nutrient requirements vary during the human lifecycle then this might suggest that certain lifecycle groups, especially rapidly growing children, might need diets that are richer in essential nutrients (more nutrient dense) than the general diet suitable for adults. Children have higher relative requirement for several essential nutrients (i.e. they need more per kg of body weight than adults) but on the same relative basis they also need more energy, i.e. need to eat more food. This was well illustrated in Chapter 10 where it was shown that young children not only require 1.5–2 times as much protein per kg body weight as adults but they also need to consume three times as many calories or three times as much food. This means that any diet with a sufficient

Table 15.2 Selected reference nutrient intakes (estimated average requirements for energy) for various UK age groups expressed as a percentage of the appropriate adult (19–50 years) value. Data from COMA (1991).

	Pregnancy	Lactation	Girls 1–3 years	Girls 4–6 years	Girls 11–14 years	Boys 15–18 years	Men 75+ years
Energy	100*	127	60	80	95	108	82
Protein	113	124	32	44	92	99	96
Vitamin A	117	158	67	83	100	100	100
Riboflavin	127	145	55	73	100	100	100
Folic acid	Supplements	130	35	50	100	100	100
Vitamin C	125	175	75	75	88	100	100
Calcium	100	179	50	64	114	143	100
Iron	100	100	47	41	100	130	100

*First two trimesters (110 per cent last trimester).

concentration of protein to meet adult needs should also comfortably provide for the needs of growing children. This principle applies more widely, even though the relative vitamin and mineral needs of a growing child may be higher than those of adults, this may be wholly or partly offset by the increased relative energy (food) requirement of the child.

Table 15.2 shows some selected reference nutrient intakes (RNI) for different nutrients expressed as a percentage of the standard adult (19–50 years) value for the same sex. It also shows the estimated average requirement (EAR) for energy expressed in the same way. Several age groups of children and other lifecycle groups have been selected to illustrate the general principle. The energy values in Table 15.2 are a general indication of the relative food intakes of the various groups. For example, if the energy value is 50 per cent this would suggest that this group should consume around 50 per cent of the energy of adults and a value of 125 per cent that they are expected to consume about 25 per cent more than the standard adult (19–50 years) of the same sex. Assuming that the same basic diet is consumed, this also means that those with a 50 per cent value in the energy box should also consume 50 per cent of the amount of nutrients consumed by adults of the same sex and those with a 125 per cent value for energy should consume 25 per cent more nutrients than standard adults. This logic would indicate that only where the value for the nutrient RNI in Table 15.2 is significantly greater than that for the energy EAR will this group need a diet that is richer in this nutrient (more nutrient dense) than that required by standard adults. There are relatively few examples in Table 15.2

where the RNI percentage is significantly higher than the energy EAR – the adolescent requirement for calcium and several of the values for lactating women are examples where it is substantially higher. In most cases though, diets that contain enough essential nutrients for standard adults will probably also be adequate for most other lifecycle groups. Often the increased relative requirement for energy in children wholly or partly cancels out any relative increase in nutrient needs. This principle justifies the traditional cultural practice of fully weaned children sharing in family meals with their parents and other adults; any 'real' extra needs can easily be met by drinking extra milk or additional nutritious snacks. This traditional family meal is now, of course, not always the norm as children often graze on self-selected foods or eat pre-prepared foods at different times to their parents; often these are high-energy, low-nutrient foods such as confectionary, cakes, biscuits, savoury snacks and sugary drinks.

Key points

- Different lifecycle groups have widely differing nutrient needs and the nutritional priorities for health promotion also vary with age, sex and reproductive status.
- Rapid growth, pregnancy or lactation may make people more sensitive to marginal nutrient deficiencies.
- Rapid growth, pregnancy and lactation would also be expected to increase the relative requirements for energy and essential nutrients.

> • In many cases increase in the relative energy requirements of children are similar to or greater than the relative increase in nutrient requirements, which means that diets that supply enough of these nutrients for adults should also be adequate for children.

NUTRITIONAL ASPECTS OF PREGNANCY

Pregnancy overview

Effects of malnutrition in pregnancy

Healthy well-fed women have the best chance of having healthy babies and of lactating successfully after the birth. This was graphically illustrated by studies of the effects of the 'Dutch Hunger Winter' of 1944–45. In October 1944, the Nazi occupiers imposed a punitive embargo on food transport in the Netherlands, which led to widespread starvation, especially in the urban areas and among the less affluent members of society. This famine was not relieved until the Netherlands was liberated in May 1945. It is estimated that 40 000 pregnant women in the Netherlands were subject to a period of starvation during this winter and the effects of this are summarized below (Diamond, 1999).

- During the winter of 1944–45, the rates of conception fell to around a third of their normal level; starvation and low body weight markedly reduces fertility in women (and also in men).
- Women who were starved during the last trimester of their pregnancy, when most fetal growth occurs, had babies that were on average over 10 per cent lighter than those born before the famine (even before the famine food supplies were low).
- Babies born 3 months after the famine ended were of normal weight.
- However, babies exposed to famine in the first trimester of pregnancy had double the rate of stillbirth and were twice as likely to have a **neural tube defect** such as spina bifida.
- Babies who were exposed to famine in the second and third trimesters had much higher mortality in the first few months of life and mortality did not normalize until they were a year old.
- The famine babies who survived into adulthood seemed to be of normal weight and intelligence.

- One interesting observation was that girls who were exposed to intrauterine starvation in the first and second trimesters had underweight babies when they became adults despite being of normal birth weight themselves.

The scale of increased nutritional needs in pregnancy

One would expect pregnancy to be a time of significantly increased nutritional needs for the mother; the phrase 'eating for two' has, in the past, been widely used to sum up this expectation. As it is a time of physiological stress, the health and well-being of many pregnant women and their babies might be adversely affected by suboptimal nutrition despite the low frequency of overt malnutrition within the population. Morning sickness affects over half of women in the early part of pregnancy and this could compound with other stresses to deplete nutrient stores in some women.

Cross-species comparisons show that human babies are much smaller than would be predicted from the size of the mother, and that gestation is also longer than would be predicted. Thus the nutritional burden of pregnancy is likely to be less in women than in other non-primate species. The small size and relatively slow postnatal growth of human babies means that similar arguments apply to lactation. This difference in the relative burdens of pregnancy and lactation in different species is illustrated in Table 15.3. An extreme comparison is between a female mouse and a woman. The mouse produces a litter that represents around 40 per cent of her pre-pregnant weight in 21 days of gestation. She then provides enough nutrients in her milk to enable this litter to double its birth weight within 5 days. A woman produces a baby that represents 6 per cent of her body weight after 9 months of pregnancy and a breastfed baby might then take 4–6 months to double its birth weight. Extrapolating or predicting the extra nutritional needs of pregnant or lactating women from studies of non-primate animals may be misleading and tend to greatly exaggerate the extra needs of these women.

Behavioural and physiological adaptations to pregnancy and the utilization of maternal nutrient stores also tend to minimize the extra nutritional needs of pregnant women. These extra nutritional needs may thus turn out to be small in comparison to the needs of non-pregnant women. 'Eating for two' implies a

Table 15.3 Species variations in the relative burdens of pregnancy and lactation

Species	Maternal weight (kg)	Litter weight (% of maternal)	Gestation length (days)	Days to double birth weight
Mouse	0.025	40	21	5
Rat	0.200	25	21	6
G-pig	0.560	68	67	14
Rabbit	1.175	19	28	6
Cat	2.75	16	64	7
Woman	56	6	280	120–180

Source: Webb (1992b).

much greater increase in need than is indicated by measurements of the actual increase in intakes that occur in pregnant women and those indicated by current DRVs for pregnant women.

Reference nutrient intake and recommended dietary allowance for pregnancy

Table 15.4 summarizes current UK and US recommendations on the extra nutritional needs of pregnant women. This table highlights some differences between the UK and US dietary standards although these are not as great as noted in previous editions of this book. The American increments are often higher than those in the UK, e.g. those for iron, zinc and niacin. As noted in Chapter 3, baseline adult values also tend to be higher in the USA. This means that for all nutrients, the absolute American recommended dietary allowance (RDA) for pregnancy equals or exceeds the corresponding UK value with the exception of vitamin D. In the UK there is no RNI for non-pregnant women but there is an RNI of 10 µg/day for pregnant women, whereas in the USA there is an RDA of 5 µg/day for both pregnant and non-pregnant women.

As noted earlier when discussing Table 15.2 where the percentage increase in the requirement for a nutrient (compared to non-pregnant women) exceeds the percentage increase in the energy value, this implies the need for increased nutrient density or supplementation. In most cases the extra increments for vitamins suggested by the British standards are relatively modest and there are no increases for the minerals. Often the average intakes of relatively affluent British women will comfortably exceed the pregnancy RNI for many nutrients prior to pregnancy and so, in practice, avoid the need

Table 15.4 Daily extra increments for pregnancy.* Values in parentheses are percentages of the value for other women

Nutrient	UK RNI[†]	US RDA
Energy (kcal)	200 (10)[‡]	340–450[¶] (14–19)
(MJ)	0.8	1.43–1.90
Protein (g)	6 (13)	25 (50)[§]
Vitamin A (µg)	100 (17)	70 (10)
Vitamin D (µg)	10**	0 (0)
Thiamin (mg)	0.1 (13)[‡]	0.3 (27)
Riboflavin (mg)	0.3 (27)	0.3 (27)
Niacin (mg)	0	4 (29)
Folic acid (µg)	400	200 (50)
	supplements)	
Vitamin B$_{12}$ (µg)	0	0.2 (8)
Vitamin C (mg)	10 (25)	10 (13)
Calcium (mg)	0	0 (0)
Iron (mg)	0	9 (50)
Zinc (mg)	0	3 (38)

RNI, reference nutrient intake; RDA, recommended dietary allowance.
*COMA, 1991; NAS, 2004.
[†] Estimated average requirement (EAR) for energy.
[‡] Last trimester only.
[¶] Last two trimesters.
[§] Last two trimesters only.
** No RNI for non-pregnant women.

for dietary change. For example, average intakes of vitamin C in British women are more than double the RNI and so the 10 per cent increase in the RNI during pregnancy looks small in relation to this. Average intakes of all vitamins in British women in 2000 were in excess of the RNI (Hoare et al., 2004) although average vitamin A intakes of younger women were only 80 per cent of the RNI. Note that even where the average intake is apparently satisfactory there may still be substantial numbers of women, particularly young women, with frankly unsatisfactory intakes. Some values, such as the American RDA for iron and the British RNI for vitamin D, require the use of supplements to be realistically achievable. Many well-nourished women take supplements during pregnancy, and the assumption is that even if they do no good then neither will they do any harm.

Apart from folic acid, which is discussed later in the chapter, there is little evidence that such supplements do any good when taken by well nourished women in affluent countries. On the contrary there is clear evidence that high levels of retinol are **teratogenic** and that concentrated protein supplements reduce birth weight. There is also some evidence that routine iron supplements can increase risk of low birth weight and risk of prematurity when given to women who do not need them. Fetal malformations in zinc-deficient animals are also more frequent when calcium supplements are given than when both minerals are deficient which suggests that supplements of one nutrient can adversely affect the absorption and metabolism of others (these studies are reviewed by Mathews, 1996). A recent controlled trial of large supplements of antioxidant supplements in women at high risk of pre-eclampsia found that they did not reduce pre-eclampsia but did reduce birth weight and the onset of pre-eclampsia was slightly earlier (Poston *et al.*, 2006).

Pregnancy outcomes

There is a strong association between infant mortality rate and birth weight. Babies who weigh less than 2.5 kg are classified as **low birth weight (LBW)** babies and they have higher mortality and morbidity rates. Thus birth weight of babies is a useful, quantitative measure of pregnancy outcome. Anything that restricts fetal growth is liable to be detrimental to the chances of the baby's survival and subsequent well-being. Many of the risk factors for having a LBW baby are listed in Box 15.1. When birth weight of babies is plotted against mortality then there is a U-shaped curve. As babies get heavier then initially mortality risk drops until an optimum birth weight is reached which is slightly higher than average birth weight of around 3.5 kg. As birth weight rises above this optimum so mortality risk starts to increase again (see Symonds and Clarke, 1996). Many LBW babies are born prematurely and

---

Box 15.1   Risk factors for having a low birth weight (LBW) baby

- Low social class of the mother
- Mother less than 18 years or over 35 years
- Previous birth of a LBW baby
- Maternal drug or alcohol misuse
- Cigarette smoking
- Mother being underweight at the time of conception
- Low maternal weight gain in pregnancy
- Dieting or restricted energy intake during pregnancy
- Poor quality of maternal diet during pregnancy
- Excessive exercise or work during pregnancy

---

gestational diabetes can be a cause of high birth weight.

The ideal outcome to pregnancy is not only a healthy baby but also a healthy mother who is nutritionally well prepared to lactate. The preparedness of the mother to begin lactation and the general well-being of the mother after parturition are not as readily quantifiable as birth weight but can be important determinants of successful reproduction. In poorer countries the presence or absence of a healthy lactating mother may be a key determinant of the baby's chances of survival.

Maternal weight gain during pregnancy may be one quantifiable measure of the mother's preparedness for lactation. In rats, there is a 50 per cent increase in maternal fat stores during pregnancy and this fat store is rapidly depleted during the subsequent lactation. This increase in maternal fat stores is a physiological adaptation to enable the female rat to provide enough milk for her large and rapidly growing litter. The increases in maternal fat typically seen in human pregnancy can also be assumed to be physiological. In women in industrialized countries who have access to an essentially unlimited food supply, this store of energy for lactation may not be critical. It may be much more important to women who are subsisting on a marginal diet and who may have limited opportunity to boost intakes to meet the extra needs of lactation.

Estimating the extra nutritional needs of pregnancy

It is possible to use factorial calculations (see Chapter 3) to predict the likely extra requirements for those nutrients that accumulate during the pregnancy, either in the mother's stores, or in the products of conception. However, it should be remembered that these are only theoretical predictions and although they may provide a useful basis for discussion, they may not truly indicate extra dietary needs because of behavioural and physiological adaptations to pregnancy.

There has, over the years, been a very considerable amount of discussion about how any extra nutritional requirements of pregnant women are distributed throughout the pregnancy. At the end of the first trimester the fetus weighs around 5 g and around 500 g at the end of the second trimester. This compares with an average birth weight of 3.5 kg. Thus fetal growth accelerates throughout pregnancy with most of the fetal weight gain concentrated in the final trimester. Should any extra nutritional allowances be concentrated in the last trimester when fetal growth rate is highest? Several adaptive mechanisms ensure that the burden is distributed more evenly throughout the pregnancy. In the first dietary standards (National Research Council (NRC), 1943), the increases in RDAs in pregnancy were generally higher than current US values but the increases in 1943 were all confined to the second half of pregnancy whereas most current increases are for the whole of the pregnancy.

Pre-conception

Maybe as few as 50 per cent of pregnancies are planned but women who are planning to become pregnant can take steps to improve the chances of successful outcome. Obesity at the time of conception is a significant risk factor for **pre-eclampsia** or pregnancy-induced hypertension and is linked to increased risk of a number of fetal abnormalities. Ideally, women intending to become pregnant should try to ensure that their body mass index (BMI) is within the normal range (20–25 kg/m²) prior to conception. Women seeking pre-conception advice can be counselled to normalize their weight before becoming pregnant. Menstruation ceases and fertility is reduced in women who are underweight, and only 10 per cent of women with a BMI of less than 18 are fertile. Underweight women who do manage to conceive have an increased risk of having a LBW baby; in general the risk of having a LBW baby decreases with increasing pre-conceptual BMI

of the mother. Some other steps that should be taken if a pregnancy is planned are listed below.

- Folic acid supplements should be taken prior to conception (discussed later in the chapter).
- Vegan women should take vitamin B_{12} supplements.
- Iron status should be checked and if necessary any anaemia treated.
- Alcohol intake should be minimized or preferably eliminated.
- A nutrient-rich diet should be selected.
- Extra care should be taken in the management of conditions such as diabetes and phenylketonuria (PKU) because poor management of these can have adverse effects on the fetus.

Key points

- Malnutrition reduces fertility and the chances of conception.
- Malnutrition in late pregnancy reduces birth weight and increases infant mortality.
- Malnutrition in early pregnancy increases stillbirths, fetal abnormalities and infant mortality, even though birth weight is normal.
- Girls born to mothers malnourished in early pregnancy have smaller babies when they themselves become mothers.
- The extra nutritional needs of pregnant women are modest and much less than the phrase 'eating for two' implies.
- Behavioural changes, physiological adaptations and utilization of maternal reserves all tend to minimize extra requirements in pregnancy and the impact of suboptimal intakes.
- The nutritional burden of human pregnancy is much less than that in non-primate species.
- American allowances for pregnancy tend to be higher than those in the UK.
- Large increases in nutrient intakes may be difficult to achieve if there is only minimal increase in total food intake in pregnancy. They may only be realistic if supplements are used.
- For many nutrients, the habitual intakes of non-pregnant women exceed the UK RNI for pregnant women.

- Apart from folic acid, there is little evidence that nutrient supplements are beneficial in pregnancy unless women are under-nourished.
- Overdoses of some nutrients are harmful during pregnancy.
- Low birth weight babies (under 2.5 kg) have higher postnatal mortality and morbidity. Some of the risk factors for LBW are listed in Box 15.1.
- Too high a birth weight increases obstetric complications and also increases mortality risk.
- A successful pregnancy should produce a healthy normal weight baby and a healthy mother who is well prepared for lactation.
- Several mechanisms may serve to distribute the nutritional burden of pregnancy more evenly than the concentration of fetal growth in the last trimester might imply.
- Obesity at conception is associated with higher risk of pre-eclampsia and fetal abnormalities.
- Women who are underweight are less likely to conceive and are at higher risk of having a LBW baby if they do conceive.
- Women planning a pregnancy should be encouraged to normalize their body weight, take folic acid supplements and generally to make sure that they enter pregnancy with good nutritional status.

Energy aspects of pregnancy

A typical British woman gains around 12.5 kg in weight during a typical pregnancy. This weight gain is made up of around 3.5–4 kg of extra maternal fat, around 6 kg as the increased weight of the uterus and contents and the remainder is due to increased body fluid. The total theoretical energy cost of this weight gain, the increase in BMR and the energy costs of moving a heavier body in a typical pregnancy has been estimated at about 70 000–80 000 kcal (around 300 MJ). In under-nourished women in developing countries total weight gain during pregnancy may be only half of this value with no net increase in maternal fat stores. Immediately prior to the 'Dutch Hunger Winter' discussed earlier, average intakes of pregnant women in the Netherlands were estimated at around 1500 kcal/day (6.3 MJ/day). These women maintained the birth weights of their babies during this period but lost weight themselves.

The theoretical energy cost of the average British pregnancy with 3.5 kg of maternal fat gain works out at just under 300 kcal (1.3 MJ) per day. If this theoretical energy cost is distributed throughout the pregnancy in proportion to the rate of fetal growth then this would amount to an extra energy cost of over 750 kcal/day (3.1 MJ/day) in the last trimester. Most of the gain in maternal fat occurs in the middle of the pregnancy and this fat store represents not only a reserve for lactation but also a potential reserve for the last trimester if intake is inadequate during this period of rapid fetal growth.

The current UK estimated average requirement (EAR) for pregnant women is only 200 kcal (0.8 MJ) above that for non-pregnant women and is for the last trimester only (Table 15.4). The UK panel on DRVs (Committee on the Medical Aspects of Food (COMA), 1991) did suggest that women who are underweight at the start of pregnancy or who remain active during their pregnancies may need more than suggested by this EAR. According to COMA (1991) several studies have suggested that pregnant women in Britain only tend to eat more than non-pregnant women in the last few weeks of pregnancy and then less than 100 kcal/day (0.4 MJ/day). These and similar findings in other industrialized countries, suggest that the spontaneous increases in energy intake during pregnancy are very small in previously well nourished women. As energy balance is physiologically regulated this strongly implies that the extra energy needs of pregnant women are also very small. Clearly, many women in industrialized countries markedly reduce their activity levels during pregnancy and so save much of the anticipated energy costs of the pregnancy. Studies on marginally nourished pregnant women, using the doubly labelled water method of measuring long-term energy expenditure, further suggest that physiological energy-sparing mechanisms operate during pregnancy (Prentice, 1989). Lack of maternal fat storage during pregnancy and energy-sparing physiological mechanisms may all but eliminate any theoretical energy costs of pregnancy in developing countries.

In the 1989 version of RDAs (NRC, 1989a) the US panel recommended an extra energy increment for pregnancy of 300 kcal/day (1.25 MJ/day) for the second and third trimesters only. These figures have since been revised by the Institute of Medicine (NAS, 2004) who recommended an increase of 340 kcal/day (1.43 MJ) for the second trimester rising to an extra 452 kcal/day (1.9 MJ) in the third trimester. These new values have been set by using estimates of the rate of energy deposition during pregnancy plus an estimate for the increase in total energy expenditure of 8 kcal/day for every week of gestation that was obtained using the doubly labelled water method.

The best practical guide to the adequacy of energy intakes during pregnancy is the maternal weight gain and the American National Academy of Sciences has published guideline values for recommended weight gains for women during pregnancy that that vary with their pre-pregnant weight, i.e.:

- underweight at conception – 12.5–18 kg weight gain
- normal weight – 11.5–16 kg gain
- overweight – 7–11.5 kg gain
- obese – at least 6 kg gain.

Any reduced energy supply to the fetus during pregnancy is likely to restrict fetal growth and thus increase the risk of LBW. There is strong evidence linking maternal weight gain during pregnancy with birth weight of the baby. Low weight gain is associated with increased risk of LBW and perinatal mortality. Excessive weight gain is associated with prolonged labour, birth injury, higher rates of death and complications in the neonatal period and increased risk of maternal obesity. In a survey of 10 000 births in the USA (summarized in Morgan, 1988), the chances of having a LBW baby was inversely related to maternal weight gain in pregnancy:

- 15 per cent of women who gained less than 7 kg had LBW babies
- 8 per cent with 7–12 kg weight gain
- 4 per cent with 12–16 kg weight gain
- 3 per cent of women who gained 16+ kg.

Restricting maternal weight gain by dieting during pregnancy may increase the risk of having a LBW baby. In animal studies, even food restriction of obese mothers during pregnancy reduced fetal weight. This suggests the need for extreme caution in the use of energy-restricted diets even if women are overweight at the start of pregnancy. Weight reduction should not be attempted during pregnancy but diet should be moderated to achieve a desirable level of weight gain.

Glucose that has been transferred from maternal blood in the placenta is the primary energy source of the fetus. The concentration of glucose in fetal blood is always lower than that in maternal blood and transfer of glucose is by facilitated diffusion down a concentration gradient. This means if the maternal blood glucose concentration is low, this can limit the availability of glucose to the fetus. Active transfer of nutrients from maternal blood makes this less likely to restrict supplies of other nutrients, like amino acids, to the fetus. Starvation or heavy exercise during pregnancy may restrict fetal growth by reducing glucose concentrations in placental blood. Fetal nutrient supply depends not only on nutrient concentration in maternal blood but also on placental blood flow; therefore anything that reduces placental blood flow may also restrict fetal growth and nutrient supply. One effect of smoking may be to reduce placental blood flow and thus retard the supply of nutrients to the fetus and fetal growth. Purely anatomical factors, such as the precise site of implantation and development of the placenta, may affect fetal blood flow and may account for some unexplained incidence of LBW babies. Uncontrolled gestational diabetes can increase the supply of glucose to the fetus and cause babies to be born too heavy.

Poverty is associated with LBW. Average weights of babies born in developing countries are lower than in industrialized countries and the proportion of LBW babies is also much higher in many developing countries. These differences are not removed by correcting for differences in maternal stature. Even in industrialized countries, social class and economic status affect birth weight. Leon (1991) found progressive increase in the percentage of LBW babies and increased postnatal mortality with decrease in the socioeconomic status of the mother. Evidence from a number of studies indicates that nutritional factors are a likely explanation for some of these differences. Women from a poor community in Britain who had a LBW baby had lower average energy intakes than those who had had babies of ideal weight. During the Dutch Hunger Winter at the end of World War II average birth weight of babies was reduced by over 300 g. Studies in Guatemala have shown that women who were marginally nourished, with typical unsupplemented intakes of 1600 kcal/day (6.7 MJ/day), had significantly heavier babies and less LBW babies when they were given food supplements prior to conception and throughout the pregnancy. A similar study in

Taiwan, with women whose unsupplemented intake was higher, typically 2000 kcal/day (8.4 MJ/day), showed no significant effect on average birth weight (both studies reviewed in Naismith, 1980). This is backed up by what was noted earlier about the Dutch Hunger Winter, i.e. that when calorie intake was restricted to approximately 1500 kcal/day prior to the food blockade fetal weight was maintained at the expense of maternal weight but when maternal food intake dropped further in the last trimester then birth weight dropped. In the Gambia there are significant differences in average birth weight between the hungry season and the harvest season. This difference can be eliminated by the use of protein-energy supplements, and the perinatal mortality is also reduced.

Dietary intervention studies generally suggest that at very low baseline levels of intake, energy supplements do favourably affect birth weight and reduce incidence of LBW babies. However, this favourable effect on birth weight is not seen at slightly higher baseline levels despite the use of very substantial supplements. A lack of measurable effect of supplements on birth weight in the less under-nourished women does not necessarily mean that supplementation had no beneficial effects because the supplements may have increased maternal fat stores and made mothers better prepared to lactate. In a review of such intervention trials, Morgan (1988) concluded that the supplements probably have a beneficial effect despite their disappointing effect on birth weight because of increased maternal weight gain and improved lactation.

> ## Key points
>
> - British women gain an average 12.5 kg in pregnancy and this represents a theoretical energy cost of 70 000–80 000 kcal (300 MJ) or 300 kcal (1.3 MJ) per day.
> - In the USA the energy standard increases by 340 kcal/day (1.43 MJ) in the second trimester and by 452 kcal/day (1.9 MJ) in the third trimester.
> - Estimates of energy expenditure in pregnancy by the doubly labelled water method suggest that it increases by 8 kcal/day for each week of gestation.
> - The US RDA rises by 300 kcal (1.3 MJ) per day for the last two trimesters.

> - Spontaneous increases in food intake by well-nourished women may rise by only 100 kcal (0.4 MJ) per day in the last few weeks of pregnancy.
> - Reduced activity and perhaps energy-sparing physiological changes may account for the difference between the theoretical energy costs of pregnancy and the apparent increases in intake; under-reporting of intakes is also possible.
> - In under-nourished women, lack of maternal fat gain and energy-sparing mechanisms may eliminate even the theoretical energy cost of pregnancy.
> - Low weight gain during pregnancy and being underweight at conception both reduce birth weight.
> - Attempts at weight reduction should be avoided during pregnancy.
> - Being overweight at conception increases risk of pre-eclampsia.
> - Being underweight reduces fertility and increases the risk of an LBW baby in women who do conceive.
> - Glucose transfer across the placenta is passive and fetal blood glucose concentration is lower than maternal.
> - Low maternal blood glucose or low fetal blood flow will restrict glucose supply to the fetus and so limit fetal growth.
> - Poverty and low social class are both associated with reduced birth size and increased postnatal mortality of babies.
> - Malnourished women have smaller babies, more LBW babies and higher postnatal mortality.
> - Energy supplements increase birth weight and reduce the incidence of LBW in women with very low baseline intakes.
> - In marginally under-nourished women, supplements do not usually have a measurable effect on birth weight but they may increase maternal weight gain and fitness to lactate.

Protein in pregnancy

The current UK RNI for protein is increased by 6 g/day throughout pregnancy. The American RDA is increased by 25 g/day which is a 50 per cent increase and represents a considerable increase on the 1989 RDA of an extra 10 g/day. If the UK RNI is expressed as a percentage of the EAR for energy in the first two trimesters (when the energy EAR is unaltered) it represents a rise from 9.3 per cent of energy to 10.7 per cent of energy as protein. Average adult intakes of protein in the UK are 1.5 times the RNI and protein represents around 16.5 per cent per cent of total energy intake (Henderson *et al.*, 2003) and so protein seems unlikely to be a limiting nutrient for pregnant women in the UK or indeed in other industrialized countries where low protein intake is likely to only occur as a secondary consequence of low total food intake. In dietary intervention studies, protein-rich supplements appeared to offer no additional benefits over and above their energy value. Even in marginally nourished women, it is energy rather than protein that seem to be the limiting factor. Amino acids are actively transported across the placenta and so adequate levels can be maintained in fetal blood even when levels in maternal blood are low. Some studies even suggest that concentrated protein supplements may depress birth weight (see Mathews, 1996).

Factorial calculations suggest a total 'protein cost' of about 925 g for a typical pregnancy. Theoretical calculations of protein accretion rates during the four quarters of pregnancy suggest rates of 0.6, 1.8, 4.8 and 6.1 g/day, respectively (NRC, 1989a). Naismith (1980) provides direct evidence that, in the rat, extra protein is laid down in maternal muscle in early pregnancy and that this is released in late pregnancy when the demands from the growing fetuses are highest. He argues that limited observations in women are consistent with these observations in the rat and may serve to distribute the extra protein need more evenly throughout the pregnancy. Measurements of nitrogen balance in pregnant women show that a small and fairly constant positive balance occurs throughout the pregnancy. Excretion of the amino acid 3-methyl histidine is taken as an indicator of muscle protein breakdown and it increases in the second half of human pregnancy.

Habitual consumption of protein in industrialized countries is almost always in excess of requirements and thus, in practice, it is unlikely that protein supply will be limiting during pregnancy. Pregnant women do not usually need to take specific steps to increase their protein intake despite their increased RNI/RDA. Even in developing countries, energy is more likely than protein to be the limiting factor in pregnancy.

Key points

- Habitual protein intakes of women in industrialized countries exceed even the slightly raised UK RNI protein in pregnancy.
- The new American RDA for pregnancy is 50 per cent higher than for other women but still represents not much more than 10 per cent of the energy intake *cf.* habitual intakes of over 15 per cent.
- Even in developing countries, the supply of energy is more likely to be limiting than that of protein.
- Physiological mechanisms may help to distribute the protein costs of pregnancy more evenly through the gestation period.
- Intervention studies with protein-rich supplements provide no evidence that they are useful and some indications that they may depress birth weight.

Minerals in pregnancy

The current RNIs for minerals in the UK indicate no routine extra increment for any mineral in pregnancy. High priority has historically been given to increased mineral intakes during pregnancy and in the USA, the RDA for most minerals are increased during pregnancy (see examples in Table 15.4). The major exception is calcium where although there is no increase in RDA for pregnancy the RDA of 1000 mg/day for adult women is 43 per cent higher than the RNI of 700 mg/day which also applies to both pregnant and non-pregnant women. Data discussed in Chapter 12 suggest that the average mineral intakes of British women are below the RNI in several cases and that the mineral intakes of many British women are unsatisfactory (below LRNI). Some examples from Chapter 12 are listed below.

- 25 per cent of women and 42 per cent of younger women have unsatisfactory iron intakes; 11 per cent show biochemical evidence of iron depletion and 8 per cent are anaemic.
- 5 per cent of women and 8 per cent of younger women have unsatisfactory intakes of calcium.
- For all of the minerals, substantial numbers of women recorded unsatisfactory intakes with higher rates in the youngest age group.

As the American RDA for pregnancy are all higher, often substantially higher, than the corresponding British values this must mean that many women in both Britain and America have mineral intakes that are well below those considered desirable by the American Institute of Medicine.

Calcium

Around 30 g of calcium accumulates in the fetal skeleton during pregnancy. This represents just over 100 mg/day when spread throughout the pregnancy. If one assumes that only a fraction of ingested calcium is retained (say 25–35 per cent) then this factorial approach suggests an increase of around 400 mg in the RDA for calcium in pregnancy; this is actually what was recommended in the 1989 version of the American RDA (although the value for non-pregnant women was lower than current values). The 'calcium cost' of pregnancy represents only around 2–3 per cent of the calcium in the maternal skeleton and there is clear evidence that the efficiency of calcium absorption in the gut increases during pregnancy. The UK panel on DRVs concluded that in most women the extra calcium cost of the pregnancy can be met by utilization of maternal stores and by improved efficiency of absorption (COMA, 1991). In certain cases (e.g. adolescent pregnancy), they suggest that some extra increment of calcium might be advisable and in America the RDA for adolescent girls (14–18 years) is 1300 mg/day whether they are pregnant or not.

Iron

During pregnancy, the plasma volume increases by around 1.5 L and the red cell mass by 200–250 mL. This means that during a normal pregnancy the large increase in plasma volume causes a fall in haematocrit and blood haemoglobin concentration despite an increase in the number of circulating red cells and the amount of haemoglobin. This physiological fall in haemoglobin concentration in pregnancy was historically interpreted as iron deficiency anaemia and iron supplements have traditionally been given to pregnant women. The American RDAs clearly suggest that universal iron supplementation in pregnancy should continue. Iron supplements often cause adverse gastrointestinal symptoms and it is likely that many of them are not actually taken.

The net iron cost of pregnancy, allowing for the savings due to cessation of menstruation, have been estimated at between 500 and 1000 mg, i.e. 2–4 mg/day throughout the pregnancy (Sadler, 1994 suggested a figure of 680 mg). The UK panel on DRVs suggested that in most women the iron requirements for pregnancy can be met by the following adaptations:

- utilization of maternal iron stores
- a considerable increase in the efficiency of iron absorption during pregnancy – the intestinal absorption of iron may rise from a normal 10 per cent to over 50 per cent in the last trimester
- the cessation of menstruation.

In the UK routine iron supplementation during pregnancy is not considered necessary although targeted supplementation (e.g. to women whose iron status is poor when they enter pregnancy) may be necessary.

Very recent evidence suggests that large unnecessary iron supplements may cause undesirable rises in maternal blood pressure.

The need for and benefits of iron supplements in pregnancy is still a matter of scientific debate. The American and UK panels have thus come up with very different practical 'recommendations' using essentially the same body of factual knowledge. Mathews (1996) drew the following conclusions from a review of the literature.

- Iron deficiency anaemia is associated with increased risk of LBW and prematurity.
- High haemoglobin and haematocrit levels are associated with similar increased risks, although this may not be a simple cause and effect relationship.
- Randomized controlled trials have shown no benefit for routine iron supplements in pregnancy.

Screening and targeted supplementation is a feasible option for industrialized countries but in developing countries where iron deficiency anaemia is very prevalent and often severe, routine supplementation may be the only practical option.

Key points

- In the UK, no routine increases in mineral reference nutrient intakes (RNIs) are considered necessary during pregnancy although they may be necessary for some individuals or groups.
- It must be borne in mind, however, that evidence discussed in Chapter 12 suggests that many

women, especially younger women, have intakes of minerals that are below the lower RNI (LRNI).

- In the USA, there are substantial increases in many mineral recommended dietary allowances (RDAs) during pregnancy and in all cases the American RDA is higher, often substantially higher, than the UK RNI.

- In the UK, it is assumed that the mineral costs of pregnancy can be met by physiological adaptation, increased efficiency of absorption and utilization of maternal mineral reserves.

Folic acid and neural tube defects

The collective term **neural tube defects (NTDs)** is used to describe a group of conditions (most commonly anencephaly and spina bifida) in which the brain, spinal cord, skull and/or vertebral column fail to develop properly early in embryonic life. In anencephaly there is almost complete absence of the brain and skull and these babies die *in utero* or shortly after birth. In spina bifida, the spinal canal in the vertebral column fails to close and in severe cases the spinal cord bulges out of the back. Babies affected by this condition have a range of physical disabilities that in severe cases include paralysis, bladder and bowel incontinence and neurological damage caused by hydrocephalus (accumulation of fluid around the brain).

About 1 in 250 UK pregnancies are affected by neural tube defects and despite screening and termination of affected pregnancies around 1 in 4000 babies born in the UK have a neural tube defect. In the 1970s, before widespread screening and termination, 1 in 700 births were affected. The risk is 10 times higher in women who have already had an affected pregnancy but most babies born with a neural tube defect are nevertheless first occurrences.

The UK DRVs published in 1991 suggested a 50 per cent increase in the RNI for folic acid in pregnancy (to 300 µg) and the latest American RDA also suggest a 50 per cent increase (but in this case to a total of 600 µg). After the British RNI were formulated, a report was published which provided strong evidence that folic acid supplements during pregnancy could reduce the risk of neural tube defects in babies. This was a randomized, double-blind prevention trial using around 2000 women identified as being at high risk of neural tube defects because of a previous affected pregnancy (Medical Research Council (MRC), 1991). There were only six affected babies in the folic acid supplemented groups but 21 in the same number of women not receiving folic acid supplements, i.e. a 72 per cent protective effect. This study convincingly demonstrated the benefits of supplements for such high-risk women.

Studies published in the 1960s indicated that women who had taken a folic acid antagonist during pregnancy had an increased risk of having a baby affected by a neural tube defect. Others had shown that women who gave birth to affected babies showed biochemical evidence of defective folic acid metabolism. In 1965 Hibbard and Smithells put forward the hypothesis that folic acid supplements might reduce the risk of neural tube defects by compensating for some defect in folic acid absorption or metabolism. In the early 1980s, intervention trials using pre-conceptual supplements showed that 400 or 4000 µg of folic acid were effective in preventing recurrence of a neural tube defect (references to these early studies may be found in Report, 1992). Since the MRC (1991) study was published, other studies have confirmed the protective effect of folic acid both in preventing the recurrence of a neural tube defect in previously affected women and also preventing primary occurrence in women with no history of a pregnancy affected by a neural tube defect (e.g. Czeizel and Dudas, 1992).

The dose of supplements (5 mg/day) used in the MRC trial represents around 25 times the current adult RNI for folic acid. At this dose some rare but possibly serious and specific side effects of folic overdose have been predicted and others are possible. In 1992, an expert advisory group in the UK recommended that all women in the high-risk category should take supplements of 5 mg of folic acid daily if they plan to become pregnant and during the first 12 weeks of pregnancy. All other women were recommended to take a more modest 0.4 mg extra folic acid when planning to become pregnant and in the first 12 weeks of pregnancy (Report, 1992). However, as many as half of all pregnancies may be unplanned and so to have maximum impact on the incidence of neural tube defects, all women of reproductive age would need to substantially increase their intake of folic acid. There has been for several years now an active campaign in the UK to increase the range and level of folic acid fortification of foods such as bread and cereals and several expert groups have recommended mandatory fortification of flour. Such fortified foods are the only realistic way that many women will reach a total target intake of 0.6 mg/day of folic acid when they first become pregnant (note average intakes of UK women were about 250 μg/day in 2000). In 1996, the US Food and Drug Administration (FDA) announced that it would require fortification of all cereal grain products with folic acid. An expert report in the UK (COMA, 2000) has also recommended that there should be universal fortification of flour with 240 μg/100 g of folic acid. It is estimated that such fortification would reduce the incidence of neural tube defect affected pregnancies by up to 50 per cent. In April 2006 the Food Standards Agency (FSA) began a public consultation exercise to determine views on the mandatory fortification of flour prior to recommending this mandatory fortification to the UK government.

Since the first edition of this book, concerns about the safety of modest increases in folic acid consumption by the general population have eased and there is increasing evidence that they may be beneficial in the prevention of heart disease. It is suggested that folic acid supplements are associated with reduced levels of homocysteine in the blood and that even moderately elevated levels of homocysteine may increase the risk of cardiovascular disease (see Ball, 2004). Large increases in blood levels of homocysteine occur in the hereditary condition homocystinuria and they are toxic to vascular endothelial cells, promote the oxidation of low-density lipoproteins (LDLs) and increase the risk of thrombosis. Progress has also been made in elucidating the mechanism by which folic acid exerts its protective effect against neural tube defects. The enzyme methionine synthase requires folic acid as a co-factor and its activity is low in women who have had an affected pregnancy. Folic acid supplements may overcome a genetic defect in the regulation of this enzyme's activity (see Eskes, 1998).

An international study by Botto et al. (2005) indicates that programmes to encourage the use of folic acid supplements before conception and in early pregnancy have been ineffective in reducing the incidence of neural tube defects. They analysed the incidence of these defects in several European countries and in Israel between 1988 and 1998 and found that there had been no measurable fall in the incidence of these conditions even though campaigns to encourage use of supplements had been started in 1992 in England and Wales, and in 1993 in Ireland. In contrast to this lack of effectiveness of

supplementation programmes, there have been very significant falls in the incidence of these defects in those countries where large-scale food fortification with folic acid has been introduced.

- In the USA fortification of enriched cereal products with folic acid became mandatory in January 1998. Incidence of neural tube defects in the period October 1998 – December 1999 was 19 per cent lower than in the period October 1995 – December 1996 (Honein et al., 2001).
- In Canada, most cereal grain products have been fortified with folic acid since January 1998. The resultant estimated increase in folic acid of 100–200 μg/day was associated with an approximate halving of the incidence of neural tube defects in the province of Ontario in the period after fortification was introduced (Ray et al., 2002).
- In Chile, the incidence of neural tube defects dropped by 31 per cent after the fortification of flour began and it reached the $P < 0.001$ level of significance in the twentieth month after fortification began (Castilla et al., 2003).

The FSA (2003) concluded that total intakes of folate of 1.5 mg/day would not be expected to have any adverse effects and this is well below what would be consumed from food even if mandatory fortification occurs. The main concerns that are now voiced about mandatory fortification of bread with folic acid are:

- high folic acid intakes could mask the haematological consequences of vitamin B_{12} deficiency and thus delay its diagnosis. This might increase the spinal and neurological damage caused by B_{12} deficiency
- high folate intakes could reduce the effectiveness of certain drugs that work by interfering with folate metabolism.

More recently evidence has been accumulating that folic acid supplements also reduce the incidence of cleft lip in babies (Wilcox et al., 2007).

Key points

- In the 1980s, around 1 in 250 UK pregnancies were affected by a neural tube defect.
- Folic acid supplements in early pregnancy and pre-conceptually reduce both the recurrence and primary occurrence of a neural tube defect.

- Supplements of 400 µg of folic acid are recommended for the first trimester of pregnancy and for those planning to become pregnant.
- Many pregnancies are unplanned and so fortification of flour and other cereal products has been recommended in the UK and has already occurred in the USA.
- High doses (>1.5 mg/day) of folic acid may have detrimental consequences in some circumstances but the whole population might benefit from moderate increases in folic acid intake.
- Folic acid supplements exert their protective effect by compensating for an hereditary low activity of the enzyme methionine synthase for which folic acid is a co-factor.
- Supplementation programmes in several European countries have made no discernible effect on rates of neural tube defects but where widespread food fortification has been introduced it has resulted in immediate and substantial falls in their incidence.
- Folic acid supplements also reduce the incidence of cleft lip.

Other vitamins in pregnancy

The increases in vitamin RNIs and RDAs in Britain and the USA were summarized in Table 15.4. The table shows that the UK RNI for vitamin A is increased by 100 µg in pregnancy. The extra increment in the USA is only 70 µg but the baseline value for American women is the same as that for pregnancy in the UK, i.e. 700 µg. Average intake of vitamin A in younger British women is only 80 per cent of the RNI and 9 per cent of women have unsatisfactory intakes rising to 19 per cent in the younger women (see Chapter 12). This would suggest that many women take in less vitamin A than is considered desirable during pregnancy. It is, however, the possible consequences of excessive doses of retinol in pregnancy rather than potential inadequacy that is the current focus of concern about vitamin A in pregnancy in the UK. Very high intakes of retinol during pregnancy are **teratogenic**, i.e. they increase the risk of birth defects. Women in the UK are currently advised not to take vitamin A containing supplements during pregnancy and are advised to avoid eating liver or products containing liver (e.g. pate) because of the high levels of retinol in animal livers

(see COMA, 1991). American women are advised not to take supplements that contain more than the RDA of any vitamin (except folic acid).

It was assumed by the UK panel on DRVs that most of the adult population obtain their vitamin D principally from endogenous production in the skin via the action of sunlight on 7-dehydrocholesterol so there is no RNI for these groups. Pregnant women are one of the groups where the panel felt that endogenous production could not be relied on and therefore an RNI was given (Table 15.4). This RNI for vitamin D is over three times average UK intakes and therefore supplements are necessary to achieve it; in the USA the same RDA of 5 µg/day is given for all women whether pregnant or not.

Increases in the RNI and RDA for most other vitamins are modest and average intakes of most of these vitamins in British women is well in excess of even the raised RNI for pregnancy even though relatively large numbers of individual women may have unsatisfactory intakes or biochemical evidence of poor status (see Chapter 12 for details).

Vitamin B_{12} interacts with folic acid in methyl transfer reactions and poor vitamin B_{12} status is a risk factor for a neural tube defect. The RNI remains unaltered in pregnancy and the American RDA only rises very slightly. For omnivorous women and even for lacto-vegetarians there is probably little need to consider B_{12}; however, vegan women would not have a natural dietary source of this vitamin and should take supplements or fortified foods to ensure their adequacy because only newly absorbed vitamin B_{12} is readily transported across the placenta.

Key points

- There is some increase in the dietary standards for several vitamins during pregnancy (see Table 15.4).
- Retinol is teratogenic so pregnant women should avoid concentrated retinol supplements. In the UK, they are advised to avoid all liver, liver products, cod liver oil and any vitamin supplements that contain retinol.
- The RNI for vitamin D in pregnancy can only realistically be achieved by taking supplements although for other adults it is assumed that they can manufacture enough if adequately exposed to sunlight.
- Vegan women should take supplements of vitamin B_{12} or eat foods fortified with this vitamin.

Alcohol and pregnancy

Fetal alcohol syndrome is a recognizable clinical entity that is caused by heavy drinking during pregnancy. Babies with this syndrome:

- are small
- have characteristic facial abnormalities
- often have learning disabilities
- are immunodeficient
- show slow postnatal growth.

This syndrome starts to occur with habitual alcohol intakes in excess of 50 g/day (4 glasses of wine) and the frequency increases as alcohol intake rises. The alcohol probably exerts a direct toxic effect on the fetus and may also increase the risk of oxygen or glucose deficit to the fetus.

Moderate amounts of alcohol in pregnancy (habitual intakes of 10–50 g/day) may increase the risk of LBW. It may be prudent to advise women to limit their alcohol consumption during pregnancy to the occasional small amount and the Royal College of Obstetricians and Gynaecologists advises that they should avoid alcohol altogether. Alcohol binges should be avoided during pregnancy.

Heavy drinking prior to conception not only reduces fertility but also affects fetal growth even if drinking stops after conception. The fetus is also most vulnerable to the harmful effects of alcohol in the early stages of pregnancy. Taken together such observations suggest that moderation of alcohol consumption should ideally begin prior to conception.

Key points

- Heavy drinking during pregnancy has serious adverse effects on the fetus – fetal alcohol syndrome.
- The effects of moderate and low alcohol intakes are less clear.
- Ideally, women should avoid alcohol during pregnancy and when planning to become pregnant.

LACTATION

Lactation is nutritionally far more demanding for the mother than pregnancy. A woman will be producing up to 800 mL of milk containing as much as 9 g of protein and 700 kcal (2.9 MJ) of energy, as

Table 15.5 Extra increments for selected nutrients for lactation in the UK and USA dietary standards.* Values in parentheses are percentages of the value for other women.

Nutrient	UK RNI[†]	US RDA
Energy (kcal)	520 (27)[‡]	330 (14)
(MJ)	2.18	1.38
Protein (g)	11 (24)	25 (54)
Vitamin A (μg)	350 (58)	500 (63)
Vitamin D (μg)	10[¶]	0
Thiamin (mg)	0.2 (25)	0.3 (27)
Riboflavin (mg)	0.5 (45)	0.5 (45)
Niacin (mg)	2 (15)	3 (21)
Folate (μg)	60 (30)	100 (25)
Vitamin C (mg)	30 (75)	45 (60)
Calcium (mg)	550 (79)	0
Iron (mg)	0	0
Zinc (mg)	6 (86)	4 (50)

RNI, reference nutrient intake; RDA, recommended dietary allowance.
*COMA, 1991; NAS, 2004.
[†] Estimated average requirement (EAR) for energy.
[‡] Average for first 3 months.
[¶] No RNI for non-pregnant/lactating women.

well as all the other nutrients necessary to sustain the growing infant. The extra increments for lactation in the American and UK dietary standards are summarized in Table 15.5.

The amounts by which the British EARs for energy exceed those of other women during the first 3 months of lactation are:

- month 1 – 450 kcal/day (1.9 MJ)
- month 2 – 530 kcal/day (2.2 MJ)
- month 3 – 570 kcal/day (2.4 MJ).

After 3 months the EAR depends on whether the breastfeeding is the primary source of nourishment for the baby or whether the baby is receiving substantial amounts of supplementary feeds. The American RDA for lactating women is increased by a set 500 kcal/day (2.1 MJ/day).

The UK EARs have been estimated by measuring the energy content of milk production and assuming an efficiency of 80 per cent for the conversion of food energy to milk energy. The contribution from the maternal fat stores laid down during pregnancy has been taken as 120 kcal/day (0.5 MJ/day). These increases in the EARs for energy during lactation are said by COMA (1991) to closely match the extra intakes observed in lactating women in affluent societies.

The RNI for protein is increased by 11 g/day throughout lactation of up to 6 months' duration. When this is expressed as a proportion of the EAR for energy then it does not rise significantly above that for other women, i.e. 9.3 per cent of energy. As in pregnancy, it seems unlikely that protein will be a limiting nutrient in lactation because habitual intakes are usually well in excess of this.

The RNIs for eight vitamins and six minerals are also increased during lactation reflecting the panel's judgement of the extra needs of women at various stages of lactation. Some of these increases are substantial proportions of the standard RNIs for adult women and the increases in the American RDAs are generally even bigger (see Table 15.5).

Moderate weight loss of around 0.5 kg per week does not affect milk output and changes in the proportions of fat, carbohydrate and protein in the maternal diet do not affect milk composition. The fatty acid profile of milk is affected by the fatty acid profile of the maternal diet. The concentration of the major minerals in milk is not affected by maternal intake; maternal stores are depleted if intake is inadequate. Maternal intake and the size of maternal stores affect milk content of selenium, iodine and the vitamins. During periods of low maternal intake, milk vitamin content is initially maintained at the expense of maternal stores.

Key points

- Lactation is nutritionally demanding and this is reflected in substantial increases in the dietary standards for energy and many nutrients (detailed in Table 15.5).
- Successful lactation is compatible with moderate weight loss.
- The macronutrient and major mineral content of the maternal diet has little effect on milk composition.
- The fatty acid profile of milk reflects that of the maternal diet.
- Maternal intake and stores of the vitamins affect milk composition.

INFANCY

Breastfeeding versus bottle feeding

The assumption of most biologists would be that through the process of natural selection, evolution will have produced, in breast milk, a food very close to the optimum for human babies. Breast milk will not be the preferred food for a baby in only a few circumstances such as:

- babies with an inborn error of metabolism, which leaves them unable to tolerate lactose or some amino acid in milk protein
- babies born to women infected with agents such as the human immunodeficiency virus (HIV) that may be transmissible in the milk
- babies of mothers taking drugs that may be transmitted in the milk.

Key point

With few exceptions, breastfeeding is the best way of feeding newborn babies.

Prevalence of breastfeeding

In the 1960s, the majority of babies born in the UK would not have been breastfed after leaving hospital. Perhaps only a quarter of babies born in the USA and parts of western Europe in the 1960s would have been breastfed for any significant time after delivery. Since then there has been some increase in breastfeeding led by women in the upper socioeconomic groups, the same groups that led the earlier trend away from breastfeeding.

Table 15.6 shows the estimated prevalence of breastfeeding in babies of different ages in England and Wales at 5-yearly intervals between 1975 and 2000. In 2000, more than two-thirds of women made some initial attempt to breastfeed their babies but only 43 per cent of babies were still being breastfed 6 weeks after delivery and by 4 months this had dropped to just over a quarter of all babies. These figures nevertheless represent major increases over the figures for 1975, but there have been no significant and sustained improvements since 1980. The substantial improvement shown between 1975 and 1980 has been maintained but not built on. The apparent increase between 1995

Table 15.6 Prevalence (%) of breastfeeding in England and Wales*

Age	Year					
	1975	1980	1985	1990	1995	2000
Birth	51	67	65	64	68	71
1 week	42	58	57	54	58	57
2 weeks	35	54	53	51	54	54
6 weeks	24	42	40	39	44	43
4 months	13	27	26	25	28	29
6 months	9	23	22	21	22	22

*Data sources: DHSS (1988) and Hamlyn et al. (2002).

and 2000 is almost entirely due to changes in the age and educational profiles of the sampled mothers. The figures in Table 15.6 understate the use of bottle feeds because data collected in the 2000 survey (Hamlyn *et al.*, 2002) suggest that by 5 weeks only around 30 per cent of women were exclusively breastfeeding their babies and this fell to 20 per cent at 9 weeks and 10 per cent at 6 months.

Most of the statistical data used in this discussion of infant feeding practices is for England and Wales or for the UK as a whole but it is intended to illustrate principles, patterns and trends that are likely to be common to several industrialized countries. The prevalence of breastfeeding in Scotland and Northern Ireland is below that in England and Wales. In 2000, only 63 per cent of Scottish babies were initially breastfed and only 40 per cent were still being breastfed at 6 weeks (corresponding figures for Northern Ireland 54 per cent and 26 per cent respectively). These Scottish and Northern Ireland figures do represent significant improvement since 1995 even when corrected for maternal characteristics.

In *Healthy People 2000* (Department of Health and Human Services (DHHS), 1992) the goal was for 75 per cent of US mothers to be breastfeeding in the immediate postpartum period by the year 2000 and for 50 per cent to continue to breastfeed for 5–6 months and these goals have remained essentially unchanged in the updated *Healthy People 2010* (DHSS, 2000). Assumed baseline figures for 1988 were that 64 per cent of women made some attempt to breastfeed while in hospital, that just 54 per cent of mothers were breastfeeding on discharge from hospital and 21 per cent breastfeeding at 5–6 months. Only 32 per cent of low-income US mothers breastfed their babies at time of discharge and less than

10 per cent were still breastfeeding at 5–6 months. American data for 2001 show that 70 per cent of mothers breastfed while they were in hospital and that 33 per cent were still breastfeeding at 6 months. The initial rates are very similar to those in the UK but the proportion of women who are still breastfeeding at 6 months is considerably higher than those recorded in the UK at around the same time (see Table 15.6 for figures for England and Wales). Much higher breastfeeding rates have been reported for Canada, the Netherlands, Scandinavia, New Zealand and parts of Australia. In Sweden in 1973 only 20 per cent of babies were being breastfed at 2 months but by 1993 this had risen to 85 per cent, which shows what can be achieved by effective promotion and facilitation measures. According to Laurent (1993) 99 per cent of Norwegian mothers breastfeed their babies at birth and 90 per cent are still at least partially breastfeeding at 3–4 months. International data on breastfeeding and the primary references can be found in Wharton (1998) and King and Ashworth (1994).

UNICEF (2004) give detailed information in many of the less industrialized countries and overall it estimates that at 4 months of age only about 37 per cent of children in the least developed countries were being exclusively breastfed and 48 per cent in developing countries. UNICEF (2004) give details of estimated rates in many of these individual countries and rates vary widely from country to country – see below for selected examples of rates of exclusive breastfeeding at 4 months:

- 2 per cent – Sierra Leone
- 9 per cent – Turkey and Albania
- 16 per cent – Kenya
- 20 per cent – Nigeria
- 36 per cent – Ghana
- 46 per cent – Cuba
- 55 per cent – India
- 63 per cent – Peru
- 67 per cent – China
- 73 per cent – Chile
- 84 per cent – Ethiopia
- 97 per cent – North Korea.

Key points

- About two-thirds of UK women start to breastfeed their babies but a third of these give up within the first 6 weeks.

- Prevalence of breastfeeding in the UK rose substantially between 1975 and 1980 but current rates (2000) are still similar to those in 1980.
- By 6 weeks of age, many breastfed UK babies have received additional feeds and only around 30 per cent are being wholly breastfed.
- There is wide international variation in the prevalence of breastfeeding.
- Rates in Scandinavia are among the highest in the industrialized world – 90 per cent of Norwegian babies are still receiving some breast milk at 3–4 months of age.
- Just over a third of babies in the least developed countries are exclusively breastfed.
- Examples of rates of exclusive breastfeeding in some less industrialized countries are given and a comprehensive list can be found in UNICEF (2004).

Factors influencing choice of infant feeding method

Choice of infant feeding method is strongly dependent on social class in the UK. In 2000, 85 per cent of UK women in the higher occupation category attempted to breastfeed their babies and 60 per cent were still breastfeeding at 6 weeks. The corresponding figures for women in the lower occupations were 59 per cent and 28 per cent, respectively. Women with higher levels of education are also much more likely to breastfeed their children in the UK and 64 per cent of those in the highest education category were still breastfeeding at 6 weeks compared to 27 per cent in the lowest educational category. The mother's choice of feeding method for her first baby is a major influence on feeding of subsequent children. Mothers who had breastfed their first babies usually breastfed subsequent children whereas women who had bottle-fed the first baby usually do not. Women with previous experience of successful breastfeeding also are less likely to stop prematurely. Incidence of breastfeeding is higher among first-time mothers. For UK women in 2000 who had solely bottle fed their first babies, only 26 per cent changed to breastfeeding for their next baby but this was nevertheless a substantial increase on the 18 per cent recorded in 1995 (Hamlyn *et al.*, 2002). Ethnicity also had a pronounced effect on choice of feeding method, with much higher rates recorded in black and Asian

women than in white women both at birth and at 6 weeks.

Many factors will have compounded to decrease the prevalence of breastfeeding but the availability of a cheap, simple and 'modern' alternative was clearly an essential prerequisite. There may have even been a temptation to think that science had improved on nature if bottle-fed babies grew faster than breastfed babies. Some other factors that have probably contributed to the decline in breastfeeding are listed below.

- Breastfeeding may be inconvenient to the lifestyle of many women, especially those who wish to resume their careers soon after birth or those women whose income is considered to be a vital part of the family budget. Statutory paid maternity leave should have decreased this influence in more recent years in the UK. According to Foster *et al.* (1997), a third of UK women who stopped breastfeeding between 3 and 4 months in 1995 gave returning to work as their reason. Only a third of women in this survey were on paid maternity leave when their babies were 6 weeks old.
- Breastfeeding prevents fathers and others sharing the burden of feeding, especially night feeds in the early weeks after birth.
- There are undoubtedly some women (and men) who find the whole idea of breastfeeding distasteful. There is a strong taboo in this country against breastfeeding in public or even among close friends or relatives. This, coupled with the poor provision of facilities for breastfeeding in many public places, can only increase the inconvenience of breastfeeding and restrict the range of activities that women can participate in during lactation.
- The figures in Table 15.6 clearly indicate that many women who initially try to breastfeed give up after a very short time. Many women experience discomfort in the early stages of lactation and many women believe that they are unable to produce sufficient milk. Delay in starting suckling (e.g. to allow the woman to rest after delivery) or any prolonged break from suckling is likely to reduce the likelihood of initiating and maintaining lactation.
- Bottle feeding is promoted in many developing countries as the modern, sophisticated, 'Western' way of feeding babies. It is promoted as the high

prestige option. Yet, in industrialized countries, breastfeeding is more common among the higher socioeconomic groups and so in these countries is, in practice, the higher prestige option.

In a 2000 survey (Hamlyn *et al.*, 2002), women in the UK gave the following as important reasons for choosing to breastfeed their babies:

- 85 per cent of women chose to breastfeed because they thought this would be best for the baby
- 34 per cent because breastfeeding is more convenient
- 23 per cent because it promotes bonding between mother and baby
- 21 per cent because it is cheaper
- 14 per cent because it is more natural
- 13 per cent because it is good for the mother
- 13 per cent because the mother loses weight more easily.

Listed below are the most common reasons given for choosing to bottle feed:

- 25 per cent because someone else can feed the baby
- 19 per cent did not like the idea of breastfeeding or would be too embarrassed to breastfeed
- 39 per cent of second or later babies were bottle fed because of the mother's previous experience.

The most common reasons given for stopping breastfeeding within the first week were:

- lack of milk or failure of the baby to suckle
- the discomfort caused by breastfeeding or dislike of breastfeeding
- too time consuming or too tiring (note that 90 per cent of feeding should occur within the first 5 minutes of suckling)
- the mother was ill.

The most common reasons given by women for stopping breastfeeding between 6 weeks and 4 months were:

- lack of milk or failure of the baby to suckle
- mother returning to work or college
- too time consuming or too tiring
- mother was ill
- painful breasts or nipples.

Early feeding experience in the hospital also strongly affects the likelihood of early cessation of breastfeeding. Mothers attempting to breastfeed but whose babies were also given some bottle feeds were more than three times as likely to give up breast feeding within a fortnight as were women whose babies received no bottle feeds. Delay in initiating breastfeeding is also strongly associated with early cessation. Early cessation of breastfeeding occurred in 30 per cent of cases where there was a delay of 12 hours or more in putting the baby to the breast but in only 16 per cent of cases where this occurred immediately after birth; even a delay of 1 hour had a significant effect (Hamlyn *et al.*, 2002). White *et al.* (1992) reported that women were almost twice as likely to continue breastfeeding if feeding on demand rather than at set times was practised in the hospital.

Hamlyn *et al.* (2002) noted that there had been some improvements in practices in UK maternity hospital practices between 1990 and 2000 (see list below).

- The number of women starting to breastfeed within 1 hour had increased from 63 per cent in 1990 to 72 per cent in 2000.
- The proportion of mothers who had their babies with them continuously in hospital rose from 63 per cent to 79 per cent.
- The proportion of breastfed babies who were given some bottles in hospital dropped from 46 per cent to 31 per cent.
- In 2000, most first-time mothers said that they had been given some useful help or advice about breastfeeding their babies.

Many UK women report that they have experienced problems in finding somewhere to feed their babies in public places and in fact almost 30 per cent of women never attempted to feed their babies outside of the home. In 2000, over a third of bottle-feeding mothers had never attempted to feed their baby outside of the home compared with just 8 per cent of those who breastfed their babies although the breastfeeding mothers were more likely to have encountered problems with feeding outside of the home (Hamlyn *et al.*, 2002).

Key points

- Breastfeeding in Britain decreases in prevalence with decreasing social class and with decreasing educational attainment of the mother.

- Women chose to breastfeed because it is good for the baby and for them, because it promotes bonding between mother and baby and because it is convenient, natural and cheap.
- Women chose to bottle feed their babies because someone else can help with feeding or because they do not like the idea of breastfeeding or are embarrassed by it.
- The feeding method used for second and subsequent births is very influenced by the mother's experience with her first baby.
- Women often give up breastfeeding prematurely because they have difficulty successfully and comfortably feeding the baby.
- Returning to work becomes more important as a factor in stopping breastfeeding as time after the birth increases.
- Delay in first putting the baby to the breast or the use of supplementary bottle feeds are both associated with early cessation of breastfeeding.
- Hospital practices in the UK are changing so as to minimize these apparent hindrances to successful lactation and most women are now given support and guidance in breastfeeding.

The benefits of breastfeeding

Table 15.7 illustrates just how different are human milk, cow milk and infant formula. Cow milk is an ideal food for rapidly growing calves but unless substantially modified is now regarded as an unsuitable food for human babies. Unmodified cow milk is now not recommended for babies until they are at least 6 months old. This table also demonstrates the scale of changes that are necessary to convert cow milk into a formula that is compositionally similar to human milk. Even though modern 'humanized' formula is closer to human milk than formulations like national dried milk that were used up until 1976 in the UK they are still quite different from the human milk that it is trying to imitate.

Cow milk has around three times the protein content of human milk. This means that babies will need to excrete substantial amounts of urea if fed on cow milk whereas when breastfed, the bulk of the nitrogen is retained for growth. Around 20 per cent of the nitrogen in cow milk and breast milk is non-protein nitrogen, e.g. urea, creatine and free amino acids; its biological significance is unclear but this fraction will be absent from infant formula. The amino acid **taurine** is present in relatively large amounts in human milk and is added to some infant formula. Taurine is normally made from the amino acid cysteine which in turn can be made from the other sulphur-containing amino acid methionine. However, premature babies have a low synthetic capacity and a relatively high requirement for both cysteine and taurine and so they are normally regarded as conditionally essential in premature babies. In breastfed infants, the principal bile acid is taurocholic acid, but in infants fed on cow milk it is

Table 15.7 The composition of human milk, cow milk and modern infant formula.* All values are per 100 mL as consumed

	Human milk	Cow milk	Infant formula	1970s formula[†]
Energy (kcal)	70	67	67	55
(kJ)	293	281	281	231
Protein (g)	1.3	3.5	1.4–1.9	2.5
Carbohydrate (g)	7	4.9	7.2–7.7	5.9
Fat (g)	4.2	3.6	3.3–3.6	2.4
Sodium (mg)	15	52	19–25	40
Calcium (mg)	35	120	51–71	83
Iron (µg)	76	50	670–680	480
Vitamin A (µg)	60	40	80	23
Vitamin C (mg)	3.8	1.5	8	2.4
Vitamin D (µg)	0.01	0.03	1.1–1.2	0.8

*Data sources: Poskitt (1988) and Wharton (1998).
[†]UK national dried milk that was withdrawn in 1976.

glycocholic acid. This may adversely affect the emulsification and therefore digestion and absorption of milk fat.

The principal proteins in milk are **casein** and **whey**. The casein:whey ratio is much higher in cow milk than human milk. Casein forms hard clots in the stomach and is also relatively low in cysteine (the usual precursor of taurine). Infant formulae vary in the extent to which the casein:whey ratio has been modified to make it closer to that of human milk. In the first few weeks after birth, **whey-dominant formula** was used by over 60 per cent of UK mothers, but use of **casein-dominant formula** becomes more prevalent in older infants because of the belief that it is more satisfying than whey-dominant formula. In casein-dominant formula the casein:whey ratio is 80:20 as in cow milk but in whey-dominant formula it is closer to the 40:60 ratio in human milk. Follow-on formulae are produced as an alternative to cow milk for infants who are over 6 months. They are not intended to be a complete diet but a component of a weaning diet and at 8–9 months were being used by just over a third of UK mothers. By 8–9 months just over half of UK mothers had introduced cow milk to their babies in one way or another (as a drink or to mix with food) and 85 per cent of these used whole milk and only 1 per cent used skimmed milk. More detailed statistical information on the use of different non-breast milks during the first 9 months can be found in the extensive survey report of Hamlyn *et al.* (2002).

Cow milk fat is poorly digested and absorbed compared to that in breast milk; it is also much lower in essential polyunsaturated fatty acids. Some or all of the butterfat will be replaced by vegetable oils by infant formula manufacturers to give a fatty acid composition closer to that of human milk. Cow milk has only around 1 per cent of energy as linoleic acid whereas the figure for human milk is up to 16 per cent depending on the diet of the mother. The differences in digestibility of cow and breast milk fat may be due to:

- differences in the nature of the fat itself. Palmitic acid is generally not well absorbed by infants but in human milk most of it is in the 2-position and is absorbed as monoacylglycerol
- breast milk contains lipase, which is activated by bile salts. Lingual lipases make a major contribution to fat digestion of bottle and breastfed babies

- the differences in bile acid secretion mentioned earlier may contribute to the better fat digestion by breastfed babies.

Breast milk is particularly high in lactose and this lactose content may increase calcium absorption and act as a substrate for lactobacilli in the lumen of the gut, thus creating an acid environment that will inhibit the growth of pathogens. Breast milk contains factors that stimulate the growth of *Lactobacillus bifidi* – small amounts of oligosaccharides and nucleotides may be important in this respect. The stools of healthy breastfed babies have a low pH and contain almost exclusively lactobacilli whereas formula-fed babies have a more mixed gut flora. Formula manufacturers increase the carbohydrate content so that it corresponds to that of human milk – they may or may not use lactose for this purpose. Oligosaccharides of glucose produced by partial hydrolysis of starch are often used.

Cow milk contains much higher concentrations of the major minerals than human milk. The sodium content is over three times higher; this is a high solute load for the immature kidney to deal with and it can precipitate **hypernatraemic dehydration**. The risk of dehydration would be exacerbated by fever, diarrhoea or by making up the formula too concentrated. High sodium content was the single most important reason why, in the UK in 1976, several formulae, including national dried milk, were withdrawn. The calcium contents of cow milk and breast milk differ by even more than the sodium content but calcium uptake is homoeostatically regulated – calcium absorption from cow milk may be poor despite the high concentration. Unabsorbed fat from cow milk or formula hinders calcium absorption whereas the presence of lactose increases it.

The vitamin and trace mineral content of formula is generally set so as to match or exceed that in human milk. The iron content of formula is higher than in breast milk even though it is normal for breastfed babies to be in negative iron balance for the first few months of their lives. The iron content of breast milk is considered insufficient for older babies (4–6 months). All formula is fortified with vitamin D.

Table 15.7 shows that formula is still very different from human milk. Even if manufacturers had succeeded in producing a formula that exactly corresponded to breast milk in its nutrient content, there would still be substantial residual benefits to be gained from breastfeeding. In many developing countries, choice of feeding method may greatly affect the chances of survival of the baby. Mortality rates of bottle-fed babies are often much higher than those of breastfed babies (Walker, 1990). Even in industrialized countries there are suggestions that deaths from sudden infant death syndrome are lower in breastfed babies (see Laurent, 1993). Sample studies from both developing and developed countries are outlined in the next paragraph. Breastfeeding can reduce risk of infection both by preventing exposure to contaminated alternatives and because of the inherent anti-infective properties of breast milk. Although the former may be the dominant benefit in some developing countries there is evidence that it also reduces gut and respiratory infection rates in industrialized countries and that the latter mechanisms are predominant here (Filteau and Tomkins, 1994).

A study sponsored by the World Health Organization (WHO, 2000) compared mortality rates for breast- and bottle-fed babies in three developing countries and found that in the first 2 months mortality rates were six times higher in the bottle-fed babies. This large difference was particularly due to a reduction in deaths from diarrhoea in the breastfed babies but deaths from acute respiratory infections were also lower. Although the differences in mortality rates between the breast- and bottle-fed babies narrowed steadily after the first 2 months, they were still apparent in the second year of life. The protective effect of breastfeeding was highest in those mothers with the lowest level of educational. Chen and Rogan (2004) have reported that in the USA, breastfeeding is also associated with a significant reduction of post-neonatal death. Mortality was just over 20 per cent lower in those babies who had been breastfed compared to those who had never been breastfed. Although it is not possible to say with certainty that this reduction in mortality in the USA is caused by breastfeeding these authors did correct for the most obvious confounding variables.

Some other benefits of breastfeeding are discussed below.

- *Bonding:* breastfeeding is thought to increase bonding between mother and baby.
- *Anti-infective properties:* breast milk contains immunoglobulin A, which protects the mucosal surfaces of the digestive tract and upper respiratory tract from pathogens. It also contains immune cells, which aid in the immunological protection of the infant gut. The iron-binding protein lactoferrin has a bacteriostatic effect. The enzyme lysozyme breaks down bacterial cell walls and oligosaccharides and nucleotides promote the growth of lactobacilli. **Colostrum**, the secretion produced in the first few days of lactation, is particularly rich in these anti-infective agents. Colostrum is quite different in its composition from mature human milk. Anti-infective agents in cow milk will probably be destroyed during processing and many are in any case likely to be species specific. There is some benefit to be gained by even a very short period of breastfeeding because at least then the infant will receive the colostrum.
- *Hygiene:* it is taken for granted in most industrialized countries that infant formula will be made up with clean boiled water, in sterile bottles, and the final mixture pasteurized by being made up with hot water. The risk of contamination in many other countries is a very serious one – the purity of the water, facilities for sterilization of water and bottles, and storage conditions for pre-mixed feeds may all be poor. This means that bottle fed babies may have greatly increased risk of gastrointestinal infections. Gastroenteritis is a major cause of death for babies in developing countries. This is a major reason why breastfeeding should be particularly encouraged in these countries. This is an important cause of the higher mortality of bottle fed babies in developing countries.
- *Restoration of maternal pre-pregnant weight:* it is generally assumed that maternal fat laid down during pregnancy serves as a store to help meet the energy demands of lactation on the mother. In countries like the UK and USA, where obesity is prevalent, the assumed effect of lactation in reducing this maternal fat after delivery may be an important one. It was noted earlier that 13 per cent of UK women quoted this as a reason for choosing to breastfeed. A recent Swedish study found that even modest weight gain after a first pregnancy increased the risk of pre-eclampsia, diabetes, stillbirth and caesarean delivery (Villamor and Cnattingius, 2006).
- *Cost of formula:* in wealthy industrialized countries, the cost of formula is usually relatively trivial. Nevertheless, modern infant formula is a high technology product and in many developing countries feeding an infant with formula will

absorb a very substantial proportion of the total household budget. This may seriously reduce resources available to feed the rest of the family or it may lead to the baby being fed over-diluted formula as an economy measure and so effectively starving it.

- *Anti-fertility effect:* although breastfeeding cannot be regarded as a reliable method of contraception, it does greatly reduce fertility. Suckling suppresses the release of pituitary gonadotrophins which are necessary for development of ovarian follicles and ovulation. In cultures where suckling occurs for extended periods rather than in discreet 'meals', then this effect may be increased. In many developing countries, prolonged breastfeeding will have an important birth spacing effect and will make a contribution to limiting overall population fertility. Full breastfeeding may be up to 98 per cent effective in preventing pregnancy in the first 6 months after birth; return of fertility will be hastened by use of supplementary formula or solid food during breastfeeding (see Picciano and McDonald, 2006).
- *Reduced risk of breast cancer:* a large case–control study in the UK has suggested that breastfeeding reduces the risk of developing breast cancer in young women. Breast cancer risk declined both with the duration of breastfeeding undertaken by the woman and with the number of babies that she had breastfed (UK National Case–Control Study Group, 1993). Several other studies in other countries have reported similar findings and also suggested a possible protective effect against ovarian cancer (see Picciano and McDonald, 2006).

- Cow milk is high in sodium and some early infant formulae were withdrawn in the UK in 1976 because of their high sodium content.
- Mortality and infection rates of breastfed babies are much lower in developing countries than those of bottle fed babies.
- Even in industrialized countries, breastfed babies have lower rates or severity of infection and reduced post-neonatal mortality.
- Breastfeeding reduces risk of infection because it reduces exposure to contaminated alternatives and because of its inherent anti-infective properties.
- Infant formula is an expensive commodity for mothers in developing countries.
- Breastfeeding decreases fertility, may help the mother to regain her pre-pregnant weight and reduces the mother's risk of breast cancer and possibly ovarian cancer.

Weaning

When to wean?

Weaning is the process of transferring an infant from breast milk or infant formula onto solid food. The process begins when the child is first offered food other than breast milk or formula. The process may be very gradual with other foods forming an increasing proportion of total energy intake over several months until breast or formula is eventually phased out completely. During weaning there is ideally gradual transition from a very high fat, high sugar liquid diet to a starchy, moderate fat, low sugar and fibre-containing solid diet. The magnitude of the compositional and textural changes involved would seem to indicate the advisability of a gradual transition to allow babies to adapt to them.

In the report *Weaning and the weaning diet* (COMA, 1994b) it was recommended that the majority of infants should not be given solid food before the age of 4 months and that a mixed diet should be offered by the age of 6 months. More recently, Morgan (1998) has suggested that 14 weeks should be the minimum age for weaning or when the infant's weight reaches 7 kg. This means that the current ideal window for weaning in the UK is between 4 and 6 months. After around 6 months, it is thought that breast milk can no longer supply all of the nutritional needs of the infant and growth is likely to be impaired if the baby receives only breast

Key points

- Breast milk is very different in composition to either cow milk or even modern infant formula.
- The casein:whey ratio is higher in cow milk and formula can either be casein dominant or whey dominant like breast milk.
- In infant formula some of the highly saturated butter fat of cow milk is replaced by vegetable oil.
- Human milk fat is much better digested and absorbed than that in cow milk.
- Breast milk has more lactose than cow milk and infant formula is supplemented with carbohydrate, which may not be lactose.

milk. Breast milk or formula may continue to make a contribution to total food supply long after weaning has begun.

The early introduction of solid foods is considered undesirable because:

- some babies do not properly develop the ability to bite and chew before 3–4 months
- the infant gut is very vulnerable to infection and allergy
- the early introduction of energy-dense weaning foods may increase the likelihood of obesity.

Full production of pancreatic amylase may not occur in human infants until 6–9 months of age. As milk contains no starch but most weaning foods are starchy, this may be a physiological indicator that a relatively late introduction of starches into the diet is desirable. Introducing starchy solid foods too early may produce symptoms similar to infectious gastro-enteritis because of poor digestion and absorption due to the lack of pancreatic amylase.

In 1975, 18 per cent of British babies had been given some food other than milk in their first month and 97 per cent by the time they were 4 months old; corresponding figures for 1995 were 2 per cent and 91 per cent, respectively (COMA, 1988; Foster *et al.*, 1997). The practice of introducing solid foods to infants very soon after birth has become much less common. Table 15.8 shows comparative figures for the age at which solid foods were introduced by mothers in the UK in 1995 and

Table 15.8 The percentage of UK babies who have been introduced to solid food at different ages in 1995 and 2000

Age of baby	Year	
	1995	2000
6 weeks	7	3
8 weeks	13	5
3 months	56	24
4 months (17 weeks)	91	85
6 months	99	98
9 months	100	100
Age at first introduction to solids		
Before 16 weeks		49
Between 16 and 26 weeks		49
After 26 weeks		2

*Data from Hamlyn et al. (2002).

2000. The figures in Table 15.8 indicate a marked and continuing trend for the later introduction of solid foods in the UK but still nearly half of mothers introduced solid food before the 16 weeks recommended by COMA (1994b) and many before the 14-week minimum (or 7 kg body weight) suggested by Morgan (1998).

What weaning foods?

In the UK, the first foods for most babies are cereals, rusks or commercial weaning foods rather than home-prepared weaning foods. At 4–10 weeks, only 9 per cent of mothers who had offered solid food to their babies had used a home made food and even at 4 months, when 85 per cent had offered some solid food, only 38 per cent of them had used home made food (Hamlyn *et al.*, 2002).

The priorities for weaning foods

Morgan and colleagues asked a large sample of British mothers for their views on good infant feeding practices and some of the findings of this survey are summarized in Table 15.9.

Table 15.9 The priorities of a sample of UK mothers for infant feeding*

	% Of mothers' responses	
	Not important	(Very) important
Wide variety of foods	3	95
Plenty to drink	1	98
Plenty of calories	20	76
Low fat intake	10	88
High fibre intake	15	83

*Adapted from Morgan (1998).

Clearly most of the women thought that a high-fibre and low-fat diet should be the priority for weaning foods and a fifth do not think that an energy-rich diet is important for rapidly growing infants. These maternal priorities are very different from the current consensus of expert nutritional opinion such as those of COMA (1994b) listed below. The numerical values in Table 15.9 represent the views of women sampled over a decade ago but they do emphasize the importance of informing pregnant women and new mothers about the different nutritional priorities for young children and the well-publicized advice to adults.

- Provision of adequate dietary energy for growth is the principal determinant of the diets of the under 5s.
- Adult recommendations on reducing fat consumption should not apply to the under 2s and should fully apply from the age of 5 years.
- The diets of the under 2s should not contain fibre-rich foods to the extent that they limit energy content and the absorption of micronutrients.

Poskitt (1998) suggested that weaning foods should be:

- rich in energy, including energy from fat
- rich in vitamins and minerals
- fed frequently
- initially used as a supplement to milk rather than a replacement
- fed in a form that develops the child's feeding skills whilst still allowing assistance.

One of the main aims of weaning is to raise the energy density of the infant's diet above that for breast milk. The weaning food should have a suitable texture, but be of high enough energy and nutrient density for the baby to meet its nutritional needs without having to consume an excessive volume of food. If very viscous foods are introduced too early in the weaning process then the infant may reject them by spitting them out. A typical developing world weaning food made up to give a suitable viscosity from a starchy cereal or root staple, such as cassava or millet flour, might contain only 0.3 kcal/g (1.3 kJ/g). This compares with around 0.7 kcal/g (3 kJ/g) for breast milk and perhaps 1.5 kcal/g (6 kJ/g) for a typical UK weaning diet (Church, 1979). At the lower extreme, the child is incapable of consuming the volume of food required to meet its energy needs. This problem may be exacerbated if the child is fed infrequently, has frequent periods of infection and anorexia, and perhaps by the poor sensory characteristics of the food itself. In industrialized countries, this could be a problem if parents mistakenly apply the recommendations for low-fat, low-sugar and high-starch diets in adults too rigorously to infants. Some strict vegetarian weaning diets in industrialized countries may also be of insufficient energy density because of their low fat and high starch content. The lower limit for the energy density of weaning foods should be 0.7 kcal/g (3 kJ/g). Pureed fruit or vegetables are not suitable as weaning foods unless they

have their energy density enhanced, e.g. by the addition of a source of fat. Skimmed and semi-skimmed milk are not suitable for very young children although Hamlyn et al. (2002) found that 14 per cent of UK mothers who were giving their babies cow milk at 9 months of age were using semi-skimmed milk and 1 per cent were using skimmed milk.

Weaning foods should be clean and not contaminated with infective agents. Poverty, poor hygiene and contaminated food precipitate much malnutrition in the developing world. Even when dietary intakes are judged sufficient to permit normal growth, infection and diarrhoea may be an indirect cause of dietary deficiency. One survey reported that 41 per cent of traditional weaning foods and 50 per cent of drinking water specimens in rural Bangladesh were contaminated with faecal microorganisms (see Walker, 1990). Although substantial progress has been made in improving sanitation and water supplies, especially in south Asia since 1990, UNICEF estimates that maybe 1.5 million children die each year around the world because they do not have access to safe water and proper sanitation.

In affluent countries, such as the UK and US, other aims are also considered important for infant feeds. They should be:

- low in salt
- low in added sugar
- perhaps should be gluten-free.

High-salt foods expose the immature kidney to a high-solute load and increase the risk of hypernatraemic dehydration and maybe increase the later risk of high blood pressure. Sugar is regarded as empty calories and is detrimental to the baby's new teeth. Over-consumption of sugar in infancy may also be creating bad preferences for the future. There is strong evidence that fluoride is protective against dental caries, the UK panel on DRVs suggested a safe fluoride intake for infants of 0.05 mg/kg/day – around 50 per cent of the amount likely to cause fluorosis. To achieve this safe intake most UK infants would need supplements and the amount of supplemental fluoride required depends on the fluoride content of the local water supply (see Chapter 14 for details). Swallowing fluoridated toothpaste is one way that many young children receive supplemental fluoride.

Although most babies will suffer no harm by early exposure to the wheat protein called gluten, those sensitive to gluten and thus at risk of coeliac disease (see Chapter 16) cannot be identified in advance. The incidence of coeliac disease in children has been falling in recent years at the same time as there have been trends towards later introduction of solid foods and towards the use of gluten-free, rice-based weaning cereals.

Key points

- Weaning should start sometime between 4 and 6 months after birth.
- Breast milk is not adequate for babies after 6 months but can usefully continue to contribute to their diets.
- Very early introduction of solid foods is undesirable and is now much less common in the UK than it was.
- Half of UK women still introduce solid foods before the baby is 16 weeks old.
- Mothers in Britain usually use some form of commercial weaning food in the early stages of weaning.
- Weaning foods should be free from contamination and should be energy and nutrient dense.
- Weaning foods should not be low in fat or too high in fibre and they should be low in salt and added sugar.
- Babies should be fed frequently during weaning.
- In 1995, many British mothers mistakenly believed that weaning foods should be low in fat and high in fibre.
- Pureed fruit or vegetables are unsuitable weaning foods unless their energy density has been increased and very young children should not be given low-fat milk.
- In many developing countries, the traditional starchy weaning foods have such low energy density that they limit energy intake and precipitate malnutrition.

CHILDHOOD AND ADOLESCENCE

Even when fully weaned, children still have nutritional needs and priorities that differ from those of adults. They need enough energy and nutrients to enable them to grow and develop, especially during the intensely anabolic adolescent period. Too heavy an emphasis on a low-fat, low-sugar and high-fibre diet may limit growth. These differing needs have to be reconciled with the need to start good dietary habits early and to prevent the development of obesity. Note that inactivity is now regarded as the key factor in childhood obesity (see Chapter 8).

Table 15.10 Selected dietary reference values (per day) for UK children and their percentage of the corresponding adult values*

Nutrient	1–3 years	% Adult[†]	4–6 years	% Adult[†]
Boys' energy (kcal)	1230 (5.15 MJ)	48	1715 (7.16 MJ)	67
Girls' energy (kcal)	1165 (4.86 MJ)	60	1545 (6.46 MJ)	86
Protein (g)	14.5	29	19.7	40
Thiamin (mg)	0.5	55	0.7	78
Riboflavin (mg)	0.6	50	0.8	50
Niacin (mg)	8	53	11	73
Folate (μg)	70	35	100	50
Vitamin C	30	75	30	75
Vitamin A (μg)	400	62	500	77
Vitamin D (μg)[‡]	7	–	–	–
Calcium (mg)	350	50	450	64
Iron (mg)	6.9	60	6.1	52
Zinc (mg)	5.0	61	6.5	79

*Data source: COMA (1991).
Note that the body weight of a 1–3-year-old is approximately 20 per cent of that of an adult and that of a 4–6-year-old is approximately 30 per cent of the adult value.
[†] In most cases this is calculated using the average of the male and female value for 19–50 year olds.
[‡] For adults and older children there are no reference values as it is synthesized in the skin when exposed to sunlight.

Table 15.10 shows selected UK RNIs for children in the 1–3- and 4–6-year-old category. The values have also been expressed as an approximate percentage of the value for adults. These values confirm that children require proportionately much more energy than do adults. Girls 1–3 years of age weigh about a fifth of an adult woman but require three-fifths as much dietary energy as a woman. The values for the other nutrients are generally in line with this proportionately higher energy requirement (much less in the case of protein). A diet that is compositionally suitable for adults should therefore contain adequate amounts of nutrients for young children provided they eat enough of it to satisfy their energy needs. Of course, children may be more sensitive to the effects of nutrient deficiencies as, for example, they may have smaller stores than adults or their growth may be impaired.

In a survey of the diets of a representative sample of UK pre-school children (1.5–4.5 years old), Gregory et al. (1995) made the following observations.

- Energy intakes of the children were less than the EARs which is probably because the EARs are set too high.
- The proportions of food energy contributed by the major nutrients was 13 per cent from protein, 51 per cent from carbohydrate and 36 per cent from fat.
- Within the major macronutrient categories, sugars provided 29 per cent of energy, non-milk extrinsic sugars 19 per cent and saturated fat 16 per cent.
- Average intakes of most vitamins and minerals were generally well above the RNI, except for vitamin A, iron and zinc.
- About half of children had intakes of vitamin A that were below the RNI and around 8 per cent below the LRNI.
- A large majority of children had iron intakes below the RNI and a fifth of the very young ones had intakes that were below the LRNI.
- Inadequate iron intakes in many of the sample were confirmed by blood analyses which showed that 10 per cent were anaemic and 20 per cent had less than satisfactory iron stores (serum ferritin below 10 μg/L).
- Intakes of vitamin D were under 2 μg/day and this is clearly an insufficient amount if children do not get adequate exposure to summer sunlight.

Although the macronutrient composition of the diets of UK pre-school children recorded in this survey was close to the guideline values for adults, the levels of added sugars and saturated fat were high. More than half of the added sugar in the diet came from soft drinks and sweets. These are practically devoid of nutrients, lower the overall nutrient density of the diet and are damaging to children's teeth. Milk and vegetables contributed about half of the vitamin A in children's diets. Liver where eaten made a major contribution to average daily vitamin A intake. Fruits and vegetables together only accounted for 16 per cent of total vitamin A intake. Cereals, which are often fortified, contributed about half of the children's iron intake and meat and fish only about 20 per cent. Milk and milk products provided about 40 per cent of the saturated fat and meat and fish about 15 per cent. Biscuits, cakes, chips and savoury snacks provided 20 per cent of the saturated fat. The message from this survey is what most parents probably would have guessed and many are trying to implement. Children's diets would be improved if they consumed less sugary drinks, sweets, cakes, biscuits and chips (French fries) and ate more fruit, vegetables, lean meat, fish, cereals and boiled potatoes.

The rate of growth of children decelerates steadily from birth until puberty. During adolescence there is a very pronounced and sustained growth spurt. Between the ages of 12 and 17 years boys gain an average 26 cm in height and 26 kg in weight, and between the ages of 10 and 15 years girls gain 23 cm in height and 21 kg in weight. Adolescence is thus an intensely anabolic period and a time when there is inevitably a relatively high demand for energy and nutrients to sustain this rapid growth. In a proportion of adolescents, high levels of physical activity because of participation in games and sports will still further increase needs for energy and perhaps other nutrients. Adolescence is also a time of major psychological changes brought on by the hormonal changes of puberty and these may have major effects on children's attitudes to food. Adolescent girls are the most common sufferers from anorexia nervosa and paradoxically, obesity is also a common nutritional problem of adolescence.

Increasing secretion of sex hormones at puberty produces a major divergence in the body composition of boys and girls. Male sex hormones cause boys to gain more muscle than fat and to adopt a more abdominal distribution of their body fat. Female sex hormones cause girls to gain more fat than muscle and to increase their deposition of fat in the hip and thigh region. This increase in fatness that is a natural part of female adolescence may be an important contributor to the unhealthy pre-occupation with body image and dieting experienced by many adolescent girls. Many adolescent girls perceive themselves as too fat when they are not and diet when it is inappropriate. They sometimes adopt unhealthy dietary and other strategies for losing weight, e.g. fasting, avoidance of meat and other staple foods and even smoking (e.g. Ryan *et al.*, 1998). Girls need to be better prepared for these changes and be reassured that they are a normal consequence of maturation.

As with rapidly growing infants, diets with very low energy density (e.g. diets very low in fat and high in fibre) may tend to limit growth during adolescence. Strict vegetarian diets tend to be bulky and have low energy density; this is indeed often cited as one of their advantages. Vegan children tend to be smaller and lighter than other children (Sanders, 1988). The phrase 'muesli belt malnutrition' has been widely used in the UK to describe undernutrition in rapidly growing children precipitated by overzealous restriction of energy dense foods by health conscious, middle-class parents.

During the 5-year period of adolescence, boys accumulate an average of around 200 mg/day of calcium in their skeleton with a peak value of about double this average. They also accumulate an average of 0.5 mg/day of iron and 2 g/day of protein during the 5 years of adolescence. The onset of menstruation represents a further major stress on the iron status of adolescent girls. Table 15.11 shows some DRVs for 11–14-year-olds, 15–18-year-olds and adults. The energy EAR for 15–18-year-old boys is 8 per cent higher than that for adult men despite the smaller size of the boys. The calcium RNI is 43 per cent higher for both age groups of boys than that for men and clearly reflects the DRV panels assumptions of the extra calcium needs required for skeletal growth. This calcium RNI would be difficult to meet without drinking good amounts milk. Similar, relatively high DRVs for girls compared with women are also shown in this table. Similar trends are also seen in the American RDAs, the relative allowance (i.e. allowing for size) is higher in adolescents than in adults. American values for all groups tend to be higher than the corresponding British values. Note particularly that the

Table 15.11 A comparison of some UK dietary reference values for adolescent boys and girls with those for adults*

		Age		
		11–14 years	15–18 years	Adult
Energy EAR (kcal)	Male	2200	2755	2550
	Female	1845	2110	1940
Energy EAR (MJ)	M	9.21	11.51	10.60
	F	7.92	8.83	8.10
Calcium (mg)	M	1000	1000	700
	F	800	800	700
Iron (mg)	M	11.3	11.3	8.7
	F	14.8	14.8	14.8
Zinc (mg)	M	9.0	9.5	9.5
	F	9.0	7.0	7.0
Niacin (mg)	M	15	18	17
	F	12	14	13

EAR, estimated average requirement.
*Data source: COMA (1991).

calcium RDAs for both ages of boys and girls are 1300 mg/day (*cf.* adult value 1000 mg/day); the calcium RDAs for American girls are thus 50 per cent higher than the corresponding UK values.

COMA (1989b) published a survey conducted in 1983 of the diets of a nationally representative sample of British girls and boys at 10–11 years and 14–15 years. The panel concluded that the main sources of energy in the diets of British children were bread, chips (French fries), milk, biscuits (cookies), meat products (e.g. sausages, burgers, meat pies), cakes and puddings. These foods together accounted for about half of the total energy intake. Mean recorded energy intakes were within 5 per cent of the EAR for all groups when interpolated from actual recorded body weights. Fat made up about 38 per cent of total energy intake of these British children, very similar to the adult figure recorded just a few years later by Gregory *et al.* (1990). Three-quarters of all children exceeded the target of 35 per cent of food energy from fat. Surprisingly, meat and meat products contributed less than 15 per cent of the total fat, marginally less than that contributed by chips (French fries) and crisps (potato chips). Average intakes of all four groups of children exceeded the current RNIs for most of the nutrients surveyed. The two main areas of concern highlighted by this study were:

- average calcium intakes of the older children were about 10 per cent below current RNI (more than 40 per cent of calcium came from milk and cheese)
- iron intakes of the older girls were only 62 per cent of the current RNI and around 60 per cent of girls had iron intakes below the RNI appropriate for the start of menstruation.

The overall impression from this survey of British children was that their diets met most criteria for adequacy although there are a few areas for concern such as the iron intakes of the adolescent girls. In terms of health education priorities, particularly dietary fats, the diets of children were, as one might expect, very similar to those of their parents at this time. These general conclusions would probably apply to most other industrialized countries.

A more recent survey of school-age (4–18 years) British children has been conducted as part of the rolling programme of National Diet and Nutrition Survey (NDNS) by Gregory *et al.* (2000). Energy intakes recorded in this more recent survey were significantly lower than those recorded 15 years earlier by COMA (1989b) even though the children in the more recent survey were bigger and heavier. This probably reflects the general decline in population activity leading to reduced energy expenditure and higher weight gain despite lower food intake; this is a major factor in the increased levels of overweight and obesity in all age groups. Information collected on activity in those children age over 7 years indicated that most young people are inactive. Generally girls are less active than boys and activity tends to fall as children get older. In this survey 40–50 per cent of the children failed to meet the recommendation that young people should participate in at least moderate activity for an hour each day.

The proportion of energy derived from fat was 35 per cent for boys and 36 per cent for girls which is close to the recommended value of 35 per cent and this suggests that the proportion of fat in children's diets has dropped in the last couple of decades just as it has done in their parents' diets (see Chapter 11). Saturated fat intakes at around 14.2 per cent of energy were still above the recommended 11 per cent. Intakes of non-milk extrinsic sugars were 16.5 per cent of energy compared to the recommended

11 per cent with fizzy drinks and chocolate confectionery being the main sources of these added sugars.

Although average intakes of most nutrients were above the RNI, a number of problems with the micronutrient intakes were highlighted by the survey and some are listed below.

- Average intakes of vitamin A were close to the RNI in younger children but below it in older children. Around 20 per cent of older girls and 12 per cent of older boys had intakes that were below the LRNI.
- A fifth of older girls had inadequate riboflavin intakes and biochemical evidence of poor riboflavin status was noted in some individuals in this survey.
- Biochemical evidence of poor vitamin D status was found in 13 per cent of 11–18-year-olds with a higher proportion in winter samples.
- Biochemical evidence of poor nutritional status in some individuals was also found for thiamin, folate and vitamin C.
- There were substantial numbers of children with mineral intakes that were below the LRNI: for zinc in all groups; potassium, magnesium and calcium in older children; and, iron in older girls.
- Some 50 per cent of older girls had iron intakes below the LRNI and low ferritin levels, indicating low iron stores, were found in 27 per cent of girls and 13 per cent of boys.

It was noted in Chapter 12, when discussing adults' micronutrient intakes, that even where average intakes appear satisfactory there may still be many individuals with unsatisfactory intakes and/or biochemical indications of poor nutrient status. Many of the adverse findings are similar to those recorded for younger age groups of adults by Hoare *et al.* (2004) and discussed in Chapter 12.

About 20 per cent of the children sampled by Gregory *et al.* (2000) reported that they took a micronutrient supplement. About 10 per cent of girls in the 15–18 year age band were vegetarian and about 16 per cent were dieting (comparable figures for boys were 1 and 3 per cent, respectively). Those children with lower socioeconomic status tended to have lower quality diets as indicated by lower recorded intakes of many nutrients and lower biochemical status for several vitamins and for iron.

Key points

- Children need enough dietary energy and nutrients to allow them to grow and develop properly.

- Young children need proportionately much more energy than adults and so good energy density is still an important priority.

- Inactivity is the major cause of child obesity.

- Diets that are adequate for adults should be adequate for young children if they meet their energy requirements.

- The average diets of young British children are high in added sugar but low in vitamin A, iron and zinc.

- 20 per cent of young British children have biochemical evidence of poor iron status.

- Young British children need regular exposure to sunlight to achieve satisfactory vitamin D status.

- Young British children should consume less sugary drinks, sweets, cakes, biscuits and chips but more fruit, vegetables, lean meat, cereals and potatoes.

- Adolescence is an intensely anabolic period and there are substantial increases in body weight, body protein and body calcium content.

- At puberty, boys increase their lean:fat ratio.

- Female sex hormones cause a substantial increase in the body fat content of girls, particularly increases in fat around the hips and thighs.

- Girls who are unprepared for the pubertal increases in body fat may be encouraged to diet inappropriately and to adopt unhealthy practices to try to lose weight.

- The average diets of British schoolchildren are similar in their macronutrient composition to those of their parents and contain adequate amounts of most essential nutrients.

- The calcium intakes of older children and more especially the iron intakes of adolescent girls are less than satisfactory.

- The diets of British schoolchildren would also be improved if they consumed less sugary drinks, sweets, cakes, biscuits and chips but more fruit, vegetables, lean meat, cereals and potatoes.

THE ELDERLY

Demographic and social trends

Much of this section is based on material in the first chapter of Webb and Copeman (1996). Table 15.12 gives an approximate breakdown of the proportion of the population of England and Wales in various age bands. The proportion of elderly people in the

Table 15.12 The percentage of the population of England and Wales in various age bands*

Age band	% of total population[†]
0–14 (children)	19.2
15–44 (young adults)	43
45–64 (middle-aged)	21.9
65+ (elderly adults)	15.9
65–74	8.8
75–84	5.4
85–89	1.2
90+	0.5

*Reproduced with permission from Webb and Copeman (1996).
[†] Total population of 51.3 million in 1992.

populations of industrialized countries rose substantially during the twentieth century and is projected to continue rising. By the end of the 1990s, around 16 per cent of the population of England and Wales were over 65 years and almost 2 per cent were over 85 years of age. At the start of the twentieth century, life expectancy at birth was around 47 years in both the UK and USA but had risen to over 76 years by the end of the century. In 1901, only 4.7 per cent of the population of England and Wales was over 65 years. The increase in life expectancy during the twentieth century has not been confined to the younger age groups:

- between 1901 and 1991 the life expectancy of a 1-year-old child rose from 55 to 76 years (38 per cent increase)
- that for a 60 year old increased from 14 to 19 more years (36 per cent increase)
- that for a 75 year old from 7.5 to 10.5 (40 per cent increase).

The ratio of females to males in the elderly population increases progressively with age and in the over 85 age group there are three times as many women as men. By 2026, the over 65s are expected to represent 19 per cent of the UK population and the over 85s almost 2.5 per cent of the population. In the USA in 1990, about 13 per cent of the population were over the age of 65 and this proportion is projected to rise to around 22 per cent by 2040.

A third of the over 65s in England and Wales live alone and the proportion living by themselves increases markedly with advancing age as a result of the deaths of spouses. Almost two-thirds of women and nearly half of men aged over 85 live alone. The number of elderly people living in residential homes for the elderly increased from around 150 000 in 1977 to around 235 000 in 1990. This 1990 figure represents around 3 per cent of all people over the age of 65 years and almost 0.5 per cent of the total population of England and Wales. The chances of an elderly person living in care accommodation rises steeply with age and the increase in the number of people living in care accommodation is entirely due to increases in the size of the elderly and very elderly population. In 1995, the number of elderly people living in all types of long-term residential care (residential homes, nursing homes and long stay hospitals) was:

- 1 per cent of 65–74 year olds
- 6 per cent of 75–84 year olds
- 27 per cent of those aged over 85 years.

Catering for the dietary and nutritional needs of the elderly is thus a topic that should warrant an increased educational and research priority.

The household income and expenditure of elderly people in England and Wales tends to be concentrated at the lower end of the range. Retired people make up a high proportion of those in the three lowest household income groups but they become progressively less well represented in the higher-income categories. Retired persons in the upper-income groups inevitably receive some income in addition to the state pension. In 1992, over 60 per cent of the households with an elderly head had an income in the lowest band compared with only about 15 per cent of young adult households. Less than 20 per cent of older households had an income in the highest band compared to about 60 per cent of young adult households. Amongst the elderly, income declines with increasing age. The average expenditure per person in households where the head was aged over 75 years, was only two-thirds of that in households where the head was aged 50–64

years. Many elderly people spend their later years in relative poverty. The increasing ratio of retired to working people in the population makes it difficult to foresee any immediate large improvement in the finances of elderly people in the UK who are largely dependent on the state retirement pension. The ongoing crisis in the private pension industry may lead to increases in the numbers of elderly people with relatively low incomes.

As income declines, so absolute *per capita* expenditure on food also declines but food accounts for an increasing share of expenditure. The proportion of income spent on housing and fuel also increases with age in Britain but the proportion spent on clothing, transport, alcohol and tobacco declines. The food expenditure of retired couples in the lowest income group in the UK is close to the minimum estimated cost of a 'modest but adequate' diet that is also broadly in line with the usual UK diet (see Chapter 2). Webb and Copeman (1996) compared the food expenditure of elderly households with other one and two adult households in the UK. They made the following observations.

- Elderly households spend less on food than the equivalent younger households.
- Elderly households get more calories for each penny of their expenditure, a general trend with lower income.
- The elderly spent less on cheese, vegetables (excluding potatoes), fruit, soft drinks and alcohol but more on sugars and fats.
- Elderly households were less likely to buy low-calorie soft drinks and low-fat milk but more likely to buy butter.

More than half of all the over 65s report being affected by some longstanding illness and the proportion rises with advancing age. Bone and joint diseases, including arthritis and rheumatism, are easily the most common group of longstanding illnesses. Other important causes of longstanding illness in the elderly include heart disease, hypertension, respiratory diseases such as bronchitis and emphysema, stroke and diabetes. Ageing inevitably leads to increasing rates of mortality, morbidity and disability. Despite this, the majority of elderly people consider themselves to be in good or fairly good general health. In 1985, about 80 per cent of men and women aged over 65 years perceived their own health as good or fairly good and even in the 85+ age group only around 27 per cent of men and 33 per cent of women described their health in the previous year as 'not good'. This suggests that some level of disability is seen by elderly people as being inevitable and does not stop many of them from perceiving their overall health as good. More than 80 per cent of elderly people still report seeing friends or relatives at least once a week and even in the over 85s this figure is still around 75 per cent. About 97 per cent of people over 65 years still either live in their own homes or with their families. The widespread image of the post-retirement years as being inevitably an extended period of poor health, disability, dependence and social isolation does not seem to be the perceived experience of the majority of older people in Britain.

As average life expectancy starts to reach its inevitable plateau, so improving the quality of life of the elderly population has become an increasing priority for health education in industrialized countries. A major goal in the USA is to 'increase the span of healthy life for Americans' and similarly in England the aim is not only to reduce premature deaths and 'add years to life' but also to 'add life to years' by increasing the years that are free from ill-health and minimizing the adverse effects of illness and disability. Bebbington (1988) calculated 'the expectation of life without disability' from self-reported rates of disability and long-standing illness recorded in the British General Household Survey together with estimates of the numbers of people living in institutions for the 'disabled'. Although total life expectancy in the UK increased over the period 1976–88 (from 70 to 72.4 years in men and from 76.1 to 78.1 in women) the 'expectation of life without disability' remained essentially unchanged. Over this same period the years of illness and disability increased by 2.1 years in men and 2.5 years in women. The main effect of the recent increases in life expectancy has been to increase the number of years spent suffering from illness and disability. A similar study in the USA (Crimmins et al., 1989) concluded that between 1970 and 1980 increases in life expectancy were largely concentrated in years with a chronic disabling illness. A good diet and an active lifestyle would contribute both to increasing total lifespan and to compressing the years of morbidity and disability at the end of the lifespan.

Key points

- Improved life expectancy during the twentieth century caused large increases in the proportion of elderly and very elderly people in the populations of industrialized countries.
- By the year 2000, 16 per cent of British people were aged over 65 years and around 2 per cent were over 85 years.
- Not only are more people surviving to 65 years but elderly people are also living longer.
- Women greatly outnumber men in the older age groups.
- Many elderly people in Britain live alone or in care accommodation and the proportions increase sharply with age.
- Elderly people are disproportionately represented in the lowest income groups in the UK.
- Elderly people spend less on food than younger adults but it accounts for a higher proportion of their spending.
- The food expenditure of many elderly British people is at, or below, that considered necessary to purchase a 'modest but adequate' diet that is broadly in line with the current UK diet.
- Many elderly people are affected by some long-standing illness, but this does not prevent most of them perceiving their general health as good or fairly good.
- Improving the quality of life in the later years, rather than simply increasing life expectancy, is now being given a higher priority in health promotion.
- Some increase in life expectancy in recent decades in the USA and UK has been achieved by increasing the years spent suffering from illness and disability.
- A good diet and an active lifestyle should help to improve life expectancy and compress the period of chronic morbidity at the end of life.

The effects of ageing

Ageing is characterized by a gradual decline in the ability of an organism to adapt to environmental stresses and an inability to maintain homoeostasis. This loss of adaptability or capacity to maintain homoeostasis results in increasing mortality, increased morbidity and increased rates of disability.

There is measurable age-related deterioration in the functioning of most systems of the body. For example, ageing of the immune system leads to a decline in the efficiency of the immune surveillance and defensive mechanisms which leads to increased incidence of infection, autoimmune disease and cancer. The absorptive area of the small intestine decreases with age and it is likely that the absorption of several nutrients decreases with age. Deterioration is usually earliest and fastest in those systems where there is no replacement of dead cells (e.g. brain, muscle and heart) than in those where continual replacement occurs (e.g. red cells and intestinal epithelium). Generally, complex functions involving co-ordination are more affected than simple ones, e.g. reaction time increases more rapidly than the slowing in nerve conduction velocity.

There is a marked change in body composition with age, the proportions of lean tissue and bone decline and the proportion of fat increases. There is also a loss of height with age from about 30 years onwards. There is a decline in the basal metabolic rate (BMR) with age, which is probably a function of the decline in lean body mass in the elderly because when the BMR is expressed per kg of lean body mass there is no decline with age (COMA, 1992). The speed of homoeostatic regulation is reduced as people become elderly. Some examples are given below.

- In response to cold stress, old people tend to start shivering later and in response to heat stress they sweat later. Old people are also more susceptible to hypothermia because of their reduced BMR and their reduced levels of physical activity.
- There is slower restoration of acid–base balance if it is disturbed. Elderly people have reduced buffering capacity, a diminished respiratory response to acid–base disturbance and a reduced ability to eliminate excess acid or base via the kidney.
- There is a decline in the efficiency of the mechanisms regulating salt and water balance. For example, there is an age-related decline in the acuity of the thirst mechanism. Rolls and Phillips (1990) found that immediately after a period of water deprivation elderly men drank much less than younger men and experienced much less thirst even though their levels of dehydration were similar.

Key points

- All body systems deteriorate during ageing and there are increasing rates of mortality, morbidity and disability in the elderly.
- The proportions of muscle and bone in the adult body decrease with age and the proportion of fat increases.
- The loss of lean tissue in the elderly leads to a fall in BMR.
- Ageing is characterized by a reduced speed of homoeostatic regulation and a reduced ability to adapt to environmental change.

Nutritional requirements of the elderly

Energy expenditure and therefore energy requirements fall as people become elderly. The two factors listed below are thought to be responsible for this decline in energy expenditure.

- Levels of physical activity decline with increasing age. This may be accelerated by retirement and is inevitable in those who are housebound or bedridden.
- BMR decreases in the elderly. This is due to the decline in lean body mass and may itself be largely a consequence of reduced levels of physical activity.

Table 15.13 shows the UK EARs and the American dietary reference intakes for energy for different age categories of men and women. These dietary standards represent quite substantial reductions in the estimated energy requirements and therefore likely total food intake of elderly people, particularly of elderly men. The UK values for younger adults are set by multiplying the BMR by a multiple of 1.4 (the **physical activity level** (PAL)) whereas that for older adults is set using a PAL multiple of 1.5. This is despite clear evidence that physical activity decreases in the elderly. The rationale for this decision was discussed in Chapter 7. The US standards clearly acknowledge the decline in average energy requirements with age because the standards drop by 10 kcal/day for men and 7 kcal/day for women for each year after the age of 19 years.

Table 15.14 summarizes differences between the dietary standards for elderly people and those for younger adults. For nutrients not listed in Table 15.14

Table 15.13 UK and US dietary reference values for energy in older adults*

Age (years)	Men		Women	
	Kcal	MJ	Kcal	MJ
UK (EAR)				
19–50	2550	10.60	1940	8.10
51–59	2550	10.60	1900	8.00
60–64	2380	9.93	1900	7.99
65–74	2330	9.71	1900	7.96
75+	2100	8.77	1810	7.61
USA†				
20	3075	12.78	2396	10.02
40	2857	11.94	2256	9.43
60	2657	11.10	2116	8.84
80	2457	10.27	1976	8.26

EAR, estimated average requirement.
*Data sources: COMA (1991); NAS (2004).
†Note that the dietary reference intakes are listed for healthy and moderately active Americans and Canadians at 19 years and then 10 kcal/day are subtracted for each year for males and 7 kcal/day for females.

the values for younger and older adults are the same. Although energy requirements and total food intakes tend to fall in the elderly, Table 15.14 suggests that there is no corresponding decrease in the requirement for most other nutrients. The UK RNIs for the elderly suggest small reductions in the RNI for:

- protein in men – due entirely to differences in the assumed body weight of young and elderly men
- thiamin and niacin, which are set according to the assumed energy expenditure
- a substantial reduction in the female RNI for iron, which reflects the cessation of menstrual blood losses. The American standards for iron in elderly women are also reduced to the same as those for men.

In young adults, endogenous production of vitamin D in the skin is the primary source of the vitamin. The UK RNI for vitamin D in older adults shown in Table 15.14 reflects the view that endogenous production can no longer be relied on in elderly people who may be housebound and inadequately exposed

Table 15.14 Differences between dietary reference values for elderly and younger adults (for other nutrients, the values are the same). Data from COMA (1991) and NAS (2004)

Nutrient	RNIs – UK			
	Male		Female	
	19–50 years	50+	19–50	50+
Protein (g)	55.5	53.3	45.0	46.5
Thiamin (mg)	1.0	0.9	–	–
Niacin (mg)	17	16	13	12
*Vitamin D (μg)**	0	10	0	10
Iron (mg)	–	–	14.8	8.7

	RDAs – USA					
	31–50 years		51–70 years		70+ years	
	Male	Female	Male	Female	Male	Female
Vitamin D (μg)†			10	10	15	15
Vitamin B₆ (mg)	1.3	1.3	1.7	1.5	1.7	1.5
Calcium (mg)	1000	1000	1200	1200	1200	1200
Iron (mg)	8	18	8	8	8	8
Chromium (μg)	35	25	30	20	30	20

*RNI applies after 65 years
†In the absence of adequate sunlight exposure.

to sunlight. In America there is also an RDA of $10\,\mu g$/day set for those aged 51–70 years (none for those aged 30–50 years) which rises to $15\,\mu g$/day for those aged over 70 years. Poor vitamin D status was identified in Chapter 14 as a major aetiological factor for osteoporosis in the very elderly.

The American standards also suggest a substantial increase in vitamin B_6 requirement in the elderly and a 200 mg/day increase in the calcium requirement, which in younger adults is already well above the UK RNI. The UK dietary standards for older adults have often been set at the same value as younger adults because at the time they were set (1991) there was a lack of data on how nutrient requirements change with ageing. It now seems probable that requirements for some nutrients (e.g. calcium and vitamin B_6) may increase in the elderly and that reduced efficiency in the gut may affect requirements more generally. The raised American standards for calcium and vitamin B_6 have occurred relatively recently and may reflect this change in attitude.

Thus elderly people are perceived as requiring intakes of most nutrients that are similar to or higher than those for other adults but requiring average intakes of energy up to 20 per cent lower than those of other adults. For many elderly people, the real fall in energy expenditure and food intake may be even greater than the figures in Table 15.13 suggest. COMA (1992) suggested that for many inactive elderly people, who only spend an hour a day on their feet, a value of 1.3 times BMR would represent their balance rather than the 1.5 times BMR used to set the EARs in COMA (1991). Of course, if very elderly people are losing weight then they are not even eating enough to maintain energy balance. This increases the risk that energy intakes can be met without fulfilling the requirements for all other nutrients. This risk increases if the nutrient density of the diet is low, i.e. if a substantial proportion of the energy is obtained from nutrient-depleted sources such as fatty or sugary foods or from alcohol. Energy intakes may be so low in many elderly people that it becomes difficult to obtain good intake of the other nutrients without substantial alterations in the nature of the diet. Elderly people, or those responsible for providing meals for the elderly, were advised in COMA (1992) to ensure that their diet is of high nutrient density so that adequate intakes of the other nutrients can be maintained despite a considerable decline in total food intake.

COMA (1992) also suggested that the intake of sugars in the elderly tend to be towards the top end of the UK range (i.e. 10–20 per cent of total energy) although this is not borne out by survey data discussed in the next section (see Table 15.16 later). The panel concluded that the general dietary guidelines suggesting limiting non-milk extrinsic sugars to 10 per cent of energy might be especially appropriate for older people to ensure a high nutrient density of their diets.

Key points

- Energy requirements fall in the elderly due to the combined effects of reduced activity and lower BMR.
- In elderly immobile people, energy expenditure may be as low as 1.3 times BMR.
- There is no fall in the estimated requirement for most nutrients to compensate for the fall in energy needs and food intake.
- The iron needs of elderly women are reduced substantially because menstruation has ceased.
- Elderly housebound people are unlikely to obtain sufficient vitamin D from their diet and should either take supplements or ensure exposure to summer sunlight.
- Very low energy requirements mean that the nutrient density of the diet needs to be good.
- The need for some nutrients probably increases in the elderly, e.g. due to reduced absorption and this is reflected in the recent substantial increase in vitamin B_6 and calcium standards for older people in the USA.

Diets and nutritional status of elderly people

Longitudinal studies of the food intakes of groups of elderly people in the UK and in Sweden indicate that the average energy intakes of elderly people do indeed fall as they get older (see COMA, 1992). Gregory et al. (1990) in a survey of 16–64-year-old British adults found a distinct trend towards decreasing energy intakes in the older age groups. The average intake of men aged 50–64 years was 5 per cent less than that of those aged 35–49 years (7 per cent less in women); however, the more recent repeat of this survey showed a much smaller drop between the 35–49 years and 50–64 years age bands (Hoare et al., 2004). Hoare et al. (2004) also found that the lowest recorded energy intakes were in men aged 19–24 years and women aged 25–34 years and the average recorded intake of women aged 50–64 years was actually slightly higher than the average for all women (19–64 years) recorded in this survey. A Danish cross-sectional study of 1000 men and 1000 women in 1982–84 found a marked decline in energy intakes across the age range 30–85 years. The average intake of 85 year olds was only 72 per cent of that of 30 years olds in men and 79 per cent in women (see Schroll et al., 1993).

A survey of 750 elderly people living in the UK in the late 1960s (Department of Health and Social Security (DHSS), 1972) indicated that only around 3 per cent of the surveyed population were malnourished and that in the great majority of cases malnutrition was associated with some precipitating medical condition. Around half of this population were re-assessed in 1972, by which time they were all aged over 70 years (DHSS, 1979). In this second survey the prevalence of malnutrition was found to be around 7 per cent but twice as high as this in the over 80s. Once again, most of the nutritional deficiencies were related to some underlying disease, certain social factors were also identified as being associated with the risk of malnutrition in the elderly, e.g. being housebound and having a low income. According to this survey the diets of elderly British people were in their general nature very similar to those of other adults.

The general impression created by the results of this survey were that if elderly people have good general health, are reasonably mobile and affluent then they tend to have few specific nutritional problems. However, as people get older they are more likely have a number of medical conditions that may precipitate nutritional problems. The elderly are also more likely to be affected by a range of social factors associated with higher risk of nutritional inadequacies, such as:

- immobility and being housebound
- social isolation
- recent bereavement and depression
- low income
- living alone
- low social class
- low mental test score.

Finch et al. (1998) conducted a dietary and nutritional survey of a representative sample of British people aged over 65 years that included both free-living elderly people and those living in care accommodation. Table 15.15 shows the average energy intakes recorded in this survey for various age groups of men and women living independently and living in care accommodation and shows for comparison that recorded in the slightly more recent survey of adults aged 19–64 years. For the elderly people who are living independently, energy intakes are significantly lower than those of younger adults and drop progressively with age in both sexes. The average intakes of those living in care accommodation are significantly higher than those of similar age living independently and in women the average for those aged 65–84 years and living in care accommodation is actually higher than that for all other categories including those aged 19–64 years. These latter figures may indicate that perhaps problems with obtaining or preparing food depress the intakes of very elderly free-living people and that they would eat more if it was easily available to them.

Table 15.15 Average recorded energy intakes (MJ) for different age groups of British adults*

Age group (years)	Free living		Institutionalized	
	Men	Women	Men	Women
19–64	9.72	6.87		
65–74	8.21	6.07		
75–84	7.75	5.88		
65–84			7.99	6.77
85+	7.20	5.77	8.22	7.14

*Data for 16–64 years from Hoare et al. (2004) and that for older adults from Finch et al. (1998).

Table 15.16 compares the sources of energy for free-living elderly adults recorded in this survey of Finch et al. (1998) with the most recent survey of adults aged 16–64 years (Hoare et al., 2004). In terms of macronutrient composition, the diets of elderly people are quite similar to those recorded for younger adults except that the alcohol intakes were notably lower in the older people. In Chapter 6 it was noted that over the period 1986/7–2000/2 there had been substantial changes in the macronutrient composition of the diets of adults aged 16–64 years towards

Table 15.16 A comparison of the macronutrient and food sources of energy recorded in samples of British adults aged 16–64 years (Hoare *et al.*, 2004) and free living adults aged over 65 years (Finch *et al.*, 1998).

	Percentage contribution to total energy intake	
	16–64 years	65+ years
Protein	15.8	15.9
Fat	33.5	35.0
Carbohydrate	45.7	46.7
Alcohol	5.2	2.4
Non-milk extrinsic sugars	13.7	12.7
Saturated fatty acids	13.3	14.7
Cereal foods	31	34
Milk and milk products	10	13
Meat, fish, eggs	21	20
Fruit and vegetables (including potatoes)	16	13
Fats and sugars (including drinks and confectionery)	21	17

the reference values suggested in COMA (1991). If similar time trends are affecting the diets of older people then the macronutrient breakdown of older adults' diets may well be as good as or better than those of younger adults in terms of these goals. Table 15.16 also shows that the elderly sample obtained less of their energy from drinks, sugar, confectionery and vegetables but more from cereals and milk; so despite the suggestion of COMA (1992) that elderly people may be heavy sugar users they in fact seem to use less sugar than younger adults.

About two-thirds of the free-living sample and just under half of the institutional sample were overweight or obese (BMI >25 kg/m²). About 16 per cent of the institution sample were underweight (BMI <20 kg/m²) as were 3 per cent of the free-living men and 6 per cent of the women. The proportions of those who were overweight and those who were obese declined markedly with age in both sexes and in the free-living sample and for women also in the institutionalized sample; for institutionalized men the proportion who were overweight increased between the two age bands but the proportion who were obese decreased. The implications of being overweight and underweight for elderly people are discussed in the next section.

Finch *et al.* (1998) generally found that the average intakes of most major vitamins and minerals were above or close to the RNI and in many cases well above it. Despite this the average intakes for most micronutrients recorded for elderly people were less than those recorded for younger adults although the vitamin A and D intakes of the older adults were exceptions and were higher than the averages recorded in the latest NDNS survey of younger adults (Hoare *et al.*, 2004). In only a few cases did more than 5 per cent of the sample record intakes that were below the LRNI, namely:

- the riboflavin intakes of those living independently
- the calcium intakes of men (5 per cent) and women (9 per cent) living independently
- the iron intakes of all women and institutionalized men (5–6 per cent)
- magnesium and potassium intakes in around a quarter of the total sample
- zinc intakes in 8 per cent of independent men (5 per cent women) and 13 per cent of institutionalized men (4 per cent women).

Despite recording lower average intakes of most nutrients than younger adults, the percentages with inadequate intakes were generally low although if this sample is truly representative, this does represent very large numbers of older individuals. Biochemical status was also measured for several nutrients and the following areas of concern were highlighted by this part of the survey.

- about 10 per cent of the total sample had serum ferritin levels that were indicative of poor iron status
- about 8 per cent of the free-living sample and 37 per cent of those living in institutions had biochemical indications of poor vitamin D status. Vitamin D intakes were only around a third of the RNI but it is difficult to achieve this RNI without the use of supplements. This reinforces the recommendation of COMA (1992) that elderly people should either get regular exposure to summer sunlight or take vitamin D supplements
- about 40 per cent of the total sample had biochemical indications of low riboflavin status although as noted in Chapter 12 this may reflect the high sensitivity of this test
- 40 per cent of the institutionalized sample had low biochemical status for folate and around 30 per cent of the independent sample

- 14 per cent of the independent sample had low biochemical status for vitamin C and around 40 per cent of the institutionalized sample
- low biochemical status for thiamin was found in 10–15 per cent of all groups
- 15 per cent of men and 7 per cent of women in institutions had biochemical indications of zinc deficiency.

The percentage of those recording poor biochemical status looks high despite the high average intakes and the generally small numbers of individuals recording inadequate intakes. This may well add weight to the case that the requirement for some nutrients increases in the elderly.

Key points

- Recorded energy intakes decline with age in middle-aged and elderly people.

- Only a few per cent of elderly Britons in the 1960s and 1970s were found to be malnourished but the prevalence did rise with age and more recent studies suggest that about 16 per cent of elderly people living in care accommodation are underweight.

- Nutritional inadequacy in elderly people is often precipitated by some illness or is associated with adverse social circumstances.

- Elderly British people who were mobile, in good health and reasonably affluent had few specific nutritional problems and had diets that were in their general character similar to those of other Britons.

- Table 15.16 shows a comparison of the dietary energy sources of elderly and other British adults as determined by separate surveys using weighed inventory.

- Around 10 per cent of elderly Britons show biochemical indications of iron and zinc deficiency.

- Many elderly people living in care accommodation show evidence of vitamin D deficiency.

- The relatively high numbers of elderly people showing biochemical indications of micronutrient inadequacy are higher than might be expected from the dietary data and suggest that requirements for some nutrients do increase with age.

Diet and disease risk in the elderly

There is an age-related deterioration in the immune system especially in cell-mediated immunity. Malnutrition has similar deleterious effects on the immune system (see Chapter 16). Malnutrition could compound with the effects of ageing in depressing the immune function of elderly, malnourished people. Indicators of nutritional deficiency have been found to be associated with reduced responses in immune function tests in disease-free, elderly people. Nutritional supplements given to these elderly subjects were associated with improvements in both the measures of nutritional status and the measures of immunocompetence (Chandra, 1985). Chandra (1992) randomly assigned free-living elderly people to receive either a micronutrient supplement or a placebo. After a year, several measures of immune function were higher in the supplemented group than in the controls and the supplemented group had fewer than half the number of days affected by infective illness as the controls. Woo et al. (1994) showed that nutritional supplements given to elderly people recovering from chest infections were effective in helping them to recover from their illness. More recently, Chandra (2004) has reviewed the effects of nutrient supplements on immune function in older people and concluded that multinutrient supplements are likely to enhance their immune responses and reduce the occurrence of common infections.

Mowe et al. (1994) assessed the diets and nutritional status of a large sample of elderly people admitted to hospitals in the Oslo area for an acute cause such as a stroke or myocardial infarction. They compared these results with those obtained from a matched sample of well elderly people living within the same area. They concluded that there were several indicators that suggested that the food and nutrient intake of the hospitalized group had been inferior to that of the well group in the 3 months prior to admission. They raised the possibility that poor food and nutrient intake might be a contributory factor in the acute illnesses that led to hospitalization.

In the Allied Dunbar National Fitness Survey (1992) ageing was associated with a substantial decline in aerobic fitness, muscle strength and flexibility. Only a relatively minor proportion of this decline seems to be due to age per se and much of it represents a form of disuse atrophy. The average aerobic fitness of the top 10 per cent of men aged 65–74 years was higher than the average of the bottom 10 per cent of men aged 25–34 years. The report's authors concluded that 'much functional disability among older people could be reversed or avoided through continued regular exercise as people grow older'. Fiatarone *et al.* (1994) found that resistance training led to significant increases in muscle strength, walking speed, stair climbing power and spontaneous physical activity even in very elderly nursing home residents (mean age 87 years).

Maintenance of a reasonable level of physical activity would seem to be strongly advisable for the elderly as a complement to sound nutrition in maximizing good health and quality of life. In addition to the general beneficial effects on the cardiovascular system, increased activity will maintain energy expenditure and help to maintain lean body mass in the elderly. Exercise and improved fitness, strength and flexibility will help elderly people to continue with the everyday activities that are essential to independent living. The general benefits of regular exercise and physical fitness are reviewed in Chapter 16. These benefits are maintained and perhaps even greater in older people.

Overweight and obesity are generally associated with excess morbidity and reduced life expectancy (see Chapter 8). However, this conclusion is less secure in older people. Lehmann (1991), in a review of nutrition in old age concluded that underweight is a more important indicator of increased mortality and morbidity risk than is obesity She suggested that, in the elderly, being moderately overweight is not associated with any excess mortality risk whereas underweight is associated with the following adverse outcomes:

- increased mortality
- increased risk of hip fracture
- increased risk of infections
- increased risk-specific nutrient deficiencies.

Being underweight and having low reserves of energy and nutrients may leave elderly people less able to survive periods of illness or injury. The combined effects of low body weight, reduced lean tissue to fat ratio and extreme inactivity may also reduce the maintenance energy requirements of these elderly individuals substantially and threaten their ability to obtain adequate intakes of the other essential nutrients.

At least in the short term, low body weight rather than high body weight may be the better predictor of mortality in the elderly; two studies, described below, illustrate this point.

- Campbell *et al.* (1990) found that anthropometric indicators of low body weight, low body fat and low muscle bulk were associated with an increased risk of death in the 4 years following measurement in those aged over 70 years. In contrast, those with a high BMI had no increased risk of death over this period.
- Mattila *et al.* (1986) found that in Finns aged over 85 years, there was a progressive increase in the 5-year survival rate as BMI increased.

An expert working party in the UK (COMA, 1992) recommended that there should be more research on the prognostic significance of BMI in the elderly. The group reviewed data from a 10-year cohort study of elderly people (65–74 years) which found that the relationship between mortality and BMI was U-shaped with a tendency for mortality to rise at the extremes of the range, i.e. at very low or very high BMI. More recent data have supported these earlier indications of an inverse relationship between BMI and mortality in older people as opposed to the positive relationship seen in younger adults and particularly in younger men (see Chapter 8). For example, Inoue *et al.* (2006) found that in a group of 370 Japanese elderly people, mortality in those with low BMI was twice that in the normal category and that there were no deaths in the high BMI category during the 5 years of follow-up. Similarly Janssen *et al.* (2005) found that after controlling for waist circumference, mortality risk decreased by 21 per cent for every standard deviation increase in BMI in a sample of 5200 men and women aged over 65 years. When waist circumference was corrected for BMI, this was associated with higher mortality risk, i.e. having a little bit of extra weight is associated with lower mortality but at any given BMI, high waist circumference was associated with higher mortality. Large stores of abdominal fat seem to have similar negative health associations to those in younger adults as discussed in Chapter 8.

The general dietary guidelines reviewed in Chapter 4 are still regarded as being appropriate for the bulk of elderly people. Despite this, the nutritional priorities for older people are different to those of younger adults. Dietary adequacy assumes a greater priority in the face of declining energy intakes. In those elderly people suffering weight loss, loss of taste perception and reduced ability to chew, maintaining high palatability and good food intake may be more important than conforming to current nutritional education guidelines. These guidelines are intended to reduce the long-term risk of degenerative diseases. It seems inevitable that, even if these preventive benefits still occur in the elderly, they are likely to be reduced. The application of several of these guidelines to the elderly is reviewed below.

- The association between increased serum cholesterol concentration and increased risk of coronary heart disease has in the past often been assumed to be less convincing in elderly people than in young and middle-aged adults. According to COMA (1992), more recent data from both the USA and the UK indicated that the predictive value of a raised serum cholesterol for increased coronary heart disease risk is maintained in later years and thus that the general cholesterol-lowering guidelines should also apply to the elderly. Table 15.16 indicates that elderly peoples' diets are close to the guideline values for fat but that the proportion of energy from saturated fat is still well above the target value of 10 per cent of total energy. Given the time trends for younger adults noted in Chapter 11, it is quite probable that in the decade since the data of Finch et al. (1998) was collected there may have been significant declines in both the fat and saturated fatty acid composition of elderly Britons' diets. Recent studies do suggest that cholesterol-lowering is effective in reducing both fatal and non-fatal heart attacks in older people. For example, Shepherd (2004) reviews the results of the PROspective Study of Pravastatin in the Elderly at Risk (PROSPER) study and this showed that this cholesterol-lowering drug (one of the statins discussed in Chapter 11) markedly improved blood lipoprotein profiles, reduced deaths from coronary heart disease and non-fatal heart attacks and strokes. Although this was a drug trial it does confirm that, as with younger people, effective management of high blood lipid levels is effective in reducing heart disease in elderly at-risk people. In a review of the treatment of high blood lipids in the elderly, Pohlel et al. (2006) concluded that modern lipid-lowering strategies have been shown to prevent or delay the progression of diseases associated with abnormal blood lipid profiles such as cardiovascular disease and cerebrovascular disease.

- Increased intakes of non-starch polysaccharides (fibre) are likely to reduce constipation and beneficially affect existing minor bowel problems such as haemorrhoids. Increased activity and prevention of dehydration would also improve bowel function. Dehydration is common among elderly people because of: reduced acuity of the thirst mechanism; reduced ability to concentrate urine; and physical problems with getting drinks or even voluntary suppression of fluid intake because of fears of incontinence or difficulties in using the toilet. Dehydration is also a cause of confusion in the elderly. Elderly people are advised to drink the equivalent of 6–8 glasses of water per day and those charged with care of the elderly should make sure that immobile patients are regularly offered palatable drinks.

- Hypertension is very prevalent among the elderly population (see Chapter 14) and COMA (1992) recommended that an average intake of 6 g/day of salt was a reasonable target for elderly people as well as other adults.

- COMA (1992) recommended that the targets for non-milk extrinsic sugars for elderly people should be the same as for the rest of the population. Moderating the intake of added sugar should help to ensure a high nutrient density of the diet. The majority of elderly people now still have some natural teeth and so the effects of sugars on the teeth and gums are still relevant to older people. According to Finch et al. (1998), the sugar intake of elderly people is fairly close to current guidelines and these results are at variance with the expectations of COMA (1992), which assumed that the sugar intakes of elderly people tended to be towards the top of the UK range.

- Like the rest of the population, elderly people are advised to eat more fruit and vegetables (five portions per day). This should increase intake of many vitamins, antioxidants, non-starch polysaccharide and some minerals including potassium.

Key points

- Immune function deteriorates with age and is also depressed by malnutrition.
- Nutrient supplements can improve immune function in some elderly people and malnutrition may contribute to the decline in immune function with age.
- Aerobic fitness, strength and flexibility all decline sharply with age in Britain, largely because of decreased activity rather than as an inevitable consequence of ageing.
- Resistance training can increase strength and performance even in people in their 80s and 90s.
- Increased activity and fitness in elderly people would increase life expectancy and improve the quality of life in the later years and so enable more elderly people to remain independent for longer.
- Underweight is a much more important indicator of mortality risk in the elderly than is overweight or obesity.
- Overweight elderly and very elderly people tend to have reduced mortality risk in the subsequent few years.
- A high waist circumference remains a positive indicator of mortality risk in the elderly,

confirming that the negative health implications of large abdominal stores of fat remain in the elderly.
- Maintaining dietary adequacy becomes an increasingly important goal as people become elderly and very elderly.
- The dietary guidelines for other adults are still generally appropriate for elderly people provided that they do not compromise dietary adequacy, i.e. lower intakes of fat, saturated fat, added sugar and salt but more non-starch polysaccharide, starch and fruits and vegetables.
- Studies with statins confirm that effective management of hyperlipidaemia yields considerable benefits even in old age.
- Dehydration is common in the elderly and it causes confusion and constipation; the equivalent of six to eight glasses of water per day is recommended for elderly people.
- Good intakes of non-starch polysaccharide, increased activity and ample fluid intakes should all contribute to improved bowel function in the elderly.

16

Nutrition as treatment

DIET AS A COMPLETE THERAPY

Overview and general principles

There are a small number of diseases or conditions where dietary change can be an effective and complete therapy. In many such diseases the patient is intolerant of a specific nutrient or component of food. **Food intolerance** has been defined as 'a reproducible, unpleasant (i.e. adverse) reaction to a specific food or ingredient, which is not psychologically based'. Where there is 'evidence of an abnormal immunological reaction to the food' then this is termed a **food allergy** (Mitchell, 1988).

The therapeutic principles in cases of food intolerance are simple.

- To identify the nutrient or foodstuff to which the patient is intolerant. In practice, it may prove difficult to pinpoint the food or foods causing the symptoms or even to establish with certainty that the symptoms are really due to food intolerance
- To devise a dietary regimen that provides a healthful and acceptable diet while either keeping intakes of the problem nutrient within tolerable limits or completely excluding the offending foodstuff. This may be difficult if the offending food is a staple food and an ingredient of many foods or dishes, e.g. flour, egg or milk. It may also be difficult if a person is intolerant to excessive amounts of an essential nutrient found in many foods, e.g. an essential amino acid such as phenylalanine.

These problems will be illustrated in the following sections which use food allergies (including **coeliac disease**) and **phenylketonuria** (**PKU**) as examples of the dietary management of food intolerances.

In addition to diseases where exclusion is the primary dietetic aim there are a few diseases that are not of primary dietary origin but can be alleviated by nutrient supplements. **Pernicious anaemia** is probably the best known example; autoimmune destruction of the parietal cells of the stomach results in a failure of vitamin B_{12} absorption. Most of the symptoms of this potentially fatal disease can be alleviated by regular injections of B_{12}. **Hartnup disease** is a rare but fatal inherited disorder with symptoms that resemble those of pellagra (niacin deficiency). The symptoms of this disease result from a failure to absorb the amino acid tryptophan (the precursor of niacin) which leads to niacin deficiency. The condition responds to niacin treatment, which reduces the dermatitis and neurological consequences of pellagra. If plenty of protein is given, tryptophan may be absorbed in di- and tripeptides.

L-Carnitine is an important cellular metabolite that does not qualify as an essential nutrient because it is normally synthesized in the body from the amino acid lysine. There are several relatively rare hereditary disorders that respond to therapy with pharmacological doses of L-carnitine, e.g. a defect in the enzyme that normally transfers carnitine across the plasma membrane and some disorders of fatty acid metabolism. There is a short discussion of L-carnitine in Chapter 12 under the heading of conditionally essential nutrients.

> ### Key points
>
> - There are a few conditions where diet can be an effective and complete therapy, and this often involves restricting the intake of a food or ingredient to which the person is intolerant.

- A few conditions, like pernicious anaemia, respond well to nutrient supplements.
- Food intolerance is an adverse reaction to a food or component that is not psychological; if there is involvement of the immune system, this is termed a food allergy.
- It may be difficult to pinpoint the precise cause of a food allergy or other intolerance.
- If someone is intolerant to a staple food or an essential nutrient then it may be difficult to devise a diet that will alleviate the symptoms and also be adequate and acceptable.

Food allergy (including coeliac disease)

Immediate hypersensitivity reactions

Most food allergies are **immediate hypersensitivity reactions** that are mediated by a class of antibodies or immunoglobulins known as **immunoglobulin E (IgE)**. In this type of reaction, symptoms begin within a few minutes of ingesting the food to which the person is allergic. The symptoms vary from case to case but can include one or more of the following:

- gastro-intestinal symptoms like abdominal pain, diarrhoea and vomiting
- eczema or urticaria (hives)
- asthmatic symptoms and laryngeal swelling
- allergic rhinitis (runny nose) and itchy, watering eyes.

In rare cases, the symptoms may be severe enough to be life-threatening, e.g. anaphylactic shock, which is widespread blood vessel dilation resulting in a fall in blood pressure and circulatory collapse.

Exposure to the allergen which is usually a food protein, e.g. in cow's milk, eggs, peanuts, tree nuts or shellfish, results in production of IgE antibodies which bind to and sensitize tissue mast cells and their circulating form, the basophils. Once a person is sensitized, then during subsequent exposures, the allergen binds to the antibodies on the mast cells causing them to release histamine and other chemical mediators that bring about the allergic symptoms.

Many people believe that they or their children are allergic to particular foods but many of these client diagnoses are inaccurate or involve too many foods. A first step towards a firm diagnosis is for patients to keep a food diary where they record everything they eat and drink and also record the severity of their allergic symptoms or the occurrence of allergic episodes. This should give an indication of likely allergens. For chronic symptoms such as dermatitis, the suspected food can be withdrawn to see if this leads to gradual easing of symptoms which, provided they are no too severe, can be re-provoked by re-introduction of the food. Provided that the symptoms are not too severe then the most reliable way of establishing an allergy to a particular food is to use a **blind challenge** or a double blind, placebo-controlled food challenge which is analogous to double-blind clinical trials discussed in Chapter 3. Neither the patient nor the clinician knows which is the real and placebo challenge until after the trial is completed. Some patients will respond to the placebo, which suggests that the symptoms may be psychological.

Skin prick tests are now widely used to identify causes of food allergy; small amounts of potential allergens are injected into the skin and the extent of any inflammatory skin reaction is then used to assess sensitivity. A positive skin test does not automatically mean that a person will have an allergic reaction to that substance when it is given by mouth although a negative response means that the substance is an unlikely cause of allergic symptoms. Skin prick tests are useful in confirming a suspected allergy and in deciding which foods might need to be considered in challenge tests. The radioallergosorbent test (RAST) is a more expensive alternative to skin prick tests; it assesses the amount of specific IgE present in a patient's blood. The patient's serum is reacted with allergen, which is adsorbed onto a solid paper matrix, and the specific IgE in the serum will compete with added radioactive IgE for binding to this antigen. The more specific IgE there is in the patient's blood the less radioactivity will remain on the paper.

Food allergies affect perhaps 3–4 per cent of the population, with shellfish being the most common sensitivity in adults. Rates of food allergies are higher in young children, perhaps double that for the population as a whole, but many of them grow out of these allergies and are able to tolerate the food later in childhood. The most common sensitivity in young children is to eggs, followed by cow milk and peanuts.

The main treatment is dietary avoidance of the offending substance although drugs such as antihistamines can alleviate the symptoms of the allergy.

Coeliac disease (gluten-induced enteropathy)

Coeliac disease results from a hypersensitivity or allergy to the gliadin component of the wheat protein, **gluten** and similar proteins are found in barley, rye and some other less well known cereals. Oats do not cause symptoms unless they have been contaminated with wheat. The disease is sometimes termed **gluten-sensitive enteropathy**. The disease is classified as a food allergy because it involves an 'abnormal immunological response to food' but it differs from classical allergy, e.g. hay fever, and does not involve production of IgE antibodies. It is an example of the other type of food allergy in which symptoms do not develop until some hours after the ingestion of the offending food and may not reach their peak until 48 hours or more after ingestion. This is known as **delayed-type hypersensitivity (DTH)**. Exposure to the allergen leads to sensitization of T cell lymphocytes and after sensitization re-exposure to the antigen causes the sensitized T cells to release inflammatory mediators and cause a localized inflammatory response. Patients with coeliac disease are also more likely to have other autoimmune diseases such as type 1 diabetes, thyroiditis, pernicious anaemia and the chronic skin condition dermatitis herpetiformis.

In people with untreated coeliac disease, the villi of the small intestine atrophy and there is excessive secretion of mucus. Diagnosis is confirmed by a biopsy of the jejunal mucosa using an endoscope. These changes in the small intestine result in severe malabsorption of fat and other nutrients leading to: fatty diarrhoea, distended abdomen, weight loss or growth failure, and other symptoms that are the result of nutrients deficiencies such as anaemia, rickets/osteomalacia and bleeding due to vitamin K deficiency. In the long term, there may be cancerous changes in the intestine induced by continued exposure to gluten-type proteins leading to small bowel lymphoma. Some patients diagnosed with this condition can tolerate some dietary gluten without overt symptoms but this may increase their later risk of small bowel lymphoma.

The aim of dietary management in coeliac disease is to avoid all gluten-containing foods and foods that contain the similar rye and barley proteins. The achievement of this goal is complicated because bread and cereals are not only staple dietary items but flour is also an ingredient of many prepared foods. Gluten-free flour and bread are available on prescription in the UK and gluten-free cakes and biscuits (cookies) are commercially available. Many food manufacturers use a 'crossed grain' symbol to indicate that a particular product is free of gluten. Debenham (1992) has reviewed the practical aspects of the dietary management of coeliac disease.

The symptoms of coeliac disease may present in early childhood or in adulthood. It has been suggested that increased use of rice-based weaning foods and thus delayed exposure to wheat has caused a delay in the onset of the disease with more adult and less childhood presentations.

Key points

- Most food allergies are mediated by IgE antibodies and are immediate hypersensitivities where symptoms appear within minutes of exposure.
- A double-blind, placebo-controlled food challenge is the most reliable method of diagnosis unless the severity of the symptoms prevent its use.
- Skin prick tests can be useful in identifying or confirming suspected allergies.
- The presence of specific IgE antibodies to suspected allergens in a patient's blood can be measured using the *in vitro* radioallergoabsorbent test (RAST).
- Perhaps 3–4 per cent of the population have IgE mediated immediate hypersensitivities to food with maybe double this frequency in young children who may grow out of their allergies.
- Shellfish is the most common sensitivity in adults whereas egg, cow milk and peanuts, in that order, are the most common in young children.
- Coeliac disease is an example of delayed-type hypersensitivity (DTH) where symptoms appear some hours after ingestion of the food.
- Sensitized T cells release inflammatory mediators when exposed to the antigen and cause local inflammation.
- Coeliac disease is a hypersensitivity to the wheat protein gluten and similar proteins in barley and rye.
- Gluten causes atrophy of the villi in the small intestine, which leads to diarrhoea, malabsorption, and a variety of abdominal symptoms.

- If untreated, the condition leads to growth failure, weight loss, a range of nutritional deficiencies and may eventually result in cancerous changes in the small bowel.
- The treatment is to exclude from the diet the wheat, barley and rye that contain the gluten-like proteins.
- Dietary compliance is made difficult by the widespread use of wheat flour in manufactured foods.
- Rice, maize and uncontaminated oats do not contain gluten and a range of gluten-free wheat products are available, some of them on prescription in the UK.

Phenylketonuria

Phenylketonuria (PKU) is an inherited disease which affects around 1:10 000 babies in the UK. Since the 1960s, all babies born in the UK have been tested for this condition within the first 2 weeks of life. The blood phenylalanine concentration is measured using the Guthrie test. Classical PKU is caused by a genetic defect in the enzyme phenylalanine hydroxylase that converts the essential amino acid phenylalanine to tyrosine.

$$\text{Phenylalanine} \xrightarrow{\text{phenylalanine hydroxylase}} \text{tyrosine}$$

Normally, excess phenylalanine, either from the diet or from endogenous protein breakdown, is metabolized via its conversion to tyrosine. In normal adults 90 per cent of the phenylalanine consumed is converted to tyrosine and only about 10 per cent is used for protein synthesis. In PKU, this route is blocked and so excess phenylalanine and unusual metabolites of phenylalanine accumulate in the blood where they seriously impair mental development. In PKU, tyrosine becomes an essential amino acid and some of the symptoms of PKU are probably associated with tyrosine deficiency. Untreated children have severe learning disabilities and are prone to epilepsy, but they grow normally and have a normal life expectancy.

The objective of dietary management in PKU is to restrict phenylalanine intake so that mental development is not impaired but to provide enough of this essential amino acid and all other nutrients to allow growth and physical development. In particular, adequate amounts of tyrosine must be provided. These objectives cannot be achieved with normal foods because all foods with good amounts of protein and tyrosine also contain high levels of phenylalanine. The tolerance to phenylalanine depends on the precise nature of the biochemical lesion and varies from child to child. The amount of phenylalanine that the child can consume while keeping their blood levels within the acceptable range for their age is first determined. The phenylalanine allowance that has been defined in this way, is taken in the form of normal foods, usually milk, cereals and potatoes. Meat, fish, eggs, cheese and pulses will be totally excluded and only sugars, fats, fruits and non-leguminous vegetables can be eaten relatively freely and even for these there will be some restrictions. The resultant diet is, by design, very low in protein and tyrosine and it is likely to provide inadequate amounts of energy. Children are therefore given medical supplements that provide amino acids, energy and other nutrients such as vitamin B_{12} that are likely to be deficient. Infant formulae that are low in phenylalanine are available prior to weaning.

The prognosis for children with PKU depends on how strictly the dietary regimen is followed but even in families where control is poor the children should still be educable. Prior to the 1960s, and the introduction of universal screening, most PKU children would have been very severely impaired (the average IQ of untreated PKU patients is about 50) and many would have spent much of their lives in institutions for the mentally handicapped. Children whose blood phenylalanine levels have been well controlled have normal IQs at 9 years (see Elsas and Acosta, 2006). Current consensus suggests that some dietary regulation needs to be maintained throughout life. Neurological changes occur in adults with PKU when their blood phenylalanine concentration is allowed to rise and these symptoms are reversed by re-introduction of a low phenylalanine diet. Special care needs to be taken over the diet of women with PKU intending to become pregnant because the developing fetus is vulnerable to high phenylalanine levels. Babies of women with uncontrolled PKU often have congenital defects that are incompatible with life and those that do survive fail to grow and develop normally. The dietary management of PKU and other inborn errors of metabolism has been reviewed by Elsas and Acosta (2006).

Key points

- Phenylketonuria (PKU) is caused by inherited defects in the enzyme phenylalanine hydroxylase.
- This leads to accumulation of phenylalanine and its metabolites which impair brain development and tyrosine becomes an essential nutrient.
- Management involves severe dietary restrictions and extensive use of medicinal dietary supplements.
- If phenylalanine levels are tightly controlled then children can develop with normal IQs.
- Pregnant women with PKU must control their phenylalanine levels to permit normal fetal development.

DIET AS A SPECIFIC COMPONENT OF THERAPY

There are many conditions in which diet does not give complete relief from symptoms, nor is it the sole treatment, but for which there is an apparently sound theoretical and empirical basis indicating a specific role for a particular dietary regimen in its management. Three examples, **diabetes mellitus**, **cystic fibrosis** and **chronic renal failure** are briefly overviewed.

Diabetes mellitus

Classification and aetiology

Diet has long been regarded as a key element of the treatment of diabetes. Diabetes mellitus results from insufficient production of the pancreatic hormone **insulin**. In the severe **type 1 diabetes**, which usually develops during childhood, there is destruction of the insulin-producing cells in the pancreas and this results in an almost total failure of insulin supply. It is envisaged that some environmental factor such as a viral infection triggers the autoimmune destruction of the cells in the pancreas that produce insulin, the β-cells in the islets of Langerhans. This type of diabetes accounts for around 10–15 per cent of all cases of diabetes. Type 1 diabetes is always treated by a combination of diet and insulin injections. Patients cannot survive long without insulin therapy and before insulin therapy was available they usually died within a few weeks of diagnosis.

In the much more common and milder **type 2 diabetes** there is no primary failure of insulin supply or any obvious β-cell pathology. The primary defect in this case is reduced target tissue sensitivity to insulin and this results in compensatory increases in insulin production. In genetically susceptible people there is an inadequate compensatory increase in insulin production resulting in a progressive shortfall of insulin and gradually increasing symptoms of diabetes. In Chapter 8 it was noted that high insulin production caused by insulin resistance leads to increases in several cardiovascular disease risk factors and to increased risk of heart disease even in the absence of overt diabetes. This insulin resistance was referred to as the **metabolic syndrome or syndrome X** and many of these individuals will go on to become diabetic. Insulin sensitivity decreases as body fat content increases and excessive weight gain is the most important trigger for the onset of type 2 diabetes in those who are genetically susceptible to it (see Chapter 8). Excessive weight gain is particularly detrimental if it associated with a high waist circumference because adipose tissue within the abdominal cavity has less sensitivity to insulin than that stored subcutaneously. A high-fat, low-fibre diet and inactivity are other important lifestyle characteristics that decrease insulin sensitivity and predispose to this type of diabetes.

Type 2 diabetes is usually treated either by diet alone or by a combination of diet and oral hypoglycaemic drugs. Insulin injections may be used to improve the management of this type of diabetes, particularly in those who have had the condition for some time. Around 5 per cent of the UK population aged over 65 years are diagnosed as having diabetes, but there may be an equal number who are undiagnosed and untreated but still at risk of the long-term complications of diabetes. The risk of this form of diabetes increases with age and so the number of people with diabetes will continue to increase as the numbers of very elderly people in the population continue to rise and also as the prevalence of obesity continues to rise. Until recently, type 2 diabetes was almost exclusively confined to adults aged 40 years or more, but cases now occur with increasing regularity in younger adults and even in children because of the increased prevalence of obesity in younger people.

Diagnosis

The normal fasting blood glucose concentration of a healthy young adult is 4–5 mmol/L and this will rise to just over 7 mmol/L in the period after a carbohydrate meal and return to the fasting level an hour or so after absorption is complete. All people with diabetes have an elevated blood glucose concentration and this is the basis for diagnosis. Traditionally, diagnosis was confirmed by a glucose tolerance test; the fasting subject was giving a 75 g oral load of glucose and blood glucose concentration monitored over the subsequent 2 hours. This is less often used nowadays and diagnosis is often made on the basis of clinical symptoms and a simple elevated blood glucose measurement. The following criteria are indicative of diabetes:

- clinical symptoms plus a casual plasma glucose concentration of 11.1 mmol/L or more
- a fasting (8-hour) plasma glucose concentration of over 7.0 mmol/L or a whole blood concentration of 6.1 mmol/L
- a 2-hour plasma glucose concentration of 11.1 mmol/L or more during an oral glucose tolerance test.

A single measurement of hyperglycaemia without clinical symptoms of diabetes would need a repeat test to confirm the diagnosis of diabetes. People with a fasting plasma glucose concentration of 6.1–7.0 mmol/L would be classified as having impaired glucose tolerance and half of these will become overtly diabetic within 10 years.

Symptoms and long-term complications

As a consequence of their high blood glucose concentration diabetics of both types excrete glucose in their urine. This is because glucose is freely filtered in the renal tubule and as blood glucose rises so the amount filtered exceeds the capacity of the re-absorption system in the proximal part of the renal tubule and the excess spills into the urine. This glucose in the urine acts as an osmotic diuretic and causes increased water loss, increased thirst and propensity to dehydration. The blood glucose concentration in an untreated diabetic may reach 10 times the normal fasting value and hundreds of grams of glucose may be lost in the urine each day. In untreated type 1 diabetes there are other severe and even life-threatening symptoms (see below):

- rapid weight loss (weight loss also occurs in type 2 and so tends to obscure the strength of the association between obesity and diabetes)
- very high blood glucose concentration and severe dehydration

- excessive production and excretion of ketone bodies leading to acidosis, electrolyte imbalance and eventually to coma and death.

The symptoms of the disease suggest that the diabetic is carbohydrate intolerant and so severe restriction of dietary carbohydrate and almost total exclusion of dietary sugar were the rule for diabetic diets for most of the twentieth century. Prior to 1975 most diabetic diets would have contained no more than 40 per cent of the calories as carbohydrates and often much less than this. These low-carbohydrate diets were inevitably high in fat. According to Leeds (1979), when insulin treatment was first used in the 1920s, diabetic diets typically contained less than 10 per cent of calories as carbohydrate and more than 70 per cent as fat. People with diabetes in Western countries have traditionally had much higher mortality from cardiovascular diseases than people without diabetes. This high rate of cardiovascular disease is not an inevitable consequence of diabetes because Japanese and black east African diabetic people have been relatively free of cardiovascular disease unlike either Japanese American or black American diabetic people (Keen and Thomas, 1988). Insulin resistance and hyperinsulinaemia lead to detrimental changes in blood lipoprotein profiles (see metabolic syndrome in Chapter 8) and a high-fat diet is an accepted risk factor for cardiovascular diseases and so the very-high-fat diet that was in the past prescribed for people with diabetes almost certainly increased their propensity to cardiovascular disease still further.

Diabetic people also develop a range of conditions that are attributed to degenerative changes in their microvasculature, i.e. capillaries. These changes in the microvasculature are responsible for the **diabetic retinopathy** that causes many people with diabetes to go blind and also for the high levels of renal disease (**diabetic nephropathy**) in diabetes. Persistent hyperglycaemia also leads to cataract and degeneration of peripheral sensory nerves (**peripheral neuropathy**). Changes in capillaries also lead to poor oxygenation of peripheral tissues and this together with the peripheral neuropathy leads to chronic ulceration in the extremities and to enhanced risk of gangrene in the toes and feet; many elderly diabetic people have lower limb amputations because of gangrene. Changes in the capillaries of diabetics are thought to stem from a chemical change in the proteins of the basement membrane of capillary cells that results from their continued exposure to high glucose levels; the proteins react abnormally with glucose and become **glycosylated**. Glycosylation probably also plays a role in the development of cataract and the degeneration of peripheral nerves seen in older diabetic people. Glycosylation of **low-density lipoproteins (LDL)** may increase their atherogenicity. The proportion of glycosylated haemoglobin is used as an indicator of average blood glucose concentration over the previous 2–3 months. In a healthy person glycosylated haemoglobin is less than 6 per cent of the total but it can rise to over 25 per cent in some people with diabetes.

Principles of management

The historical aim of diabetic therapy was to alleviate the immediate symptoms of the disease, which are at best unpleasant and incapacitating and at worst acutely life threatening. Despite the availability for many years of therapies that are effective in this limited aim for almost all people with diabetes, the life expectancy of diabetic people remains considerably less than that of non-diabetics. Also, people with diabetes have continued to have a high level disability in their later years for the reasons discussed in the previous section. A major additional objective of modern diabetic therapy is to increase the life expectancy and to reduce the long-term morbidity of people with diabetes. From the previous discussion the two major considerations that seem to be important in this respect are:

- the hyperlipidaemia that is associated with diabetes (and high-fat diets) and the consequent increase in risk of atherosclerosis
- the persistent hyperglycaemia of diabetes.

Modern diabetic management seeks to reduce these longer-term complications by:

- achieving and maintaining a more normal body weight
- minimizing hyperlipidaemia and hyperglycaemia.

The modern diabetic diet is almost the complete opposite of that recommended prior to 1970. It is a low-fat diet that is high in complex carbohydrate and fibre. More than half of the energy should come from carbohydrate with the emphasis on unrefined foods high in complex carbohydrate and fibre. It has moderate levels of fat and saturated fat, ideally less

than 35 per cent of energy as fat and less than 10 per cent as saturated fat. The very strict avoidance of sugar has been relaxed provided it is a component of a meal. The general avoidance of isolated sugary foods except for hypoglycaemic emergency is still recommended. A diet considered ideal for diabetics with type 2 diabetes is very similar to that recommended for the population as a whole. The matching of carbohydrate to insulin dose in type 1 diabetes is a specialist topic beyond the scope of this text but the overall dietary strategy is as outlined here. Note that overdose of insulin causes blood glucose level to fall below normal, hypoglycaemia, and this fall in blood glucose can lead to a variety of symptoms ranging from confusion and disorientation through to coma and even death. Hypoglycaemia is treated by consuming a sugary snack or by infusion of glucose if the patient is unconscious. It occurs, for example, if the patient misses or unduly delays a meal or takes too much insulin.

As was seen in Chapter 8, obesity is a major risk factor for type 2 diabetes and normalization of body weight and regulation of caloric intake to match expenditure improves the symptoms of type 2 diabetes. Much of the success of traditional low-carbohydrate diabetic diets may have been due to their regulation of energy intake rather than carbohydrate restriction *per se*. Provided the diabetic person is in energy balance, the proportions of energy that come from fat and carbohydrate do not really affect short term diabetic control. A raised carbohydrate intake increases peripheral sensitivity to insulin and thus does not increase the need for insulin. This adaptation cannot occur in the absence of insulin, and so carbohydrate does have adverse effects in untreated severe diabetes, thus explain-ing the past assumption that carbohydrate was inevitably bad for diabetic people. The well-documented effects of fibre in improving glucose tolerance are discussed in Chapter 9. An increase in the proportion of energy from carbohydrate, together with an increase in dietary fibre, has a generally favourable effect on blood glucose control in both type 1 and type 2 diabetes. The moderate levels of fat and saturated fat in diabetic diets would be expected to reduce blood lipid levels and contribute to a reduction in atherosclerosis.

There is now firm evidence from the Diabetes Control and Complications Trial (DCCT, 1993) that people with type 1 diabetes, who achieved good long-term glycaemic control, have reduced risk of nephropathy, retinopathy and neuropathy than those with poor glycaemic control. Data from the UK Prospective Diabetic Study (UKPDS) show very convincingly that better glycaemic control considerably reduces the macrovascular and microvascular complications of type 2 diabetes (Stratton *et al.*, 2000). This group used the mean concentration of glycosylated haemoglobin as the indicator of glycaemic control in over 4000 people with type 2 diabetes in the UK. The authors found that there was a highly significant and progressive improvement in all measured outcomes with each 1 per cent reduction in glycosylated haemoglobin. Reduced diabetes-related mortality, incidence of heart attacks, amputations, retinal degeneration and cataract were all found in those with better glycaemic control (as indicated by lower glycosylated haemoglobin concentration) and the best outcomes were seen in those patients whose glycosylated haemoglobin levels were within the normal range for non-diabetics.

Jenkins *et al.* (1981) coined the term **glycaemic index** to describe in a quantitative way the rise in blood glucose that different carbohydrate foods produce. It is the rise in blood glucose induced by 50 g of carbohydrate present in a test food expressed as a percentage of that induced by the same amount of a standard carbohydrate source (discussed in Chapter 9). For example, bread and cornflakes have high glycaemic index, porridge oats and All Bran moderate values and pulses have low values. It is generally accepted that foods with low glycaemic index would be beneficial for glycaemic control in diabetes management.

Table 16.1 shows examples of the glycaemic index of several foods compared with that of white bread. (See Chapter 9 for further discussion of the glycaemic index.)

Table 16.1 The glycaemic index of sample foods. The glycaemic response to 50 g of carbohydrate in the test food is compared with that of 50 g of white bread (designated GI 100)*

Food	Glycaemic index (GI)
White bread	100
Spaghetti (boiled)	67
Parboiled rice (boiled 15 minutes)	54
Cornflakes	121
Shredded wheat	97
Baked beans	70
Frozen peas	85
Dried lentils	38
Orange	59
Sugar	83
Milk†	approximately 45
Wholemeal bread	100
White rice (boiled 10–25 minutes)	81
All Bran	74
Porridge	88
Boiled new potatoes	80
Butter beans	46
Red kidney beans (dried)	43
Apple	62
Orange juice	71
Honey	126
Potato crisps	77

*Data taken from Shils et al. (2006).
†Values for whole or skimmed milk are very similar.

Key points

- Diabetes mellitus is caused by insulin deficiency.
- In type 1 diabetes there is β-cell destruction in genetically susceptible children which results in an absolute insulin deficiency.
- In type 2 diabetes, the primary change is reduced sensitivity to insulin which precipitates a relative insulin deficiency.
- Type 2 diabetes is triggered in genetically susceptible people by excessive weight gain (particularly increased abdominal fat), a high-fat, low-fibre diet and inactivity.

- The acute symptoms of type 2 diabetes are relatively mild whereas those of type 1 are acutely life-threatening and insulin therapy is an absolute requirement.
- 85 per cent of diagnosed diabetics are type 2, many more remain undiagnosed and the numbers are rising with the growth in the elderly population and the increasing prevalence of obesity.
- Cases of type 2 diabetes are now starting to occur in obese young adults and even children.

- Both types of diabetes lead to hyperglycaemia, glucose in the urine, increased urine flow and increased thirst.

- Diagnosis of diabetes is by detection of hyperglycaemia with various threshold values used depending on whether a random sample, a fasting sample or one obtained after glucose challenge are used.

- In untreated type 1 diabetes there is rapid weight loss, severe dehydration and ketoacidosis, which will eventually result in coma and death.

- Diet is a key part of the treatment of both types of diabetes.

- Diabetic people are particularly prone to heart disease, strokes, renal failure, blindness, peripheral nerve degeneration and gangrene.

- Good control of body weight, blood lipids and blood glucose are important for reducing the long-term complications of diabetes.

- Obesity reduces insulin sensitivity, high blood lipids increase atherosclerosis and hyperglycaemia induces the excessive

- glycosylation of proteins which is responsible for many of the long-term complications.

- Modern diabetic diets are low in fat and saturated fat but high in fibre and complex carbohydrate.

- High carbohydrate diets improve glycaemic control because they increase insulin sensitivity.

- Dietary fibre slows carbohydrate digestion and absorption and so improves glycaemic control.

- Low saturated fat intake reduces atherosclerosis.

- Better glycaemic control has been shown to reduce mortality and all of the complications associated with both type 1 and type 2 diabetes.

- The blood concentration of glycosylated haemoglobin is used as a measure of glycaemic control.

- The glycaemic index is a measure of the rise in blood glucose produced by individual carbohydrate foods.

- Increased use of foods with low glycaemic index (such as pulses) should facilitate better glycaemic control in people with diabetes.

Cystic fibrosis

Cystic fibrosis (CF) is an inherited disease caused by an autosomal recessive gene and it affects around 1:2400 live births in the UK. According to Dodge *et al.* (1997) in 1992 there were 6500 people with this condition living in the UK, and two-thirds of these were under 16 years. However, because of increasing life expectancy births were then outnumbering deaths by around 160 per year which suggests UK prevalence in 2007 of around 9000 people. Screening for the CF gene is offered to potential parents in the USA and if both parents carry the gene then prenatal screening of the baby is available with the option of terminating affected pregnancies. Many people with CF now survive into middle-age and early detection and treatment improves the long-term prognosis – since 2003 all newborn babies in Scotland have been screened for the disease.

The genetic lesion results in the production of a sticky mucus which blocks pancreatic ducts and small airways in the lungs. In the pancreas, this blockage leads to formation of cysts and progressive fibrosis and loss of function as these cysts are repaired. Similar changes occur in the lungs; there are repeated chest infections and progressive fibrotic damage to the lungs. In the past, affected children would have been unlikely to survive into adulthood but improved therapy is steadily increasing the life expectancy of affected patients. The increasing prevalence is evidence of increased survival of affected patients into adulthood.

Regular physiotherapy to clear the lungs of the thick secretions and the availability of antibiotics to treat lung infections have been key factors in the improved survival and quality of life of those affected, and lung transplants may further extend the life expectancy. Improved dietetic management has also been an important factor in improving the prognosis for CF patients. The fibrosis of the pancreas leads to a failure to produce pancreatic juice and as a consequence there is poor digestion and absorption of fat and protein and poor absorption of fat-soluble vitamins. Untreated CF patients are at high risk of general malnutrition, fat-soluble vitamin deficiencies and perhaps even essential fatty acid deficiencies. Evidence of vitamin A deficiency has frequently been found in untreated CF patients and in some cases

xerophthalmia (due to vitamin A deficiency) has been the presenting symptom. Anorexia is often seen in CF patients, especially associated with infection, and there is also increased energy expenditure which compound to increase the risks of malnutrition.

The principal dietetic objective in this condition is to maintain the nutritional adequacy of the patient. Dietetic management should prevent the wasting, the deficiency diseases and the fatty diarrhoea of untreated CF. There is also evidence of interaction between nutritional status and the pulmonary manifestations of CF which ultimately determine survival. Malnourished patients are more prone to respiratory infections whereas well-nourished patients have fewer episodes of pneumonia. Experience of other sick and injured patients suggests that weak, malnourished people have an impaired ability to cough and expectorate (KFC, 1992). The strategies employed to meet this objective of maintaining dietary adequacy are summarized below.

- Pancreatic supplements containing the missing digestive enzymes are given with food. These are now in the form of coated microspheres that are protected from destruction in the stomach but disintegrate in the small intestine (duodenum).
- CF patients are prescribed a diet that is high in energy and protein and, with the more effective pancreatic supplements, this need not now be low in fat.
- Vitamin supplements (particularly fat-soluble vitamins) are given.
- Dietary supplements or artificial feeding are given when patients cannot take adequate food by mouth.

Dodge (1992) has reviewed the dietary management of cystic fibrosis.

Key points

- Cystic fibrosis is an inherited condition that results in progressive fibrotic damage to the lungs and pancreas.
- A combination of effective physiotherapy, antibiotic treatment of lung infections and improved dietary management allows many CF patients to now survive into middle age.
- Failure of pancreatic secretion leads to malabsorption of fat, protein and fat-soluble vitamins.

- Anorexia and malabsorption reduce energy and nutrient supply and raised energy expenditure increases energy requirements.
- The aim of dietary management is to prevent the wasting and deficiency diseases that CF can precipitate.
- Improved nutrition may slow pulmonary deterioration and certainly maintains muscle strength and the ability to cough and expectorate.
- Oral supplements of pancreatic enzymes ensure proper digestion of food and allow patients to eat a normal diet.
- Vitamin supplements are a precautionary measure.
- Supplements or artificial feeding should be used during bouts of infection and anorexia.

Chronic renal failure

The weight of the kidney and the number of functional units (nephrons) both decline with age. There is also an age-related decline in measures of renal function such as glomerular filtration rate. In large numbers of elderly people, renal function declines to the point where the **chronic renal failure (CRF)** becomes symptomatic. Incidence of CRF is five times higher in the those over 60 than in those aged 20–49 years and 10 times higher in those over 80.

As the kidney fails, there is reduced excretion of the urea produced by breakdown of excess dietary protein (or body protein in wasting subjects). Levels of creatinine and urea in the blood rise and increased blood urea (**uraemia**) produces unpleasant symptoms such as headache, drowsiness, nausea, itching, spontaneous bruising, vomiting and anorexia. As the condition progresses the patient will eventually lapse into a coma and die unless they receive either dialysis or a kidney transplant. A diet that minimizes urea production would be expected to reduce the symptoms of uraemia, and low-protein diets have long been used in the symptomatic treatment of CRF.

There is a widespread belief that a low-protein diet is not only palliative but that if started in the early stages of renal failure actually slows the pathological degeneration of the kidney. It thus extends the period in which conservative management can be used before either dialysis or transplantation become essential. It has even been argued that chronic over-consumption of protein in early adult life may be a contributory factor in the aetiology of CRF (e.g. Rudman, 1988). This benefit of low-protein diets in slowing the progression of CRF is still a matter of dispute. Many of the early studies that claimed a benefit for low-protein diets were small, improperly controlled or short term. Even if very restrictive diets have some effect this may be outweighed by effects they have on the patient's quality of life and general nutritional status. Locatelli *et al.* (1991) reported only marginal benefits from a low-protein diet and a controlled but 'normal' protein diet on the progression of CRF in a large sample of Italian patients with renal disease. They concluded any extra benefits of the low-protein diet did not justify the restrictions imposed on the patients. Compliance with the low-protein diet was acknowledged to be poor in this study. A large and long-term American cohort study suggested that moderate protein restriction slowed the progression of CRF in patients with moderate renal insufficiency. More severe restriction of protein intake in those with more advanced renal failure did not appear to offer any additional benefits compared with moderate restriction (Klahr *et al.*, 1994).

Low-protein diets for chronic renal disease aim to restrict protein intake to around 40 g/day (and phosphorus intake to around 600 mg/day) and to give a high proportion of this protein in the form of high-quality animal protein. The typical protein intake of British men is 84 g/day. Intakes of lower-quality cereal proteins with their attendant relatively high nitrogen losses are restricted and the diet also aims to be high in energy to prevent the breakdown of endogenous protein as an energy source. The overall aim is a high-energy, low-protein but high-protein-quality diet. A range of high-energy but protein-reduced foods such as protein-reduced flour, bread, pasta and crackers are available not only as direct low sources of low-protein calories but also to act as vehicles to carry fats and sugars, e.g. butter and jam (jelly). High-energy, low-protein supplements may also be used. In the past, dietary restriction was often initiated in asymptomatic patients based on biochemical evidence of mild insufficiency but there was little evidence to support use of this early intervention.

Key points

- Renal function declines with age and in many, usually elderly, people chronic renal failure (CRF) becomes symptomatic due to high blood urea concentrations.

- Blood levels of urea and creatinine increase as the capacity of the kidney to excrete them declines.
- Low-protein diets reduce production of urea and give symptomatic relief in CRF.
- Maintenance of good nutrient and energy intakes is necessary as wasting will increase urea production from endogenous protein breakdown.
- Moderate restriction of protein probably also slows the progress of CRF and so extends the time that the patient can be maintained without resort to dialysis or transplantation.

MALNUTRITION IN HOSPITAL PATIENTS

Overview

Every careful observer of the sick will agree in this, that thousands of patients are annually starved in the midst of plenty, from want of attention to the ways which alone make it possible for them to take food

Florence Nightingale (1859) Notes on nursing. *Reprinted 1980 Edinburgh: Churchill Livingstone*

Many people with severe illness are at risk from an unrecognised complication – malnutrition ... Doctors and nurses frequently fail to recognise under-nourishment because they are not trained to look for it.

Kings Fund Centre report (1992) A positive approach to nutrition as treatment (KFC, 1992)

Malnutrition is both a cause and consequence of disease; it predisposes to and delays recovery from illness ... the problem often goes unrecognised and untreated ... . Yet there is no consistent or coherent framework in place to deal with this problem.

Press release, Malnutrition Advisory Group of the British Association for Parenteral and Enteral Nutrition (11 November 2003)

These three quotations are separated by almost a century and a half but all three suggest a high prevalence of malnutrition among hospital patients that is partly the result of inadequate care. Despite much research and writing about this problem since 1980, the conclusions of the 2003 quote are strikingly similar to those of 1859.

Several examples of conditions where diet is a specific part of the therapy have been discussed earlier in the chapter and in such patients there is likely to be careful monitoring of their intake and early recognition of nutritional problems. However, good nutrition is no less important to all long-stay hospital patients and is a vital, if non-specific, complement to their medical or surgical treatment. General medical and nursing staff are likely to be less vigilant in monitoring the food intake and nutritional status of the general hospital population. Historically, nutrition has been given low priority in medical and nursing education. Many doctors and nurses are neither trained to recognize signs of inadequate nutrition nor educated about the key importance of good nutrition in facilitating recovery. The key to improving the nutritional status of hospital or community patients is heightened awareness among all medical staff of the importance of sound nutrition to prognosis and their increased vigilance in recognizing indications of poor or deteriorating nutritional status. A specialist nutrition team can only personally supervise the nutritional care of a small number of patients. This team must rely on other medical and nursing staff to identify nutritionally 'at-risk' patients and refer them quickly to the team. The general nutritional care of those patients not specifically at risk also depends on non-nutrition specialists.

Budgetary pressures may encourage hospital managers to economize on the 'hotel' component of hospital costs and to concentrate resources upon the direct medical aspects of care. However, pruning the catering budget is likely to be a false economy if it leads to deterioration in the nutritional status of patients. Any deterioration in nutritional status will lead to higher complication rates, longer hospital stays and to increased costs in spite of maintained or even improved surgical, medical and nursing care. In the report of an expert working party it was estimated that the potential financial savings in the UK from a nationwide introduction of nutritional support for under-nourished patients amounted to over £250 million at 1992 prices (KFC, 1992). In a major report for the British Association of Parenteral and Enteral Nutrition (BAPEN), Elia *et al.* (2003) estimated that the healthcare costs of malnutrition, specifically under-nutrition, in the UK in 2003 was around £7.3 billion. Compared with well-nourished people, malnourished patients had more general practitioner visits, more hospital admissions, a longer hospital stay and more admissions to care homes. Of this total of £7.3 billion, more than half was for the treatment of malnourished patients in hospital. This total represents about 10 per cent of the total health budget and so even modest fractional savings would have a significant impact on resources within the health system.

Key points

- Malnutrition is still prevalent among hospital patients, nearly 150 years after Florence Nightingale first highlighted this problem.
- Nutrition has traditionally been inadequately covered in medical and nursing education and so hospital staff are neither trained to monitor nutritional status nor aware of its importance to successful treatment.
- Improving the nutritional support for hospital patients could generate considerable financial savings.
- Under-nutrition and its consequences may well cost the healthcare system more than those associated with obesity.

Prevalence of hospital malnutrition

Two papers published in the 1970s are widely credited with focusing attention on the problem of hospital malnutrition. Bistrian *et al.* (1974) in the USA and Hill *et al.* (1977) in the UK reported that up to 50 per cent of surgical patients in some hospitals showed indications of malnutrition, both general protein energy malnutrition and vitamin deficiencies. Since these landmark publications, there have been reports of high prevalence of suboptimal nutrition in children's wards, medical and geriatric wards and in hospitals in other countries. For example, almost 1 in 6 children admitted to a Birmingham (UK) hospital were stunted or severely wasted – at least a quarter of children admitted with chronic respiratory, cardiac and digestive problems were short for their age (see KFC, 1992 and Powell-Tuck, 1997 for further examples and references). More recently, Elia *et al.* (2000) have estimated that up to 60 per cent of patients in hospitals are clinically malnourished.

Key points

High prevalence of malnutrition has been reported in most hospital specialities from medical to surgical and from paediatrics to geriatrics.

Consequences of hospital malnutrition

Following a general review of the relationship between nutritional status and outcome in hospital patients, an expert committee in the UK concluded that malnutrition is associated with increased duration of stay, increased hospital charges, increased requirements for home health care after hospital discharge, increased rates of complications and increased mortality (KFC, 1992). Some of the specific consequences of under-nutrition in hospital patients are summarized in Box 16.1 (see KFC, 1992 and Powell-Tuck, 1997).

Box 16.1 Possible consequences of undernutrition in hospital patients

- Higher rates of wound infections because of slow healing and reduced immunocompetence
- Increased risk of general infections, particularly respiratory infections and pneumonia
- Muscle weakness – which means that patients take longer to re-mobilize and weakness of the respiratory muscles will impair the ability to cough and expectorate and predispose to respiratory infections
- Increased risk of pressure sores because of wasting and immobility
- Increased risk of thromboembolism because of immobility
- Malnutrition will reduce the digestive functions of the gut and probably also increase its permeability to bacteria and their toxins
- Increased liability to heart failure because of wasting and reduced function of cardiac muscle
- Apathy, depression and self-neglect

Wasting of muscles and fat is one of the most obvious outward signs of starvation but there is also wasting of vital internal organs like the heart and intestines. In the classical starvation studies of Keys *et al.* (1950), chronic under-nutrition in healthy subjects was also found to cause apathy and depression. This would clearly hinder the recovery of malnourished hospital patients.

It is a general observation that in famine areas, malnutrition is associated with high rates of infectious disease, with increased severity and duration of illness and ultimately with higher mortality. Providing medicines and medical personnel has limited impact if the underlying problem of malnutrition is not addressed. Chandra (1993) reviewed the effects of nutritional deficiencies on the immune system. He concluded that there were a number of demonstrable changes in immune responses as a consequence of malnutrition (see below).

- **Delayed-type cutaneous hypersensitivity** responses to a variety of injected antigens are markedly depressed even in moderate nutritional deficiency. In this type of test the antigen is injected into the skin and the inflammatory reactions occurs some hours after injection. The best known of these reactions is the **Mantoux reaction** in which individuals immune to the organism that causes tuberculosis respond to a cutaneous tuberculin injection with a DTH reaction. These DTH reactions are a measure of the cell-mediated immune response which deals with pathogens that have the capacity to live and multiply within cells, e.g. the bacilli that cause tuberculosis and leprosy, some viruses such as the smallpox virus and parasites such as that responsible for the disease toxoplasmosis.
- Secretion of **immunoglobulin A (IgA)**, the antibody fraction that protects epithelial surfaces such as those in the gut and respiratory tract, is markedly depressed. This would make malnourished patients more prone to respiratory, gut and genito-urinary infections.
- Circulating antibody responses (**IgG**) are relatively unaffected in protein energy malnutrition although the response may be delayed.
- White cells kill bacteria after they have ingested them by generating an oxidative pulse of superoxide radicals. Their capacity to kill ingested bacteria in this way is reduced in malnutrition.

Note that trauma also has an immunosuppressive effect and the degree of immunosuppression is proportional to the amount of trauma (Lennard and Browell, 1993). This means that, for example, the immune systems of poorly nourished patients undergoing major and traumatic surgery will be doubly depressed. Minimizing surgical trauma with modern techniques should lessen the immunosuppressive effect of surgery.

Key points

- Malnutrition of hospital patients increases their duration of stay, their risk of complications, their requirements for medical care after discharge and their mortality risk.
- Malnutrition decreases immune function and predisposes hospital patients to infection.
- In malnutrition the cell-mediated immune response is reduced, there is reduced secretion of IgA, and white cells have a reduced capacity to generate an oxidative pulse to kill ingested bacteria.
- Some specific consequences of malnutrition for hospital patients are summarized in Box 16.1.

The causes of hospital malnutrition

Hospital malnutrition is not solely or even primarily a consequence of things that happen in the hospital environment. Up to 40 per cent of patients are already malnourished when they are admitted. For example McWhirter and Pennington (1994) surveyed the nutritional status of 100 consecutive admissions to each of five areas of a major Scottish acute teaching hospital. They found that about 40 per cent of patients were malnourished at the time of admission. A study by Mowe et al. (1994) suggests that at least in the elderly, malnutrition may be one factor in precipitating the illnesses that necessitate hospital admission. They made a nutritional assessment of a large sample of elderly patients admitted to an Oslo hospital because of an acute illness (e.g. stroke, myocardial infarction and pneumonia). They also assessed the nutritional status of a matched sample of older people living within the hospital catchment area; 50–60 per cent of patients were under-nourished at the time of their admission to hospital and the nutritional status of the hospital group was much worse than that of the home group. Using several measures of nutritional status the authors found that 86 per cent of the home subjects showed no sign of malnutrition compared with only 43 per cent of the hospital group. They found that poor food intake in the month prior to admission was much more common in the hospital group than the home group. In the period prior to admission many more of the hospital group had:

- inadequate energy intakes in the month before admission

- intakes of vitamins and trace elements below 66 per cent of the US recommended dietary allowance
- problems with buying and preparing foods
- eating difficulties and reduced enjoyment from eating.

They suggested that reduced nutrient intakes and deteriorating nutritional status in the period prior to admission could cause an increased risk of hospitalization. Note that in the third quotation at the start of this section, this expert group stated that 'malnutrition is both a cause and a consequence of disease'.

Although many patients are already malnourished when they reach hospital, there is a tendency for any under-nutrition to worsen during hospitalization (Powell-Tuck, 1997). In their survey of 500 Scottish hospital admissions, McWhirter and Pennington (1994) reported that two-thirds of patients lost weight during their stay and that this weight loss was greatest amongst those patients identified as most malnourished on admission. Very few patients were given any nutritional support but those who were showed a substantial mean weight gain. Those selected for nutritional support obviously tended to be the most severely malnourished on admission. The deterioration in nutritional status that often accompanies hospitalization can usually be avoided with appropriate care. Less than half of the malnourished patients in this survey had any nutritional information documented in their notes. The authors concluded that 'malnutrition remains a largely unrecognised problem in hospital and highlights the need for education on clinical nutrition'. In their earlier study Hill et al. (1977) also found that only 20 per cent of patient notes contained any reference to their nutritional status, and then only a brief note such as 'looks wasted'. Only around 15 per cent of the patients they surveyed had been weighed at any stage during their hospital stay.

Depressed intake is usually the main cause of nutritional inadequacy during illness or after injury. Several factors that may depress food intake in the sick and injured are listed below.

- Physical difficulty in eating, e.g. unconsciousness, facial injury, difficulties in swallowing, oral or throat infection, lack of teeth, arthritis and diseases affecting co-ordination and motor functions.
- Anorexia induced by disease or treatment. Severe anorexia is a frequent consequence of malignant

disease but anorexia is a symptom of most serious illnesses and a side effect of many treatments. It is likely in anyone experiencing pain, fever or nausea.

- Anorexia resulting from a psychological response to illness, hospitalization or diagnosis. Starvation itself may lead to depression and apathy and may thus reduce the will to eat in order to assist recovery.
- Unacceptability of hospital food. This is most obvious in patients offered food that is not acceptable on religious or cultural grounds but equally, low-prestige, unfamiliar and just plain unappetizing food may severely depress intake in people whose appetite may already be impaired.
- Lack of availability of food. Patients may be starved prior to surgery or for diagnostic purposes, or they may be absent from wards at meal times. This may help to depress overall nutrient intake.

In general, the more specific and more obvious these influences are the more likely they are to be addressed. It will be obvious that particular measures are needed to ensure that someone with a broken jaw can eat but a patient who lacks teeth and has a sore mouth and throat is more likely to be overlooked. More allowance is likely to be made for a Jewish patient known to require Kosher food than for a patient who simply finds hospital food strange and unappetizing. Some service provision factors that may help to depress the food intake of hospital patients are listed in Box 16.2.

A recent survey of over 2200 patients in 97 English hospitals highlighted and quantified several problems that tend to depress food intake in hospital patients (Commission for Patient and Public Involvement in Health (CPPIH), 2006). This survey reported that:

- 40 per cent of patients had their hospital food supplemented by their visitors
- 37 per cent left their meal because it smelt, looked or tasted unappetizing
- 26 per cent did not receive the help they needed in feeding themselves
- 22 per cent of meals were served at the incorrect temperature
- 18 per cent of patients did not get their choice of meal.

In addition to the myriad of factors that tend to depress intake, the factors listed below may also

---

Box 16.2 Service provision factors that may depress energy and nutrient intakes in hospital patients

- Timing of meals. Meals may be bunched together during the working day with long enforced fasts from early evening to morning
- Prolonged holding of food prior to serving leads to deterioration of both nutritional quality and palatability
- Inherently unappetizing food and limited choice
- Failure to allow choice, e.g. patients may initially be given meals selected by the previous occupant of the bed
- Providing patients with portions of food that are insufficient for their needs perhaps because staff underestimate the needs of bedridden patients
- Plate wastage not monitored or recorded by staff, and so very low intakes are not recognized early
- Inadequate amount of time allowed for slow feeders to finish their meals
- Lack of staff help for those who need help with eating. Staff shortages may mean that by the time help is provided, the food is cold and unappetizing

Adapted from Webb and Copeman (1996).

---

increase the nutrient requirements of many sick and injured patients.

- Increased nutrient losses, e.g. loss of blood, the protein lost in the exudate from burned surfaces, loss of glucose and ketones in the urine of people with diabetes and protein in the urine of patients with renal disease.
- Malabsorption of nutrients, e.g. due to diseases of the alimentary tract or simple age-related deterioration in the efficiency of absorption. Malnutrition itself produces adverse changes in gut function with reduced efficiency of digestion and reduced absorption of several nutrients.
- Increased nutrient turnover – illness and injury lead to hypermetabolism, the **metabolic response to injury**.

In a classical series of studies that began in the 1930s, Cuthbertson demonstrated that in patients with traumatic injury the initial period of shock after injury was followed by a period of hypermetabolism. He coined the term **ebb** to describe the period of depressed metabolism or shock in the first 12–24 hours after injury and the term **flow** to describe the state of hypermetabolism that occurs once the initial period of shock is over. The flow phase is characterized by increased resting metabolism and oxygen consumption and an increased urinary loss of nitrogen associated with increased muscle protein breakdown, increased gluconeogenesis and increased fat breakdown and fatty acid oxidation. Cuthbertson found that the magnitude of this flow response was greater the more severe the injury and the better nourished the patient. Long-bone fractures may increase resting metabolic rate by 15–25 per cent and extensive burn injuries can double the metabolic rate. In severe trauma, sepsis or advanced disease nutritional support can only partly ameliorate the severe depletion of body fat and protein reserves that this hypermetabolic state produces (see Cuthbertson, 1980).

Following a traumatic injury, Cuthbertson found that the flow response generally reached its peak 4–8 days after injury and that the total loss of body protein could exceed 7 per cent of total body protein within the first 10 days after injury. The increased metabolism was a consequence of the increased rate of body protein turnover and the use of body protein as an energy-yielding substrate. Cuthbertson regarded this catabolic response as an adaptive mechanism to provide a source of energy when incapacitated by injury (traumatic or infective) and a means of supplying amino acids for the synthesis of new tissue and for the functioning of the immune system. The aim of nutritional management during this phase is to supply sufficient energy and protein to prevent or minimize use of endogenous protein and energy reserves and to maintain an adequate intake of essential micronutrients. Some nutrients, in particular the amino acid glutamine, may become conditionally essential during this phase and there is likely to be increased turnover of other micronutrients, especially zinc and vitamin A.

This catabolic response is partly mediated through hormonal responses to the stress of injury or illness. Levels of cortisol and catecholamine hormones from the adrenal glands rise in the flow phase but induced hormone changes in healthy subjects are not able to reproduce the magnitude of protein catabolism seen in severe injury. Levels of inflammatory mediators known as cytokines are elevated during the hypermetabolic phase and several of these have clearly identified metabolic effects that contribute to the multiple metabolic changes seen during the metabolic response to injury.

A patient who is well nourished and able to mount a bigger flow response is enabled to recover more quickly (see Cuthbertson, 1980; Richards, 1980). This would suggest that improving nutritional status prior to planned major surgery should improve the acute recovery from surgery although studies designed to test this hypothesis have produced variable results (KFC, 1992).

Key points

- The high prevalence of hospital malnutrition is largely explained by high prevalence of malnutrition among new admissions.

- In some cases, malnutrition is a contributory factor to the illness that necessitates hospitalization.

- However, many patients lose weight during their hospital stay and any under-nutrition at the time of admission tends to worsen.

- Much of the deterioration in nutritional status during hospitalization can be avoided if there is effective nutritional support.

- There is inadequate monitoring and recording of nutritional status in many hospitals.

- Weight loss is due to depressed food intake and sometimes to increased requirements.

- Intake of hospital patients is depressed for many reasons including:
  - eating difficulties
  - anorexia due to illness treatment or anxiety
  - unacceptability of hospital food
  - enforced periods of fasting
  - some more specific service provision factors are listed in Box 16.2.

- Nutritional requirements may be increased if there are increased nutrient losses in urine or from the site of injury or if absorption of nutrients is impaired.

- Major trauma, sepsis and serious illness induce a hypermetabolic state in which there is increased metabolic rate and protein catabolism leading to rapid wasting of muscle and adipose tissue.

Improving the nutritional care of hospital patients

Aims of dietetic management of general hospital patients

The two main aims of dietetic care of hospital patients are:

- to assess and monitor the nutritional status of all patients and where necessary take measures to correct nutritional inadequacy. Where feasible, the nutritional status of poorly nourished patients should be improved prior to planned surgery
- to ensure that after injury, surgery or during illness the input of energy, protein and other essential and conditionally essential nutrients should be sufficient to maintain body reserves or even to increase them in under-nourished patients. In grossly hypercatabolic patients it may only be possible to partly compensate for losses caused by this hypercatabolism.

The basal energy requirements of a patient can be estimated from their body weight (see Chapter 3). The following additional allowances can then be added to this basal figure to estimate their total requirements.

- An amount to allow for the hypermetabolism of illness and injury, which will depend upon the exact nature of the condition. It might range from +5–25 per cent in postoperative patients, those with long-bone fractures or mild to moderate infections up to as much as +90 per cent in patients with extensive burns.
- An amount to allow for the mobility of the patient ranging from +20 per cent in the immobile, 30 per cent in the bed bound but mobile to 40 per cent in those able to move around the ward.
- An increment to allow replenishment of stores if the patient is already depleted.

Protein allowances will also need to be increased in line with the extent of the calculated hypermetabolism.

Aids to meeting nutritional needs

The simplest and cheapest way of satisfying the nutritional requirements of sick and injured persons is to encourage and facilitate the consumption of appetizing and nutritious food and drink. In some patients, additional support measures may be needed (see list below).

- *Nutritional supplements.* Concentrated energy and nutrient sources that are usually consumed in liquid form and are readily digested and absorbed.
- *Enteral feeding.* The introduction of nutrients directly into the stomach or small intestine by use of a tube that is introduced through the nose and into the stomach or intestine via the oesophagus. Tubes may be introduced directly into the gut by surgical means particularly if there is likely to be an extended period of enteral feeding.
- *Parenteral feeding.* The patient may be supplied with nutrients intravenously, either as a supplement to the oral route or as the sole means of nutrition, **total parenteral nutrition (TPN)**. In TPN the nutrients must be infused via an indwelling catheter into a large vein. In some cases of extreme damage to the gut, patients may be fed for years by TPN. A major factor that has enabled patients to be maintained indefinitely with TPN was the development of a means of safely infusing a source of fat intravenously.

When supplementary feeding is being given via the gut, either as nutritional supplements or enteral feeds, it is important that they really do increase total nutritional intake and that they do not suppress voluntary intake and thus simply replace what the patient would voluntarily consume. Systematic reviews and meta-analyses of the use of oral nutritional supplements indicate that they do increase total energy and nutrient intakes in a variety of types of patients and that these supplementary feeds have little depressing effect on voluntary food intake. In post-surgical patients they may even increase appetite and voluntary food intake. Experimental studies with healthy subjects suggest that quite substantial supplementary enteral feeds when given by slow continuous infusion have almost no appetite suppressing effect and substantially increase total energy intake. Clinical trials also report that enteral feeding in this way does increase total nutritional intake in patients when used as a supplement to normal oral feeding. If the supplement is given as a bolus or 'meal', it does depress voluntary food intake (reviewed by Stratton, 2005).

When patients are being fed totally by the parenteral route because normal food intake is contraindicated by the patient's condition, e.g. severe intestinal disease, the parenteral feed ideally should not only supply the patient's needs for energy and essential nutrients but also satisfy their hunger and reduce the desire to eat normal food. However, even though the parenteral nutrition supplies all of their nutritional needs and maintains their body weight within the normal range, three-quarters of these patients report that they feel hungry and almost half report that they are distressed by hunger. Almost all such patients report a desire to eat and two-thirds report specific food desires. The presence of hunger in people being maintained on long-term parenteral nutrition is clearly an unpleasant consequence of their therapy, akin to intractable pain experienced by many other people with chronic conditions.

Ideally a specialist nutrition team should supervise these artificial feeding methods; TPN, in particular, requires specialist management and is usually only used where the oral route is ruled out, e.g. in patients who have had a large part of the intestine removed or have severe inflammatory disease of the intestine. Infection of the intravenous lines can be a major problem in TPN but with skilled specialist management can be largely eliminated (KFC, 1992). KFC (1992) estimated that at that time around 2 per cent of hospitalized patients in Britain received some form of artificial feeding and that in three-quarters of cases an enteral tube was the method used. Its analysis of the workload of a nutrition team at one general hospital suggested that the number of patients receiving dietary supplements was similar to those being fed artificially. A minority of patients may continue to receive long-term enteral or parenteral nutrition at home. KFC (1992) estimated that at that time well in excess of 1000 patients were receiving enteral nutrition at home and 100–150 parenteral nutrition. Comparison of these figures with those of Stratton (2005) show that there has been a very steep rise in the home use of these artificial feeding regimens since then. At the end of 2003 it was estimated that at that particular point 25 000 patients in the UK were using enteral feeding at home and that 600 patients per year were using parenteral feeding at home.

Use of oral supplements costs just a few pounds per week but the cost of artificial feeding rises steeply the more sophisticated the method; enteral feeding is

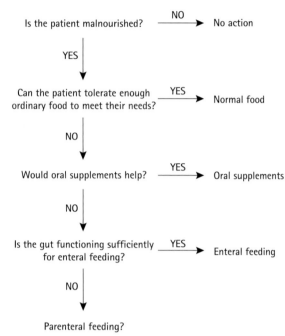

Figure 16.1 *A scheme for deciding the appropriate level of nutritional support for a patient (based on a scheme in RCN, 1993).*

many times more expensive than oral supplements and total parenteral nutrition many times more expensive than enteral feeding. It is therefore important that patients receive a level of intervention that is appropriate for their needs. Figure 16.1 shows a scheme that could be used to select the appropriate level of nutritional support for a given patient.

Measures that could improve the nutritional status of hospital patients

- Improved nutrition education for doctors and nurses and heightened awareness of the importance of adequate nutrition for patient recovery. Staff must be aware of the effect of illness and injury on nutritional needs and must be able to carry out simple nutritional monitoring and to interpret the results.
- Inclusion of a nutritional assessment as part of the standard admissions procedure. KFC (1992) suggested that this should include information about appetite, recent weight changes, oral and dental health, social characteristics and physical indicators of nutritional status such as body mass index (BMI) or arm circumference. Many hospitals do now include such information in their admission

forms and have developed simple scoring schemes to screen for those people who are nutritionally 'at risk'. In Scotland all patients entering hospital are nutritionally screened. In 2003 the Malnutrition Universal Screening Tool (MUST) was launched as a screening tool that could be used to simply and quickly assess nutritional status in hospitals, the community or in other care accommodation and is simple enough to be used by any care worker (Elia *et al.*, 2003). This is briefly discussed at the end of the chapter.

- Regular monitoring of patients' food intake and weight or any other simple anthropometric indicator. This would facilitate early identification of patients with depressed food intake and deteriorating nutritional status.
- Provision of appetizing, acceptable and nutritious food that reaches patients in good condition and ensuring that they receive the correct level of assistance with feeding. Ways of minimizing the adverse impact of the service provision factors listed in Box 16.2 should be sought and proper provision should be made for patients with special cultural needs. There should be formal procedures to record absences from wards at meal times and active measures to provide food for patients who are absent for meals and after a period of enforced fasting. In 2000 the UK National Health Service recruited a celebrity chef (Loyd Grossman) to lead a team of experts who were charged with improving the menus and the food in Britain's hospitals. This initiative received extensive publicity at the time and was heralded by the popular media as an important step to improving hospital food and the nutritional well-being of hospital patients. However, as discussed earlier in this chapter, a recent large survey of English hospitals still found very high levels of patient dissatisfaction with the hospital food and high levels of wastage (CPPIH, 2006).
- Rapid referral of patients with poor or deteriorating nutritional status to a nutrition specialist. These patients can then be given the appropriate level of nutritional support by a specialist nutrition team. Several authors who have conducted surveys and have reported high prevalence of malnutrition in hospitals have also noted that few of the malnourished patients had received any nutritional support (e.g. Hill *et al.*, 1977 and McWhirter and Pennington, 1994).

In many acute conditions, nutritional support can substantially reduce mortality. A number of controlled studies on the effects of supplementary feeding in hospital patients have been conducted. Reduced complication rates, decreased length of hospital stay and reduced mortality are general findings from such studies (KFC, 1992; Pennington, 1997; Powell-Tuck, 1997). Larsson *et al.* (1990) carried out a randomized study of the effects of energy supplements using 500 patients admitted to a long stay geriatric ward of a Swedish hospital. The supplements reduced the deterioration in nutritional status following admission and reduced mortality. Two studies on the effects of supplementation in patients with hip fractures suggest that oral or enteral supplements improve both the nutritional status of the patients and measures of outcome. Supplementation was associated with reduced hospital stay, more rapid mobilization, reduced rates of complications and lower mortality (Bastow *et al.*, 1983; Delmi *et al.*, 1990). A recent review (Stratton, 2005) reported that several systematic reviews had indicated that, compared with those receiving routine care, patients receiving oral supplements or tube feeding had significantly lower mortality, significantly lower rates of complications like wound infections and pneumonia, greater respiratory and skeletal muscle strength, improved wound healing and other physical and psychological benefits.

The Malnutrition Universal Screening Tool

MUST is a new screening tool for malnutrition that is said to be simple enough for use by any care worker and suitable for use in almost any setting – in hospitals, care homes, doctors' surgeries and outpatient clinics, and in other community settings. It was developed by Elia *et al.* (2003) for BAPEN. The basic protocol and explanatory notes can be downloaded from the BAPEN website (www.bapen.org.uk/must_tool.html). It involves a five-step process.

- **Step 1** – measure height and weight and calculate the body mass index (BMI). If BMI is:
  - under 18.5 kg/m^2 – score 2
  - 18.5–20 – score 1
  - over 20 – score 0
  - over 30 – score 0 (but classify as obese).
- **Step 2** – record amount of unplanned weight loss in past 3–6 months:
  - less than 5 per cent – score 0

- 5–10 per cent – score 1
- over 10 per cent – score 2.
- **Step 3** – if patient is acutely ill and it is likely that there has been no nutritional intake for more than 5 days:
  - score 2.
- **Step 4** – add scores from steps 1, 2 and 3:
  - total score – 0 low risk
  - total score – 1 medium risk
  - score 2 or more – high risk.
- **Step 5** Management guidelines:
  - low risk – routine care with regular repeat screening
  - medium risk – monitor intake for 3 days; if improved or adequate then there is little clinical concern but if intake is poor or not improved – clinical concern and follow local management policy. Continue to monitor regularly
  - high risk – treat by reference to a nutrition specialist or team, improve and increase intake and monitor and review treatment plan regularly.

Alternatives are also given for patients for whom the required measurements cannot be obtained:

- If height cannot be measured then either (a reliable) self-reported height can be used or knee height, demispan or ulna length can be used and tables are given for estimating height from these measures.
- If neither height nor weight can be measured then mid upper arm circumference (MUAC) can be used and guideline values are given.
- Subjective evaluations can also be used as an alternative to an objective BMI measure/estimate.
- Subjective indicators of recent weight loss can also be used where numerical values/estimates cannot be made, e.g. loose fitting clothes or jewellery or a history of low food intake or feeding problems.

Key points

- The nutritional status of all patients should be routinely monitored and all appropriate measures taken to minimize any deterioration in nutritional status.
- The new 'MUST' screening tool developed for BAPEN is simple to use and suitable for almost any clinical or community setting including hospital patients.
- 'MUST' consists of a five-step process whereby height, weight, body mass index, recent weight loss and recent clinical condition are used to produce a score which classifies patients as low, medium or high risk.
- Where necessary special nutritional supplements can be given orally or patients can be fed by an enteral tube or parenterally (intravenously).
- Feeding costs increase steeply with increasing sophistication of nutritional support and so the minimum effective level of support should be used (see Figure 16.1).
- Controlled trials and systematic reviews have shown that nutritional support can lead to significant patient benefits including:
  - lower mortality
  - reduced complications such as local infections and pneumonia
  - improved muscle strength including respiratory muscles
  - improved healing
  - faster re-mobilization
  - psychological benefits.
- Some measures that could improve the nutritional status of hospital patients:
  - improved nutrition education for medical and nursing staff
  - nutritional screening of patients at admission and regular monitoring during hospitalization
  - improvements in catering and the delivery of food to patients
  - rapid referral of patients identified by screening as 'at risk' to a nutrition specialist or team.

17

Some other groups and situations

VEGETARIANISM

A strict vegetarian, or **vegan**, avoids consuming any animal products, i.e. meat, fish, eggs, dairy produce and perhaps even honey. Others are less strict in their avoidance and although they do not eat meat, they may eat dairy produce, eggs or fish or any combination of these three. The prefixes **lacto**, **ovo** or **pesco** are used alone or in combination to describe these degrees of vegetarianism, e.g. one who avoids meat and fish but eats eggs and dairy produce is an ovolactovegetarian. Johnston and Sabate (2006) have written a wide ranging and extensively referenced review of health aspects of vegetarianism and most of the uncited references for statements made in this section can be found in this review.

An American survey conducted in 1994 suggested that about 7 per cent of Americans called themselves vegetarians. Only a small fraction (approximately 4 per cent) of self-styled vegetarians are vegans and many of them occasionally eat meat and many more eat poultry or fish. The term vegetarian clearly has a variety of different meanings to different consumers. People who consume little meat and poultry but are not strictly vegetarian are sometimes referred to as semi- or demivegetarians. Detailed analysis of the questionnaires from this 1994 survey suggested that only about 1 per cent of Americans actually refrained from eating any meat, fish or poultry at this time. A similar poll conducted in 2000 concluded that 2.5 per cent of the American population could then be classified as vegetarian using this criterion.

Surveys conducted by Gallup for the Vegetarian Society in Britain show that in 1999, 5 per cent of those sampled (approximately 4000 adults) reported being vegetarian and this was twice as many as in a similar survey conducted in 1985 (www.vegsoc.org/info/realeat.html). Almost half of those surveyed in 1999 reported that they were eating less meat and almost 9 per cent reported that they were avoiding red meat. Vegetarianism was twice as common in women as in men and was particularly prevalent among women in the under 35 age groups. In the latest National Diet and Nutrition Survey (NDNS) of British adults (Hoare *et al.*, 2004), 5 per cent of adults reported that they were vegetarian or vegan with rates in women more than three times those in men. The prevalence of vegetarianism was also age dependent: 11 per cent of women aged under 35 but only around 4–5 per cent of those aged over 35. As in the American data discussed previously there was some variation in the extent of avoidances of animal products and less than 30 per cent of vegetarians claimed to avoid all animal products.

The major reasons cited for adopting vegetarianism in the USA and UK are:

- health reasons – the vegetarian lifestyle may reduce the risk of several chronic diseases and there have been several major alarms about the safety of animal foods such as the bovine spongiform encephalopathy (BSE) crisis in Britain (see Chapter 18)
- ecological and environmental reasons – in Chapter 2 it was noted that it requires between 3 and 10 kg grain to produce 1 kg of meat
- animal welfare and cruelty concerns
- not liking the taste of meat.

Several major religions restrict or discourage the consumption of meat, e.g. Buddhism, Hinduism and

Seventh Day Adventism. In the UK, many members of the large south Asian community are lactovegetarians, and these people probably represent the biggest group of vegetarians in the UK. Religious considerations and lack of meat availability mean that many people in developing countries eat little or no meat.

Traditionally, nutritionists have been concerned about the adequacy implications of vegetarian and particularly vegan diets. From an adequacy viewpoint, any major restriction of the categories from which food may be selected cannot be regarded as ideal. The greater the degree of restriction the greater are the chances of the diet being inadequate and also of any toxicants in food being consumed in hazardous amounts. Paradoxically, most recent interest has been shown in vegetarian diets as a possible means to increasing wellness. There have been numerous reports of low incidence of chronic disease among vegetarian groups. This change has been reflected in the focus of scientific research about vegetarianism; between 1966 and 1975, 48 per cent of scientific papers about vegetarianism were concerned with their nutritional adequacy and only 24 per cent about their possible role in disease prevention or treatment but in 1986–95 these figures were almost reversed at 24 per cent and 40 per cent, respectively. Indeed, the possible health benefits is now frequently cited as the reason for adopting vegetarianism in the UK and USA.

A recurring theme of the dietary guidance offered in this book has been to encourage diversity of food choice. The avoidance of whole groups of foods runs contrary to that theme and is therefore regarded by the author as suboptimal. Paradoxically, another recurring theme has been to encourage adults in industrialized countries to reduce their consumption of meat and other animal foods and to increase their consumption of cereals, fruits and vegetables, i.e. to move towards a more vegetable-based diet. It is clear that a thoughtfully constructed vegetarian or even vegan diet is compatible with nutritional adequacy and may well be more diverse and adequate than the current diets of many omnivores. When people decide for cultural, religious, ethical or ecological reasons to adopt some degree of vegetarianism then the role of the nutrition educator should be to facilitate the healthful implementation of that personal choice. Nutritionists should only try to discourage practices that are irrevocably dysfunctional.

Key points

- Only a small proportion of vegetarians are vegans who avoid all animal products.
- Most vegetarians consume milk and dairy produce (lactovegetarian); many consume eggs (ovo) and/or fish (pesco).
- Some people classify themselves as vegetarian despite eating some poultry or meat and could be termed demivegetarian.
- Several major religions encourage vegetarianism but many affluent Western vegetarians choose to be vegetarian for health, ecological or ethical reasons or simply because they claim not to like the taste of meat.
- Vegetarianism restricts dietary choice and so theoretically increases the risks of dietary inadequacy.
- Most dietary guidelines in Western countries imply that a move towards a more vegetable-based diet would have health benefits.
- Vegetarians in Western countries often have lower rates of chronic disease and lower mortality than omnivores.
- The potential health benefits of partial or complete vegetarianism is now the predominant theme of research rather than its potential to cause dietary inadequacies.

Adequacy of vegetarian diets

Animal-derived foods are the only, or the major, sources of some nutrients in typical UK and US diets. The possibility that supplies of such nutrients might be inadequate in vegetarian or vegan diets needs to be considered and, where necessary, remedial measures identified that are consistent with maintaining the chosen diet. The degree to which less strict vegetarians are threatened by these potential inadequacies will depend upon the extent of individual restrictions. Many vegetarians make liberal use of dairy produce and in some cases also of eggs and fish and so most of the theoretical deficiencies of totally vegetable-based diets will not apply to them.

Vegan diets theoretically contain no vitamin B_{12}, no vitamin D and no retinol. They are also likely to contain less total energy, protein, calcium, zinc, riboflavin and available iron. Several studies do indeed suggest that intakes of vitamin B$_{12}$, vitamin D, retinol, calcium and zinc are lower in vegetarians. Vegan and probably other vegetarian diets are likely to be less energy dense than omnivorous diets because they have less fat and more starch and fibre. Total energy intakes are, as a consequence, also likely to be lower than those of omnivores. Indeed, the reduced energy density of vegetarian diets is perceived as one of the major advantages of such a diet for affluent adult populations where overweight and obesity are common. There is a general consensus that Caucasian vegans have lower energy intakes than omnivores and are lighter and have a lower proportion of body fat. Most studies also suggest that other vegetarians are lighter than omnivores and are less likely to be overweight or obese although the difference is smaller than that between vegans and omnivores. As discussed later, this does not necessarily mean that meat avoidance *per se* will prevent excessive weight gain or be an effective strategy for weight loss in those who are already overweight or obese.

A less positive view of the low energy density of vegetarian diets is usually taken when children are the consumers. A diet that has too low an energy density could impair their growth. Studies in the USA, the Netherlands and the UK have found that younger vegan children tend to be lighter and smaller in stature than omnivorous children. The differences are, however, generally small and the growth patterns and growth curves of vegan children are usually within normal limits and they tend to catch up this growth later in childhood, i.e. by the age of 10 years. In a sample of British vegan children, Sanders (1988) found that energy intakes were below the then recommended dietary allowances (RDAs) and that fat intakes were, on average, low but very variable (ranging from only 16 per cent to 39 per cent of calories). Sanders concluded that low-fat intake and the low energy density was probably the major determinant of the low energy intakes. In turn, the low energy intakes were probably responsible for the anthropometric differences between vegan and omnivore children rather than any differences in dietary quality. American Seventh Day Adventist children who are ovolactovegetarians grow similarly to other children and have no greater evidence of nutritional deficiencies.

Vegan diets are likely to be lower in protein than omnivorous or lactovegetarian diets. Individual plant proteins are also generally of lower quality than individual animal proteins. Thus one of the traditional concerns of vegetarians has been about the protein adequacy of their diets. The priority attached to protein deficiency as a likely cause of human malnutrition has declined very sharply in recent decades (see Chapter 10). Mutual supplementation also means that the overall protein quality of a good mixed vegetable meal or diet may not be substantially different from an omnivorous one. This means that, according to current estimates of requirements, vegetarian and even vegan diets are likely to be more than adequate both in terms of their overall protein content and in their ability to supply the essential amino acids.

Vitamin D (cholecalciferol) is naturally present only in foods of animal origin (see Chapter 13). Vitamin D is added to soya milk, many infant foods and several breakfast cereals and to margarine and other spreading fats in the UK. American milk is also often supplemented with vitamin D. Average intakes of vitamin D in the UK are generally well below estimated requirements but even intakes of British vegans do not differ substantially from those of omnivores provided that they eat vitamin D supplemented foods. Endogenous production (via the action of sunlight upon the skin) rather than dietary intake is regarded as the principal source of vitamin D for most adults and children. Endogenous production should therefore ensure adequacy of vitamin D status in strict vegetarians even if they avoid supplemented foods. In some lifecycle groups, endogenous production cannot be relied upon as a source of vitamin D (COMA, 1991) and so supplements of vitamin D may be necessary. In such groups and in anyone who has limited exposure to summer sunlight, the case for supplements is even stronger if they are vegan, especially if they avoid supplemented foods.

Retinol (vitamin A) is only present in animal foods but ample supplies of carotene in fruits and vegetables will make the total vitamin A content of many affluent vegetarian diets higher than those of typical omnivorous diets.

In strictly vegetarian diets there is no apparent vitamin B$_{12}$. Symptoms of megaloblastic anaemia and the neurological manifestations of vitamin B$_{12}$ deficiency might thus be expected to be prevalent among vegans. However, the human requirement for vitamin B$_{12}$ is extremely small (UK reference nutrient intake (RNI) – 1.5 μg/day) and stores of the vitamin in the liver are large and could amount to several years supply in an omnivore. In the UK, meat substitutes must be supplemented with B_{12} and many vegans take B_{12} supplements. Even in the absence of such alternative dietary sources, cases of clinical B_{12} deficiency among Caucasian vegans are rare. There are indirect sources of B_{12} even for those who consume no animal products or supplemented foods such as:

- from micro-organisms and moulds contaminating plant foods
- insects or insect remains consumed with plant foods
- absorption of vitamin produced endogenously by gut bacteria although most of this is produced below the point of absorption in the ileum and is excreted in faeces
- from fermented foods or yeast extracts
- from faecal contamination of foods like seaweed.

A combination of the large stores, extremely low requirement and incidental consumption from the sources listed above means that the practical hazard of B_{12} deficiency is less than might be expected even for vegans who take no active measures to ensure the adequacy of their B_{12} supply. Even though overt vitamin B_{12} deficiency is rare even in strict vegans, their serum concentrations are generally lower than those of omnivores and other less strict vegetarians have intermediate values. Vegans who do not take effective supplements may well have suboptimal status for the vitamin even though they may not show the usual overt symptoms. High intakes of folic acid in vegans tend to mask the haematological consequences of B_{12} deficiency and thus if symptoms do occur it is the neurological symptoms that are more likely to be manifested. The low incidence of B_{12} deficiency is some developing countries where a largely vegan diet is the norm may be because of higher levels of contamination of food and water with bacteria. It is now clear that in some products marketed and used as B_{12} supplements by vegans, the vitamin is present in an inactive form. The blue-green algae, *Spirulina*, for example, contains an analogue of vitamin B_{12} which is detected by the microbiological assays used to measure vitamin B_{12} but it is not biologically active (Watanabe *et al.*, 1999). Some of these analogues may actually worsen the effects of B_{12} deficiency by interfering with metabolism or absorption of the active form.

Dairy produce and eggs are major sources of riboflavin in UK and US diets and thus intakes of riboflavin are likely to be low in vegan, although not lactovegetarian, diets. Carlson *et al.* (1985) found average intakes of riboflavin in vegans of only 75 per cent of the then RDA compared with 140 per cent of the RDA in ovolactovegetarians. There is no evidence of overt riboflavin deficiency among strict vegetarians in affluent countries although it is generally one of the more prevalent micronutrient deficiencies. Plant sources of riboflavin are leafy vegetables, nuts and pulses.

Milk and dairy produce, including soya milk, are major sources of dietary calcium. Strict vegetarians who avoid these foods are likely to have lower calcium intakes than omnivores. High fibre and phytate intakes might also be expected to hinder the absorption of calcium from the gut. However, vegans apparently adapt to low calcium intakes and have reduced faecal losses of calcium. Low prevalence of osteoporosis has frequently been reported in vegetarian groups, like Seventh Day Adventists. Very few studies have looked specifically at vegans and this has been highlighted as a possible area of concern; note that leanness is also a risk factor for osteoporosis and vegans are often leaner than other groups. In general, many largely vegetarian populations in developing countries have very low calcium intakes by American and British standards but also have very low rates of osteoporosis (see Chapter 14).

Haem iron is the most readily absorbed form of dietary iron. Hazel and Southgate (1985) found that between 12 and 25 per cent of the iron in meat and fish was absorbed compared with 2–7 per cent from a variety of vegetable sources. Rice and spinach were at the bottom of the vegetable range and soya at the top. The higher fibre and phytate content of vegetarian diets would also tend to reduce non-haem iron absorption although high levels of vitamin C in vegetarian diets is an important promoter of inorganic iron absorption. Several groups have reported lower iron stores in lactovegetarians although there is little evidence of increased clinical anaemia. Some studies have reported lower haemoglobin levels in lactovegetarian children and adults despite their having higher iron intakes than omnivores. This would suggest that poor iron absorption may be a particular problem with some vegetarian diets. The latest NDNS surveys of both British adults (Hoare *et al.*, 2004) and of schoolchildren

(Gregory *et al.*, 2000) have both highlighted low iron intakes and poor biochemical iron status as particular problems for girls and young women generally. Gregory *et al.* found that 27 per cent of girls had low serum ferritin levels and Hoare *et al.* found that this was also true of 16 per cent of young women. One might expect, given the increased theoretical risks of iron deficiency in vegetarians, that the figures for vegetarian women and girls would be even higher. In a follow-up analysis of data from a survey of schoolchildren, Thane *et al.* (2003) reported that adolescent girls who were vegetarians had significantly poorer iron status than meat eaters and they suggested that increased consumption of enhancers of non-haem iron, such as fruit and fruit juice, was a possible way of reducing this problem.

Over 40 per cent of the zinc in omnivore diets comes from meat and fish and another 20 per cent comes from dairy foods. The overall zinc intake of vegetarians is similar to that of omnivores but it is less well absorbed. Many British girls have zinc intakes that are below the lower RNI (LRNI) as do around 5 per cent of younger women. There is as yet, however, no persuasive evidence of greater prevalence of unsatisfactory zinc status among vegetarians.

Key points

- The risk of dietary inadequacy in vegetarians is partly dependent upon the level of dietary restriction.
- Well-planned vegetarian diets are more varied and have higher levels of adequacy than the diets of many omnivores.
- Vegetarian diets are likely to be less energy dense than omnivorous diets and Western vegetarians tend to be lighter and leaner than omnivores.
- A vegan diet can restrict the growth of children although the effect is usually small and temporary.
- Vegan diets reduce growth rates in children because they are low in fat and of low energy density rather than because of protein or other nutrient deficiency.
- If energy intakes are adequate then most diets, even vegan diets, should have ample supplies of protein and essential amino acids.
- If plenty of coloured fruits and green vegetables are consumed then vegetarian diets should have

ample vitamin A in the form of carotenoids even though retinol is only found in animal foods.
- Plant foods theoretically contain no vitamin B_{12}.
- Overt vitamin B_{12} deficiency is rarely seen, even in vegans, although there may be suboptimal status in some who do not take supplements.
- The vitamin B_{12} in some algal supplements, e.g. *Spirulina*, is not biologically active and may even interfere with normal B_{12} metabolism.
- Dietary deficiency of B_{12} is uncommon because:
  - requirements are extremely small
  - omnivores have stores sufficient for several years
  - many vegetarians take supplements or eat supplemented foods
  - many plant foods contain some B_{12} as a contaminant, e.g. from microbes.
- Vitamin D is not naturally present in vegetable foods although some are supplemented.
- For most people the principal source of vitamin D is endogenous synthesis in the skin when it is exposed to summer sunlight.
- Vegetarians, especially those who do not eat supplemented foods, are more reliant than omnivores on sunlight as their primary source of vitamin D.
- Vegetarian diets lack haem iron, which is the most readily available form of dietary iron.
- The iron in vegetarian diets is likely to be less well absorbed than in omnivorous diets, and several surveys suggest that vegetarians have lower body iron stores than omnivores.
- Vitamin C is an important promoter of non-haem iron absorption.
- Animal foods are important dietary sources of riboflavin, calcium and zinc, but there is no persuasive evidence of a specific problem of inadequate status for these nutrients in vegetarians or vegans.

Vegetarian diets and nutritional guidelines

A vegetarian diet has been reported by a variety of authors and using a variety of vegetarian groups to be associated with:

- lower body weight and reduced prevalence of obesity
- lower blood pressure

- lower prevalence of osteoporosis (not specifically reported in vegans)
- reduced risk of coronary heart disease
- reduced risk of developing type 2 diabetes
- reduced incidence of certain cancers, particularly bowel cancer
- lower all-cause mortality.

It is very difficult to determine to what extent these associations are wholly or partly due to lack of meat consumption *per se*. Caucasian vegetarians in the UK tend not to be from the lower social groups, many of them adopt vegetarianism for health reasons and thus they are likely to pay particular attention to the healthiness of their diet and their lifestyle in general. Those who are vegetarian for cultural or religious reasons, also tend to adopt other practices that are considered healthful, e.g. avoidance of alcohol and tobacco. American Seventh Day Adventists are a frequently studied group because many are vegetarians. They do indeed have lower rates of the diseases listed above but they also tend to avoid alcohol and tobacco and are perhaps different in many other lifestyle characteristics to Americans in general. Several studies have compared the health of meat eating and non-meat eating Seventh Day Adventists and these have found that the vegetarians have increased life expectancy, lower rates of coronary heart disease, bowel cancer and a reduced risk of diabetes. A study is currently underway with 125 000 American and Canadian Adventists – the Adventist Health Study-2 which is centred on Loma Linda University in California, an Adventist university (details of this study may be found at www.llu.edu/llu/health/about.html). As already discussed in Chapters 3 and 9 the European Prospective Investigation into Cancer and Nutrition (EPIC) found strong support for the hypothesis that consumption of red and processed meat increases the risk of colorectal cancer whereas dietary fibre and fish consumption decreases the risk.

Compared with the UK population in general, Caucasian vegetarians in the UK would probably tend to:

- be more health conscious
- drink less alcohol
- make less use of tobacco
- take more exercise
- be lighter and less likely to be overweight or obese

- be less likely to come from the lower manual social classes
- be more likely to be female.

Compared with omnivores, the diets of vegetarians, and vegans in particular tend to be lower in fat, saturated fat, cholesterol and alcohol but higher in fruits and vegetables and their associated antioxidants and phytochemicals and also higher in complex carbohydrates, fibre and polyunsaturated fatty acids.

To assume that any differences in mortality or morbidity patterns of vegetarians are largely due to the avoidance of meat or animal foods *per se* is probably premature. Non-dietary risk factors may be very different in vegetarian and non-vegetarian groups. There are also numerous compositional differences between the diets of vegetarians and omnivores. Some of these are almost inevitable but a thoughtfully constructed omnivorous diet could match even a good vegan diet in many respects. The key question is not whether vegetarians are healthier than omnivores but 'how would the health records of vegetarians compare with omnivores of similar racial and social backgrounds who have similar smoking, drinking and activity patterns and who take equal care in the selection and preparation of a healthy diet?' The point of this discussion is to suggest to those reluctantly contemplating vegetarianism on health grounds alone, that giving up meat or 'red meat' may well, by itself, be ineffective but that adopting some of the lifestyle and dietary practices characteristic of vegetarians will almost certainly be beneficial. This point is even more important for nutrition educators seeking to influence the behaviour of others. The discussion in the next section on the health of British Asians makes the point that vegetarianism and good health statistics are not invariably linked. Thorogood (1995) has reviewed epidemiological studies of the relationship between vegetarianism and chronic disease.

Key points

- Affluent Western vegetarians tend to be:
  - leaner than omnivores
  - have reduced levels of several risk factors and lower prevalence of several chronic diseases
  - have reduced all-cause mortality.

- There are numerous social, lifestyle and dietary differences between affluent vegetarians and the rest of the population that may contribute to the observed health differences between them.

- Studies with Seventh Day Adventists do suggest that those of them who avoid meat have higher life expectancy, reduced rates of bowel cancer, heart disease and diabetes.

- Adopting a more vegetarian diet and lifestyle should produce more health benefits than simple meat avoidance.

RACIAL MINORITIES

Overview

Williams and Qureshi (1988) and Bush *et al.* (1997) have reviewed nutritional aspects of the dietary practices of racial minorities in the UK. Davey Smith *et al.* (2000) have published a detailed review of the variations in disease incidence and causes of mortality in different minority ethnic groups within the UK. Several topics and issues discussed in Chapter 2 are also of relevance when considering the nutrition of racial minorities:

- the effects of migration on dietary habits and nutrition
- economic influences on food choices
- cultural and religious factors that influence food selection and dietary practices.

Those offering dietary or other health education advice to people from a different cultural background need to carefully identify the particular needs and priorities of the target group and the reasons for them. This should enable them to determine what advice is appropriate from the scientific viewpoint. However, before they attempt to translate these scientific goals into practical advice and recommendations they need to assure themselves that they are aware of, and understand, the cultural and social determinants of the group's practices. Only by doing this can they then ensure that their advice is compatible with the beliefs and normal practices of the group.

There is a general tendency for the health of racial minority groups living in industrialized countries to be inferior to that of the majority population. Indeed, one of the health promotion goals set for the American nation in 1992 was to 'reduce the health disparity among Americans' (Department of Health and Social Security (DHHS), 1992). If improved nutrition is credited with being a major factor in the improving health and longevity of the majority population, then one would have to assume that some of this disparity is due to nutritional improvements lagging behind in minority groups. Racial minorities often tend to be economically and socially disadvantaged as compared with the majority population and this is almost certainly an important factor in some of these ethnic disparities in health. One of the most striking inequalities in health of Americans is that between low income groups and all other groups (DHHS, 1992) and when the mortality statistics of black Americans are adjusted for socioeconomic factors the differences between white and black largely disappear. Socioeconomic disadvantage has also been highlighted as a major barrier to sound nutritional health in ethnic minorities in the UK (Bush *et al.*, 1997).

The health and nutrition of particular minority groups

The health record of Native Americans is particularly poor, with two nutrition-related risk factors, alcohol misuse and obesity, clearly identified as important. Death rates from accident, homicide, suicide and cirrhosis of the liver are all much higher in Native Americans than in other Americans and are all associated with alcohol misuse. Rates of diabetes are also very high among Native Americans with more than 20 per cent of the members of many tribes affected by the disease; diabetes and the metabolic syndrome are acknowledged as major determinants of coronary heart disease risk (see Chapter 8). The increasing rates of diabetes in Native Americans have paralleled increasing rates of obesity; the proportion of overweight adults varies between a third and three-quarters depending on the tribe. In Chapter 8 it was noted that Pima Indians living in Mexico have much lower rates of obesity and diabetes than those living in the USA: adults in the USA are on average 25 kg heavier than those living in Mexico. Clearly nutritional factors, including alcohol misuse, are major determinants of the poor health statistics of this minority group (DHHS, 1992).

In 1987, black Americans had a life expectancy of 69.4 years compared with 75 years for the American population as a whole and this gap widened during the first half of the 1990s. Mortality rates for heart disease are considerably higher for black Americans than white Americans. The poverty rate among black people is also three times that of white people and when heart disease rates of black and white people are compared within income levels, then the rates for black people are actually lower than those for white people. A good proportion of the poor health record of some American racial groups seems to result from their generally lower socioeconomic status (DHHS, 1992).

In the UK, the two largest racial minority groups are African Caribbeans and British Asians. The African Caribbeans originated from the former British colonies in the West Indies and large-scale immigration of this group started in the 1950s. British Asians are a racially and culturally mixed group and most of the immigration has occurred since 1960. They originate from the countries of southern Asia (India, Pakistan, Bangladesh and Sri Lanka) or from the Asian communities of east Africa. In their review, Bush *et al.* (1997) also identified the Irish as a large minority ethnic group with particular evidence of nutrition-related health disadvantages including low stature, high rates of coronary heart disease, cancer and high overall mortality, which persists among those who are British born. They identified poverty and solitary living as barriers to nutritional health in older Irish people living in Britain, especially Irish men. In future editions it may be necessary to consider the nutritional health of the very large numbers who have recently migrated to Britain from the countries, especially eastern European countries, that have recently been admitted into the European Union.

British Asians are made up of three major religious groups – Hindus, Sikhs and Muslims. Rates of vegetarianism are high. Hindus are usually lactovegetarians and they do not usually eat Western cheese. Sikhs do not eat beef and rarely eat pork and many are lactovegetarian. Muslims should not eat pork or consume alcohol and any meat or animal fat should have come from animals slaughtered and prepared according to Islamic ritual. The potential health problems of vegetarianism, discussed earlier in the chapter, would thus apply to many within this group. For example, Robertson *et al.* (1982) suggested that nutritional deficiencies of folic acid and vitamin B_{12} were virtually confined to the Asian population in the UK. They suggested that the practice of boiling milk with tea leaves when making tea destroys much of the B_{12} present in the milk and strict

Hindus would have no other apparent source of B_{12} in their lactovegetarian diet. They also suggested that prolonged gentle heating of finely cut-up foods also destroys much of the folic acid initially present in some Asian diets.

Mini-epidemics of rickets and osteomalacia occurred in the 1960s and 1970s among Asian children and women in the UK. For example, a 5-year-old Asian child living in Glasgow between 1968 and 1978 had a 3.5 per cent chance of being admitted to hospital with rickets before the age of 16 years whereas the equivalent risk for a white child was negligible (Robertson *et al.*, 1982). Vitamin D deficiency has also been reported as common among pregnant Asian women in the UK and this has serious implications for the health of the baby. Several factors probably contribute to this high prevalence of vitamin D deficiency (see list below).

- Avoidance of those few foods that contain good amounts of vitamin D, e.g. fatty fish, liver, fortified margarine and infant foods and eggs.
- A cultural tendency not to expose the skin to sunlight, perhaps coupled with pigmentation of the skin, would be expected to reduce endogenous vitamin D synthesis. This endogenous synthesis is normally regarded as the primary source of vitamin D.
- High levels of fibre and phytate in chapattis (a traditional unleavened bread) might impair calcium absorption and perhaps also prevent entero-hepatic recycling of vitamin D (Robertson *et al.*, 1982).

Robertson *et al.* (1982) suggested that the problem is particularly associated with new immigrants and diminishes in those who are well established because of acculturation and partial adoption of a Western diet. They concluded that the most practical way of addressing the problem was by increased awareness through health education campaigns and by the provision of vitamin D supplements to those 'at risk'. Note, however, that biochemical evidence of high prevalence vitamin D deficiency has recently been reported in all children, adults and the elderly in Britain (see Chapters 12 and 15). Bush *et al.* (1997) still recognized rickets/osteomalacia as an area where intervention was needed in south Asians. At least one local health authority in the UK with a large south Asian community (Bradford) was so concerned about rickets and poor vitamin D status among its children that in 2006 it offered free supplements for young children. Zipitis *et al.* (2006) in a study in Burnley, England, found that clinical rickets was re-emerging as a problem in Asian children in the town. Although the number of clinical cases was small, almost all of them had occurred in the second half of the 10-year study period, suggesting a rising trend. If these results are typical of British Asian children then it points to a significant and growing problem and, of course, clinical cases of rickets are likely to represent 'the tip of the iceberg' with many more children having poor vitamin D status and impaired functioning. This group recommended that health authorities should provide supplements of vitamin D for Asian children for at least the first 2 years of life.

The relative prominence of the different causes of mortality also varies quite considerably between different ethnic groups in the UK. The incidence of hypertension and strokes is high in the African Caribbean population of the UK. It is also high among black Americans with stroke mortality among black American men almost twice that in the total male population. Africans and African Caribbeans may have an ethnic predisposition to hypertension due to a hypersensitivity to salt (Law *et al.*, 1991a).

The rates of coronary heart disease among the Asian groups in the UK are higher than in the white population despite the high prevalence of vegetarianism among British Asians. Age-standardized mortality is around 50 per cent higher for Asians in England and Wales than for the general population and mortality in those aged under 40 years is up to three times higher. A similar trend has been reported for Asians living in other industrialized countries. This problem was first highlighted in the UK by McKeigue *et al.* (1985) who compared the dietary and other risk factors for coronary heart disease among Asians and non-Asians living in London. They confirmed that rates of coronary heart disease were much higher among the Asians and that the excess morbidity and mortality was common to the three major religious groups despite considerable differences in dietary and lifestyle characteristics between the three. They found that the diets and lifestyles of Asians differed from their white neighbours in the following ways.

- The Asians had lower intakes of saturated fat and cholesterol and had lower serum cholesterol concentrations.
- The Asians smoked fewer cigarettes and drank less alcohol.

- Vegetarianism was much more common among the Asians.
- The Asians had had lower rates of bowel cancer than the white population even though high rates of bowel cancer and coronary heart disease tend to go together in populations.

McKeigue *et al.* (1991) reported high levels of insulin resistance among British Asians and the prevalence of diabetes was more than four times higher than in the population as a whole. They also reported very high incidence of central obesity in this Asian population (i.e. with a high waist-to-hip ratio). Vegetarianism among the Asian population does not seem to protect against overweight and obesity as it usually does for Caucasian vegetarians. McKeigue *et al.* (1991) suggested this insulin resistance was associated with high caloric intake and inactivity. They therefore proposed that these Asian groups are adapted to life in environments where high levels of physical activity and frugal use of food resources have been traditionally required. When these groups migrate to countries where levels of physical activity are low and caloric intakes are high this leads to insulin resistance, central obesity and other associated metabolic disturbances (see The metabolic syndrome in Chapter 8), including maturity onset diabetes. This in turn predisposes them to coronary heart disease. A major recent report on heart disease in south Asians (Department of Health/British Heart Foundation (DH/BHF), 2004) confirmed that the increased risk applies to all of the major ethnic and religious groups encompassed by the broad term south Asian. A high genetic susceptibility to insulin resistance and diabetes is triggered by inactivity and abdominal obesity leading to low plasma high-density lipoprotein (HDL) levels, increased plasma triglycerides, hypertension, and hyperglycaemia (the metabolic syndrome) or frank diabetes which in turn leads to increased risk of coronary heart disease. In a prospective cohort study in south London, Farouhi *et al.* (2006) assessed conventional cardiovascular risk factors and those associated with insulin resistance in Asian men. They confirmed the very high heart disease mortality in Asian men and the high prevalence of diabetes but from a multivariate analysis they concluded that conventional risk factors, insulin resistance and the metabolic syndrome criteria could not fully explain the high heart disease mortality in Asian men; unmeasured risk factors contributed to this risk.

Most authors who write about this topic assume that south Asians in Britain are less active than the rest of the population and that this contributes to their increased levels of obesity, diabetes and heart disease. In a systematic review of the literature, Fischbacher *et al.* (2004) found evidence of substantially lower levels of activity among all south Asian groups in the UK. Although there were methodological flaws in the 17 studies that they reviewed (12 adult studies and 5 with children) they did nevertheless confirm the general assumption of high levels of inactivity contributing towards their diabetes and heart disease risk.

Dietary comparison of ethnic groups in Britain

The household Food and Expenditure Survey (Department for Environment, Food and Rural Affairs (DEFRA), 2006) now publishes comparisons of the food and drink purchases of families classified into different ethnic groups according to the ethnicity of the household reference person (HRP). The results of this comparison need to be treated cautiously because 95 per cent of the families were classified as white and because there are some differences in average family composition and age structure between the ethnic groups. Table 17.1 shows a

Table 17.1 A selective comparison of the food purchases and expenditure of British families where the household reference person is classified as white, Asian or black British*

Household purchases (all g or mL/pp/week)	Asian	Black	White
Milk and cream	1948	1319	2031
Cheese	48	44	117
All meat and products	605	919	1073
Fats and oils	275	203	182
Potatoes	460	485	875
Confectionery	70	61	135
All alcohol (home and outside)	337	507	1496
Average gross weekly household income (£ per week)	640	424	565
Expenditure (pence/pp/week excluding alcohol)			
All household food and drink	1423	1520	2149
All eating out	478	429	765

*Data source: DEFRA, 2006.

very selective comparison of the purchases and expenditure of families classified as white, Asian or black British; examples of substantial differences between these groupings have been selectively included in this table. Compared with the majority white category, the Asia families purchased:

- slightly less milk and cream and much less cheese
- much less meat and meat products
- more fats and oils
- less potatoes
- less confectionery
- much less alcohol.

The Asian grouping also spent much less per head on both household food and eating out than the white majority, despite having a higher average gross household income. Compared with the white majority the black grouping purchased:

- much less milk and cream and much less cheese
- slightly less meat and meat products
- slightly more fats and oils
- much less potatoes, confectionery and alcohol.

The black grouping also spent much less per head than the white majority on both household food and eating out, and they also had a much lower gross weekly household income. Some of these differences are very predictable in light of cultural differences between the three groups such as:

- the low meat purchasing of Asians because it includes a large number of vegetarian Hindus
- the high potato consumption of the white grouping reflects the importance of potatoes as a staple in the traditional British diet
- the low alcohol consumption of the Asian group because it contains many Muslims who should not drink.

Table 17.2 shows selected comparisons between these groups of nutrient intakes estimated from the recorded food purchases. In general, the estimated micronutrient intakes of the Asian and black groupings are less than that of the white majority. In several cases the average intakes of micronutrients fall below the RNI in one or both of the non-white groups, e.g. for calcium in the black grouping and for iron, zinc and vitamin A in both the black and Asian groupings. The low calcium intakes are in line with the low milk and cheese purchases of the two non-white groups and the iron and zinc are in line

Table 17.2 A selective comparison of nutrient
intakes in British families where the household
reference person is classified as white, Asian or
black British. Nutrient intakes have been estimated
from food purchases*

Nutrient intake as % RNI	Asian	Black	White
Total energy (% EAR including alcohol)	93	85	98
Calcium	109	89	130
Iron	84	87	106
Zinc	86	89	104
Folate	113	120	139
Vitamin A	90	88	127

Macronutrient as % food energy (excluding alcohol)			
Fat	36.3	35.9	37.8
Saturated fatty acids	11.9	11.7	15.0
Carbohydrate	51.9	50.7	48.0
Non-milk extrinsic sugars	12.7	15.6	15.7
Starch and intrinsic sugars	39.2	35.2	32.3

RNI, reference nutrient intake; EAR, estimated average
requirement.
*Data source: DEFRA, 2006.

with the lower meat intakes of the non-white
groups. When macronutrients are expressed as a
percentage of food energy (excluding alcohol) then
the white group has the highest total fat intake,
highest added sugar intake and the lowest carbohydrate intake. The saturated fat intake of the white
group is much higher than the other two (reflecting
their lower use of meat, cheese and milk and
cream). The Asian group has a much higher intake
of starch than the white group. These differences in
macronutrient content between the Asian and
white groups are, as noted earlier, superficially at
odds with the high rates of coronary heart disease
and high obesity rates recorded in British Asians.

Key points

- The health statistics of racial minorities are
  often worse than those of the majority
  population.
- Native Americans are much more likely to be
  obese and to develop the metabolic syndrome
  and type 2 diabetes than other Americans.
- Obesity and alcohol-related problems are major
  contributors to the generally poor health record
  of Native Americans.

- Black Americans have shorter life expectancy
  and higher heart diseases mortality than white
  Americans.
- The relatively poor health statistics of black
  Americans can be largely attributed to their
  relative poverty and this probably applies to
  other minority groups in industrialized countries.
- African Caribbeans and south Asians are the
  largest racial minority groups in the UK.
- The potential problems of a lactovegetarian diet
  are relevant to many British Asians who are
  lactovegetarian for religious reasons.
- Rickets and poor vitamin D status are prevalent
  among British Asians due to the combined
  effects of low dietary availability and low
  endogenous synthesis because of inadequate
  exposure of the skin to sunlight.
- People of African and Caribbean origin have
  high prevalence of hypertension because they
  are genetically sensitive to the hypertensive
  effects of salt.
- Coronary heart disease is very prevalent among
  British Asians even among those who are
  lactovegetarian and even though they generally
  have lower exposure to several established risk
  factors than the white population.
- High rates of inactivity and abdominal obesity
  leading to insulin resistance among British
  Asians probably accounts for their susceptibility
  to coronary heart disease.
- Despite some methodological problems there is
  a substantial body of evidence which suggests
  that all south Asian groups are more inactive
  than the rest of the UK population.
- Insulin resistance and abdominal obesity of
  British Asians leads to frank diabetes or the
  metabolic syndrome which in turn predisposes
  them to premature heart disease.
- Rates of type 2 diabetes are around five times
  higher in British Asians than in the rest of the
  population.
- Dietary comparisons between white, Asian
  and black British families suggest substantial
  differences in the food purchasing and
  expenditure of these three groupings (see
  Table 17.1 for examples).
- Asian and black families purchase much less
  alcohol than white British families.
- Asian and black families' food purchases contain
  less essential micronutrients per person than

those of white families and in several cases the estimated average intakes of the non-white groups are well below the RNI.

- Compared with white families the purchases of Asian families contain less fat, much less saturated fat, more carbohydrate and much more starch (similar but slightly lower trends are seen in the black families).
- These dietary comparisons between British Asians and white Britons are superficially inconsistent with the high rates of obesity and heart disease recorded in British Asians.

NUTRITION AND PHYSICAL ACTIVITY

Fitness

It does not require scientific measurement to convince most of us that regular exercise leads to increased levels of physical fitness. Any sedentary person, who undertakes a programme of regular vigorous exercise, will soon notice that they can perform everyday activities such as garden and household chores, climbing stairs, walking uphill or running for a bus with much less breathlessness and pounding of the heart than previously. Simple personal monitoring would show a reduction in resting heart rate and smaller increases in pulse rate in response to an exercise load.

Scientific appraisal of the benefits of physical activity on long-term health or the effects of different training schedules on fitness requires a precise definition of fitness and an objective method of measuring it. This allows changes in fitness levels to be monitored during training and allows the fitness levels of different individuals or populations to be compared. The scientific criterion normally used to define fitness is the **aerobic capacity** or the rate of oxygen uptake of the subject when exercising maximally – **the VO$_{2max}$**. This VO$_{2max}$ is a measure of the functional capacity of the cardiopulmonary system to deliver oxygen to the body muscles and other tissues. Direct measurement of oxygen uptake in maximally exercising subjects is feasible but it requires relatively sophisticated laboratory equipment and trained personnel. It also requires subjects to perform sustained exercise to the limit of their capacity and this may be undesirable and sometimes dangerous in untrained people. The heart rate measured at several submaximal exercise levels is

therefore often used to derive a measure of aerobic capacity. In one widely used test, subjects cycle on a static bicycle ergometer at defined work loads. The external work performed by the subject is calculated from the speed of cycling and the resistance applied to the bicycle fly-wheel. In the steady state, heart rate is assumed to equate with oxygen uptake. Three graded levels of work are performed and the steady state heart rate is measured at each. The calculated work rate is then plotted against the heart rate on a graph and the best straight line drawn through the three points (see Figure 17.1). By extending this straight line, the graph can be used to predict the work rate at:

- the predicted maximum heart rate (220 – age in years) for the subject, **the maximum physical work capacity (PWC$_{max}$)**
- at a defined heart rate, e.g. the physical work capacity at 170 beats per minute, the **(PWC$_{170}$)**.

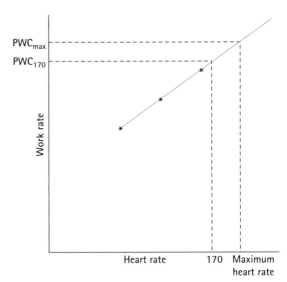

Figure 17.1 *A graph of work load against heart rate. The straight line through the three measured points can be used to predict the physical work capacity (PWC)$_{170}$ or the PWC$_{max}$.*

The rate of 170 beats per minute is approximately 85 per cent of the maximum heart rate in young adults and using this value involves less extrapolation than predicting to maximum heart rate. In older subjects a lower defined heart rate would be used. Similar tests are available that involve walking or running on a treadmill rather than the use of a static bicycle. Conditioning of the cardiopulmonary system to produce measurable improvements in aerobic capacity requires that the system be significantly exerted for sustained periods, i.e. three sessions each week in which heart rate is raised to 60–70 per cent of maximum for at least 20 minutes' duration.

Regular exercise not only produces measurable increases in aerobic capacity but also produces other rapid and readily demonstrable benefits in the short term, such as those listed below.

- Training increases muscle strength.
- Training increases endurance, i.e. the maximum duration that one is able to sustain a particular activity. Both the endurance of individual trained muscle groups and the endurance of the cardiopulmonary system are increased.
- Training improves or maintains joint mobility or flexibility, i.e. the range of movements that subjects are able to safely and comfortably perform is increased.
- Training increases or at least maintains muscle mass. During bouts of sustainable activity like aerobics, jogging or walking the supply of oxygen to the muscles is sufficient for the muscle to produce energy by the normal **aerobic** (oxygen-requiring) processes, hence **aerobic exercise**. The most effective exercises for increasing muscle mass are high intensity, short duration activities where the effort involved is close to the maximum, e.g. lifting a heavy weight, pushing against a resistance, press ups, jumping, climbing stairs or sprinting. Such exercises are so intense that the oxygen supply to the muscle is insufficient to produce all the energy needed for the intense activity and so the muscle temporarily 'tops up' the energy supply by switching to energy-producing processes that are **anaerobic** (not requiring oxygen) hence **anaerobic exercise.**
- Training leads to measurable increases in psychological wellbeing, including less depression.

Several of these latter benefits of exercise accrue at intensities and durations of activity that are considerably below those necessary to produce measurable changes in aerobic capacity. These latter effects of increased strength, endurance and flexibility may be of even greater importance to some subjects than increases in aerobic fitness, e.g. in the elderly. Note that in Chapter 15 it was suggested that much of

the loss of physical capacity and functional disability associated with ageing is not a result of the ageing process *per se* but is largely the result of inactivity. Even in extreme old age resistance training resulted in measurable increases in strength and functional ability (Fiatarone *et al.*, 1994). A 40-minute walk, three times a week, increased the aerobic fitness of a group of Texans in their 70s and after 6 months they had aerobic capacities that were typical of 50-year-old Texans.

There is also a substantial body of evidence suggesting that participation in regular physical activity produces psychological as well as physiological benefits. It improves the general sense of wellbeing and self-confidence, improves the ability to cope with stress and may even reduce the frequency and severity of personality disorders. Some of these psychological benefits may well be a consequence of the physiological conditioning (see Hayden and Allen, 1984; Fentem, 1992; Bowen *et al.*, 2006).

It is now recognized that setting activity targets for the general population based on the 20 minutes of vigorous exercise (60–70 per cent of maximum heart rate) is probably unrealistic. In both the UK and USA, encouraging moderate physical activity is seen as a more realistic health promotion goal and offers the prospect of greater health benefits for the population as a whole (see Table 17.3 for a quantitative grading of activity levels). The latest Health Education Authority guidelines for adults in the UK is that they should aim for at least 30 minutes of moderate activity on at least five occasions each week and that this 30 minutes can be accumulated in up to three shorter 10-minute activity sessions (see Sproston and Primatesta 2004).

In the *Health of the nation* (DH, 1992), the stated intention of the British government is 'to develop detailed strategies to increase physical activity' in the light of the activity and fitness levels found in the Allied Dunbar National Fitness Survey (1992). In the follow-up document *Saving lives – our healthier nation* the benefits of increased physical activity are mentioned several times and there is general encouragement to increase levels of physical activity and fitness.

Healthy people 2010 in the USA (DHHS, 2000) set a number of specific targets for increasing physical activity by 2010 including:

- to reduce to 20 per cent the proportion of adults engaging in no leisure-time physical activity.

Table 17.3 Variation by age and sex in the percentage of English adults who reported engaging in different periods of 30 minutes of at least moderate-level activity

Weekly occasions	Age in years					Total
	16–24	25–44	45–64	65–74	75+	
5 or more						
Male	53	43	35	17	8	37
Female	30	29	27	13	3	24
1–4 sessions						
Male	29	36	30	32	20	31
Female	39	44	35	31	14	36
None						
Male	18	22	35	52	72	32
Female	31	27	38	56	82	40

Vigorous activity is that where the energy expenditure is at least 7.5 kcal (30 kJ)/min
Moderate activity is 5–7.5 kcal (20–30 kJ)/min
Light is 2–5 kcal(8–20 kJ)/min
Inactive <2 kcal(8 kJ)/min
Moderate activities: walking a mile (1.6 km) at brisk or fast pace; heavy gardening work such as digging or cutting large areas of grass by hand; heavy do-it-yourself work such as knocking down walls or breaking up concrete; heavy housework such as walking with heavy loads of shopping or scrubbing/polishing floors by hand. Vigorous activities: running or jogging; playing squash; several other sporting activities if it caused the subject to breathe heavily or sweat a lot such as aerobics, tennis, weight training or swimming.

- 30 per cent of adults should be engaging in 30 minutes of daily moderate activity
- 30 per cent of adults should engage in 20 minutes of vigorous physical activity of 20 minutes' duration on at least three occasions each week
- to increase the number of adults who engage in physical activities that enhance and maintain flexibility, muscle strength and endurance.

Current levels of physical activity and fitness

The average levels of physical activity of the populations of the wealthy industrialized countries have, by general agreement, declined in recent decades. Car ownership, workplace automation and labour saving aids in the home and garden have drastically reduced the amount of obligatory physical exertion that most people are now required to undertake. Any increases in voluntary leisure-time activities have not been enough to offset this reduction in obligatory activity. The average Briton now watches twice as much television as they did in the 1960s and many people spend more time watching television than they do at work or school. Between 1975

and 1995 the average distance walked by British adults fell by about 20 per cent.

The increased levels of overweight and obesity in the UK and USA in recent decades have occurred despite a sharp decline in average energy intakes and this gives indirect evidence of the scale of this reduction in activity (discussed in Chapter 8). Energy expenditure (i.e. activity) has been declining faster than the decline in energy intake.

There are estimates of activity levels of the American population in *Healthy People 2010* (DHHS, 2000). The examples listed below were estimates for 1997.

- 40 per cent of American adults engaged in no leisure-time physical activity (i.e. no activity that substantially increased the rate of energy expenditure). Rates of inactivity were higher in black and Hispanic Americans and rates decreased substantially with increasing educational attainment and increased steadily with advancing age. Similar racial, educational and age trends were seen in the other measures of activity listed below.

- Only 15 per cent of adults engaged in 30 minutes of moderate activity on 5 or more days each week rising to 31 per cent if the criterion is reduced to 20 minutes of moderate activity on 3 or more days per week.
- 23 per cent of adults engaged in sufficient vigorous physical activity to improve cardiorespiratory fitness.

Table 17.3 summarizes activity levels determined by interview in a health survey of English adults (Sproston and Primatesta, 2004). Only just over a third of the men and a quarter of the women reported engaging in the recommended five 30-minute periods of moderate activity each week. Well over a third of adults recorded no 30-minute periods of moderate activity each week rising to more than half of those aged 65–74 years. As with the American data discussed earlier, activity levels declined markedly with increasing age and people with higher educational qualifications were more active.

The Allied Dunbar National Fitness Survey (1992) also found very low levels of reported physical activity and low levels of aerobic fitness among a representative sample of 4000 English adults. This survey report suggested that 70 per cent of men and 80 per cent of women had lower levels of physical activity than would be necessary to achieve aerobic fitness. For around a third of men and two-thirds of the women, walking at 4.8 kmph (3mph) up a gradient of 1:20 would be difficult, with even higher proportions in the over 65s. A large number of women over 35 years would find even walking at 4.8 kmph on the flat severely exerting and would need to rest or slow down after a few minutes. Many elderly women do not have enough strength in their legs to rise from a chair without using their arms. Many elderly and even middle-aged people do not have enough shoulder flexibility to allow them to wash their own hair in comfort.

There is also convincing evidence that activity levels of children in Britain have decreased sharply in recent decades. As previously noted in Chapter 8, Durnin (1992) has suggested that average energy intakes of teenagers were up to a third higher in the 1930s than in the early 1990s. Several other studies have also found a reduction in recorded energy intakes of various age groups of children in recent decades. Over these same decades British children have got taller and fatter and this must indicate a decrease in their energy expenditure via physical activity. It was argued in Chapter 8 that the rising prevalence of childhood obesity is primarily a result of declining activity rather than dietary changes *per se*. There was a 20 per cent decrease in walking among British children in the 10 years up to 1995 and a 25 per cent decrease in the amount of cycling. Between 1975 and 1995 the annual distance walked by children in the 11–15-year category dropped a third from 399 km (248 miles) in 1975 to 320 km (199 miles) in 1994. In the NDNS survey of British schoolchildren (Gregory *et al.*, 2000) it was reported that children were taller and heavier than in a similar study conducted in 1982–83 but had lower energy intakes. This clearly points to a decline in energy expenditure, i.e. activity over this period. Data on activity *per se* were collected for those children aged over 7 years and this indicates that young people in Britain are inactive. Some of these findings are summarized below.

- Girls were generally less active than boys.
- A third of boys aged 7–14 years did not participate in at least 1 hour of moderate activity each day (the Health Education Authority recommendation for young people) and this rose to half of those aged 14–18 years.
- In girls, over half of 7–14 year olds and over a third of the older group failed to meet the Health Education Authority recommended activity level.

In *Healthy People 2010* evidence is also presented of the current levels (1999) of activity of American children with targets set for 2010. Some of these are:

- to increase the proportion of adolescents who participate in at least five weekly sessions of 30 minutes of at least moderate activity from 27 per cent to 35 per cent
- to increase the proportion of adolescents who engage in three weekly sessions of activity vigorous enough to promote cardiorespiratory fitness from 65 per cent to 85 per cent
- to increase the proportion of schools that require daily physical education for students and to increase the proportion of children who participate in them
- to increase the proportion of adolescents who watch television for fewer than 2 hours on school days from 57 per cent to 75 per cent.

Key points

- Scientific assessment of fitness uses some measure of aerobic capacity such as the maximum oxygen uptake (VO_{2max}).
- Aerobic capacity is usually extrapolated from pulse rates measured at submaximal exercise loads.
- Measurable increases in VO_{2max} require regular and significant exertion for sustained periods, typically three weekly sessions of 20-minute duration when heart intake is raised to 60–70 per cent of maximum.
- Training also maintains muscle mass, increases strength, endurance and flexibility and produces beneficial psychological effects.
- These other benefits of exercise are discernible at lower intensities than that required to produce increases in VO_{2max}.
- The overall activity levels of affluent populations have decreased substantially in recent decades.
- Increasing mechanization has greatly reduced occupational energy expenditure and the energy required to perform the tasks of everyday living.
- The Allied Dunbar National Fitness Survey and the Health Survey for England have confirmed the extreme inactivity and low levels of aerobic fitness, flexibility and strength of many adult Britons.
- Children are also much less active than they were even 20 years ago.

Long-term health benefits of physical activity

In the short term, increased physical activity improves aerobic capacity, endurance, strength, flexibility and various aspects of psychological wellbeing. Over a period of weeks or months it also leads to changes in appearance and body composition; increased lean to fat ratio and improved muscle tone. It is inevitable that low levels of physical activity will lead to reduced energy requirements and predispose people to becoming overweight and obese. In the longer term, regular exercise contributes to reduced morbidity and mortality from several of the diseases of industrialization and therefore increases both life expectancy and years of healthy life. Some the health benefits of regular exercise and increased fitness are summarized in Box 17.1.

Box 17.1 Some of the demonstrable benefits of regular exercise and increased physical fitness

- Increased activity and fitness is associated with increased bone density in children and younger adults (e.g. Pocock et al., 1986) and reduced levels of osteoporotic fracture in elderly people (e.g. Wickham et al., 1989). More examples are given in Chapter 13.
- Increased physical activity (Paffenbarger et al., 1986) and high level of aerobic fitness (Blair et al., 1989) are associated with reduced all-cause mortality in men and women. These benefits are detectable even in the elderly and may even become more pronounced with age.
- Although most early studies of the benefits of exercise were conducted in men, it is clear that the same dose-dependent benefits on all-cause mortality are also seen in women (Oguma et al., 2002).
- Middle-aged male civil servants who participated in vigorous leisure-time activities had reduced risk of coronary heart disease as compared with those who do not (Morris et al., 1980).
- Men with active jobs have less heart attacks than those in similar but less active jobs (see Leon, 1985).
- There are psychological benefits resulting from increased physical activity (Fentem, 1992; Bowen et al., 2006). These may be direct effects of the physical activity, or indirect effects caused by the improved physical capabilities and conditioning that increased activity brings with it.
- Exercise maintains the ability to perform the activities of daily living as people become elderly and so maintains the morale, self-esteem and quality of life of older people (see Bennet and Morgan, 1992).
- Increased activity leads to increased energy expenditure, both directly and as a result of the associated higher lean body (muscle) mass (particularly important in the elderly).
- Exercise increases the anti-atherogenic HDL-cholesterol concentration in blood (Macnair, 1994).
- Those who are physically fit seem to be protected against the consequences of being overweight or even mildly obese (Lee et al., 1998). Discussed in Chapter 8.
- Regular moderate exercise reduced the frequency of colds in post-menopausal women in a study lasting for 1 year (Chubak et al., 2006).

Regular, sustained and moderate (aerobic) activity should aid in the long-term control of body weight. Inactivity undoubtedly predisposes to becoming overweight and obese. Regular physical activity is more likely to be effective as a preventative measure rather than as a relatively short-term measure to cure established obesity. An exercise programme is nonetheless an important adjunct to dietary management of obesity. It increases the chances that any short-term weight losses will be sustained in the longer term (see Chapter 8 for a discussion of the role of inactivity in causing obesity and the role of exercise in its treatment).

Exercise increases and maintains bone density and therefore protects against osteoporosis. For example, Pocock et al. (1986) found physical fitness to be a major determinant of bone density in two regions frequently associated with osteoporotic fracture, the neck of the femur and the lumbar spine. Other examples of studies that indicate positive benefits of weight-bearing exercise and physical fitness on bone health can be found in Chapter 14. Note, however, that extremes of physical exercise in women that are accompanied by very low body weight and amenorrhoea almost certainly accelerate bone loss and predispose to osteoporosis (see Chapter 14).

Regular physical activity is protective against cardiovascular disease. This may be a direct effect, e.g. by strengthening heart muscle or an indirect consequence of its effects on other risk factors. Physical activity reduces the tendency to overweight, insulin resistance and maturity-onset diabetes, it lowers blood pressure and has beneficial effects on blood lipid profiles (e.g. Blair et al., 1989). As far back as 1980 Morris et al. found that middle-aged men who participated in vigorous leisure-time activity had lower rates of both fatal and non-fatal coronary heart disease than those who did not. This was based upon an 8.5-year cohort study of 18 000 middle aged, male British civil servants. This apparent protective effect of exercise was maintained in all age groups and in subgroups classified according to smoking behaviour, family history of coronary heart disease and even in those with existing hypertension and subclinical angina. They concluded that vigorous exercise has 'a protective effect in the ageing heart against ischaemia and its consequences'.

Several studies have looked at the comparative mortality of different occupational groups with differing levels of work-related activity (reviewed by Leon, 1985). Farmers and farm labourers have been the subject of several such studies because of the perception that their work required considerable activity. Studies in California, North Dakota, Georgia and Iowa have all found lower levels of heart disease among farm workers than other inhabitants of these regions (Pomrehn et al., 1982). Less smoking and higher levels of activity were identified as differences between farmers and non-farmers in these studies. Pomrehn et al. (1982) analysed all death certificates in the state of Iowa over the period 1964–78 for men aged 20–64 years. They compared death rates of farmers and non-farmers in Iowa over that period. They found that farmers had lower all-cause mortality and mortality from heart disease than non-farmers. They also compared the lifestyle and dietary characteristics of a sample of farmers and non-farmers living in Iowa in 1973. They found that the farmers were significantly less likely to smoke (19 per cent vs 46 per cent of non-farmers), were more active, were fitter and drank less alcohol. The farmers in their sample also had significantly higher total serum cholesterol levels. They concluded that the reduced total and heart disease mortality of farmers could be attributed to a lifestyle that included regular physical activity and much less use of alcohol and tobacco than non-farmers.

In a 16-year cohort study of 17 000 Harvard graduates, ranging in age from 35 to 74 years, Paffenbarger et al. (1986) found that reported exercise level was strongly and inversely related to total mortality. They used reported levels of walking, stair climbing and sports play to calculate a relative activity index. The relative risk of death of those with an index of around 3500 kcal (14 MJ) per week was around half that of those with an index of less than 500 kcal (2 MJ) per week. They found that mortality among the physically active was lower with or without consideration of other confounding factors, such as hypertension, cigarette smoking, body weight or weight gain since leaving college and early parental death.

In an 8-year cohort study of over 13 000 men and women, Blair et al. (1989) found a strong inverse correlation in both sexes between measured fitness level and relative risk of death from all causes. The apparent protective effect of fitness was not affected by correcting for likely confounding variables. In Chapter 8 there is a discussion of the data of Blair and his colleagues (Lee et al., 1998) which suggests that people who are overweight or mildly obese but have high levels of aerobic fitness do not have excess mortality as compared those who have similar fitness but are lean. Aerobic fitness seems to offset the usual health risks associated with being overweight or obese.

Most expert reports dealing with strategies for reducing chronic disease and improving long-term health emphasize the importance of increased physical activity and often highlight its role in maintaining normal body weight, e.g. COMA (1994a) report of cardiovascular disease and COMA (1998) dealing with dietary aspects of cancer prevention.

Key point

Some of the long-term benefits of regular exercise and increased fitness are summarized in Table 17.3.

Diet as a means to improving physical performance

Body weight, athletic performance and energy intake

Athletes in training expend considerably more energy than the average person for whom the dietary reference values are intended. Their total energy expenditure during training and competition may be well over twice their basal metabolic rate (BMR) as compared with the 1.4 or 1.5 times BMR assumed when dietary reference values (DRVs) are set. During the 10 days of the Tour de France cycle race, athletes may expend 3.5–5.5 times their BMR (see Wilson, 1994). One would also therefore expect that the energy and nutrient intakes of those in training would be considerably higher than those of the average person. Even though requirements for some nutrients may be increased by heavy exercise, one would therefore expect that athletes should still be unlikely to have problems of dietary inadequacy.

In some events, where performance is judged on aesthetic appeal (e.g. gymnastics, ice skating and dancing) thinness may be seen to increase the chances of a favourable verdict by judges. In some sports (e.g. middle- and long-distance running, jumping and cycling) being light may improve performance. In some sports, competitors are divided up into weight categories and competitors of both sexes

may starve themselves to make the weight or even dehydrate themselves. These pressures may cause some athletes to consume much less than one would expect. Many female athletes in particular have much lower energy intakes than might be expected from their activity levels. According to Wilson (1994) average recorded intakes of female runners in several studies were only about 100 kcal (420 kJ)/day higher than those recorded in non-athletes. This means that unless their diets are nutrient dense then even small increases in nutrient requirements due to exercise may become significant in athletes with such unexpectedly low energy intakes.

Many female athletes have such low body weights that they cease to menstruate and have low levels of circulating sex hormones. This may adversely affect their bone health. It may make them more prone to stress fractures and increase their risk of developing osteoporosis in later life. Several studies have suggested that there is high prevalence of eating disorders among female athletes competing in events where low body weight might be considered advantageous (Wilson, 1994). The female athlete triad is a condition in which there are no menstrual periods, disordered eating and osteoporosis brought on by inadequate energy intake.

Energy and nutrient requirements

Adequate intakes of dietary energy and of micronutrients are prerequisites for maximum athletic performance. There is, however, no convincing evidence that any particular vitamin or mineral supplements boost performance in already well-nourished individuals. There may be small increases in the requirements for some water-soluble vitamins in those undertaking vigorous training schedules, e.g. vitamin C, thiamin, niacin and riboflavin. Nevertheless a well-balanced diet should contain sufficient of these vitamins, especially as total food intake will be higher during training. Some vitamins are toxic in excess (e.g. vitamins A and D) and excesses of some others may actually impair performance (e.g. niacin).

In their joint position statement, the American College of Sports Medicine and two other North American organizations stated that athletes who obtain adequate energy from a variety of sources will get adequate amounts of vitamins and minerals from their food. Supplements may, however, be required by athletes who restrict their energy intake, use severe weight-loss practices, restrict whole food groups from their diet or consume a high-carbohydrate diet with low micronutrient density (American College of Sports Medicine, American Dietetic Association, Dietitians of Canada (ACSM, ADA and DC), 2000).

Iron status has frequently been reported to be low and iron requirements to be increased in athletes, particularly endurance athletes. This situation with regard to iron is complicated because endurance training produces a haemodilution effect similar to that described in pregnancy in Chapter 15. Training increases plasma volume and total circulating red cell mass but the relatively larger increase in plasma volume causes blood haemoglobin concentration to fall. True anaemia (low circulating haemoglobin) and iron deficiency (low amounts of iron stored as **ferritin**) in athletes are usually due to low dietary intake. This would be particularly likely in athletes, often female athletes, who restrict their energy intake to keep their body weight low. Exercise may increase iron losses and it may impair the increase in iron absorption that normally occurs when iron stores are low. Training may thus slightly increase iron requirements and poor iron intakes during training may precipitate iron deficiency or even anaemia in some athletes, especially female ones. Anaemia would certainly impair athletic performance particularly in endurance events. Indeed artificially boosting blood haemoglobin levels is used as an unfair way of trying to boost performance.

The protein requirements and optimal protein intakes of athletes and bodybuilders has been the subject of hundreds of studies stretching back over several decades. Although a detailed analysis of these studies is beyond the scope of this book, a few general conclusions are listed below.

- Prolonged heavy exercise does increase protein losses slightly as amino acids start to be used as substrates.
- Habitual protein intakes are almost always well in excess of requirements.
- If athletes consume sufficient energy and carbohydrate, any specific measures to boost protein intakes are unnecessary even in ultra-endurance events.
- The large protein supplements taken by many athletes are almost certainly ineffective either

in increasing muscle mass or boosting athletic performance.
- It was noted in Chapter 10 that excess protein intakes have been speculatively suggested to have adverse long-term consequences, e.g. increased risk of chronic renal failure.

Contrary to the conclusions of several other expert groups, the ACSM, ADA and DC (2000) position statement does conclude that protein requirements are higher in very active persons and suggest that protein intakes should be raised to 1.6–1.7 g/kg body weight in resistance athletes and 1.2–1.4 g/kg in endurance athletes. These quantities of protein can be obtained from normal food in athletes who are eating enough to meet their raised energy requirements.

Substrate utilization during exercise and its implications

In explosive events like short sprints, jumping or throwing, the energy supply of the muscle during the event is mainly from **creatine phosphate** plus a contribution from the anaerobic metabolism of glycogen. Creatine phosphate is the muscle's short-term energy reserve and it can be used to convert ADP to ATP by transfer of a phosphate moiety:

$$\text{Creatine P} + \text{ADP} \rightarrow \text{ATP} + \text{creatine}$$

Creatine is present in the diet in meat and fish and can be synthesized in sufficient quantities for normal circumstances from other amino acids even if a vegetarian diet is eaten. Some athletes do take supplements of creatine, which do elevate the stores of creatine in muscles. In the longer sprints and other events when there is more sustained and very intense activity, then energy supply comes from creatine phosphate, anaerobic metabolism of glycogen plus a contribution from the aerobic metabolism of glycogen. The build-up of lactate from the anaerobic metabolism of glycogen will produce fatigue and limit performance.

In endurance events then the aerobic metabolism of glucose plus a contribution from the metabolism of fat are the major sources of energy. In any endurance event or competitive sport (or even a long training session for a more explosive event), the depletion of muscle glycogen is a factor that potentially limits sustained high performance. One would expect glycogen stores in liver and muscle to be depleted after 1.5–2 hours of vigorous exercise and depletion of muscle glycogen leads to fatigue – the so called 'wall' that affects marathon runners. Training for endurance events increases muscle glycogen stores. Training also increases the aerobic capacity of muscles enabling them to use fatty acids more effectively. As the duration of exercise increases, so the contribution made by fatty acids to the total energy supply of the muscle increases. Once glycogen reserves have been used up then running speed is limited by the speed at which fatty acids can be metabolized aerobically.

Maximizing the glycogen stores in muscle and liver are now seen as a key element in the preparation for competition in endurance sports (i.e. longer than 1 hour of sustained heavy exercise). In some endurance sports it may also be possible to take in extra carbohydrate during the event. In experimental studies, the maximum duration for which heavy exercise (75 per cent of VO_{2max}) can be sustained is directly proportional to the glycogen content of the muscle at the start. Exhaustion occurs when the muscle glycogen reserves are completely depleted. High-carbohydrate diets (70 per cent of energy) during training increase the muscle glycogen content and so increase the maximum duration that heavy exercise can be sustained. In their position statement ACSM, ADA and DC (2000) suggested that in diets for athletes, fat should provide 20–25 per cent of the energy (i.e. 75–80 per cent from protein and carbohydrate) but that less than 15 per cent of energy from fat offered no health or performance benefits. This moderate level of fat should provide adequate amounts of essential fatty acids and fat-soluble vitamins and help provide adequate energy for weight maintenance. Many endurance athletes manipulate their diets and exercise schedules prior to competition in an attempt to increase their body glycogen stores – **carbohydrate loading**. This extra carbohydrate also increases muscle water content which may not be advantageous for those in explosive events where the size of muscle glycogen stores is not critical.

There are several theories about the best way to increase muscle glycogen stores – one regimen that is not associated with any obvious side effects is for the athlete to eat a normal high-carbohydrate diet during heavy training up to a week before the event. Then in the week before competition, a mixed diet (50 per cent carbohydrate) is eaten for the first 3 days followed by a very-high-carbohydrate diet (75 per cent carbohydrate) during the rest of the week. Training intensity is wound down in the second half of the week with a complete rest on the day before the competition. A high-carbohydrate diet should be continued during the week following competition to replenish carbohydrate stores. Carbohydrate taken in the first hour or two following the completion of the event seems to be most effective in replenishing muscle glycogen stores.

The need to prevent dehydration

A marathon runner competing in a warm environment may expect to lose up to 6 L of sweat during the run and, even in a more temperate climate, sweat losses will often be in the range 3–4 L. Prolonged exercise, particularly in a hot environment, can lead to dehydration which produces fatigue and reduces work capacity. Profuse sweating and an inability to dissipate excess body heat in a warm, humid environment may lead to a combination of dehydration and hyperthermia, **heat stroke**, which can have serious, even fatal, consequences. Ideally, marathon runners should drink 0.5 L of fluid 15–30 minutes before competition and then take small, regular drinks (say every 4.8 km (3 miles)) although competitive rules may prevent drink stops in the early part of the race. Ideally the athlete should take in enough water to replace that which is lost rather than simply drink enough to satisfy thirst. These principles apply not just to marathon runners but anyone participating in events that involve long periods of heavy exertion and sweating, e.g. tennis players, long-distance cyclists and soccer players.

The ACSM, ADA and DC (2000) recommend that athletes should be well-hydrated before starting to exercise and should drink enough during and/or after exercise to balance fluid losses. They suggest that the consumption of sports' drinks containing carbohydrates and electrolytes during exercise will help to maintain blood glucose, maintain fuel supplies to the muscles and prevent dehydration and sodium depletion.

The following referenced reviews about nutrition for exercise and sport may be useful for further reading: Eastwood and Eastwood (1988), Powers and Howley (1990) and Williams (2006).

Key points

- Athletes in training expend much more energy than the average person for whom dietary reference values (DRVs) are intended.

- Low body weight and consequent amenorrhoea are common among female athletes who restrict their energy intake to enhance performance or because judges favour lean competitors.

- Amenorrhoea reduces bone density in female athletes and can make them more susceptible to stress fractures and to osteoporosis in later life.

- Requirements for some nutrients may be increased slightly by prolonged training.

- A balanced diet should provide sufficient nutrients even during training unless total energy intake is severely restricted.

- There is no convincing evidence that micronutrient supplements improve performance in those who are not deficient but large excesses of some nutrients can be toxic and hinder performance.

- The iron stores of some athletes are low and this is largely due to poor iron intake.

- Endurance training produces a haemodilution effect, which may exaggerate the apparent prevalence of iron deficiency anaemia among athletes.

- Prolonged heavy exercise may increase protein requirements slightly but habitual intakes are almost always well in excess of even these increased requirements.

- The ACSM, ADA, DC position statement did recommend protein intakes that were substantially above normal DRV but these amounts can still be obtained from normal food.

- There is no evidence that the large protein supplements taken by many athletes either increase performance or increase muscle mass.

- In explosive events, creatine phosphate is the principal source of muscle energy.

- Creatine is present in meat and fish and can be made from amino acids, nevertheless creatine supplements can increase creatine stores in muscle.

- In endurance events, depletion of muscle glycogen limits performance and so maximizing glycogen stores prior to competition is an important goal for endurance athletes.

- A high-carbohydrate diet increases muscle glycogen stores.

- Manipulating diet competition and training schedules during the week before competition can significantly increase glycogen stores – carbohydrate loading.

- Enormous amounts of fluid can be lost from the body during sustained heavy work or exercise.

- Dehydration produces fatigue, reduces work performance and can lead to potentially fatal heat stroke.

- Maintaining hydration during prolonged heavy exercise enhances performance but thirst is an insensitive indicator of dehydration in these circumstances.

- Sports drinks consumed during exercise can help maintain glucose supplies and prevent dehydration and sodium depletion.

PART FIVE

THE SAFETY AND QUALITY OF FOOD

18

The safety and quality of food

AIMS OF THE CHAPTER

This chapter provides an overview of factors that influence the safety and quality of food in industrialized countries and of the legal framework that has been designed to try to ensure food safety and quality. The major aims of this chapter are to give readers:

- enough understanding of the sources of potential hazard in their food to enable them to take practical measures to improve the safety and quality of their own food
- make a realistic evaluation of the real hazards posed by potential threats to food safety, i.e. to identify priorities for improved food safety
- a realistic appraisal of the likely benefits of regularly consuming the major categories of functional foods which are heavily marketed on their supposed health benefits.

CONSUMER PROTECTION

Food law

The webpages on UK and European food law prepared by Dr David Jukes of Reading University are recommended for anyone seeking further information on this topic (www.foodlaw.rdg.ac.uk). A discussion of US food legislation can be found in Tompson *et al.* (1991), and Fisher *et al.* (2006) is a more recent source for information on legal regulation of food and supplement labelling in the USA.

Food law has traditionally had three major aims.

- *To protect the health of consumers.* To ensure that food offered for human consumption is safe and fit for people to eat.
- *To prevent the consumer from being cheated.* Food laws try to ensure that verbal descriptions, labels and advertisements for food describe it honestly, and that manufacturers and retailers do not dishonestly pass off some substitute or inferior variant as the desired product.
- *To ensure fair competition between traders.* To prevent unscrupulous traders from gaining a competitive advantage by dishonestly passing off inferior and cheaper products as more expensive ones or by making dishonest claims about the merits of their product.

Another aim could be added for some current legislation governing the labelling of foods.

- *To facilitate healthy consumer choices.* To give consumers enough information about the nutritional content of foods to allow them to make informed food choices that increases their compliance with nutrition education guidelines and also warns them of the presence of ingredients they may wish or need to avoid.

In the UK, the first comprehensive food legislation was passed in the middle of the nineteenth century and there have been regular revisions and additions to this legislation ever since. The 1990 Food Safety Act is the latest version. The first food legislation was introduced in an attempt to combat widespread adulteration and misrepresentation of foods designed to cheat the consumer but also on occasion resulting in a product that was directly injurious to health. The sweetening of cider with sugar of lead (lead acetate) and addition of red lead to cayenne pepper are examples of practices with serious health repercussions for the consumer. The watering of milk (often with dirty water), addition of alum and bone ash to flour, dilution of pepper with brick dust and the bulking out of tea with floor sweepings are all examples of practices designed to cheat the consumer. The sale of meat from diseased animals slaughtered in knackers' yards and the passing off of horseflesh as beef has also occurred. Below are some of the main provisions of the UK 1990 Food Safety Act that illustrate a formal legal framework designed to achieve the aims listed above.

- It is illegal to add anything to food, take any constituent away, subject it to any treatment or process, or use any ingredient that would render the food injurious to health.
- It is forbidden to sell food not complying with food safety regulations. Food does not comply with food safety regulations if:
  - it has been rendered injurious to health by any of the above
  - if it is unfit for human consumption (e.g. food that contains high levels of food-poisoning bacteria)
  - if it is contaminated, e.g. by dirt, insect bodies, metal or glass fragments.
- It is illegal to sell any food not of the nature, substance or quality demanded by the purchaser. Customers are given a legal right to expect to be given what they ask for and to expect certain minimum standards for any food product.
- It is an offence to describe, label or advertise a food in a way that is calculated to mislead about its nature, substance or quality. This is an additional requirement on top of any specific food labelling requirements.

The 1990 Food Safety Act also empowers government ministers to issue, with parliamentary approval, specific regulations to ensure food safety, e.g. setting maximum permitted levels of contaminants. There are many such specific regulations or statutory instruments. For a successful prosecution under this act, it is not necessary to prove intent on the part of the manufacturer or retailer. The main defence against prosecution is for the defendant to show that they took all reasonable precautions and 'exercised due diligence' in trying to prevent the defect in the food.

Over the past couple of decades or so there have been a series of highly publicized alarms in Britain about the safety of food, most notably the bovine spongiform encephalopathy (BSE) crisis discussed later in the chapter. This undermined public confidence in the safety of British food and in the ability of the old Ministry of Agriculture, Fisheries and Food (MAFF) to balance the interests of farmers and food producers against those of consumers when dealing with food safety issues. As a consequence of these concerns, an independent **Food Standards Agency** (FSA) was established and began operating in 2000. This agency is charged with ensuring public health in relation to food. The Agency is expected to consult widely, assess scientific information impartially and give advice to ministers on legislation and controls that should ensure and improve food safety. The Agency is expected to take into account the costs and consequences of any proposed actions so that they are proportionate to the risks involved. MAFF has also been replaced by the **Department of Food, Environment and Rural Affairs**.

Enforcement of food legislation is, in the UK, primarily the responsibility of trading standards officers (TSOs) and environmental health officers (EHOs) employed by local authorities. The EHOs mainly deal with issues relating to food hygiene and the microbiological safety of food; they are involved in investigating food-poisoning outbreaks. The TSOs primarily deal with food labelling, advertising and the chemical safety of food. These officials do not just police the food safety laws but also give guidance and advice to local businesses relating to food safety issues.

The **Codex Alimentarius Commission** is an international body that was set up by the United Nations in 1962 in an attempt to establish international food standards. Over 160 countries are members of this commission. Membership of the commission does not oblige members to accept the international standards and most industrialized countries have retained their own national standards. This means that so far the commission has been a useful forum for international debate of food standards and safety issues, but the direct impact of its standards has been limited.

Key Points

- Food law exists to protect consumers' health and to try to ensure high standards of honesty and responsibility in food manufacturing and retailing.
- The 1990 Food Safety Act in UK makes it illegal to:
  - do anything to food that would make it harmful to health
  - sell food that is unfit to eat or does not comply with food safety regulations
  - dishonestly describe a food
  - sell food that is of unacceptable quality.
- UK ministers are also empowered by the 1990 Act to make specific food regulations subject to approval by parliament.
- An offence can be committed under the 1990 Act even if there is no intent, unless the defendant took all reasonable measures and care to try to avoid the defect in the food or its description.
- An independent food standards agency has been set up whose brief is to ensure public health in relation to food.
- Enforcement of food safety legislation in the UK is usually the responsibility of local government.
- The Codex Alimentarius Commission is an international body that sets international food standards.

Food labelling

Labelling in the UK

Most packaged foods in Britain must contain the following information on the label:

- the name of the food
- a list of ingredients
- an indication of its minimum durability
- an indication of any special storage conditions or conditions of use that are required (e.g. refrigerate, eat within 3 days of opening, etc.)
- most foods must be marked with a 'lot' so that they can be identified in the case of a problem that requires them to be withdrawn from sale

- the name and address of the manufacturer or packer of the food.

If a food is perishable and likely to become microbiologically unsafe after a relatively short storage period then it carries a **use by** date and it is illegal to offer for sale any food that is past its use by date. Such foods usually need to be stored in a refrigerator or chill cabinet and these foods should not be eaten after their use by date, e.g. cooked meats, ready meals, sandwiches, meat pies, etc. Other foods that are unlikely to become hazardous on storage are labelled with a **best before** date. Although unlikely to represent a hazard after that date, their eating quality may be impaired, e.g. biscuits (cookies), cakes, bread, chocolate. Foods may be legally offered for sale after their best before date provided they have not become unfit for human consumption.

In Britain and the European Union (EU) the ingredients of packaged foods must be listed in order of their prominence, by weight, in the final product. All additives must be listed and their function given. Certain foods are exempted from the requirement to carry a list of ingredients such as fresh fruit and vegetables, cheese, butter, alcoholic drinks and any food composed of a single ingredient. In Britain, the great majority of packaged foods also carry nutritional information on the labels. Most manufacturers voluntarily choose to include some nutritional information on their labels, and such nutrition labelling is compulsory if the manufacturer makes any nutritional claim for the product, e.g. low fat or high fibre. The minimum nutritional information the food must carry is the energy, protein, carbohydrate and fat content per 100 g together with the amount of any nutrient for which a claim is made.

The FSA has developed a new system for labelling foods that is intended to help consumers make healthier food choices based on the red, amber and green colours of traffic lights. It would like this **traffic light system** to be used on a range of processed foods, i.e. ready meals, pizzas, sandwiches, breakfast cereals, sausages, burgers, pies, and foods products with breadcrumb coatings. Many of the major British retailers and food manufacturers have started to use this system although each has adopted its own slightly different style of presentation. The system is intended to give information about four nutrients that we have been advised to

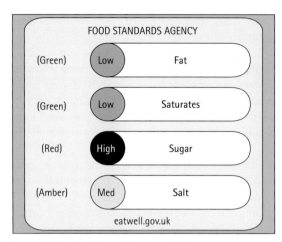

Figure 18.1 *The 'traffic light' food labelling system recommended by the Food Standards Agency in the UK.*

consume less of, namely: fat, saturated fat, sugar and salt (it is also sometimes used to indicate energy content). The red, amber and green lights on the label indicate the amounts of these four nutrients per 100 g of the food (see Figure 18.1):

* red = high
* amber = medium
* green = low.

This means that when comparing alternative versions of similar products consumers can see at a glance which is the healthier choice with respect to these four nutrients. Consumers are advised by the FSA that foods with a red light should be eaten occasionally or as a treat but that generally we should eat less of these. A green light means that the food is low in the nutrient and so the more green lights the healthier the choice. Amber light foods have moderate amounts of the nutrient and so are a reasonable choice most of the time, although consumers might wish to choose some foods with a green light for that nutrient on some occasions. When assessing overall food choices, consumers are advised to choose more green lights and not too many red lights (details of this traffic light system with illustrated examples can be found at the FSA's Eat well, be well webpage (www.eatwell.gov.uk/foodlabels/trafficlights/).

As at March 2007 some major retailers have actively chosen not to implement this system partly because of fears that red lights on a food may make consumers resist buying the food at all. An alternative

system based on **guideline daily amounts (GDAs)** has been developed and is favoured by some retailer (some use both the traffic light and the GDA system on their labels). GDAs are the approximate amounts of a nutrient that should be consumed each day in a healthy diet. They have been developed for men, women, adults and children for calories, fat, saturated fat, carbohydrate, total sugars, protein, fibre, salt and sodium. These GDAs are calculated by using the approximate energy estimated average requirement (EAR) for the group in question and the dietary reference values (DRVs) for macronutrients and fibre in the Committee on the Medical Aspects of Food (COMA, 1991) and the Scientific Advisory Committee on Nutrition (SACN, 2003) recommendation for salt and sodium. There are separate GDAs for both sexes and different age groups of children and a generalized set of GDAs for children aged 5–10 years. The decision about which GDAs to include on any given food label will depend on space available and on the likely consumers of the food. This system is much more complex than the traffic light system recommended by the FSA, and is essentially very similar to that used on American food labels as outlined below. Further details of this system including tables of numerical values can be found in IGD (2006).

Labelling in the USA

American food labelling regulations underwent a major revision in the Nutrition Labelling and Education Act of 1990 (NLEA). Many food 'activists' would regard this very formal and detailed set of regulations, amounting to 4000 pages, as an ideal model for other countries to follow. This short review is offered to readers from outside the USA as an illustration of the complexity involved when statutory regulation of full nutritional labelling of food is attempted.

The stated aims of the US legislation were to produce a simple, understandable label that clears up confusion and helps consumers to make healthy choices and also:

> To encourage product innovation, so that companies are more interested in tinkering with the food in the package, not the word on the label.
>
> *D A Kessler*, FDA Commissioner (1991)

Ironically, one of the original purposes of food law was to stop producers 'tinkering with the food in the package'! This brief summary of these American food labelling regulations illustrates the complexity of trying to frame food labelling rules that cover every eventuality. They have tried to ensure that all labels contain all the useful information, in a clear, comprehensible and truly informative form and are free from misleading information and claims. Shortly after these regulations were introduced in 1992, it was suggested in the influential journal *Nature* (volume 360 p. 499), that the resulting labels were 'all but incomprehensible' and 'leaving the consumer in need of a mainframe computer to translate it all into practical terms'. Listed below are a sample of the important provisions introduced in NLEA (source Food and Drug Administration (FDA), 1992).

- *Range of foods.* Nutrition labelling is mandatory on almost all packaged foods. Food stores are also asked to display nutrition information on the most frequently consumed raw fruits, vegetables, fish, meat and poultry.
- *List of ingredients.* A full list of ingredients is required on all packaged foods, even those made according to the standard recipes set by the FDA such as mayonnaise, macaroni and bread. The ingredients must be listed in descending order of weight in food and a number of additional specific requirements are listed, e.g. all colours must be listed by name, caseinate (used in non-dairy coffee whitener) must be identified as being from milk and the source of any protein hydrolysate must be indicated (e.g. hydrolysed milk protein). One purpose of these specific rules is to assist people with food allergies.
- *Serving sizes.* These have to be stated and for many products the serving size is laid down so as to properly reflect what an adult actually eats, e.g. the 'reference amount customarily consumed' for a soft drink is 8 oz (about 250 g). There are detailed regulations about what happens if packages contain less than two statutory servings, e.g. if the carton also contains less than 200 g/200 mL then the whole package should be treated as one serving. This measure has been introduced to prevent producers misleading consumers as to, for example, the fat, sugar or energy content of their product by using unrealistically small portion sizes.
- *Nutritional information.* The label must contain the amounts of the following per serving: calories; calories from fat; total fat; saturated fat; cholesterol; sodium; total carbohydrate; complex carbohydrate; dietary fibre; sugars; protein; vitamins A and C; calcium; and iron. Other nutritional information that can be voluntarily listed (e.g. B vitamins) is also specified. The label must not only give the amount of the nutrient in absolute terms but must also put it into the context of an average ideal diet, e.g. if a serving contains 13 g of fat this is equivalent to 20 per cent of the total fat in the ideal 2000 kcal diet. Not only the content of the label but also its format is laid down. A nutrition information panel from a sample label is shown in Figure 18.2.
- *Descriptive terms.* Several of the descriptive terms that are frequently used on food labels are formally defined and the food must comply with this statutory definition, e.g. 'free' as in say 'fat free' or 'sugar free', 'low' as in 'low calorie' or 'low sodium', and 'less' as in 'less fat'. Other descriptive terms are light, lite, reduced and high. Low-fat versions of products such as butter, sour cream and cheese need no longer be called imitation or substitute but may be called simply low fat, provided they comply with certain specified criteria. This is aimed at improving the image of low-fat foods.
- *Health claims.* As at November 2004, 12 relationships between nutrients and disease were regarded as well enough established to be allowed to be used in health claims on food labels. They are:
  - calcium and osteoporosis
  - sodium and hypertension
  - saturated fat and cholesterol and coronary heart disease
  - fat and cancer
  - folic acid and neural tube defects
  - fibre-containing food and cancer
  - fruits and vegetables and cancer
  - foods that contain fibre, especially soluble fibre, and coronary heart disease
  - soy protein and risk of coronary heart disease
  - phytosterols and phytostanols and the risk of coronary heart disease (discussed at the end of this chapter).

Only foods that meet the compositional criteria specified for each claim can carry the claim and the suggested wordings for such claims are also laid

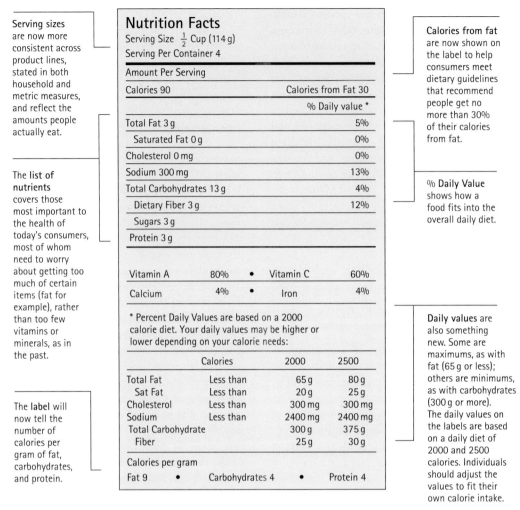

Serving sizes are now more consistent across product lines, stated in both household and metric measures, and reflect the amounts people actually eat.

The **list of nutrients** covers those most important to the health of today's consumers, most of whom need to worry about getting too much of certain items (fat for example), rather than too few vitamins or minerals, as in the past.

The **label** will now tell the number of calories per gram of fat, carbohydrates, and protein.

Nutrition Facts

Serving Size $\frac{1}{2}$ Cup (114 g)

Serving Per Container 4

Amount Per Serving	
Calories 90	Calories from Fat 30
	% Daily value *
Total Fat 3 g	5%
Saturated Fat 0 g	0%
Cholesterol 0 mg	0%
Sodium 300 mg	13%
Total Carbohydrates 13 g	4%
Dietary Fiber 3 g	12%
Sugars 3 g	
Protein 3 g	

Vitamin A	80%	Vitamin C	60%
Calcium	4%	Iron	4%

* Percent Daily Values are based on a 2000 calorie diet. Your daily values may be higher or lower depending on your calorie needs:

		Calories	2000	2500
Total Fat	Less than		65 g	80 g
Sat Fat	Less than		20 g	25 g
Cholesterol	Less than		300 mg	300 mg
Sodium	Less than		2400 mg	2400 mg
Total Carbohydrate			300 g	375 g
Fiber			25 g	30 g

Calories per gram		
Fat 9	Carbohydrates 4	Protein 4

Calories from fat are now shown on the label to help consumers meet dietary guidelines that recommend people get no more than 30% of their calories from fat.

% Daily Value shows how a food fits into the overall daily diet.

Daily values are also something new. Some are maximums, as with fat (65 g or less); others are minimums, as with carbohydrates (300 g or more). The daily values on the labels are based on a daily diet of 2000 and 2500 calories. Individuals should adjust the values to fit their own calorie intake.

Figure 18.2 *A typical nutrition information panel from an American food label.*

down. See the next section for an overview of health claims in Britain and the USA.

When these regulations were first introduced in 1992, the FDA estimated the cost of these labelling changes at US$1.4–2.3 billion (£1–1.5 billion) over 20 years. They assumed that these costs would be more than compensated for by the improvements in the diet that they facilitate and the resultant reduction in healthcare costs! Up-to-date information on American food labelling regulations may be found in Fisher *et al.* (2006).

Overview of health claims

Health claims is an issue that is addressed several times in this book, i.e. in Chapter 12 in the section dealing with dietary supplements, at the end of this

chapter in the section dealing with functional foods, and here in this section dealing with food labelling. As supplements and functional foods are legally classified as foods, the regulations that apply to food also apply to these. In the UK it is not permitted to make claims that a food can prevent or cure a disease (even if true) although general health claims like 'may help to maintain healthy joins' are permitted (several examples or permissible and non-permissible claims are given in Chapter 12). The situation in the USA is similar to that in Britain although the health claims listed in the previous section are additionally allowed in the USA. In order to prevent a legal challenge to health claims restriction being an unconstitutional restriction on freedom of speech the FDA in the USA further allows a number of 'qualified health claims' that do not meet the criterion of significant scientific agreement (SSA) and these may be printed on foods or supplements along with a suitable qualifying disclaimer, e.g. 'the evidence supporting the claim is not conclusive' (see Fisher *et al.*, 2006 for further details).

Key Points

- In the UK, most packaged foods must have on their label the food's name, ingredients, shelf life, storage requirements, batch number and the name and address of the packer.
- A 'use by' date on a food in the UK indicates that the food is likely to be microbiologically unsafe after that date.
- A 'best before' date indicates that a UK food's quality may have deteriorated after that date but it is unlikely to have become unsafe.
- Most British foods carry some nutritional information on the label and they must do so if they make any nutritional claim for the product.
- If nutritional information is used on a British label then it must include the energy and macronutrient content per 100 g and the amount of any nutrient for which a claim is made.
- The Food Standards Agency (FSA) has devised a traffic lights system of nutritional labelling which is designed to indicate whether a food is high, moderate or low in fat, saturated fat, sugar and salt.
- Many UK retailers and manufacturers have adopted the FSA 'traffic light' system although each has used their own design.
- Some retailers have opted to use a more complex system of nutritional labelling based on guideline daily amounts which are similar to the American system.
- There are now very detailed and complex regulations controlling food labelling in the USA.
- Almost all packaged foods in the USA must have a label which must:
  - contain a full list of ingredients
  - use prescribed serving sizes for nutritional information
  - give detailed nutritional information according to prescribed rules

  - only use descriptive terms such as high or low if the food meets certain prescribed criteria
  - only make permitted health claims and then only if the food meets the prescribed criteria.
- In the UK, foods (including dietary supplements and functional foods) may only carry general claims about health and not claims that they cure or prevent disease.

FOOD POISONING AND THE MICROBIOLOGICAL SAFETY OF FOOD

There cannot be many readers of this book who have not experienced several bouts of microbial food poisoning. There seems to be a general acceptance that the incidence of microbial food poisoning has risen sharply in recent decades in many industrialized countries. For example, the number of officially recorded and verified cases of food poisoning in England and Wales rose throughout the 1980s and 1990s from under 15 000 in 1982 to more than 100 000 by the end of the 1990s. Since then the number of such cases has started to fall, to around 80 000 in 2005. Food poisoning is rarely serious enough to cause death but it can be fatal in the very young, very old and those people whose immune system is suppressed by drugs or disease. One to two hundred people die each year in the UK as a consequence of food poisoning. To put this figure for deaths from food poisoning into perspective, in the 1940s, prior to the introduction of general pasteurization of milk, 1500 people died in the UK each year from bovine tuberculosis contracted from drinking contaminated milk. Bovine tuberculosis has now been all but eradicated in the UK.

The number of officially recorded and verified cases of food poisoning will, almost inevitably, only represent the 'tip of the iceberg' because only a minority of sufferers will even consult a doctor. Reported cases have been variously estimated as representing between 1 and 10 per cent of all cases. The Health Protection Agency estimated that in 2000 there may have been as many as 1.3 million cases of foodborne disease in England and Wales of whom around 370 000 consulted a doctor and yet in that year only 87 000 cases of food poisoning were notified and a figure of 5.5 million cases of foodborne illness is widely accepted, which is 1 person in 10 of the population. Even though recorded cases represent only a small and indeterminate fraction of actual cases, it seems probable that real cases have risen in line with the number of recorded ones. It is also likely that infections that produce a relatively mild or relatively short-lasting illness will probably be underrepresented in the recorded data as compared to their true incidence. The relatively high incidence in children may again be because parents are more likely to consult a doctor about food poisoning in a child.

Key points

- Recorded cases of food poisoning rose sharply during the 1980s and 1990s to a total of around 100 000 cases annually in England and Wales but have been dropping since then to under 80 000 in 2005.
- Recorded food-poisoning cases only represent a small fraction of total cases of foodborne disease with perhaps as many as 1 in 10 of the population being affected each year.
- Food poisoning is seldom fatal and most of the 100–200 annual deaths in the UK are in vulnerable groups like the elderly, infants and those with impaired immune function.

Causes of foodborne diseases

Causative organisms

Textbooks of food microbiology usually list more than 10 organisms or groups of organisms as significant causes of food poisoning. In classical food poisoning, large numbers of organisms generally need to grow in the food to cause illness and this usually presents as acute gastro-enteritis. There are a number of other foodborne (or waterborne) diseases, e.g. typhoid, cholera, and infections with *Campylobacter* and *Shigella* species, that usually require relatively few organisms to cause illness and in these cases there is usually no need for the organism to grow in food as there is in classic food poisoning. Several organisms that are now important causes of food poisoning require only a few organisms to cause illness and so there is no need for them to multiply in the food to cause illness (e.g. *Campylobacter* and *Escherichia coli* O157).

The relative importance of the various organisms in causing food poisoning varies in different countries and communities, and depends on the diet and food practices of the population. For example, food poisoning caused by the organism *Vibrio parahaemolyticus* is associated with consumption of undercooked fish and shellfish. In Japan, where consumption of raw fish (sushi) is widespread, food poisoning due to this organism is the most common cause of food poisoning. It is, however, a relatively uncommon causative agent in the UK and US where sushi bars and Japanese restaurants are frequently the source of infection.

Roberts (1982) analysed over a 1000 outbreaks of food poisoning that occurred in England and Wales. She found that four organisms or groups of organisms accounted for almost all of these outbreaks: the salmonellae, *Clostridium perfringens*, *Staphylococcus aureus* and *Bacillus cereus*. Similar analyses of US outbreaks had also identified the first three on this list as the most common causative agents (Bryan, 1978).

During the 1980s the incidence of food poisoning in the UK caused by *Salmonella* increased dramatically mainly due to increases in infection with *S. enteritidis* from poultry and eggs. As a group, the salmonellae now account for over a third of all recorded cases of bacterial food poisoning in England and Wales, and are the second most common cause of food poisoning. *Campylobacter jejuni* was only recognized as a general cause of food poisoning in the late 1970s when techniques for its isolation and identification became available. The organism is difficult to grow on standard laboratory media and does not usually multiply in food. *Campylobacter* are now the organisms most frequently causing acute bacterial gastro-enteritis in the UK and account for over half of all recorded cases. *Campylobacter* were not mentioned in the Roberts report of 1982. It requires only a few of these organisms to cause illness and they can be spread from person to person, and in this respect it is more like the other group of foodborne diseases such as typhoid and cholera. *C. perfringens* is now the third most common cause of bacterial food poisoning whereas *B. cereus* and *S. aureus* each represent less than 1 per cent of recorded food poisoning cases.

Listeriosis was also not mentioned in the earlier report of Roberts (1982), neither is it mentioned in textbooks of food microbiology published well into the 1980s. It has, however, been a cause of great public concern in the UK and USA in recent years, with the demonstration of the causative agent (*Listeria monocytogenes*) in many supermarket chilled foods.

It has been of particular concern because it may cause miscarriage, birth defects and death of new-born infants if pregnant women are infected.

E. coli O157 is another food-poisoning organism that has attracted much media and public attention in the past few years. This bacterium was associated with an outbreak of food poisoning in Scotland that affected hundreds of people and killed 20 elderly people. This is one of a group of bacteria that produces a verocytotoxin that damages cells in the gut and the endothelium of blood vessels. These vero-cytotoxin-producing E. coli (**VTEC**) only emerged as a cause of food poisoning in the early 1980s but reached a peak of over 1000 cases per year in the late 1990s (down to around 700 cases in 2004). They have attracted a lot of attention because a proportion of those affected develops renal complications and even acute renal failure, which can be fatal. It has significant mortality especially in children and the elderly.

How bacteria make us ill

Food poisoning organisms produce their ill effects in one of the following three ways.

- Some organisms cause illness by colonizing the gut when they are ingested, e.g. the salmonellae, *Campylobacter* and *V. parahaemolyticus*. They produce an infection.
- Some organisms produce a toxin when they grow in the food, and it is the ingestion of this toxin that is responsible for the illness associated with the organism, e.g. *S. aureus*, *B. cereus* and *C. botulinum*. The illness is caused by chemical intoxication.
- Some organisms like *C. perfringens*, *E. coli* O157 and the other VTEC infect the gut and produce a toxin after ingestion that is responsible for the food-poisoning symptoms.

Some cases of gastro-enteritis cannot be attributed to bacteria or bacterial toxins and many are caused by foodborne viruses. Some of the major food poisoning organisms and their characteristics are listed in Table 18.1.

Circumstances that lead to foodborne illness

For foodborne disease to occur, the food must have been contaminated with the causative organism at

Table 18.1 Some characteristics of important food-poisoning bacteria

Bacteria	Effect of 75°C	Incubation	Infective dose	Mode of Pathology	Likely source	Other point
Campylobacter	Killed	2–10 days	Low	Infection	Meat, poultry	
Salmonella	Killed	12–48 hours	High	Infection	Meat, poultry, eggs	
Clostridium perfringens	Spores resist	8–12 hours	High	Toxin in food	Meat, poultry	
Escherichia coli O157	Killed	1–14 days	Low	Toxin in gut	Cattle	Can be lethal
Staphylococcus aureus	Killed	2–6 hours	High	Toxin food	Food handler	Heat-resistant toxin
Bacillus cereus	Spores resist	1–16 hours	High	Toxin in food	Rice	
Clostridium botulinum	Spores resist	18–36 hours	High	Lethal toxin in food	Improperly canned or bottled food	Rare Often fatal Anaerobic
Listeria monocytogenes	Killed	2 days–7 weeks	Low in pregnancy and vulnerable groups	Infection	Chilled foods, pate, soft cheese	Grows at 3°C Tolerates salt and sugar
Vibrio parahaemolyticus	Killed	2–48 hours	High	Infection	Fish, shellfish	

some stage prior to ingestion. There are many possible means by which the food can be contaminated with micro-organisms. Some examples are listed below.

- The organism may be widespread in the environment, e.g. in the soil, water, dust or air.
- The organism may be present in the animal carcass at slaughter or transferred from contaminated carcasses during processing.
- Eggs and meat may become contaminated with animal faeces.
- Fish and shellfish may become contaminated by sewage in seawater – particularly important in filter-feeding molluscs like mussels.
- Fruits and vegetables may become contaminated by being washed or watered with dirty water.
- The food handler can be a source of contamination.
- Insects, like flies, may serve as mechanical vectors for contamination.
- Food may be cross-contaminated from contact with another food – particularly important if cooked food that is to undergo no further heat treatment is contaminated by raw meat or poultry.
- Contamination in the kitchen, e.g. from contaminated work surfaces or dish cloths.

With some bacteria (e.g. those causing foodborne diseases such as *Shigella* dysentery, typhoid, paratyphoid and cholera), illness can result from the consumption of small numbers of organisms (say 10–10 000) and thus contamination of any food with these organisms may in itself be sufficient to cause illness. Such organism are said to have a low **infective dose** and in these cases infection may well result from drinking contaminated water or in some cases may spread from person to person. Of the major food-poisoning bacteria both the *Campylobacter* and *E. coli* O157 also have a low infective dose.

Foreign travel and gastro-enteritis – **traveller's diarrhoea** – seem to be frequently associated. Some of these cases may be due to a wide variety of food-poisoning organisms including those listed earlier but a high proportion are probably due to strains of *E. coli* to which the traveller has not acquired any immunity. Cook (1998) has suggested that up to 80 per cent of cases of acute diarrhoea amongst travellers may be due to strains of *E. coli* that are much less virulent than the potentially fatal infection of *E. coli* O157. Faecal contamination of drinking water,

bathing water or perhaps contamination of water used to irrigate fruits or vegetables is the likely source of the organisms. The lack of immunity means that foreigners may have a much lower infective dose than the indigenous population and so foreigners become ill but the local population is untouched. Low infective doses from water, ice in drinks, or raw fruit and salad vegetables washed in contaminated water may be a source of infection. Those on short visits to foreign countries, especially where the water supply may be suspect, would be well advised to consume only drinks made with boiled or purified water, to avoid ice in drinks, to peel, or wash in purified water, any fruits or vegetables that are to be eaten raw.

Many common food-poisoning organisms (including salmonellae) need to be ingested in higher numbers (often in excess of 100 000) to cause illness in a healthy adult. These organisms have a high infective dose and they do not usually cause illness as a result of the consumption of contaminated water because of dilution and because water does not have the nutrients to support bacterial proliferation. Similarly, with many organisms that cause illness by producing a toxin in the food, once again a large bacterial population usually needs to have accumulated before sufficient toxin is produced to cause illness. For food poisoning to occur in healthy adults, not only must food be contaminated with these organisms but the following conditions also usually need to be met.

- The food must support growth of the bacteria (and allow production of toxin if relevant).
- The food must at some stage have been stored under conditions that permit the bacteria to grow (or produce toxin).

Note that even within a group of healthy young adults there will be variation in the susceptibility to any particular infective organism. In highly vulnerable groups, infective doses are likely to be at least an order of magnitude smaller. Babies are vulnerable because their immune systems are not fully developed and the functioning of the immune system also declines in elderly people (see Chapter 15). Others who are at increased risk of food poisoning are those people whose immune system has been compromised by illness, starvation, immunosuppressive drugs or radiotherapy. Not only is the infective dose lower in such vulnerable groups but the severity of the illness is likely to be greater, perhaps even life-threatening, and the speed of recovery slower. Most food-poisoning deaths occur in these vulnerable groups.

Key Points

- At least 10 groups of bacteria are important potential causes of bacterial food poisoning.
- Classic food-poisoning bacteria require large numbers to be present in the food to produce illness, i.e. they have a high infective dose.
- Some organisms produce illness when only a few are present in the food, i.e. they have a low infective dose.
- A group's diet and dietary practices determine the relative importance of different food-poisoning bacteria.
- In the early 1980s, the salmonellae, followed by *C. perfringens*, *S. aureus* and *B. cereus* accounted for almost all recorded outbreaks of food poisoning.
- In recent years, *Campylobacter* have risen from being unrecognized as a cause of food poisoning to being the most common cause in Britain.
- Other organisms that have attracted particular attention in recent years are:
  - *S. enteritidis* because it became the most common cause of salmonella food poisoning, and its presence in British poultry and eggs was very widespread
  - *L. monocytogenes* because it is present in may chilled foods and can cause miscarriage, birth defects and stillbirth if consumed by pregnant women
  - *E. coli* O157 because it may lead to acute and potentially fatal renal complications in children and elderly people.
- Food-poisoning bacteria produce illness by infecting the gut or by producing a toxin either in the food or in the gut after ingestion.
- Initial contamination of food with the organism is a prerequisite for all foodborne diseases.
- If organisms have a high infective dose, the bacteria must have multiplied in the food prior to ingestion and so the food and storage conditions must have been suitable for bacterial growth.

- Traveller's diarrhoea is often caused by strains of *E. coli* to which the traveller is more susceptible than the local population.
- Contaminated water may be directly or indirectly responsible for many cases of traveller's diarrhoea.

Principles of safe food preparation

The safe preparation of food involves measures and practices that attempt to do some or all of the following.

- Minimize the chances of contamination of food with bacteria.
- Kill any contaminating bacteria, e.g. by heat or irradiation.
- Ensure that food is stored under conditions, or in a form that, prevent bacterial proliferation.

Some bacteria produce changes in the flavour, appearance and smell of the food that reduces its palatability, i.e. they cause **spoilage**. The growth of spoilage organisms serves as a warning that the food is stale or has been the subject of poor handling procedures, inadequate processing or poor storage conditions. Food-poisoning organisms, on the other hand, can grow in a food without producing changes in palatability. Thus, the absence of spoilage is no guarantee that the food is safe to eat, otherwise food poisoning would be a much rarer occurrence.

Requirements for bacterial growth

Many bacteria must actively grow in food before they are numerous enough or have produced enough toxin to cause illness in healthy people. In order to grow in food, bacteria need the following conditions to be met.

- *Nutrients.* Many foods are ideal culture media for the growth of micro-organisms. The same nutrients that people obtain from them can also be used to support bacterial growth. One reason why meat, meat products, eggs, seafood and milk products are so often the causes of food poisoning is because they are nutrient-rich and generally support bacterial growth.
- *A suitable temperature.* Bacterial growth slows at low temperature and growth of most pathogens ceases at temperatures of less than 5°C. At the

temperatures maintained in domestic freezers ($-18°C$) all bacterial growth will be arrested even though organisms can survive extended periods at such freezing temperatures. Growth of food-poisoning organisms will also not occur at temperatures over $60°C$ and most will be slowly killed. At temperatures over $73°C$ non-spore-forming bacteria will be very rapidly killed, although those capable of forming spores may survive considerable periods even at boiling point. Note also that, for example, *S. aureus* produces a heat-stable toxin and so foods heavily contaminated with this organism remain capable of causing food poisoning even if heat treatment or irradiation kills all of the bacteria.

- *Moisture.* Bacteria require moisture for growth. Drying has been a traditional method of extending the storage life of many foods. High concentrations of salt and sugar preserve foods by increasing the osmotic pressure in foods and thus making the water unavailable to bacteria, i.e. they reduce the **water activity** of the food. Moulds generally tolerate much lower water activities than bacteria and grow, for example, on the surface of bread, cheese and jam (jelly).

- *Favourable chemical environment.* A number of chemical agents (preservatives), by a variety of means, inhibit bacterial growth. They create a chemical environment unfavourable to bacterial growth. Many pathogenic and spoilage organisms only grow within a relatively narrow pH range, they will not, for example, grow in a very acid environment. Acidifying foods with acetic acid (pickling with vinegar) is one traditional preservation method. Fermentation of food using acid-producing bacteria (e.g. the *lactobacilli*) have also been traditionally used to preserve and flavour foods such as yoghurt, cheese and sauerkraut.

- *Time.* The contaminated food needs to be kept under conditions that favour bacterial growth for long enough to allow the bacteria to multiply to the point where they represent a potentially infective dose. Note that under favourable conditions, bacteria may double their numbers in less than 20 minutes and so a thousand organisms could become a million in 2 hours.

- *Oxygen.* Food-poisoning organisms do not require oxygen for growth although it may hastens their growth. *C. botulinum* is an anaerobe that is killed by oxygen.

Some specific causes of food-poisoning outbreaks

Roberts (1982) identified the factors that most often contributed to outbreaks of food poisoning in England and Wales (see Table 18.2). Bryan (1978) had earlier concluded that the factors contributing to food-poisoning outbreaks in the US and UK were similar. Hobbs and Roberts (1993) suggest that factors contributing to outbreaks of food poisoning are unlikely to have changed significantly since that time. Such analyses give a useful indication of practices that are likely to increase the risk of food poisoning and so indicate some of the practical measures that can be taken to reduce risk. It must be borne in mind that Roberts' (1982) analysis would not have included cases of infection with those bacteria that have relatively recently attracted attention as important causes of food poisoning and have a low infective dose, e.g. *Campylobacter* and *E. coli* O157.

Table 18.2 Factors most often associated with 1000 outbreaks of food poisoning in England and Wales*

Factor	% Of outbreaks
Preparation of food in advance of needs	61
Storage at room temperature	40
Inadequate cooling	32
Inadequate heating	29
Contaminated processed food	19
Undercooking	15
Inadequate thawing	4–6
Cross-contamination	4–6
Improper warm holding	4–6
Infected food handler	4–6
Use of leftovers	4–6
Consumption of raw food	4–6

*After Roberts (1982).

In her analysis of food-poisoning outbreaks, Roberts (1982) found that two-thirds of outbreaks could be traced to foods prepared in restaurants, hotels, clubs, institutions, hospitals, schools and canteens. Less than 20 per cent of outbreaks were linked to food prepared in the home. In a later review of these figures Hobbs and Roberts (1993) suggested that they were seriously distorted due to the low rate of inclusion of home-related incidents because of lack of epidemiological data on these outbreaks. Nevertheless, outbreaks of food poisoning that originate from home-prepared food will usually generate far fewer individual cases than outbreaks associated with commercial and institutional catering:

> Situations where food is prepared in quantity for a large number of people are most likely to give rise to most food poisoning
>
> Hobbs and Roberts (1993)

For example, a flaw in the pasteurization process of a major US dairy resulted in over 16 000 confirmed cases and around 200 000 suspected cases of food poisoning in Illinois in 1985 (Todd, 1991).

In the vast majority of the outbreaks investigated by Roberts (1982), meat and poultry were identified as the source of the infection. Eggs, as well as poultry, are now also recognized as a source of the organism causing the most common type of salmonella food poisoning (*S. enteritidis*). The size of this problem was such that a series of reduction measures were introduced such as mass vaccination of egg-producing flocks.

Certain foods, such as those listed below, are associated with a low risk of food poisoning:

- dry foods like bread and biscuits or dried foods – the low water activity prevents bacterial growth
- high sugar or salted foods like jam because of the low water activity
- fats and fatty foods like vegetable oil lack nutrients and provide an unfavourable environment for bacterial growth
- commercially canned foods because they have been subject to vigorous heat treatment and maintained in airtight containers
- pasteurized foods like milk because they have been subjected to heat treatment designed to kill likely pathogens
- high acid foods like pickles
- vegetables generally do not support bacterial growth. They can, however, be a source of contamination for other foods, e.g. if used in prepared salads containing meat, eggs or mayonnaise. Fruit and vegetables contaminated by dirty water may be a direct source of infection if the infecting organism has a low infective dose.

Canned or pasteurized foods cannot be assumed to be safe if they may have been contaminated after opening or, in the case of dried foods, after rehydration. This information may be particularly useful if one is obliged to select food in places where food hygiene seems less than satisfactory.

Key points

- Spoilage organisms adversely affect the taste, smell and appearance of food but food poisoning organisms generally do not.
- Safe handling and preparation of food requires that the risks of contamination and bacterial proliferation are minimized and/or that the killing of bacteria during preparation is maximized.
- In order to grow, bacteria require nutrients, moisture, warmth, time and a suitable pH.
- Safe storage of food involves depriving likely pathogens and spoilage bacteria of one or more of their requirements for growth.
- Table 18.2 lists some of the factors most often linked to outbreaks of food poisoning due to mainly high infective dose bacteria in the early 1980s.
- Institutional and commercial catering is responsible for most large outbreaks of food-poisoning.
- Meat, poultry and eggs are the sources of most food-poisoning outbreaks in the UK.
- Some foods that are seldom associated with food poisoning are:
  - foods with low water activity, i.e. dry, salted or high sugar foods
  - fats and oils
  - newly opened canned or pasteurized foods
  - pickled foods
  - fruits and vegetables unless they act as vehicles for contaminated water.

Some practical guidelines to avoid food poisoning

Minimize the risks of bacterial contamination of food

Some specific steps for reducing the risk of food contamination are listed in Box 18.1. Much of the meat, poultry and eggs that we purchase must be assumed to be already contaminated when they are purchased. It will require improvements in farming and slaughtering practices to reduce the initial contamination of these foods. For example, there has been a

Box 18.1   Tips for reducing the risk of food poisoning

Reducing bacterial contamination of food

- Buy food that is fresh and from suppliers who store and prepare it hygienically

- Keep food covered and protected from insect contamination

- Wash hands thoroughly before preparing food and after using the toilet or blowing one's nose

- Cover any infected lesions on hands

- Ensure that all utensils and surfaces that come into contact with food are clean

- Ensure that any cloth used to clean utensils and surfaces or to dry dishes is clean and changed regularly

- Avoid any contact between raw food (especially meat) and cooked food

- Do not store raw meat in a position in the refrigerator where drips can fall onto other foods that will not be heat treated before being eaten

- Wash utensils, hands and surfaces in contact with raw food before they are used with cooked food

Maximize killing of bacteria during processing

- Cook meat, poultry and eggs thoroughly so that all parts of the food reach a minimum of 75°C

- Defrost frozen meat and poultry thoroughly before cooking

- Re-heat food thoroughly so that all parts of it reach 75°C

Minimize the time that food is kept in conditions that allow bacteria to grow

- Prepared food as close to the time of consumption as is practical (prolonged holding of food also leads to loss of nutrients)

- When food is prepared well in advance of preparation, it should be protected from contamination and should not be stored at room temperature

- Discard foods that are past their 'use by' dates or show evidence of spoilage (e.g. 'off' flavours and smells or discoloration)

- Food that is kept hot should be kept at 65°C or above

- Food that is kept cool should be kept below 5°C

- When food is cooked for storage it should be cooled quickly

- Leftovers or other prepared foods that are stored in a refrigerator should be covered and used promptly

- Store eggs in a refrigerator and use them within 3 weeks of purchase

---

sharp fall in the number of infections with *S. enteriditis* in the UK following the introduction of stringent new safety measures for egg production and handling including a massive hen vaccination programme.

Most of the tips for reducing bacterial contamination in Box 18.1 are common sense measures that require little amplification or explanation but carelessness can cause us to overlook them, even though they seem obvious when written down. Most people would require no prompting to avoid a butcher who kept his meat in a warm place where flies could crawl over it or to avoid buying food that is obviously spoiled or past its 'use by' date. Lax hygiene can allow the cook's hands to become a source of faecal organisms or of *S. aureus* which is frequently present in skin lesions and in the nasal passages of many people. It is vital to avoid cross-contamination of ready-to-eat foods with raw foods like meat which are usually contaminated with bacteria. The bacteria in the raw food will probably be killed during cooking but if the bacteria multiply in the ready-to-eat food, there is no further heat treatment to eliminate them. There are very strict food hygiene regulations that are intended to ensure that raw and cooked meats are separated in supermarkets and butchers' shops and staff should be trained to avoid cross-contaminating cooked meats.

Maximize killing of bacteria during home preparation of food

Some tips for maximizing the killing of bacteria during home preparation are listed in Box 18.1. Even though many raw foods may be contaminated when bought, if they are thoroughly cooked then almost all of them should be made safe by this cooking. Most of the common food-poisoning organisms are killed rapidly at temperatures over 73°C. Meat that is eaten 'rare' will not have undergone sufficient heat treatment to kill all bacteria and represents a hazard if contaminated prior to cooking. Poultry should always be well cooked. Note that this is especially important for hamburgers and other minced meat. With a joint or slice of meat most of the contaminating bacteria will be on the outside and these will be killed even if the centre of the meat is pink and underdone. However when meat is minced, the bacteria are spread throughout the meat so that the centre of a hamburger contains as many bacteria as the outside.

Raw eggs (e.g. in homemade mayonnaise) and undercooked eggs represent a potential hazard, especially to the elderly, the sick and the very young. People in Britain have been officially advised to only eat eggs that are thoroughly cooked, e.g. not soft boiled eggs.

Minimize the time that food is stored under conditions that permit bacterial multiplication

Some tips for minimizing the time that food is stored under conditions that allow bacteria to multiply are listed in Box 18.1. The time between food preparation and consumption should be as short as is practically reasonable. Where food is prepared well in advance of serving it should be protected from contamination and should not be stored at room temperature. Buffets, where prepared food may be left uncovered at room temperature for some hours before consumption, are particularly hazardous.

Most bacteria only grow between 5°C and 65°C and are slowly killed at temperatures of over 65°C. This means that food that is kept hot should be kept above 65°C and any food that is to be re-heated should be thoroughly re-heated so that all parts of it reach 75°C (the temperature at which non-spore forming bacteria are rapidly killed). Food that is to be kept cool should be kept below 5°C because most food poisoning bacteria will not grow below this temperature. Food that has been cooked but is to be stored cool should be cooled rapidly so that it spends the minimum time within the growth range of bacteria. Leftovers, or other prepared foods, that are stored in a refrigerator should be covered and used promptly; care should be taken to ensure that they do not come into contact with raw food, especially flesh foods.

The principal aim of this chapter has been to encourage greater care and awareness in the home preparation of food. In order to effect reductions in the rates of food poisoning produced outside the home there needs to be improved training of catering workers and regulatory changes that lead to improvements to commercial and institutional catering practices. Food hygiene laws and regulations are complex, often extremely detailed, and vary from nation to nation (recent attempts to harmonize food hygiene laws within the EU have highlighted this latter point). Food hygiene laws must remain the province of specialist texts of food microbiology and food technology (e.g. see Jacob, 1993). Note, however, that in principle, food hygiene laws represent attempts by governments to enshrine the safety principles and practices outlined for home food preparation into a formal legal framework so as to ensure that they are carried through into mass catering situations.

A note about treatment of foodborne disease

Most cases of food poisoning go unrecorded because the symptoms are not severe enough or prolonged enough to prompt people to consult their doctor. The best way of treating simple food poisoning is to maintain the patient's fluid and electrolyte levels with oral rehydration fluids containing glucose and salts. In severe cases intravenous infusion of fluid may be necessary. In simple food poisoning, antibiotics are not used because they do not affect the course of the disease and their use may simply encourage the development of antibiotic resistance in bacteria. As a general rule, self-medication with preparations that stop diarrhoea by inhibiting gut motility should not be used, especially with children, because they increase retention of the bacteria and increase exposure to any toxin. These antimotility agents may, for example, increase the risk of renal damage in cases of infection with E. coli O157. They may be helpful in relatively mild cases of traveller's diarrhoea.

Key Points

- Many practical measures that will reduce the risk of food poisoning are listed in Box 18.1.
- It should be assumed that meat, poultry, eggs and raw milk are likely to be contaminated when purchased.
- Heat will kill bacteria but some heat-resistant spores may survive boiling and some bacterial

toxins may be heat resistant and remain in food even when all the bacteria have been killed.

- Most cases of food poisoning can be treated by simple supportive measures aimed at body fluid balance.
- Antibiotics do not generally affect the course of a bout of food poisoning.
- Compounds that stop diarrhoea by inhibiting gut motility are generally contraindicated because they may prolong the infection.

Pinpointing the cause of a food-poisoning outbreak

Identifying the cause of food-poisoning outbreaks should highlight high-risk practices and thus may be useful for improving food handling. If a single event (e.g. serving a contaminated dish at a buffet) is the cause of an outbreak, a time distribution of cases like that shown in Figure 18.3 would be expected. Each food-poisoning organism has a characteristic average incubation period from time of ingestion to the onset of symptoms. Incubation times in individuals will vary around this average, a few people develop symptoms early, most towards the middle of the range and a few towards the end of the range as in Figure 18.3. The variation in the speed of onset of symptoms is influenced by all sorts of factors, such as:

- the dose of organism or toxin consumed
- the amount of other food consumed and thus the dilution and speed of passage through the gut
- individual susceptibility.

The organism causing the illness can be identified from the clinical picture and/or laboratory samples and then, knowing the incubation period, the approximate time at which all of the victims were exposed to the organism and the meal at which the organisms were consumed pinpointed (see Figure 18.3). Sampling of leftovers or circumstantial evidence can then identify the responsible food and hopefully the unsafe practice that led to the outbreak.

Board (1983) gave an illustrative case history of an outbreak of food poisoning among the passengers and crew of a charter flight. More than half of the passengers on this flight developed food poisoning, a few at the end of the flight and large numbers at the airport within 2 hours of landing. The clinical picture (the symptoms, the rapid onset and short

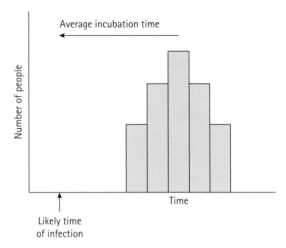

Figure 18.3 *Theoretical time course of first experiencing food poisoning symptoms after infection.*

duration) indicated that the illness was probably due to ingestion of toxin from *S. aureus*. The time distribution of cases indicated that the breakfast served on the plane 90 minutes before landing was the likely source of the illness and samples of uneaten breakfasts confirmed the presence of this organism in ham omelette. The food had been contaminated by infected sores on the hands of one of the cooks at the catering company that had supplied the breakfasts to the airline. A long time (3 days) had elapsed between the initial preparation of the food and its eventual serving to the passengers and the food had not been kept cool for much of the time between preparation and serving.

If no food samples are available for analysis then the responsible food can often be implicated by calculation of **attack rates**. All of those participating in the meal identified as the point of infection are asked to complete a questionnaire about which foods they consumed and whether they became ill. The attack rate is the percentage of persons becoming ill. For each food the percentage of those who became ill is calculated for those who did and those who did not consume that food, i.e. the **food-specific attack rates**. A statistically significantly higher attack rate for those consuming a particular food as compared to those not consuming it indicates that it was the likely source of the infection. In the example in Table 18.3, eating food A significantly increased the attack rate whereas eating food B significantly reduced it. Food B appears protective because A and B were alternative choices on the menu

Table 18.3 Food-specific attack rates for people present at a social function identified as the point of infection for an outbreak of food poisoning*

Food	Ate			Did not eat		
	Ill	Not ill	Attack rate (%)	Ill	Not ill	Attack rate (%)
A	30	131	19	0	51	0[†]
B	0	27	0	30	154	16[†]
C	8	49	14	21	125	14
D	21	95	18	9	84	10
E	8	69	10	22	107	17
F	13	60	18	17	121	12

*After Hobbs and Roberts (1993).
[†]Statistically significant difference between the attack rates of those who did and did not consume that particular food.

and so people who ate food B did not eat food A. It would thus seem almost certain that food A was the source of the infection.

The time distribution of people reporting symptoms of food poisoning may not follow the bell-shaped model shown in Figure 18.3. For example, there may be multiple peaks or the number of new cases may tend to plateau rather than fall away. Such distributions would indicate either person-to-person spread or a continuing source of infection, e.g. a processing fault, an infected food handler, continuing use of a contaminated ingredient or continued sale of a contaminated processed food. If the incubation period of the causative organism is known, a questionnaire should establish what all of the victims were doing (and eating) within the window of time when infection is predicted to have occurred. It should then be possible to identify a common factor, e.g. all victims ate a particular processed food, ate at a particular place or bought a processed food from a particular source during the period when they were likely to have become infected.

Key Points

- Food-poisoning bacteria each produce a characteristic set of symptoms and have characteristic incubation times.
- Incubation times will vary between individuals depending on dose consumed, its dilution with other food and drink and the susceptibility of the person.
- If the time distribution of cases in an outbreak is 'normal' as in Figure 18.3 then this indicates a

single point of infection and one can predict when this occurred from the average incubation period of the organism.

- One can identify which specific food was responsible because there will be a higher 'attack rate' among those who ate this food than among those who did not.
- If there is a continuing source of infection or person-to-person spread then the time distribution of cases will show multiple peaks or a tendency to plateau rather than the single peak seen in Figure 18.3.
- Even with a continuing source of infection, it should still be possible to identify a factor common to all victims during the window of time when they were likely to have been infected.

A review of some common food-poisoning organisms and foodborne illnesses

Campylobacter

Campylobacter were only recognized as a general source of foodborne disease in 1977. The organisms do not grow in food at room temperature and do not grow readily on normal laboratory media. This means that suitable methods needed to be developed for their identification. From being almost totally ignored as a cause of food poisoning 30 years ago, this organism is now the most common cause of acute bacterial gastro-enteritis in the UK with around 40 000–50 000 cases recognized each year.

The illness has a relatively long incubation period (2–10 days) and it produces a quite severe and prolonged illness. It initially produces flu-like symptoms and abdominal pain, which last for 1–2 days and this is followed by profuse, sometimes bloody, diarrhoea lasting for 1–3 days. It may take a week or more for complete recovery. *Campylobacter* may contaminate water, unpasteurized milk, meat and poultry and it may reside in the intestines of domestic animals. It has a low infective dose and thus is potentially transmissible through water, through the hands of children playing with or near domestic animals, or even from person to person. Undercooked poultry is the most common cause. Poultry or meat that has been inadequately cooked on garden barbecues has been blamed for many cases in the UK. The organism has a high optimum growth temperature but is killed rapidly at temperatures of 75°C.

Salmonellae

Many different types of the salmonella group of bacteria are responsible not only for common food poisoning but also for the more serious food- and waterborne illnesses, typhoid and paratyphoid. The common food-poisoning organisms usually need in excess of 100 000 bacteria to represent an infective dose. These latter organisms produce diarrhoea, stomach pain, vomiting and fever about 12–48 hours after ingestion and the illness lasts for between 1 and 7 days. Intensive farming methods and slaughtering practices mean that raw meat, poultry, eggs and raw milk should be regarded as potentially contaminated with these organisms. These organisms grow at temperatures between 6°C and 46°C. They are relatively heat sensitive and are killed slowly at 60°C and very rapidly at 75°C. They are not tolerant of very acid conditions, i.e. pH less than 4.5.

Meat and especially poultry has long been regarded as food with a high potential to cause salmonella food poisoning but in recent years the contamination of eggs with *S. enteritidis* has been a major cause for concern in the UK. Many thousands of hens were slaughtered in an apparently unsuccessful attempt to eradicate these organisms from the laying flock. Incidence of *S. enteritidis* infection has fallen sharply in the UK in the past few years because of changes in egg production and handling and a mass vaccination programme for hens.

Eggs have a number of natural barriers that tend to reduce the risk of bacterial entry but they are sold in millions, so even if only a very small proportion are contaminated this can represent, in absolute terms, a large number of potentially infected meals. Eggs also have a number of systems that inhibit bacterial growth (bacteriostatic systems) by making nutrients unavailable to the bacteria. The likelihood of a single fresh egg containing an infective dose for a healthy adult is thus low. However, if eggs are stored at room temperature and kept for long periods then a small number of original contaminating bacteria can multiply to the point where they represent an infective dose. Eggs should be stored in a refrigerator and they should not be kept for more than 3 weeks. Fresh and well-cooked eggs should represent no hazard at all and Britons are currently advised to eat only well-cooked eggs. Any potential hazard from eggs is increased significantly if uncooked egg is added to other foods, e.g. mayonnaise or cheesecake, and then the mixture stored under conditions that allow bacterial proliferation, e.g. at room temperature.

C. perfringens

C. perfringens has a high infective dose of between a hundred and a thousand million organisms. Illness is due to a toxin produced by bacteria within the gut. The disease has an incubation period of 8–12 hours and lasts for up to 24 hours. The symptoms are diarrhoea and abdominal pain but not usually vomiting or fever. The organism grows at temperatures of up to 53°C and the temperatures of 100°C are needed to kill spores. Food poisoning from this organism is usually associated with meat and poultry consumption and the organism is of widespread distribution in the gut of animals and people and also in soil and dust. When food is inadequately cooked these organisms may continue to grow during the initial heating of the food; some will survive at high temperatures by forming spores. Surviving spores may start to grow as the food cools and during storage of the cooked food. The organism grows very rapidly at temperatures, towards the top end of its tolerable range.

E. coli *O157 and the VTEC bacteria*

Media and public awareness of *E. coli* O157 was increased sharply in the UK by an outbreak of food poisoning in Lanarkshire, Scotland, in November 1996 that affected around 500 people and caused the deaths of 20 elderly people. Interviews with the initial cases established that all of them had eaten cooked meat products from a single butcher or had attended a lunch at which a steak pie supplied by this butcher had been served.

Cattle are almost always the source of infection with *E. coli* O157. Undercooked beef and more especially beef products such as burgers, raw milk and cheese made from unpasteurized milk are the potentially infective foods. The organism has a low infective dose and so cases have occurred due to contact with farm animals (e.g. children visiting farms), contamination of drinking water and even person-to-person spread.

E. coli O157 is one of a group of bacteria that produce toxins that have potentially fatal effects, the VTEC. These toxins damage gut cells and cells in the vascular endothelium. The onset time is typically 3–4 days after exposure but can range from 1 to 14 days. The symptoms are abdominal cramps, vomiting and diarrhoea but a proportion of sufferers will go on to develop more serious complications including kidney failure, which can be fatal in some children and elderly people. It is one of the major causes of acute renal failure in children.

S. aureus

The illness caused by this organism is due to a toxin present in food where this organism has grown. Greater than 5 million bacteria are usually regarded as necessary to produce enough toxin to evoke illness. The symptoms are vomiting, diarrhoea, abdominal pain but no fever. Symptoms are rapid in onset (2–6 hours) and of short duration (6–24 hours). The organism is heat sensitive. It grows within the range 8–46°C and is killed at temperatures in excess of 60°C but the toxin, once formed in food, is very heat stable and will not be eliminated by further heat treatment or irradiation of the food.

Food handlers are an important source of contamination. Many people carry the organism in their nasal passages and this can lead to contamination of hands and thence food; infected lesions on the hands may contain this organism. The organism needs foods rich in protein to produce toxin but it is comparatively tolerant of high salt and sugar concentrations, e.g. as found in ham or custard. *S. aureus* does not compete well with other bacteria present in raw food but if essentially sterile, cooked food is then contaminated by the handler then, without any competition, the organism is able to grow even in foods with relatively high salt or sugar contents.

B. cereus

This organism is commonly found in soil and thus on vegetables. It grows in starchy foods and, in the UK and USA, poisoning due to this organism is usually associated with consumption of rice. The organism produces heat-resistant spores which may survive cooking of rice. If the cooked rice, containing viable spores, is stored at temperatures that permit growth of the organism (7–49°C) then an infective dose will accumulate. Boiling rice in bulk and then storing it at room temperature prior to flash frying, e.g. in Chinese restaurants, is a common scenario for food poisoning due to this organism. The resultant illness is acute in onset (1–16 hours) and of short duration (6–24 hours), and it is caused by toxins produced by the organism in food. An infective dose is in excess of 100 000 organisms in the food. The symptoms depend on the particular toxin involved but may include diarrhoea, abdominal pain, nausea or vomiting.

C. botulinum

This organism grows under anaerobic conditions in low acid foods. Canned or bottled meats, fish or vegetables (but not acidic fruit) are potential sources of illness. The organism is killed by oxygen and thus the storage of these foods in airtight containers allows growth. The organism may also occasionally grow deep within non-canned flesh foods or meat products. Commercial canning processes involve a heat treatment that is specifically designed to ensure that all of the heat-stable spores of this organism are killed, the so-called **botulinum cook**. Cured meats and meat products contain nitrate, nitrite and salt, which are effective in preventing growth of this organism, and the addition of these preservatives is legally required in the UK for meat products such as sausages. Home canning or bottling of vegetables results in significant numbers of cases of botulism in the USA each year because the heat treatment is insufficient to kill the *Clostridium* spores. The very rare cases in the UK have usually been traced to occasional rogue cans of imported meat or fish, e.g. after heat treatment, contaminated water might be sucked into the cooling can through a damaged seam. The most recent UK outbreak in 1989 was traced to a can of nut puree that was subsequently used to flavour yoghurt. In the USA, honey is regarded as a potential source of small amounts of toxin, and so honey is not recommended for young children.

The organism produces an extremely potent toxin within the food. This toxin is destroyed by heat so danger foods are those eaten unheated (e.g. canned salmon or corned beef) or those that are only warmed. The toxin, although a protein, is absorbed from the gut and affects the nervous system, blocking the release of the important nerve transmitter acetylcholine. A dry mouth, blurred vision and gradual paralysis are the symptoms, and death will occur due to paralysis of the respiratory muscles. With rapid treatment, including artificial ventilation, about 75 per cent of those affected survive. In those victims who survive, recovery may take weeks or months. The incubation period is usually 18–36 hours. This organism is included in this review even though it rarely produces illness in the UK because the symptoms are frequently fatal, and because the imperative to avoid contamination of food with this organism has had a great influence on food-processing practices.

L. monocytogenes

Chilling of food has been a traditional method of storing food, it reduces both microbial growth and the rate of chemical deterioration. An enormous range of chilled foods are now available in supermarkets, e.g. fresh meat and fish, cheese, cooked meals, sandwiches, pies, etc. Such foods are susceptible to the development of infective doses of pathogenic bacteria that continue to grow slowly at low temperatures. Small variations in temperature within the low range (0–8°C) can have marked effects on the rate at which these low temperature organisms grow. Strict temperature control is therefore of great importance in ensuring safe storage of chilled foods. For foods that are to be eaten without further cooking, or just re-warming, current UK legislation requires that they be stored below 5°C, e.g. cook-chill ready meals, sandwiches, cured meat and fish.

The organism *L. monocytogenes* is one of these low-temperature organisms and it has attracted much media attention and public concern in the UK and USA in the past few years. This organism will grow slowly at temperatures as low as 3°C and it will tolerate a salt concentration of 10 per cent and a pH down to 5.2. Soft cheeses and pâté, which have a relatively long shelf-life, are considered to be at particular risk from this organism. Its presence has been reported in many cook-chill ready meals and it is likely to survive the mild re-heating in a microwave oven recommended for many of these foods.

The organism causes a disease known as listeriosis in vulnerable groups such as the elderly, infants, pregnant women and immunodeficient people, although it does not usually cause illness in healthy people. Symptoms range from those resembling mild flu to severe septicaemia and occasionally meningitis. If infection with this organism occurs during pregnancy then abortion, fetal abnormality or neonatal death may result. In the UK, pregnant women are currently advised to avoid those foods that are liable to harbour *Listeria* (e.g. pâté and soft cheese made with unpasteurized milk) and to thoroughly re-heat cook-chill foods. Increased use of chilling led to an increase in recorded cases of listeriosis from around 25 per year in the early 1970s to around 300 per year by 1988. In 1988 there were 26 deaths of newborn babies, 52 total deaths and 11 abortions caused by listeriosis. By the late 1990s, recorded cases of listeriosis had fallen to just over 100 cases per year as a result of increased awareness and measures to reduce it. The rise in the prominence of listeriosis with increased use of food chilling is a good illustration of how changing eating habits and processing methods can lead to changes in the prominence of different types of food-poisoning organisms.

BOVINE SPONGIFORM ENCEPHALOPATHY

When I completed the first edition of this book in 1994, there was no evidence that **BSE** would directly affect human beings. It is now clear that the human form of this disease (**variant Creutzfeldt-Jakob disease (vCJD)**) has affected people (with 158 deaths up to February 2007) and that most of these people acquired this disease by eating contaminated beef products (a very small number may have acquired it through blood transfusions). When I wrote the second edition of this book in 2001 it was estimated that anywhere between a few hundred and 135 000 people in Britain would eventually die as a result of this foodborne disease. In the intervening years it has become clear that many of the wildest predictions about the likely scale of this human epidemic were much too pessimistic; there were suggestions that 'hospices would be overflowing with terminally ill disease sufferers'. Even allowing for a small number of infections from blood transfusions or surgical transmission, the total number of deaths from the vCJD will probably gradually edge up over the coming years to around 200 in total (see Ghani *et al.*, 2003). A wealth of reliable information on this disease is available through the internet, and three recommended websites are listed below. Prusiner (1995) has written a review of the **prion** diseases of which BSE is an example.

- The Department for Environment, Food and Rural Affairs website. Bovine spongiform encephalopathy (www.defra.gov.uk/animalh/bse/index.html).
- The CJD surveillance unit website (www.cjd.ed.ac.uk/index.htm).
- The archive website of the official UK government inquiry into BSE (www.bseinquiry.gov.uk).

This disease has had massive economic and political effects and has had devastating effects on British farming and consumer confidence. For several years, media articles and broadcasts about the possible human consequences of BSE engendered fear, almost amounting to panic, in large sections of the population and certainly affected the mood of the whole nation. The 'BSE crisis' was a stimulus to the establishment of the **FSA** and to the restructuring and renaming of the ministry of agriculture (MAFF has been replaced by the **DEFRA**). It is now reasonable to suggest that the cattle epidemic of BSE is all but over and that the much smaller human epidemic of vCJD will continue to peter out over the coming years and cause only a very small number of further deaths. The impact of this disease has been enormous considering the low number of human deaths (about 160 since 1995 compared to over 45 000 deaths in road accidents over the same time period). The total cost to Britain of the BSE epidemic has been many billions of pounds. Some of these costs are still ongoing (e.g. research costs, testing of slaughtered animals, removal of **specified bovine offal (SBO)** from cattle destined for consumption, tagging and tracking of cattle, costs to the blood transfusion service, etc.).

Overview

BSE is an apparently new disease of cattle that first appeared in British cattle in 1985. The affected animals are excitable, aggressive, easily panicked, have an abnormal gait and a tendency to fall down. These symptoms gave rise to the popular name 'mad cow disease'. Up to February 2007 around 180 000 British cattle have developed this disease and millions more have been slaughtered and burnt in an attempt to eradicate it. Over 80 per cent of cases of

BSE have been in dairy cows and most of these in older cows. Only a handful of symptomatic cases have been recorded in cattle under 3 years old. The cattle epidemic peaked in 1992 when around 37 000 confirmed cases were recorded. Figure 18.4 charts the rise and fall of the BSE epidemic in cattle, which now seems to be almost over, with just a handful of confirmed cases in 2006. In addition to those that have developed the disease, millions of cattle have been culled and their carcasses incinerated to try to eradicate the disease from the national herd.

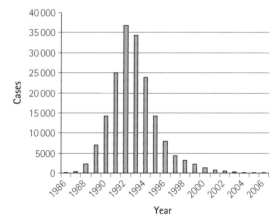

Figure 18.4 *Annual number of confirmed cases of bovine spongiform encephalopathy (BSE) in British cattle.*

The symptoms of BSE and the spongiform lesions seen in the brains of affected animals are similar to those seen in other **transmissible spongiform encephalopathies (TSEs)** such as those listed below. These diseases are all inevitably fatal.

- *Scrapie* of sheep and goats, which has been endemic in British sheep since the eighteenth century without any apparent effect on human health.
- *Creutzfeldt Jakob disease (CJD)* – a rare disease that kills around 30–70 elderly people in the UK each year.
- *Kuru* – a disease that was prevalent among the Fore tribe in Papua New Guinea.

All of these diseases are potentially transmissible by injecting extracts of diseased brain into healthy animals. The 'infective agent' is resistant to heat and radiation and, unlike any other infective agents or any living organism, appears to contain no nucleic acid. Stanley Prusiner proposed that transmission was caused by an infective protein or prion; he was awarded a Nobel Prize for this work.

TSEs can be acquired in the three ways listed below.

- *Spontaneous sporadic cases.* Most cases of conventional CJD fall into this category. CJD affects around one in a million people in most populations. It almost always occurs in elderly people. It is unrelated to the presence of scrapie in the sheep flock.
- *Genetic.* A few cases of CJD are familial.
- *Transmission.*
  - Experimentally induced by injecting infected brain into healthy animals.
  - Iatrogenically induced (caused by medical treatment), e.g. by injections of contaminated growth hormone or gonadotrophins extracted from the pituitary glands of human cadavers, by the use of contaminated surgical instruments or by transplants of infected corneal tissue and more recently perhaps by transfusions of infected blood.
  - Through eating infected tissue – kuru is thought to have been caused by eating infected human brains in cannibalistic rituals.

The incubation period of all of these transmissible encephalopathies is long. In Kuru and iatrogenic CJD the average time from exposure to onset of clinical symptoms is thought to be around 20 years.

In 1996 it was formally announced that a new variant of CJD (**vCJD**) had been identified in Britain. It now seems certain that it was caused by eating contaminated beef products. The symptoms of vCJD are different from sporadic CJD; it also has different histological characteristics, a different time course, a different EEG pattern and most significantly it affects much younger people. Sporadic CJD rarely affects people under 60 years but almost all cases of vCJD have been in younger age groups including teenagers.

What caused the epidemic of BSE in British dairy cattle?

Since the 1920s, cattle and especially dairy cows have been fed a protein supplement made by rendering animal remains including cattle remains. It is now seems certain that this feed was the cause of the epidemic but it is unclear how this feed initially became contaminated with the BSE agent. A once popular theory was that a change in the rendering process of this feed in the late 1970s/early 1980s allowed large amounts of sheep scrapie prion to remain in the feed. This scrapie prion then triggered some cows to develop BSE. The disease was then spread by recycling of BSE-infected cattle material in the feed. This theory offered much reassurance because scrapie had been around for hundreds of years and not been transmitted to people by eating sheep products. Although the scrapie prion had apparently crossed the species barrier it was to another ruminant.

The official inquiry into BSE concluded that this theory was incorrect and that BSE was probably present in cattle several years before 1985 but went undetected and that recycling of infective cattle material in feed spread the disease. It was suggested in this report that the original source of the epidemic may have been a single animal with a mutation in the prion protein gene.

In 1988 the inclusion of ruminant protein in feeds for ruminants was banned and this should have eliminated the source of infection in cattle. However, some animals born long after this feed ban came into force still developed BSE and there are several reasons for this, as listed below.

- Existing stocks of banned feed were used up on some farms.
- Use of ruminant protein remained legal for pig and poultry feed and this allowed cross-contamination of ruminant feeds to occur during production. The feed ban was extended in 1996 and it became illegal to feed mammalian meat and bone meal (MBM) to any farm animal or to fish. The primary purpose of this reinforced ban was to prevent cross-contamination of cattle feed.
- There is some vertical transmission (from cow to calf) of the disease. It is estimated that a calf born within a year of the mother developing clinical symptoms of BSE has a 10 per cent chance of being infected by the mother. Infection either occurs in the womb or during delivery. There is no transmission from paternal semen. There is no evidence of any significant horizontal transmission, i.e. from cow to cow.
- A very small number of cattle born after the reinforced MBM feed ban came fully into force have developed BSE and this is probably due largely to cross-contamination of feed occurring outside the UK. In 2001 an EU-wide ban on

feeds containing MBM was introduced although those new member states joining in 2004 may not have implemented this ban until later.

The infective agent in TSEs

The dominant theory is that the infective agent in these TSEs is an infective protein or prion (Prusiner, 1995). This prion protein PrP is a normal protein found in the brains and other tissues of animals. It is suggested that in normal healthy animals the normal PrP protein is present largely in α-helical form and this is easily broken down by proteases. In TSEs large amounts of this PrP protein is present in a different configuration (β-pleated sheet form) and this is extremely resistant to proteases. It is also very resistant to heat and radiation. When the abnormal PrP comes into contact with the normal form it causes the normal form to change shape and a chain reaction is established and a large amount of abnormal protein accumulates and destroys brain cells leading to the clinical symptoms and spongiform lesions in the brain. According to Prusiner there are three likely ways in which TSEs can develop (see below).

* *Spontaneous.* Some spontaneous production of abnormal PrP can occur and this will occasionally trigger the chain reaction as in spontaneous CJD in elderly people.
* *Genetic.* A mutation in the PrP gene may occur which makes the protein more likely to flip to its abnormal structure. There are rare examples of a familial form of CJD in people. It may be that brain tissue from a cow with such a PrP mutation, which when fed back to other cows, triggered off the BSE epidemic.
* *Transmission.* If abnormal PrP protein is introduced into the brain via the diet or via direct injection of infected brain material, this can trigger the chain reaction.

Transmission of BSE to humans

Scrapie has long been prevalent in British sheep but is not transmitted to humans via the diet and it is hard to transmit sheep scrapie to rodents. There was a general belief in the 1980s and early 1990s that BSE would probably not jump the species barrier and affect humans. This view was encouraged by the widespread belief that BSE was scrapie that had been transmitted to cows. In 1990 cases of BSE-like diseases were reported in several exotic species in

zoos and these had been given feed containing ruminant protein. More disturbingly, the first of several cases of a TSE in domestic cats was identified. These observations suggested that BSE had jumped the species barrier and affected species other than ruminants and even carnivores. It is this 'species barrier' that has limited the spread of BSE to humans and even though millions of people (and cats) may have been exposed to some bovine prion, the number of cases of vCJD (and feline spongiform encephalopathy) has remained low.

In general, the more differences there are in the amino acid sequences of the prion proteins of two species, the more difficult it is to transmit the disease experimentally. Cow prion protein has about 30 amino acid differences to the human protein and it is already clear that normal genetic variation in the human prion protein affects susceptibility to vCJD. It is also clear that transmission of TSEs is most efficient when infective material is injected directly into the brain and less efficient when it is given orally.

In experimental transmission studies, only some tissues in Kuru and BSE contain infective quantities of abnormal PrP, i.e. brain, spinal cord and lymphatic tissues. Milk and muscle meat do not contain infective quantities of prion protein in such studies. Steaks and joints of beef from young beef cattle should have been unlikely sources of human infection, even at the peak of the BSE epidemic. Concern has focused on meat products, including baby foods, which often included the potentially infected tissues and were often made from meat obtained from elderly dairy cows. A number of measures were introduced by the British government to protect the human population from BSE. The most important of these measures are listed below.

* In 1988 it was ordered that all clearly infected animals should be destroyed and their carcasses incinerated. Milk from infected animals was also removed from the food chain. All animals are now inspected before slaughter to make sure they do not show symptoms of BSE.
* In 1989 a ban on SBO entering the human food chain was introduced. It was required that all of the likely infective tissues should be removed from all cattle at slaughter, i.e. the brain, spinal cord, spleen, thymus, tonsils and intestines. This measure, if properly enforced, should have afforded almost complete protection to people eating beef. It has been claimed that until 1996

the enforcement of this measure was not rigorous enough and that significant amounts of these tissues entered the human food chain between 1989 and 1996 (largely by contamination of edible meat with SBO during the removal process). In 1997 these controls were extended to cosmetics, pharmaceuticals and medical products.

- In 1996 it was made illegal to sell cattle aged over 30 months (OTM) for human consumption. Very few young animals have developed BSE and so this measure ensured that little infective material actually reached the slaughterhouse. Animals up to 42 months old could be sold if they came from specialist beef producers whose animals had only been fed on grass and who met very strict criteria under the Beef Assurance Scheme. In November 2005 this OTM rule was replaced by compulsory testing of the carcasses of slaughtered animals over 30 months of age and the meat from these older tested animals can now be legally sold.
- For a time it was forbidden to sell beef with bone in it largely because of concerns that it might have nervous tissue adhering to it.

The measures listed above taken together with the very low and still declining incidence of BSE in cattle should afford complete consumer protection at this point in time. In 1996, the EU instituted a worldwide ban on British beef exports. This ban was lifted in 1999 but the recovery in British beef exports has been slow.

The human 'epidemic' of vCJD

It was in the spring of 1996 that the British government formally announced that a new variant of CJD (vCJD) had been discovered and that this was probably linked to eating contaminated beef before the bovine offal ban was introduced in 1989. Figure 18.5 shows the annual numbers of deaths from vCJD since 1995. Experience with Kuru and iatrogenic CJD suggests that incubation period of vCJD may be much more than 20 years in some individuals and so a gradually diminishing trickle of cases may continue to occur for some years yet. It is not possible to say when exactly this mini-epidemic will be over. Some possibilities that may extend the epidemic of vCJD are listed below.

- Transmission by non-food means, e.g. by transfusion of contaminated blood, transplantation of infected tissue or use of contaminated surgical instruments. Note that since 1999 all blood for transfusion has had the white blood cells removed (leucodepletion) which should greatly reduce the risk of transmission of vCJD. More recently anyone who has themselves received a blood transfusion after January 1980 is prevented from donating blood for transfusion. These measures have considerably increased the costs of supplying blood for transfusion.
- All of the early cases of vCJD have occurred in people with a particular variant of the human prion protein, which about 40 per cent of people have (they are homozygous for a methionine code at codon 129 of the prion protein gene). It is just conceivable that a second epidemic will occur in those with other genotypes because they have a longer incubation period. It seems reasonable to expect that if these genotypes substantially delay the onset of the disease then they are also likely to reduce the chances of acquiring the disease at all and thus any second wave of cases, if it occurs, will probably be markedly smaller than the first wave illustrated in Figure 18.5.

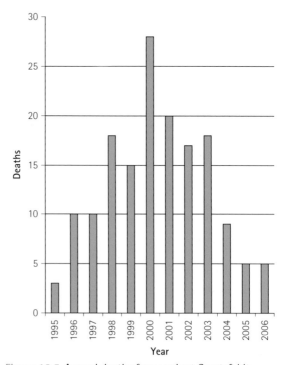

Figure 18.5 *Annual deaths from variant Creutzfeldt–Jakob disease in the UK.*

Key points

- Bovine spongiform encephalopathy (BSE) or 'mad cow disease' is a new and inevitably fatal neurological disease of cattle.

- BSE produces spongiform lesions in the brain similar to those seen in sheep scrapie and human Creutzfeldt–Jakob disease (CJD) and kuru.

- The British cattle epidemic appears to be almost over but it has affected 180 000 cattle mostly in dairy herds and especially older cows.

- Around 160 people have died from a new form of CJD (vCJD) which is the human form of BSE contracted through eating contaminated beef products.

- BSE and vCJD belong to a group of so-called prion diseases that can be transmitted by injecting or eating infected tissue.

- The infective agent (prion) in these prion diseases is thought to be a normal protein that has undergone a conformational change from α-helix to β-pleated sheet.

- When abnormal prion protein is introduced into the brain it causes other normal prion protein molecules to change shape and this begins a chain reaction which ultimately destroys large areas of brain tissue.

- The abnormal prion protein is resistant to protease enzymes and to heat and radiation so it is not destroyed by cooking or by the body's natural defences.

- Contaminated animal feed made from rendered ruminant remains was almost certainly the source of the cattle epidemic.

- It was at first thought that the initial trigger for BSE was sheep scrapie protein that had survived the rendering process.

- The belief that BSE was essentially scrapie in cows was reassuring because scrapie has been endemic in British sheep for centuries without affecting human health.

- It is now thought likely that BSE is a completely new disease that may have been propagated by the recycling of the infected remains of a single animal with a mutant prion protein.

- The initial source of the infection is not, and may never be, definitely established.

- The British government banned the use of ruminant protein in ruminant feed in 1988 but some incidentally contaminated feed continued to be fed to cattle until 1996 and this prolonged the cattle epidemic.

- The use of all meat- and bonemeal-containing feeds to farm animals and fish was banned in the UK in 1996 and later banned in the rest of the EU.

- There is occasional transmission of BSE from cow to calf but not apparently from cow to cow or bull to calf.

- Milk and meat from symptomatic animals has been destroyed since 1988 and all cattle are inspected at slaughter for signs of the disease.

- All beef sold after 1989 in the UK should have had all of the infective tissues (the SBO) removed but there are claims that this measure was not enforced rigorously enough prior to 1996.

- Between 1996 and 2005 only cattle under 30 months and free from SBO have been permitted to be sold in the UK (with a few specified exceptions). This over-30 months rule has now been relaxed and meat from older animals can be sold if the carcass is tested for BSE.

- Current measures, coupled with the low and declining incidence of BSE in cattle, should guarantee the safety of current beef sales.

- A great deal of infected cattle material probably entered the human food chain prior to 1996 and millions of people may have been exposed to it.

- The human epidemic of vCJD has been at the very low end of earlier predictions; it peaked in 2000 and is now reduced to a small trickle of new cases each year (<5).

- The 'species barrier' has limited the spread of the cattle disease to humans who have eaten contaminated beef products.

- It is possible that a second wave of cases of vCJD will occur in people whose prion protein structure has delayed the onset of the disease; it seems reasonable to expect that if this second wave does materialize it will be even smaller than the first wave.

FOOD PROCESSING

Some general pros and cons of food processing

This term food processing covers a multitude of processes to which food may be subjected. These processes may be traditional or modern and they may occur in the home, catering unit or factory. Unless one eats only raw, home-grown foods, it is impossible to avoid 'processed foods'. It would be impossible to feed a large urban industrial society without some commercial processing of foods. For example, around 50 per cent of the value of all food purchases in the UK are frozen or chilled. Processing includes cooking, smoking, drying, freezing, pasteurizing, canning, irradiation, etc.

Processing of foods, particularly preparation of ready-to-eat foods 'adds value' to the ingredients and increases their commercial potential for retailers and processors. Food processors and retailers represent some of the most commercially successful businesses in developed countries. This high profitability has tended to politicize food processing issues, sometimes to the detriment of constructive critical debate. The term 'processed food' is often used to convey very negative connotations about modern food and food suppliers. However, it is such an all-embracing term, covering foods across the whole spectrum of composition, that its use in this way is unhelpful and probably warns of the prejudice or political motivation of the critic. Each processed food should be judged on its own merits and should be considered within the context of the whole diet rather than purely in isolation.

Commercial processing of food has several objectives in addition to the obvious commercial ones, such as those listed below.

- Processing reduces or prevents the chemical deterioration and microbial spoilage of foods. It thus increases the shelf-life of foods and increases food availability, reduces waste and may reduce the cost of food.
- By destroying pathogens or preventing their growth, processing lowers the risk of foodborne diseases.
- It can increase the palatability of foods.
- Processing enables new varieties of foods to be created.

- Commercially prepared food products reduce the time that individuals need to spend on food preparation. Even those unable or unwilling to spend much time on food preparation can eat an interesting and varied diet if they can afford to buy high-quality prepared foods.

Commercial processing usually, but not always, has some negative effects on the nutrient content of the unprepared food. These losses may be very similar to, or even less than, those involved in home preparation of food. These losses may not be very significant in the diets of many North Americans and western Europeans who have ample intakes of the essential nutrients. Imbalance of selection from the major food groups is a more significant threat to dietary adequacy in Western industrialized countries. In many cases the nutrient content of processed foods (e.g. vitamins in frozen vegetables) may actually be higher than stale versions of the same food bought 'fresh'. It is often argued that food processors encourage people to consume foods high in fat, sugar and salt but low in complex carbohydrate and thus are partly responsible for the increased prevalence of the diseases of industrialization. It seems probable, however, that even without the encouragement of food processors, our natural inclination to consume such a diet would have prevailed. Nevertheless, it is true that, for example, most of the salt in the UK diet is added by food manufacturers and reductions in the salt of commercially processed foods would have a major impact on total salt intakes. Although sales of sugar have dropped considerably in recent years in the UK, there has been a smaller fall in total sugar intake because more sugar is consumed within commercially prepared foods. Commercial processing tends to reduce the consumer's ability to monitor and regulate their intakes of sugar, salt, fat, etc., despite attempts at making the composition of processed foods more transparent by improved food labelling.

Commercial processors and food retailers provide what they think they can profitably sell. They have, for example, been quick to recognize the commercial opportunities offered by the demand for 'healthy foods'. Many highly processed foods have a very healthy image, e.g. some margarine and low-fat spreads, some breakfast cereals, low-fat salad dressings, low-fat yoghurts, low-calorie drinks and certain meat substitutes of vegetable or microbial origin. Some of the modern **functional foods** that are marketed on their proposed health benefits are the products of modern food processing, e.g. margarine with high levels of plant sterols that lower blood cholesterol.

Key points

- The term 'processed food' covers a huge and diverse range of food products and so general discussion of their merits and flaws is of limited usefulness.

- Commercial processing often extends the shelf-life of foods and may increase their microbiological and chemical safety.

- Commercial processing can improve the palatability of individual foods and increase variety by making foods more accessible and even allowing the creation of new foods.

- The availability of commercially prepared foods decreases the time individuals need to spend on food preparation, although this may increase food costs.

- Nutrient losses during commercial processing of foods may be comparable to losses during home preparation.

- Many commercially prepared foods are high in fat, salt and/or sugar but low in complex carbohydrate.

- Food manufacturers will, at least superficially, respond to consumer demands for healthier processed foods if it is profitable for them to do so.

- Many highly processed foods are marketed on their image as healthier options.

Specific processing methods

Canning

This is a very good method for the long-term preservation of food. The food is maintained in sealed containers and thus protected from oxidative deterioration or growth of aerobic micro-organisms. The food is subjected to a vigorous heat treatment after canning that is designed to ensure that there is no practical possibility that even heat-resistant bacterial spores will survive. The so-called botulinum cook ensures the destruction of all spores of the potentially lethal toxin-producing, anaerobic organism C. *botulinum* in at-risk foods. If commercially canned food is consumed soon after opening, there is negligible risk of it being associated with food poisoning.

Pasteurization

Mild heat is applied to a food that is sufficient to destroy likely pathogenic bacteria and to reduce the number of spoilage organisms without impairing the food itself. It is usually associated with milk but other food such as liquid egg, liquid ice cream mix and honey may be pasteurized. Pasteurization of milk traditionally involved holding it at 63°C for 30 minutes. This was designed to ensure the destruction of the organism responsible for tuberculosis but it also kills salmonellae and the other heat-sensitive pathogens usually found in milk. The same result can be achieved by the modern **high-temperature short time** method in which the milk is raised to 72°C for 15 seconds (see under UHT in the next section for the theoretical basis for this change).

Ultra high temperature treatment

Once again, ultra high temperature (UHT) treatment is most often associated with milk but is also applied to other foods like fruit juice. Traditionally, milk was sterilized by heating it to temperatures of 105–110°C for 20–40 minutes. Such severe heat treatment causes marked chemical changes in the milk that impair its flavour, appearance, smell and nutrient content. The UHT method relies on the principle that the rate of chemical reactions only doubles with a 10°C rise in temperature whereas the rate of bacterial killing increases about 10-fold. Thus full sterilization can be achieved by holding the milk at 135°C for 2 seconds with little chemical change in the milk. Two seconds at 135°C has approximately the same bacterial killing effect as 33 minutes at 105°C but results in chemical changes equivalent to only 16 seconds at this lower temperature. After UHT treatment the milk is placed aseptically into sterile containers and will keep for up to 6 months. Chemical deterioration rather than microbial spoilage limits the duration of storage of UHT products.

Cook-chill processing

With the cook-chill process, foods are cooked separately as they would be in the home kitchen.

Bacterial cells will be killed by this process but spores will survive. The food is then chilled rapidly to temperatures below 5°C to minimize growth of the surviving spore-forming bacteria. The food is then divided into portions and packaged. Rigorous standards of hygiene are required during this portioning and packaging stage to prevent re-contamination with spoilage and food poisoning organisms. Most cook-chill foods have a maximum permitted shelf life of 6–8 days partly because of the difficulty of preventing contamination by the ubiquitous *Pseudomonas* group of spoilage organisms. The introduction of cook-chill foods into hospitals is an area of particular concern. Many groups who are vulnerable to organisms such as *Listeria* are concentrated in hospitals, e.g. pregnant women and infants in maternity units, people whose immune systems have been suppressed by disease (e.g. acquired immune deficiency syndrome (AIDS)) or by treatment (e.g. immunosuppressant drugs) and those weakened by injury, disease or old age.

Food irradiation

Irradiation involves exposing food to ionizing radiation which can either be X-rays or more usually gamma rays emitted from a radioactive source such as cobalt-60 (reviewed by Hawthorn, 1989 and key issues summarized in FSA, 2007). There is no contact between the radioactive source and the food and so the irradiated food does not itself become radioactive. The irradiation of food is not a new idea; its potential was recognized and demonstrated over 100 years ago. It is only in recent years, however, that the widespread application of irradiation in food processing has become economically viable because of the ready availability of gamma emitters such as cobalt-60. Many countries have now approved the use of irradiation for some categories of foods.

In the USA, irradiation is classified with the food additives because it causes chemical changes in food. Its use is permitted for use on a wide range of foods including onions, potatoes, herbs and spices, nuts and seeds, wheat, fish, poultry and meat. Irradiated food must be clearly labelled as having been irradiated.

In the UK prior to 1990, irradiation was forbidden for all foods with the exception of herbs and spices. At the beginning of 1991 this ban was withdrawn and irradiation of a wide range of foods is now theoretically permitted in properly licensed centres, e.g.

fruit, vegetables, cereals, fish, shellfish and poultry may all now be legally irradiated in the UK. There is, however, currently only one site in the UK licensed to irradiate human food and they are only licensed to irradiate spices and condiments. The only source of radiation permitted for food irradiation in the UK is gamma rays from cobalt-60. Irradiated foods must be labelled as such. EU regulations mean that even where a prepared food contains only a small amount of irradiated ingredient this must be declared on the label. The only foods that can be freely traded across EU boundaries are those within the categories currently licensed for irradiation in the UK.

The effects of irradiation on the food vary according to the dose used (see Figure 18.6). Some of these changes are used to extend the shelf-life of foods, such as the inhibition of sprouting, delay in ripening and reducing the numbers of spoilage organisms. The killing of insect pests reduces losses and damage to food from this cause, and reduces the need to fumigate with chemical insecticides. The elimination of food-poisoning organisms should reduce the risks of food poisoning, and sterilization of food by irradiation may be particularly useful in ensuring the safety of food intended for immunosuppressed patients. Despite these apparent advantages of food irradiation, its introduction has been vigorously opposed by certain pressure groups within the UK. It has been suggested that the full effects of irradiation are not yet well enough understood to be totally confident of its safety. However, the FSA (2007) stated unequivocally that properly irradiated foods are safe and that irradiation is a consumer choice and food labelling issue rather than a safety issue.

Some potential problems of irradiated foods are listed below (note that these are potential hazards suggested by those who oppose irradiation rather than the views of the author).

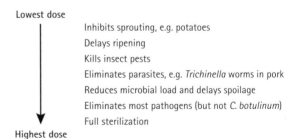

Figure 18.6 *The effects of varying doses of ionizing radiation on food.*

The ionizing radiation induces certain chemical changes within the food, it increases free radical production and chemical species known as radiolytes (see Chapter 12 for a discussion of free radicals and antioxidants). The free radicals and radiolytes produced by irradiation are short-lived species and they are responsible for the killing of micro-organisms produced by irradiation. Although there may be natural concern that these chemical changes may have detrimental effects on health, it must be added that all processing methods produce some chemical changes in food, e.g. smoking and barbecuing lead to production of small amounts of potentially carcinogenic chemicals in food. The chemical changes induced in food by irradiation are less than those produced by heat processing. The low level of chemical change induced by irradiation is illustrated by the extreme difficulty in chemically identifying whether or not a food sample has been irradiated. FSA (2007) states that methods have been validated for the detection of different irradiated foods including herbs and spices, meat and poultry containing bone and foods containing fats, and methods for detecting other irradiated foods are under development.

- Some bacterial and fungal toxins will not be destroyed by irradiation so if irradiation is used to compensate for earlier poor hygiene then food poisoning from these toxins may result.

- At the doses usually used on foods, spores will survive and may later grow in the food. Irradiation is known to increase mutation rates and so conceivably new and dangerous mutants of micro-organisms might be produced in food.

- At high doses, e.g. those required to achieve sterilization, there may be adverse effects on the palatability of the food and major losses of some nutrients such as thiamin and vitamin E. At dose levels likely to be used for 'pasteurization' of food, irradiation produces almost no change in flavour or nutrient content, unlike other methods of food processing and preservation.

- There is concern about the safety of workers at establishments where food irradiation takes place. There is thus a clear need to regulate and license facilities for food irradiation and only one site in the UK is currently (early 2007) licensed for food irradiation and this is subject to stringent regulation and inspection by the FSA.

Key points

- Rigorous heat treatment and sealed containers ensure that properly canned food will often remain in good condition and microbiologically safe for many years.

- The mild heat treatment of pasteurization should eliminate likely pathogens and reduce levels of spoilage organisms without significant adverse effects on the flavour or nutrient value of the food.

- Sterilization using ultra high temperature (UHT) for very short periods results in far less chemical change than traditional sterilization techniques and so has much less effect on flavour and nutrient loss.

- Cook-chill processing does not kill all spore-forming bacteria, and food may also be contaminated with other spoilage and pathogenic organisms during packaging.

- *Listeria monocytogenes* can still grow in chilled foods and this can have serious consequences for pregnant women and other vulnerable groups.

- Irradiating foods with varying doses of X-rays or gamma rays has a variety of potential uses (summarized in Figure 18.6).

- Consumer resistance has limited the marketing of irradiated foods although many countries permit irradiation of many foods.

- In the UK, only one site is currently licensed for food irradiation, and only to irradiate herbs, spices and condiments.

- Irradiation can extend the shelf-life of many foods and/or improve their microbiological safety.

- High doses of radiation do induce potentially adverse chemical changes in food and can reduce palatability and lead to significant losses of nutrients.

- Mild irradiation produces imperceptible changes in flavour or loss of nutrients and it is difficult to chemically detect whether or not a food has been irradiated.

- Some microbial toxins will survive irradiation.

- Some micro-organisms will survive mild irradiation and it has been argued that theoretically this might increase mutation rates in organisms that survive the irradiation process.

CHEMICAL SAFETY OF FOOD

Overview of chemical hazards in food

There are three potential sources of chemical hazard in food and these are listed below.

- *Food additives* – chemicals that are deliberately added to food during processing.
- *Natural toxicants* – compounds naturally present in the food that may have toxic effects.
- *Contaminants* – substances that are incidentally or inadvertently added to foods during agricultural production, storage or processing, e.g. residues of drugs given to food animals; pesticide or fertilizer residues; contaminants leeching into food from packaging or containers; and fungal toxins.

One dilemma that increasingly faces those trying to ensure the chemical safety of food is to decide at what level in the food the presence of any particular chemical substance represents a real hazard to consumers. Total absence of all traces of potentially hazardous chemicals from all foods is, and always has been, an impossible ideal. Almost all chemicals, including most nutrients, are toxic if the dose is high enough. More substances are being subjected to rigorous safety tests, which usually involve exposing animals to high doses of the chemical for prolonged periods. Many chemicals that are ubiquitous in our environment can be shown to have toxic potential by such tests. Analytical procedures are also becoming increasingly sophisticated and sensitive, making it possible to detect infinitesimally small amounts of potentially hazardous chemicals in foods. This combination of factors, especially when distorted by popular journalists, can lead to the impression that the chemical hazards in our food are increasing at an alarming rate. At least some of this apparent increase in chemical danger from food is an artefact caused by increased awareness of the potential hazards of chemicals and increased ability to detect small amounts of these chemicals.

In a report by the Institute of Food Technologists (IFT, 1975), the panel distinguished between **toxic**, which was defined as 'being inherently capable of producing injury when tested by itself', and **hazard**, which was defined as 'being likely to produce injury under the circumstances of exposure' as in food. Food naturally contains thousands of toxic substances, including many nutrients, but very few of these represent real hazard. For example, the average US consumer ingests around 10 000 mg of **solanine** from potatoes each year. This is enough of this atropine-like alkaloid to kill him or her if consumed in a single dose. The same average US consumer ingests about 40 mg of lethal hydrogen cyanide in their annual kilogram of lima beans and 14 mg of arsenic from seafood.

Most natural toxins are present in low concentrations in natural foods and they do not usually accumulate. They are usually metabolized and/or excreted by a variety of mechanisms that are also involved in the disposal of ingested man-made chemicals such as food additives, drugs and residues of agricultural chemicals. There are a variety of mechanisms and sites through which the different toxicants induce their effect and so generally the effects of small amounts of many individual toxicants are unlikely to be additive. Thus 1 per cent of a toxic dose of 100 different toxins almost certainly will not produce ill effects (IFT, 1975).

Key points

- Natural toxicants, contaminants and food additives must all be considered potential sources of chemical hazard in food.
- Sensitive analytical techniques can detect numerous substances in food that have toxic potential but few of them represent a real hazard to consumers who eat a varied diet.

Natural toxicants and contaminants

Circumstances that may increase chemical hazard

The chances of toxic potential becoming a real hazard is likely to be increased if there is exaggerated consumption of one food for a prolonged period. This is true whether the toxin is naturally present, a contaminant or a deliberate additive. This is yet one more reason for encouraging diversity in the diet. Examples of natural toxicants in food producing serious illness may occur when abnormally high amounts of a particular food are consumed. The plant *Lathyrus sativa* has been widely grown in Asia and north Africa, and the seeds (chickling peas or khesari dhal) regularly consumed. However, during very dry seasons it was consumed in large quantities because the plant is drought resistant. When consumed in large quantities it can produce a severe disease of the spinal cord, **lathyrism**, which can lead to permanent paralysis. When only small quantities are consumed as part of a mixed diet they do not constitute a hazard and are nutritious.

Chemical hazard from food may arise if individual susceptibility causes increased sensitivity to a particular toxin. The common broad bean *Vicia faba* contains a substance that causes haemolysis (red cell breakdown). This can lead to a severe anaemia called **favism** in those who are genetically susceptible because they are deficient in a particular enzyme (glucose 6-phosphate dehydrogenase). As many as 35 per cent of some Mediterranean peoples and 10 per cent of American blacks have this particular genetic deficiency. Vomiting, abdominal pain and fever are the acute symptoms; jaundice and dark-coloured urine may occur as a result of the haemolysis with eventually severe anaemia a possibility.

Traditional methods of preparing, processing and selecting foods often minimizes any potential hazard they may represent. Cassava is one of the most important staple foods for millions of people in the tropics; it may, for example, provide up to 60 per cent of the calorific intake in Nigeria. Cassava contains certain alkaloids that release cyanide when acted on by an enzyme in the cassava. The traditional method of preparing cassava involves peeling and soaking for several days and most of the cyanide is lost due to fermentation. Cases of sometimes fatal cyanide poisoning are associated with inadequate processing of the cassava (particularly shortening of the fermentation time) and increased use of lower quality 'bitter' cassava which has a higher cyanide content (see Akintowa and Tunawashe, 1992). As another example, polar bear liver contains toxic concentrations of retinol. Inuit avoided eating the liver but unwary polar explorers have been poisoned by eating it.

Some natural toxicants in 'Western' diets

Few natural toxicants are thought to represent significant hazards to Western consumers. In her analysis of over a thousand recorded outbreaks of food poisoning in England and Wales, Roberts (1982) found that 54 outbreaks (about 5 per cent) were due to chemical toxicity – 47 due to **scombrotoxin** from fish and seven from a **haemagglutinin** in red kidney beans. Some potential natural chemical hazards in UK food are listed below.

- Scombrotoxic poisoning is caused by heat-stable toxins liberated by the action of bacteria on fish protein during spoilage. The toxin is thus produced by bacterial action but is not in itself a bacterial toxin. Symptoms occur shortly after eating the contaminated fish and include a peppery taste in the mouth, flushing of the face and neck, sweating and sometimes nausea and diarrhoea.
- Eating raw red kidney beans leads to short-lasting symptoms of nausea, vomiting and diarrhoea. These symptoms are thought to be due to a toxin that cause red cells to agglutinate (stick together), a haemagglutinin. The symptoms are probably due to damage to intestinal cells caused by this toxin. The haemagglutinin is destroyed by vigorous boiling but it may persist if the beans are cooked by prolonged gentle heating in a slow cooker. These beans should always be subjected to 10 minutes of vigorous boiling before being eaten. Roberts (1982) found that all of the outbreaks she investigated were due to eating the beans in an uncooked or undercooked state. As a general rule, raw or undercooked beans should not be eaten as they contain several mildly toxic factors and factors that interfere with the proper digestion of protein.
- Some cheeses contain the substance **tyramine**, which can cause a rise in blood pressure. This may be dangerous for those taking certain antidepressant drugs because they sensitize the individual to the effects of tyramine (note that these drugs called monoamine oxidase inhibitors are the oldest type of antidepressant and have largely been replaced by more modern drugs which do not sensitize people to tyramine).
- Solanine is an atropine-like substance found in potatoes. In high enough doses it will cause headache, vomiting and diarrhoea and may perhaps even result in circulatory collapse and neurological disturbances. Levels of solanine in potatoes are rarely enough to produce illness and established outbreaks of potato poisoning are rare.
- Many species of Brassicae (cabbage family) contain goitrogens, chemicals that induce goitre. These do not represent a real hazard at levels of consumption normally found in industrialized countries.
- Mussels that have ingested the plankton species *Gonyaulux tamarensis* may contain hazardous

amounts of a heat-stable neurotoxin – **saxitoxin**. At certain times the sea may turn red, 'red tides', due to large numbers of *Gonyaulux* in the water. These red tides may occasionally occur even off the coasts of Britain and the US and at such times it is dangerous to eat mussels.

- Some fungi produce toxic chemicals, **mycotoxins**. Some mycotoxins represent a hazard to the inexperienced gatherer of wild fungi and some fungal toxins are deliberately consumed because they contain hallucinogenic agents. The death cap mushroom *Amanita phalloides* is responsible for the majority of fatal cases of mushroom poisoning. This mushroom is similar in appearance to some edible species, it is reported to have a pleasant taste and symptoms do not occur until 8–24 hours after ingestion by which time irreparable liver damage may have occurred and death typically occurs after 7–10 days. Around half a cap (30 g) is enough of this mushroom to kill a human being and even with modern medical care (including liver transplants in some cases) the death rate from accidental poisoning is still around 10–15 per cent and many of the survivors have permanent liver damage. Moulds also grow on many foods that will not support the growth of bacteria because fungi are more tolerant of low water activity and low pH than bacteria. Dry foods such as nuts and bread, sugary foods such as jam (jelly) and salty foods such as cheese may all go mouldy. Several of the toxins produced by moulds are potent carcinogens. **Aflatoxins** produced by *Aspergillus flavus* have been responsible for outbreaks of fatal poisoning in Taiwan, India and Uganda. It causes gastrointestinal bleeding, liver damage and pulmonary oedema. It has been shown to cause liver cancer in animal studies. Mouldy nuts would be a likely source of aflatoxin in the USA and UK. Mouldy grain may contain the toxin **ergot** which is produced by the ergot fungus (*Claviceps purpurea*) and this has caused serious outbreaks of poisoning in the past and still does in some countries, a condition referred to as St Vitas Dance or St Anthony's Fire. The symptoms of ergot poisoning include hallucinations, nervous spasms, convulsions, psychotic delusions and spontaneous abortion. The well-know psychedelic drug LSD or lysergic acid is made from ergot and ergot has been used in the past to induce abortions. The last recorded outbreak of ergot poisoning in Europe was in a village called Pont St Esprit in France in 1951 when contaminated bread from the village bakery caused 135 people to be hospitalized and resulted in six deaths. Mouldy food should therefore be regarded as potentially hazardous and should be discarded. In the early 1990s, the detection of very small amounts of the mycotoxin **patulin** in some brands of apple juice received great publicity in the UK.

Mould growth is deliberately encouraged in the production of some foods such as blue cheese and mould-ripened cheese. These are not thought to represent hazard at usual levels of consumption.

Residues of agricultural chemicals

Expert opinion is that the residues of agricultural chemicals in foods represent no significant hazard to consumers when current regulations are adhered to, and most cases of acute poisoning resulting from ingestion of agricultural chemical have arisen because of their misuse, including the examples listed below (after Taylor, 2006).

- Confusion of an agricultural chemical with a common, harmless food ingredient such as sugar or salt.
- Eating of seeds intended for planting and treated with a fungicide – most fungicides are of low toxicity to people but those containing mercury and a substance called hexachlorobenzene are exceptions to this general rule. In the late 1950s more than 3000 people in Turkey were affected by hexachlorobenzene poisoning after eating seed grain intended for planting. The symptoms included hair loss, ulcerated skin lesions, liver and thyroid enlargement and there was 10 per cent mortality.
- Agricultural misuse of a chemical – in 1985 in the USA, almost 1400 people became ill after eating watermelons which had been treated with an insecticide called aldicarb, resulting in symptoms that included nausea, diarrhoea, headache, blurred vision and disturbances of balance. It is actually illegal to use this insecticide on watermelons because it is known to become concentrated in the edible part of the fruit.

Although most toxicologists assert that these chemicals pose no threat to long-term health, these assurances have been insufficient to convince a significant minority of the population who are willing to pay considerably higher prices for organic produce that has been grown without the aid of modern agricultural chemicals which include insecticides, herbicides, fungicides, fertilizers, and antibiotics and other drugs given to farm animals. These consumers are also willing to accept the less than perfect appearance of their fruits and vegetables that organic farming practices sometimes produce. Many producers and suppliers have been quick to recognize the commercial opportunities afforded by this new market. People who can afford it clearly have the right to choose food grown in this way but the practicability of supplying the whole population with organic food is doubtful and there are no scientifically quantifiable health benefits. There may well be more convincing environmental arguments for farming in this way. Organic growers may well use different varieties of fruits and vegetables and factors such as slower growth, longer maturation/ripening may have effects on texture and flavour. Strain or variety differences, variation in access to sunlight and exercise space may also have some effects on the taste, appearance or texture of milk, meat, eggs and even farmed fish.

Key points

- Food naturally contains small amounts of many toxic substances that because they are eaten in such small doses do not cause illness.
- The risk of a natural toxicant causing illness is increased by:
  - abnormally high consumption of the toxin-containing food
  - increased susceptibility to the toxin, e.g. genetic
  - inadequate removal of the toxin during processing.
- Some toxins present in many Western diets are:
  - scombrotoxin produced by bacterial action on fish protein
  - haemagglutinins and other toxins in raw or undercooked beans
  - tyramine in cheese which interacts with older antidepressant drugs
  - an atropine-like alkaloid, solanine, normally present in minute amounts in potatoes
  - goitrogens present in minute amounts in plants of the cabbage family

  - mussels contaminated with a neurotoxin produced by the red plankton *Gonyaulux tamarensis*
  - mycotoxins produced by fungi and by mould growth on food.
- Most but not all scientists believe that when used in permitted amounts, residues of agricultural chemicals do not represent a significant hazard to consumers.
- Acute cases of poisoning caused by agricultural chemicals (insecticides, herbicides, fungicides, fertilizers and veterinary drugs) have arisen because of accidents or misuse of the chemical.
- Most scientists therefore do not believe that more expensive organic food produced without agricultural chemicals is healthier.
- Many consumers do not accept the scientific consensus about organic food, and there may well be stronger ecological arguments for less chemical-dependent food production methods.
- Variety differences and other incidental differences between 'mass produced' food and that produced by smaller organic producers may have effects on the taste, texture or appearance of organic food.

Food additives

Around 300 food additives are used in the UK together with another 3000 flavourings. The average British person probably consumes several kilograms of these in a year.

Uses

Chemicals are deliberately added to food for a variety of purposes, such as:

- processing aids, e.g. emulsifiers, flour improvers and anti-caking agents
- to improve the sensory appeal of foods, e.g. colours, flavours and sweeteners
- to improve the nutritional value of foods, e.g. vitamins and/or minerals added to bread, breakfast cereals and drinks
- to prevent the growth of food poisoning and spoilage organisms, e.g. nitrites and nitrates in meat products
- to inhibit the growth of moulds, e.g. propionic acid or vinegar in bread
- to inhibit the chemical deterioration of foods, e.g. antioxidants like vitamins C and E.

Some arguments against the use of food additives

Those who are opposed to the use of food additives or the scale of their current usage have used all of the arguments below to criticize them.

- They are dangerous chemicals *per se;* in particular, that chronic exposure to them will lead to an increase in cancer risk.
- That they can be used to disguise faulty or inferior products and thus deceive the consumer. Colourings, flavouring and emulsifiers can disguise the high-fat and low-grade meat used in some meat products. Colourings and flavourings can disguise the lack of fruit in 'fruit' drinks and yoghurts. Polyphosphates can be used to artificially increase the weight of meat and poultry by increasing its water content.
- Even generally safe additives may trigger adverse reactions in some individuals, e.g. allergy to the yellow food colourant tartrazine and to sulphites (sulphur dioxide) used to preserve many foods.
- Preservatives can be used by manufacturers to compensate for poor hygiene standards.
- That many of the cosmetic additives are unnecessary or perhaps even imposed on the consumer by food producers and retailers.

Some counter-arguments

Additives with food-preserving functions are a necessity if large urban populations are to be supplied with a variety of safe, nutritious and affordable foods. Traditional preservatives have long been used for these purposes, e.g. salt, sugar, woodsmoke, vinegar, alcohol, nitrites and nitrates. When evaluating the safety of modern preservatives or when judging the merits of foods claiming to be 'free from all artificial preservatives' it should be borne in mind that most of these traditional preservatives have been implicated in disease. For example, salt has been linked to hypertension, nitrites lead to the generation of potentially carcinogenic nitrosamines and small amounts of potential carcinogens are found in smoked foods.

Some additives are essential as processing aids or otherwise necessary for the manufacture of a considerable number of supermarket foods. Some of these foods are considered to be 'healthy foods' and seen as important in helping consumers to comply with current nutrition education guidelines. Emulsifiers and stabilizers are essential for the production of many 'reduced fat' products such as low-fat spread

and polyunsaturated margarine. Anti-caking agents are needed for the manufacture of many powders that are to be instantly rehydrated like coffee whitener. Artificial sweeteners or **sugar replacers** are necessary for the production of many 'low-calorie' and 'reduced-sugar' foods.

The additives that are most vulnerable to criticism are those that serve cosmetic purposes, i.e. that are there to enhance the appearance or palatability of the food. These may even be claimed to be doing a positive disservice to Western consumers by encouraging over-consumption and obesity. If a purely scientific model of food function is used then appearance and palatability of food could almost be regarded as a decadent irrelevance. Few people would, however, really want to regard positive sensory appeal of food as an optional extra. Although, as already noted, these do have the potential to allow manufacturers to dupe the public into buying prepared foods made from lower-quality ingredients.

Food additive regulation

Different countries have differing regulations governing the use of food additives but the common purposes of such regulations are to ensure that they are used safely, effectively, honestly and in the minimum amounts necessary to achieve their objectives.

The **FDA** regulates the use of food additives in the USA. In order to get approval to use a new additive, a manufacturer is required to provide evidence that the additive is effective, safe and can be detected and measured in the final product. The approval of the additive is then considered after a public hearing at which experts testify for and against the use of the additive. Very few new additives have been submitted for approval in recent years because of the considerable costs involved in acquiring the extensive safety data required by the FDA; only for substances such as new artificial sweeteners (e.g. **sucralose**) or calorie-free fat substitutes (e.g. **olestra**) does the potential scale of use justify the costs involved. Additives that were in use before this procedure was adopted in the 1950s were put onto a list of substances **generally recognized as safe (GRAS)**. The GRAS list is subject to a continuing process of review and revision. More than four decades ago, Congress approved the so-called **Delaney clause** 'no additive shall be deemed to be safe if it is found to induce cancer when ingested by man or animal'. This requirement is now regarded as unreasonably absolute in its prohibition and the

FDA deems additives to be safe if the risk of human cancer is less than 1 in 1 000 000. Saccharin is a permitted sweetener in the USA despite being reported to cause bladder cancer when administered in very large doses to animals, i.e. although shown to be toxic it is not thought to represent a hazard to the US consumer.

In the UK, the responsibility for regulating the use of food additives lies with the FSA although the European Food Safety Authority is responsible for evaluating food additive safety across the whole of the EU. This European committee consists of independent experts and they have to consider and advise on any proposed new additive or new usage of an additive. They consider whether this new additive or additive use is necessary and safe. Grounds for necessity are factors such as:

- increased shelf-life of a product
- reduced cost
- an improved product for the consumer
- necessity for the manufacture of a new product or for the introduction of a new manufacturing process.

EU law states that food additives can only be used if:

- they present no hazard to health at the levels used in foods
- a reasonable need for the additive can be demonstrated (as examples above)
- they do not mislead the consumer.

E numbers, have been used to designate food additives in Britain and the rest of the EU. They were introduced as part of efforts to harmonize legislation within the EU and to overcome language barriers. They were originally envisaged as something that would help to engender consumer confidence. If an additive had an E number then the consumer could be totally assured of its safety. In reality, however, the effect was quite the opposite; E numbers on food labels evoke suspicion and have been used to epitomize everything that is unwholesome about 'modern, adulterated and artificial food'. A full listing of E numbers can be found in the webpages of Dr David Jukes (www.foodlaw.rdg.ac.uk). A quick perusal of this extensive list shows that it includes several familiar nutrients and compounds (and perhaps less threatening by name):

- E101 is riboflavin
- E300 is vitamin C
- E302 is calcium carbonate
- E307 is vitamin E
- E120 is cochineal
- E140 is chlorophyll
- E150 is caramel
- E160a is carotene
- E260 is acetic acid (vinegar)
- E553b is talc
- E901 is beeswax.

In the UK there are three sets of regulations (incorporated into UK law in 1995) dealing with the regulation of sweeteners, colours and miscellaneous food additives, the latter covering additives not covered by the first two categories. These regulations are designed to incorporate EU legislation into national legislation and they stipulate:

- which additives are permitted for use in food (and for direct sale to the consumer)
- the purity specifications for permitted additives
- conditions of additive use including in many cases setting the maximum level of use.

Flavourings are not included in these particular regulations. The regulation for all types of additives other than flavourings could be described as a 'positive list system' – only things listed as being approved can be used under the conditions specified in the regulations and other additives within these categories are by default not therefore permitted. In the case of flavourings the regulation could be said to be a 'negative list' approach whereby certain things are not permitted or restricted but there is no list of specified, approved flavourings. The long-term objective within the EU is to produce a positive list for flavourings. Many flavours are natural extracts or synthetic versions of substances within natural extracts that are 'nature identical'.

There are a few examples of food additives causing acute adverse symptoms, such as those listed below.

- Sorbitol is an alcohol of glucose and together with some other hexose alcohols is used as a sweetener for drinks, sweets and chewing gum that is non-cariogenic (does not cause dental decay). These substances are absorbed relatively slowly from the gut and so if large amounts are consumed they can remain within the gut and cause diarrhoea due to their osmotic effects. Foods containing these sugar alcohols usually carry a warning that high consumption can cause diarrhoea.

- Sulphites are added to foods for a variety of reasons such as bleaching, prevention of browning and as antimicrobials. Under acid conditions these produce sulphur dioxide in the food. A small number of people are sensitive to this sulphur dioxide and it produces asthma-type symptoms in them. Many foods carry warnings that they contain a source of sulphur dioxide to help those liable to sulphite-induced asthma.
- Tartrazine is a yellow dye and it has been claimed to cause asthma and hives in some sensitive people although this has not been established with absolute certainty.
- Olestra is a synthetic substance used as a calorie-free fat substitute for frying certain savoury snacks in the USA (although not as at February 2007 permitted in the EU). It can cause a number of gastro-intestinal symptoms in some people; symptoms such as anal leakage, oily stools, urgency of defecation, etc.

Testing the safety of food additives

Four potential sources of information that can be used to evaluate the safety of food additives are:

- human experiments
- human epidemiology
- *in vitro* tests
- animal experiments.

One of the major concerns relating to the safety of food additives is that life-time exposure to an additive may increase the risk of chronic disease and especially of human cancer. Human experiments are inevitably either short term or small scale and subject to ethical restrictions that would preclude heavy and prolonged exposure to an additive. Such human experiments can be of no real use in identifying even relatively large increases in cancer risk due to particular additives. Neither can epidemiology be expected to pinpoint harmful effects of individual additives. Epidemiology involves relating exposure to changes in disease rates, yet we are all exposed to hundreds of additives in amounts that would be difficult to quantify on an individual basis and even on a 'worse-case scenario' the increased cancer rate due to the additive is likely to be small. It proved difficult to show convincingly with epidemiological methods that smoking causes lung cancer even though the association is strong, the level of exposure is relatively easy to establish and

there is an identifiable matched but unexposed population.

In vitro tests involve the use of isolated mammalian cells or micro-organisms. The best established of these test are those, like the **Ames test**, that use the ability of compounds to cause mutation in bacteria as an indicator of their likely carcinogenicity in mammals. Mutagenesis, carcinogenesis and teratogenesis (causing fetal abnormalities) may all be caused by damage to the genetic material, DNA. Such tests are a useful way of screening out some potential carcinogens or teratogens and thus to reduce the number of compound that need to undergo full animal testing. *In vitro* tests are, however, not able to provide positive assurance that a compound or one of its metabolites is going to be safe in higher animals. Such tests are, in any case, validated by comparison of the mutagenic effects of chemicals with their carcinogenic effect when used in animal tests.

Animal tests on food additives can be categorized under four main headings: acute and subacute toxicity tests; absorption, distribution, metabolism and excretion tests; teratogenicity tests; and long-term carcinogenicity tests.

Acute and subacute toxicity tests

These tests seek to establish just how much of the additive is required to produce acutely toxic and fatal effects. In the subacute tests, animals are exposed to very high doses for 3 months and tissues are examined microscopically at autopsy for signs of damage.

Absorption, distribution, metabolism and excretion tests

These seek to establish how much of the additive is absorbed, where it goes after absorption, how it is chemically processed after absorption and how quickly it is excreted. Such studies can give important pointers to the dangers likely to be associated with consumption of the additive (see examples below).

- If the compound is not absorbed from the gut then any adverse effects are likely to be confined to the gut.
- If a water-soluble substance is absorbed and then excreted unchanged in the urine then the bladder is the likely danger organ if the substance is carcinogenic.

- If the substance is absorbed but only slowly excreted or metabolized, it will tend to accumulate. Chronic low intakes may lead to build-up of high levels.
- If the substance is metabolized then metabolites need to be identified and their potential toxicity also needs to be assessed.
- If substances are absorbed and detoxified in the liver, and then excreted in the bile or urine, the liver may be likely to be affected if the compound is carcinogenic.

Teratogenicity testing

This involves feeding large amounts of the compound to pregnant animals to see if the compound causes birth defects or in any way harms the developing fetuses.

Long-term carcinogenicity testing

This usually involves exposing test animals to relatively high doses of the additive over their whole lifespan. The tumour rates in exposed animals are then compared with those of control animals who have been maintained under identical conditions but have not been exposed to the additive. Such controlled experiments mean that experimenters are able to confidently attribute any increased tumour rate in the test group to the carcinogenic effect of the additive. There are a number of potential criticisms of these tests, such as those discussed below.

- Substances that are not carcinogenic in laboratory animals may be carcinogenic in people.
- The controlled conditions of testing are very different to those of use. In the tests, genetically homogeneous animals are used, animals are usually fed single additives and are not usually exposed to other chemicals (e.g. drugs, cigarette smoke or alcohol). Animals are also maintained on defined laboratory diets. In use, the additive will be fed to genetically diverse people – perhaps only certain genotypes will be sensitive to its toxic effects. In use, there is the possibility that the additive may only become toxic if it interacts with other chemicals or perhaps it becomes harmful under particular dietary or environmental conditions, e.g. deficiency of antioxidant vitamins or minerals.
- Laboratory animals have relatively high background tumour rates. This means that the additive

needs to produce relatively large increases in tumour rate to be detected with the comparatively small numbers of animals used in the tests. The signal (increase due to additive) must be large to detect it against the background noise (spontaneous tumours not due to additive and occurring randomly in both groups). Thus these tests may be insensitive indicators of carcinogenicity and even small increases in risk can be significant if hundreds of millions of people are to be exposed.

Safety testing of additives depends very much on animal experiments because they are the only practical methods available. To ensure safety in use, despite the potential flaws discussed, wide safety margins are used. A **no observable effect level** is identified in animal experiments, i.e. a dose of lifetime exposure that produces no detectable effects in any species used. This no effect level is then divided by a safety factor (usually 100) to determine an **acceptable daily intake (ADI)** for people. It is, of course, difficult to control the additive intakes of individuals by regulating the maximum amounts permitted in particular foods. The difficulty of converting dosages between species of different sizes has already been discussed in Chapter 3.

Most food additives have been subjected to extensive safety testing. Many substances naturally present in foods would probably fail such tests and of course a number of additives are naturally present in some foods. Nevertheless, the inevitable flaws in the testing procedures do suggest the need to use the minimum effective amounts and for there to be a continuing critical review of which additives are to continue to be recognized as safe. Millstone (1985) critically reviewed the testing and regulation of food additives from a British perspective and although this paper is now over 20 years old the arguments and principles are essentially unchanged.

Key points

- Hundreds of food additives and thousands of flavourings are in general use.
- Additives are used:
  - as processing aids
  - to preserve food and increase its microbiological safety
  - to improve its taste, texture or appearance
  - to increase its nutrient content.

- Some criticisms applied to food additives are as follows.
  - They may be toxic or have carcinogenic potential.
  - They can be used to disguise low-quality ingredients or poor standards of hygiene.
  - Idiosyncratic reactions may occur even with additives that are generally safe.
  - Flavourings and colourings are unnecessary.
- However:
  - preservatives are necessary for safe mass production of food and even traditional preservatives have their problems
  - food additives are necessary to produce some modern foods that are marketed as healthy options.
- In the USA, use of food additives is regulated by the FDA and in the UK by the Food Standards Agency although the European Food Standards Agency has an EU-wide role in this respect.
- Regulatory authorities try to ensure that additives are necessary, used in minimum amounts to achieve their purposes and that they are safe when used in permitted amounts.
- In the EU, all additives have a designated E number to be used on food labels.
- Even if huge doses of a chemical produce adverse effects in laboratory animals it does not necessarily mean that small amounts represent a hazard to people.
- Safety testing of additives is inevitably dependent on animal tests.
- Differences between species, the defined conditions of laboratory tests and the high spontaneous tumour rates in laboratory animals all tend to reduce confidence in the validity of these as tests of human safety.
- A large safety margin is used when the dose that is demonstrably safe in animals is translated into an acceptable intake for people.

FUNCTIONAL FOODS

Functional foods can be defined as those that have components or ingredients incorporated into them in order to give a specific medical or physiological benefit in addition to their purely nutritional value. These foods often carry some form of health claim on the packaging or in their advertising. They are also sometimes referred to as nutraceuticals, a term

that implies that they have both nutritional and pharmaceutical functions. The term functional food could encompass some ordinary foods that have been fortified with a nutrient, such as bread or breakfast cereals fortified with high levels of folic acid. Folic acid supplements taken by pregnant women reduce the risk of their babies being affected by a **neural tube defect** (see Chapter 15). Many of the 'active' ingredients of functional foods are found in ordinary foods such as the **secondary plant metabolites** found in fruits and vegetables (see Chapter 12). This section is based on a chapter in Webb (2006) and an extended discussion of these topics and further references can be found in this source.

Functional foods are legally classified as foods rather than medicines. In Britain, they are not permitted to carry claims that they are able to prevent or cure specific diseases – only substances legally classified as medicines are permitted to carry such claims. It would be acceptable to say that a food 'provides calcium, which is important for strong bones' but not that it 'provides calcium which helps prevent osteoporosis'. The rules are essentially the same for dietary supplements and functional foods. Permitted health claims on American food labels were discussed earlier in the chapter.

In 1999, the European and American markets for functional foods that made a specific health claim was estimated at well over £1 billion each and growing strongly. In Europe, **probiotics** account for over 70 per cent of the functional food market. In this short section I am going to restrict discussion to just three categories of functional foods as listed below.

- Probiotics, **prebiotics** and **synbiotics**. Probiotics are fermented dairy products that commonly contain living cultures of *Lactobacillus* or *Bifidobacterium* which alter the microbial balance of the gut. Prebiotics are food ingredients (like the plant polysaccharide inulin) that selectively promote the growth of some bacteria within the gut and thus have similar effects to probiotics. Synbiotics are a combination of the previous two.
- Margarine and other products which contain plant sterols (**phytosterols**) that are said to lower blood LDL concentrations when used in place of butter, margarine and other 'dairy' products.
- Foods made from soybeans or a few other foods that contain substantial amounts of substances called phytoestrogens, which although not

steroids (they are categorized as isoflavones) do have significant oestrogenic activity and are marketed on that basis.

Note that in each of these examples it is also possible to buy similar products in the form of dietary supplements to be taken in pill or potion form and I will not attempt to differentiate between these modes of consumption.

Apart from the comments made in the next paragraph, I will not include in this discussion a whole range of products that have been modified to enhance their nutritional content, e.g. foods fortified with vitamins and minerals, foods fortified with omega-3 polyunsaturated fatty acids or with enhanced level of some phytochemical, low-calorie or low-fat foods where sugar or fat have been replaced by artificial sweeteners or synthetic fats such as olestra. Some of these have been discussed in earlier chapters.

When foods are fortified with an essential nutrient or other substance, everyone consuming that food gets the extra nutrient and this can be viewed both negatively and positively. It can be argued that this is medication without consent, particularly if all foods of a type are fortified as in the universal fortification of white flour with B vitamins, calcium and iron in the UK. Many people who consume the fortified food will get no benefit from the added nutrient and there is always the possibility that some consumers may consume enough to do net harm. Any new fortification thus needs to be considered carefully before it is introduced; there needs to be strong evidence that the supplementation will yield real benefits and that active consideration of potential hazards has been undertaken. Take the example of folic acid. It has been established in controlled trials that folic acid supplements, when given pre-conceptually and in early pregnancy, substantially reduce the risk of the baby being born with a neural tube defect. However, advising fertile women to take folic acid supplements has had negligible effects on rates of neural tube defect in the UK and elsewhere. This is because the majority of pregnancies are not specifically planned and generally supplements are taken by those whose food intake of nutrients is highest. In the USA, Canada and Chile, fortification of foods with folic acid resulted in immediate falls in the prevalence of neural tube defect with no apparent negative effects (see Chapter 15 for more detailed discussion and references).

Probiotics, prebiotics and synbiotics

Probiotics are live cultures of micro-organisms that are intended to survive passage through the gut and then to adhere to and colonize the large intestine. By colonizing the large bowel they favourably alter the microbial balance, e.g. by displacing potential pathogens and creating an acid environment that is unfavourable to pathogen growth. They are mainly so-called lactic acid bacteria like the lactobacilli, bifidobacteria and some streptococci which produce lactic acid as an end-product of their metabolism. Over 20 bacteria and a few fungi have been used as probiotics and they are consumed in the form of fermented milk drinks, yoghurts and some other foods or in capsules. Prebiotics are indigestible oligosaccharides that enter the large bowel where they are fermented and enhance the growth of the types of bacteria used as probiotics. Several of these prebiotics are oligomers of fructose (fructo-oligosaccharides (FOS) and the slightly larger fructose polymer inulin). Gibson *et al.* (1995) were able to show that when taken by volunteers for 15 days as a replacement for sucrose in a controlled diet, FOS increased the proportion of bifidobacteria in the faeces from 17 per cent to 82 per cent and halved the proportion of clostridia. Inulin has a similar effect. Synbiotics contain probiotic bacteria and prebiotics, and this is aimed at improving the survival and colonization of the lactic acid bacteria. The rest of the discussion refers largely to probiotics but if prebiotics produce similar changes in gut flora to probiotics then they might be expected to have similar general effects.

Goldin (1998) has suggested that a good probiotic has the following characteristics:

- compatibility with the host
- ability to survive gut transit and reach the colon in a viable state
- good ability to adhere to the intestinal epithelium
- rapid rate of multiplication
- not pathogenic
- good survival in foods or supplements
- production of antimicrobial agents that will inhibit or kill potential pathogens
- anti-mutagenic, anti-carcinogenic effects, e.g. by reducing production of mutagens by other organisms in the intestine.

Many suggestions and claims have been made about the potential benefits of regular long-term consumption of probiotics and several of these are listed below.

- They may increase nutrient availability by fermentation within the gut or even produce available vitamins within the gut. According to Gibson (1998) probiotics increase weight gain in young animals and bottle-fed babies and increased nutrient availability may be a contributing factor to this extra weight gain.
- They may reduce the symptoms of lactose intolerance. Bacterial lactase may contribute to lactose breakdown in the intestine even if viable bacterial cells do not survive passage though the stomach.
- They may reduce the number and severity of intestinal infections and so reduce diarrhoea.
- They may reduce plasma low-density lipoprotein (LDL)-cholesterol although in a review of this topic, Taylor and Williams (1998) concluded that any effect, if it exists, is very weak and difficult to detect.
- They may reduce the prevalence of vaginal infections caused by the yeast *Candida albicans* (thrush). Lactic acid bacteria in the normal microflora of the vagina create an acid pH which protects against colonization by *C. albicans*. There is little evidence to support their effectiveness but oral consumption of probiotics does influence the vaginal micro-flora (Reid *et al.*, 2004).
- It has been claimed that long-term consumption might reduce the risk of bowel cancer.
- When taken by pregnant women and infants it is claimed that probiotics can reduce the prevalence of atopic (allergic) disease especially childhood eczema.

Three of the above suggestions, the effects on intestinal infections and diarrhoea, bowel cancer risk and childhood eczema are briefly discussed below.

The normal gut micro-flora protects against colonization by pathogenic organisms that cause diarrhoea. In breastfed babies up to 99 per cent of the bacterial population in the gut may be bifidobacteria whereas bottlefed babies have a much more diverse gut microflora, including some organisms which are potential pathogens or some that may produce potential mutagens or increase intestinal putrefaction. The stools of breastfed babies are paler, looser, have a less offensive odour and have a much lower pH than those of bottlefed babies. Rates of intestinal infections and mortality from diarrhoeal diseases are lower in breastfed than in bottle-fed babies (see Chapter 15). These observations are suggestive of a protective effect of lactic acid bacteria against colonization of the gut by potential pathogens.

Several potential mechanisms by which lactic acid bacteria might protect against gut infection have been suggested:

- production of an acid environment
- competition with other bacteria for key nutrients
- secretion of substances that kill or inhibit growth of other bacteria
- competition with pathogens for intestinal adhesion sites
- provoking of an immune response
- breakdown of toxins produced by pathogens.

A major problem with trying to assess the efficacy is that there are many types and causes of diarrhoea and there are also many different probiotic bacteria. Although the evidence is by no means conclusive there are grounds for believing that some probiotics may be beneficial in treating and/or preventing at least some types of diarrhoea. Szajewska and Mrukowicz (2001) did a systematic review of controlled trials of probiotic use in the treatment of infectious diarrhoea in infants and young children. The 10 trials they reviewed did suggest that probiotics significantly reduced the duration of diarrhoea especially that caused by rotavirus (a very common cause of infant diarrhoea). Their analysis of studies testing for a preventive benefit of probiotics found that the evidence was inconclusive and conflicting. More recently, Saavedra *et al.* (2004) gave formula containing live probiotic bacteria to babies for up to a year and they found reduced reports of colic, irritability and less antibiotic use in the group receiving the probiotic compared to those receiving the placebo.

The organism *Clostridium difficile* has attracted much media attention in the past few years and is responsible for more deaths than the much better known MRSA (methicillin-resistant *Staphylococcus aureus*). In 2005 it caused around 3800 deaths in the UK – more than double the number attributed to MRSA. It is often present in the gut without producing symptoms but after antibiotic treatment it may proliferate and cause severe diarrhoea and inflammation of the bowel. In a meta-analysis of nine randomized controlled trials, D'Souza *et al.* (2002) concluded that probiotics did help to prevent this type of antibiotic-associated diarrhoea. The lacto-bacilli and the yeast *Saccharomyces boulardii* were seen as particularly promising probiotics for this purpose.

Earlier in the chapter it was noted that diarrhoea is frequently experienced by those who travel abroad on holiday or business. Studies of the preventive effects of probiotics have yielded very mixed results with some studies reporting no benefits and others suggesting marked benefits. Mixed results are probably to be expected given the range of organisms that can cause 'traveller's diarrhoea' and the wide range of potential probiotics (see Webb, 2006 for further details).

The evidence that probiotics may have some short-term benefits on diarrhoea and gut health has helped to encourage speculation that they may afford some longer-term protection against bowel cancer. There are some animal studies that suggest that probiotics can reduce the incidence of chemically induced cancers in animal models (e.g. Reddy, 1998) but there is little direct evidence as yet for a protective effect in humans. There are several theoretical mechanisms by which probiotics might help to reduce bowel cancer risk (see examples below) but at present they are merely speculative suggestions.

- The acid conditions produced in the bowel by probiotics might reduce the production of mutagens from food breakdown and/or bile acid degradation.
- Fermentation products like butyrate may have an anti-proliferative effect which might inhibit tumour development.

The incidence of childhood eczema has doubled in Britain in the past 40 years and there have also been large increases in the incidence of other atopic (allergic) diseases such as hay fever and asthma. It has been hypothesized that optimizing the gut micro-flora might help prevent such diseases by preventing the increases in gut permeability and thus antigen penetration that occurs during infection or by stimulating anti-allergenic responses. In a large double-blind, placebo-controlled trial involving over 150 women, Kalliomaki *et al.* (2001) gave a probiotic bacterium in capsule form to women with a history of atopic disease from 2–4 weeks before their due date until 6 months after delivery. In those babies who were bottle fed the probiotic was added to the formula. Frequency of atopic eczema was halved in those receiving the probiotic compared with those receiving the placebo and this was a highly statistically significant effect. Follow-up studies have indicated that the benefits on eczema were still apparent at 4 years although there was no evidence of benefit for other atopic conditions, i.e. asthma and hay fever (see Webb (2006) for details). In a related Italian study, Moro *et al.* (2006) looked at the effect of supplementing infant formula of bottle-fed babies with a prebiotic mixture made up of several oligosaccharides. Just over 200 babies identified at being at risk of atopy completed the double-blind, randomized placebo-controlled trials. After 6 months, rates of atopic dermatitis in the placebo group were 23 per cent whereas in the prebiotic group they were only 10 per cent. The prebiotic also significantly increased the numbers of bifidobacteria in the babies' faeces.

The phytoestrogens

There are some substances in plants called phytoestrogens that have oestrogenic activity. These bind with the human oestrogen receptor and exert a weak oestrogen-like effect and they are thus termed partial agonists; they have less than 1/10 000 of the activity of the body's main endogenously produced oestrogen. Agonists are compounds that bind to a receptor and mimic the effect of the normal ligand whereas those that bind to the receptor and exert no effect are termed antagonists and these therefore block the effects of the normal ligand by competing with it for the receptor binding sites. The phytoestrogens, as partial agonists, may increase total oestrogen activity when endogenous levels are very low (e.g. after the menopause); even though their activity is very low they can be eaten in substantial quantities and so the oestrogenic effect is significant. Paradoxically, they may decrease total oestrogen activity when it is high by competing with endogenous oestrogen for the receptor sites but exerting a much lower oestrogenic effect.

The isoflavones in soya products with the most oestrogenic activity are called daidzein and genistein. These are found at levels of 2–4 mg of isoflavone per gram of soya protein and they are found in other legumes but at levels that are orders of magnitude less than the amounts in soybeans. Clover and alfalfa sprouts contain coumoestrol which is also a phytoestrogen. The chemical structures of daidzein, genistein and coumoestrol and the main mammalian oestrogen (oestradiol) are shown in Figure 18.7. Other classes of phytoestrogens are lignans found in wholegrains, vegetables, fruits and flaxseeds; these are structurally similar to the isoflavones and although usually only present in small amounts in individual foods they may be consumed in substantial amounts because of their wide distribution in plant foods.

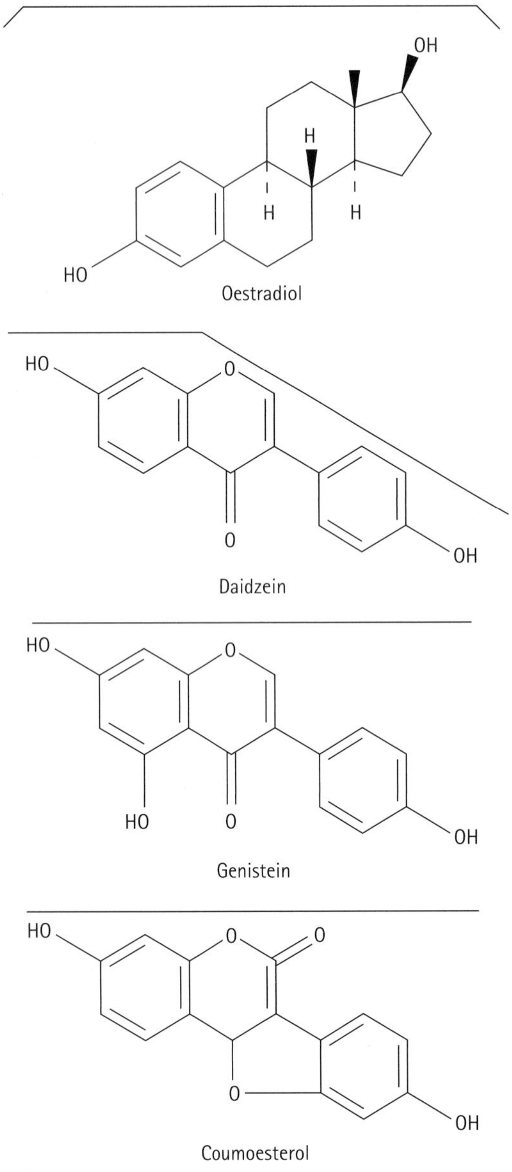

Figure 18.7 *The structures of oestradiol, the major mammalian oestrogen, and three phytoestrogens.*

The approximate amounts of phytoestrogens in some soya foods are:

- soya flour – 5 mg/g of soya protein
- tofu – 2 mg/g
- soya milk – 2 mg/g
- textured soya protein used as a meat substitute – 5 m/g
- soya sauce – none.

Phytoestrogens may be consumed in several ways:

- as soya foods
- as dietary supplements containing extracts of soya protein
- as other dietary supplements, particularly extracts of red clover and black cohosh
- as other phytoestrogens in foods, e.g. lignans in wholegrains, fruits, vegetables and flaxseeds and as isoflavones found in alfalfa sprouts.

Phytoestrogens have been claimed to offer the following potential benefits:

- Relief of acute menopausal symptoms in older women.
- Reduction in the bone loss (and consequently reduced risk of osteoporosis) in elderly women that is associated with the menopausal decline in oestrogen production.
- Reduced rates of breast cancer and possibly other cancers when consumed by younger women.
- Reduced levels of LDL-cholesterol in the blood. Clinical trials do suggest that large supplements of some soya protein extracts do reduce LDL-cholesterol but that this is not due to the phytoestrogen content as purified phytoestrogens are ineffective (see Webb, 2006).

Hormone (oestrogen) replacement therapy (HRT) is an accepted and effective way of reducing the unpleasant acute symptoms caused by declining oestrogen production at the menopause. These symptoms include hot flushes, night sweats, insomnia, depression and vaginal dryness. Several reports have highlighted concerns about the safety of HRT (e.g. Nelson *et al.*, 2002; Beral, 2003) and so many women have sought to use phytoestrogen-containing supplements of soya, black cohosh or red clover as 'natural' alternatives to HRT. Vincent and Fitzpatrick (2000) found evidence that these supplements do cause reductions in symptoms like hot flushes although they are less effective than conventional HRT. The reported reductions in some trials are quite high but they are often not substantially higher than that caused by a placebo even though in some cases they are statistically significant. The 'placebo effect' is often very high in any trial in which the outcome is a patient's subjective perception of changes in symptom severity.

Hormone replacement therapy has also been widely used to reduce post-menopausal bone loss in older women and thus to reduce the prevalence of fractures due to osteoporosis (this is discussed more fully in Chapter 14 in the section on calcium). Once again it has been suggested that phytoestrogens might offer a 'natural and safer' alternative to HRT. Most of the evidence supporting a positive effect of phytoestrogens on bone health has come from *in vitro* studies, animal experiments and epidemiological associations. Branca (2003) and the Committee on Toxicology on Phytoestrogens (COT, 2002) summed up the various lines of evidence as listed below.

- Genistein seems to reduce bone resorption by osteoclasts and stimulate bone formation by osteoblasts in *in vitro* studies.
- Soybean feeding increases bone density in female rats who have had their ovaries surgically removed.
- In high soya-consuming areas, cross-sectional studies suggest that women with the highest soya intakes have higher bone densities. This effect is not seen in areas where soya consumption is generally lower suggesting that perhaps a relatively high threshold dose is needed before any effect is detectable.
- Short-term trials (about 6 months) lend some support for a positive influence of phytoestrogens on bone mineral density in the lumbar spine.

The suggestion that high intakes of phytoestrogens might reduce the risk of breast cancer when consumed by younger women is probably the most speculative of their suggested benefits and evidence currently available is far from conclusive or even persuasive. Rates of breast cancer are low in Far Eastern countries such as Japan and China where average intakes of soya foods are around 15–20 times higher than in Western countries with high rates of breast cancer. In women who migrate from high soya-consuming areas to low soya-consuming areas the rates of breast cancer tend to remain low in the migrants but rise in subsequent generations. This

has been interpreted as indicating that exposure to soya products (i.e. phytoestrogens) early in life or even *in utero* affords later protection against breast cancer. Note also that migrants may take time to acculturate and to adopt the dietary and lifestyle patterns of their new homeland. Recent epidemiological studies that have attempted to relate phytoestrogen intakes to breast cancer risk have been inconclusive and contradictory. There is some evidence that phytoestrogens may afford some protection against chemically induced breast tumours in animals. The present state of evidence does not support the use of phytoestrogen supplements or even support the use of phytoestrogen-rich foods for this purpose. Further discussion may be found in COT (2002) and Limer and Spiers (2004).

Concerns about the safety of foods and supplements high in phytoestrogens were first raised in the 1940s when it was observed that some Australian sheep grazing on red clover became infertile. Babies fed on soya-based infant formula have the highest exposure to dietary phytoestrogens; their daily consumption is around 4 mg/kg body weight which is at least four times higher than that consumed by adults in the high soya-consuming countries of the Far East. Soya-based formula has been in use for around 80 years without any obvious harmful effects, although there are few published studies that have specifically addressed this issue. As a precautionary measure, COT (2002) recommended that soya-based infant formula should only be fed to UK babies when it is clinically indicated, e.g. allergy to cow milk would be a clinical indication if the baby could tolerate soya milk.

Another theoretical concern about high intakes of phytoestrogens is that they might exert a proliferative effect on existing oestrogen-sensitive breast tumours. There is limited evidence from animal studies that phytoestrogens can exert such an effect. It is paradoxical that this concern coexists with the suggestion that phytoestrogens may help prevent breast cancer. The safety of phytoestrogens has been reviewed by COT (2002) and Barnes (2003).

Plant sterols or phytosterols

Plants do not produce cholesterol but they do produce a range of steroids which are very similar in chemical structure to cholesterol and are collectively termed phytosterols. The most prevalent of these plant sterols are called β-sitosterol and campesterol, which make up over 80 per cent of total dietary phytosterols. Other phytosterols include stigmasterol and the fungal steroid ergosterol which, when irradiated with UV light, yields vitamin D_2. The average daily intake of these plant sterols is normally around 100–300 mg in the UK with the highest intakes naturally recorded in vegetarians. These plant sterols are structurally very similar to cholesterol, e.g. the only difference between cholesterol and β-sitosterol is that the latter has an extra ethyl (CH_3CH_2) group attached to carbon 24 of cholesterol. Cholesterol and most plant sterols have a double bond in one of the rings of the steroid nucleus (between carbons 5 and 6). A tiny proportion of the plant sterols in the diet do not have this double bond and are sometimes termed the saturated phytosterols or the (phyto) stanols – these structures are exemplified in Figure 18.8, which shows the structures of cholesterol, β-sitosterol and β-sitostanol. All phytosterols, whether saturated or not, are poorly absorbed from the gut; up to 5 per cent of the majority of unsaturated plant sterols and less than 1 per cent of the saturated phytostanols (the terms phytosterol or plant sterol are used from this point to refer to both the saturated and unsaturated forms). While poorly absorbed themselves, plant sterols do inhibit the absorption of cholesterol (both cholesterol present in food and that secreted into the gut in bile, much of which is normally reabsorbed). These plant sterols increase faecal losses of both ingested cholesterol and biliary cholesterol and thus have the potential to lower blood cholesterol levels, specifically plasma LDL-cholesterol (see Chapter 11).

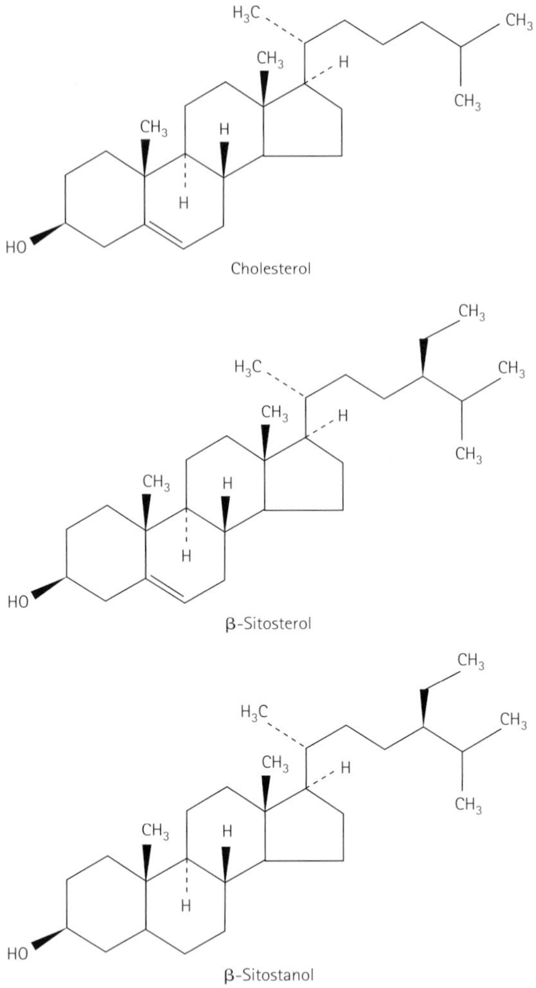

The science of this has been established for decades and β-sitosterol was used as a cholesterol-lowering drug as far back as the 1970s. In 1995, a new brand of margarine was launched in Finland that contained large amounts (about 12 g per 100 g margarine) of β-sitostanol esters which can be produced from by-products of the wood pulping and paper-making industries (see Webb (2006) for further details). This margarine has since been marketed in many other countries and a number of rival margarines and other foods containing plant sterols have been launched. There have been a series of controlled trials of these plant sterols (Law listed 14 in 2000) and these studies confirm their potential to lower blood cholesterol levels by clinically significant amounts. According to Law (2000), intakes of

Figure 18.8 *The chemical structures of cholesterol, β-sitosterol and β-sitostanol.*

2–3 g/day of these phytosterols in margarine or other functional foods lead to a significant reduction in plasma LDL-cholesterol within weeks, both in men and women. Law (2000) suggested that universal consumption of this amount of plant sterol might reduce heart disease risk by up to 25 per cent.

Webb (2006) discusses issues that make this level of consumption improbable and the scale of the effect on heart disease rates dubious, including those listed below.

• There is a limited supply of phytosterols and the products fortified with them are accordingly relatively expensive. Law (2000) estimated that at that time available sources of phytosterols could only supply around 10 per cent of people in Western countries.

- While the evidence of the cholesterol-lowering effects of phytosterols in controlled trials is persuasive, the impact of casual product replacement is not clear.
- There is as yet no substantial evidence that any fall in cholesterol levels due to casual consumption of phytosterol-containing products will ultimately translate into significant reductions in total mortality or even to a substantial fall in death rates from coronary heart disease.
- Phytosterols may interfere with the absorption of some other lipid-soluble substances such as β-carotene and vitamin E.
- Some people with rare genetic defects may be adversely affected by large phytosterol intakes.

Key points

- Functional foods or nutraceuticals have components that are intended to confer specific health benefits.

- Functional foods usually carry some health claim on their packaging, although in the UK they cannot claim to cure of prevent a specific disease.

- The worldwide market for functional foods is growing rapidly and 1999 sales in Europe and the USA each amounted to over £1 billion.

- Probiotics are fermented dairy products containing live bacteria.

- Probiotics accounted for 70 per cent of the European market for functional foods in 1999.

- Probiotics are intended to alter the microbial balance in the intestine and hinder the growth of pathogens.

- Prebiotics are indigestible food components that are intended to enhance the growth of certain bacteria within the gut.

- It has been proposed that probiotics may alleviate or help prevent gut infections and diarrhoea.

- There is a body of evidence to support probiotics reducing the duration of infantile diarrhoea due to human rotavirus and to reduce antibiotic-associated diarrhoea due to *Clostridium difficile*.

- Conclusive evidence of beneficial effects of probiotics on diarrhoea is hindered by the large number of organisms that can cause diarrhoea and the wide range of organisms that have been used as probiotics.

- There are speculative grounds for suggesting that probiotics may reduce bowel cancer risk but little direct evidence to support this proposition.

- Probiotics create an acid environment in the intestine, which may hinder pathogen colonization and prevent production of mutagens from food and bile acids.

- Probiotic bacteria may also compete with potential pathogens for adhesions sites in the intestine and again reduce risk of colonization.

- Probiotics taken in late pregnancy and during breastfeeding (or added to bottle feeds) have been reported to significantly reduce the later risk of the baby developing eczema.

- Phytoestrogens are plant substances such as daidzein and genistein from soya products that have very weak oestrogenic activity; they are partial oestrogen agonists.

- In post-menopausal women large intakes of phytoestrogens may enhance total oestrogen response and thus may possibly reduce menopausal symptoms and reduce post-menopausal bone loss.

- In younger women it is claimed that large intakes of phytoestrogens might reduce breast cancer risk by moderating the response to endogenous oestrogen.

- There is a theoretical possibility that phytoestrogens might have a proliferative effect on existing breast tumours and limited evidence to suggest that this possibility needs to be taken seriously.

- Infants fed on soya-based formula receive the highest exposure to phytoestrogens.

- Several expert groups have recommended that as a precaution, soya-based formula should not be given to infants unless this is clinically necessary (e.g. cow milk allergy), although there is no evidence of harm to babies over 80 years of use.

- Phytosterols are cholesterol-like sterols produced in plants and fungi that are very poorly absorbed from the gut.

- Phytosterols inhibit the absorption of dietary cholesterol and the reabsorption of biliary cholesterol.

- In controlled trials phytosterols have been convincingly shown to have an LDL-cholesterol-lowering effect.

- Any long-term benefits of prolonged casual use of phytosterol-containing margarine and other foods have yet to be demonstrated.

- Phytosterol-containing foods are relatively expensive and at present production capabilities are limited so they could only be used by a relatively small proportion of people in affluent countries.

Glossary

Acceptable daily intake – the daily intake of a food additive judged to be safe for lifetime consumption.

Acculturation – the cultural changes that occur when two cultures interact, e.g. when immigrants adopt the cultural practices of the indigenous majority.

Activity diary – a system for measuring the activity level. A detailed diary is kept of activities in each time block (e.g. 5 minutes) of the measurement period. Energy expenditure can be crudely estimated from the assumed energy costs of the individual activities.

Acute hypersensitivity – *see* **Immediate sensitivity reactions**.

Adaptive thermogenesis – an increase in heat production whose supposed function is to burn off surplus calories and prevent excessive weight gain. It is suggested to occur in **brown fat**.

Adenosine triphosphate (ATP) – an important short-term intracellular energy store. Energy released during the metabolism of foodstuffs is 'trapped' as ATP. ATP energy drives synthetic and other energy-requiring cellular processes.

s-Adenosyl methionine – abbreviated to SAMe. A natural metabolite synthesized from the amino acid methionine. Involved in many methyl transfer reactions and sometimes taken as a dietary supplement to alleviate depression, arthritis or liver disease.

β_3-Adrenoreceptor – a receptor found specifically on **brown fat**. Drugs that stimulate this receptor should increase heat production and burn off surplus calories.

Aerobic capacity – the capacity of the cardiopulmonary system to supply oxygen to the tissues – one definition of fitness. It can be measured by the VO_{2max}, the PWC_{max} or the PWC_{170}.

Aerobic exercise – (*aerobic* – using oxygen) moderate exercise in which the oxygen supply to the muscles is sufficient to allow it to generate the required energy by normal aerobic means.

Ames test – a test that assesses the carcinogenic potential of a chemical from its tendency to cause mutation in bacteria.

Amino acids – the units that make up proteins. They have an **amino group** (NH_2) and a **carboxyl** or acid group (COOH).

α-Amylase – a starch-digesting enzyme present in saliva and pancreatic juice.

Amylopectin – the greater part of dietary starch with the sugar residues in branched chains.

Amylose – a starch with the sugar residues in largely unbranched chains.

Anaemia – a low concentration of haemoglobin in blood. **Iron-deficiency anaemia** is characterized by small red blood cells (**microcytic anaemia**). Anaemia due to folic acid or vitamin B_{12} deficiency is characterized by large, unstable red cells (**macrocytic anaemia**); also called **megaloblastic anaemia** after the immature red cell precursors, megaloblasts, in the bone marrow.

Anaerobic exercise – (*anaerobic* – not using oxygen) intense exercise in which the supply of oxygen is insufficient to generate all of the required energy and so some is generated by other non-oxygen-requiring methods (e.g. weight lifting).

Anorexia nervosa – a potentially fatal, psychological disease principally seen in adolescent girls. It is characterized by an obsessive desire to be thin and self-starvation.

Anthropometry – measurement of the human body, e.g. measurements of weight and body dimensions.

Appestat – a collective name for the brain centres that monitor and maintain body energy stores by regulating the feeding drive; analogous to a thermostat regulating temperature.

Appetite – the desire to eat.

Arachidonic acid, $20:4_{\omega\text{-}6}$ – a fatty acid of the ω-6 (n-6) series, the main precursor of the **eicosanoids**.

Artificial sweeteners – intensely sweet chemicals that can be used to sweeten foods but are not carbohydrate and are essentially calorie free, e.g. saccharin, aspartame and the newly licensed sucralose.

Atherosclerosis – degeneration of arterial walls that is triggered by a build-up of fatty deposits (hardening of the arteries).

Attack rates – in food poisoning, the proportion of people who become ill after exposure to a food-poisoning 'incident'. **Food-specific attack rate** – the proportion of people eating a particular food who become ill.

Available carbohydrate – **sugars** and **starches**, the digestible carbohydrates. Non-starch polysaccharides are **unavailable carbohydrates** because they are indigestible by gut enzymes.

Balance – the difference between intake and losses of a nutrient. If intake exceeds losses – **positive balance**; if losses exceed intake – **negative balance**. Note particularly **energy balance** and **nitrogen balance**.

Basal metabolic rate (BMR) – the rate of energy expenditure (metabolic rate) in the resting state, i.e. lying down in a warm room and some time after eating. The minimum metabolic rate in a conscious person.

Behaviour therapy – a psychological approach to the treatment of, for example, obesity. Subjects modify behaviour to avoid situations that trigger inappropriate eating behaviour and reward appropriate behaviours, e.g. taking exercise.

Beriberi – a deficiency disease due to lack of thiamin.

Best before – the date marked on UK foods that are unlikely to become microbiologically unsafe but whose eating qualities may have deteriorated by this time.

Bioelectrical impedance – a method of estimating body fat content. It relies upon the principle that the resistance to an alternating current (impedance) passed between two electrodes on the body will depend on the body composition.

Bitot's spots – white spots on the surface of the cornea caused by clumps of epithelial cells; a symptom of vitamin A deficiency.

Blind challenge – a diagnostic procedure used to confirm food intolerance. The subject is offered foods that do and do not contain the suspected cause but is unaware of which is which.

Body mass index (BMI) – the weight in kilograms divided by the height in metres squared. It is used as an indicator of overweight or obesity. Ideal range for adults is 18.5–25 kg/m^2.

Bomb calorimeter – a device for measuring the heat released when food is burned; a crude indication of its dietary energy value.

Botulinum cook – vigorous heat treatment applied to canned foods to ensure the destruction of spores of *Clostridium botulinum*.

Botulism – a rare but potentially fatal form of food poisoning caused by the toxin of *Clostridium botulinum*. It causes paralysis, including paralysis of the respiratory muscles.

Bovine spongiform encephalopathy (BSE) – a new disease of cattle. One of a group of fatal degenerative brain infections (**transmissible spongiform encephalopathies, TSEs**) that result in 'spongiform lesions' in the brain. Other spongiform encephalopathies are **scrapie**, in sheep and goats, and **kuru**, which is associated with cannibalism in New Guinea. **Creutzfeld–Jakob disease (CJD)** is a rare disease, normally confined to elderly people, but a new variant (**vCJD**) linked to eating BSE-contaminated beef has killed more than 150 young and middle-aged people in the UK.

Bran – the outer layer of the cereal grain containing most of the fibre (**non-starch polysaccharide, NSP**); it may be removed during milling. White flour has had the bran removed, but in wholemeal flour it remains.

Brown adipose tissue (BAT) or brown fat – literally, adipose tissue that appears brown. It is prominent in small mammals and babies, where it is the principal site of non-shivering thermogenesis. Postulated as a site for **luxoskonsumption** or **adaptive thermogenesis**.

Bulimia nervosa – an eating disorder characterized by alternating periods of bingeing and compensatory behaviour such as fasting, intense exercise, induced vomiting or purging.

C-terminal – the end of a protein that has a free carboxyl group.

Cafeteria feeding – a method of increasing fatness in laboratory animals by allowing them access to a variety of tasty and 'fattening' foods; a model of human obesity.

Calcitriol – the active hormone produced from vitamin D (cholecalciferol) in the kidney – 1,25-dihydroxycholecalciferol.

Calorie – used to mean **kilocalorie (kcal)** in nutrition: a unit of energy defined as 'the heat energy required to raise the temperature of a litre of water by 1°C. 1 kcal = 4.2 kJ.

Cancer cachexia – weight loss associated with malignant disease.

Carbohydrate loading – training and dietary regimens that attempt to boost muscle glycogen stores.

L-Carnitine – a natural metabolite synthesized from the amino acid lysine and found in foods of animal origin. Long-chain fatty acids can only enter mitochondria as carnitine esters. Sometimes taken as a dietary supplement and may be **conditionally essential** for infants, people with certain inherited disorders and perhaps in patients on long-term dialysis.

β-Carotene – a plant pigment found in many coloured fruits and vegetables that acts as a vitamin A precursor and an antioxidant.

Carotenoids – a group of plant pigments that includes β-carotene, lycopene and lutein. Some have vitamin A activity, but all are thought to have antioxidant potential.

Case–control study – a type of epidemiological study. Cases of a disease are matched with unaffected controls and the diet or some other exposure of the two groups compared. Differences may suggest the cause of the disease.

Casein – a milk protein; the dominant protein in cow milk.

Casein-dominant formula – infant formula with casein as the dominant protein.

Catalase – an iron-containing enzyme involved in free radical disposal.

Centile – hundredths of the population, e.g. the fifth centile for height would be the height below which would be found 5 per cent of a population. Note also **quintile** (division into fifths), **quartile** (division into quarters) and **tertile** (division into thirds).

Chemical score – a measure of protein quality; the amount of the limiting amino acid in a gram of test protein as a percentage of that in a gram of reference protein, e.g. egg.

Cholecalciferol – vitamin D_3.

Cholecystokinin (CCK) – a hormone released from the gut after feeding that stimulates bile production. It may also act as a **satiety signal**. CCK is also found in the brain, where it acts as a nerve transmitter.

Chronic renal failure – progressive loss of renal function associated with uraemia. Low-protein diets give symptomatic relief of uraemia and may slow down progression of the disease.

Chylomicrons – **triacylglycerol**-rich lipoproteins found in plasma after feeding. The form in which absorbed fat is transported away from the gut.

Codex Alimentarius Commission – an international body set up by the United Nations in 1962 that seeks to set international food standards.

Coeliac disease – allergy to the wheat protein, gluten, causing damage to the absorptive surface of the gut. It is characterized by malabsorption, various gastrointestinal symptoms and malnutrition.

Coenzyme/cofactor – a non-protein substance needed for an enzyme to function; many are derivatives of vitamins.

Coenzyme Q_{10} – a lipid-soluble natural metabolite that is a component of the electron transport system in mitochondria and is present in the lipid phase of membranes where it may act as an antioxidant. Widely distributed in food and synthesized in most human tissues but nonetheless sometimes taken in supplement form as an antioxidant.

Cohort study – a type of epidemiological study. Measurements are recorded on a sample or cohort of people and are subsequently related to mortality or morbidity.

Collagen – the most abundant protein in the human body. A key structural component of muscle, bone, heart muscle and connective tissue.

Colostrum – fluid rich in protein and antibodies that is secreted from the breast in very early lactation.

Committee on Toxicology (COT) – the UK committee that advises upon the safety of food additives.

Conditionally essential nutrient – a nutrient that is not normally required in the diet but must be supplied exogenously to certain groups or individuals who do not synthesize it in adequate amounts, e.g. infants or those with certain diseases or genetic defects.

Confounding variable – an epidemiological term: an association between a dietary variable and a disease may be an artefact caused because both test variables are influenced by a third 'confounding' variable, e.g. a relationship between alcohol intake and lung cancer might be because smoking causes lung cancer and smokers drink more alcohol than non-smokers.

Creatine phosphate – short-term energy store in muscles; the principal source for energy used in explosive activities such as short sprints.

Cretinism – a condition in young children caused by under-secretion of thyroid hormones, e.g. in iodine deficiency. Physical and mental development can be severely impaired.

Cultural relativism – the opposite of **ethnocentrism** – trying to regard all different cultural practices as normal.

Cultural superfood – a food that has acquired a cultural significance that goes beyond its purely nutritional or dietary importance, e.g. rice in Japan.

Cystic fibrosis – an inherited disease that results in progressive fibrosis and loss of function of the lungs and pancreas. Failure of pancreatic secretion reduces the digestion and absorption of fat and protein and leads to poor fat-soluble vitamin absorption.

Cytokines – proteins produced as part of the immune response. They may be responsible for some of the anorexia and metabolic derangements seen in **cancer cachexia**.

db/db mouse – a genetically obese mouse that has a mutation in the **leptin** receptor gene and so fails to respond to leptin.

Death rate – **crude death rate** is the number of deaths per year per 1000 people in the population. **Age-specific death rate** is the number of deaths of people within a specified age range per year per 1000 people in that age range. It may also be for a specified cause.

Decayed, missing and filled teeth (DMF) – a measure of dental health, usually of children.

Deficiency disease – a disease caused by lack of a nutrient.

DEFRA – Department for Environment, Food and Rural Affairs, the UK government department that replaced the Ministry of Agriculture Fisheries and Food.

Delaney clause – passed by the US Congress: 'no additive shall be deemed to be safe if it is found to induce cancer when ingested by man or animal'. Nowadays, it is regarded as unreasonably absolute in its prohibitions.

Delayed-type cutaneous hypersensitivity (DTH) – a functional test of cell-mediated immune function. Antigen is injected into the skin and a reaction occurs after several hours' delay, e.g. the **Mantoux reaction** to a cutaneous tuberculin injection.

Demi-span – the distance from the sternal notch to the web between the middle and ring fingers when the arm is stretched out horizontally. It is used as an alternative to height in the elderly and disabled.

Demiquet index – the body weight (kg) divided by the demi-span (m) squared, used as an alternative to body mass index (BMI) in elderly people.

Diabetes mellitus – a disease caused by lack of the pancreatic hormone insulin. It is characterized by high blood glucose, glucose loss in urine and, in severe cases, ketosis. Severe **type 1 diabetes** usually presents in childhood and requires insulin replacement; the milder **type 2 diabetes** usually presents after middle age, does not usually require insulin therapy and is triggered by a decline in insulin sensitivity.

Diabetic nephropathy – progressive loss of renal function associated with diabetes.

Diabetic retinopathy – progressive degeneration of the retina that may cause blindness in diabetics.

Diet–heart hypothesis – the suggestion that high dietary saturated fat increases low-density lipoprotein (LDL)-cholesterol, leading to increased atherosclerosis and ultimately increased risk of coronary heart disease.

Dietary fibre – plant material in the diet that resists digestion by human gut enzymes – 'roughage'. It is almost synonymous with **non-starch polysaccharide**, but includes **resistant starch** and lignin.

Dietary reference values (DRVs) – a general term to cover all UK dietary standards. It includes the RNI (listed separately), the **estimated average requirement (EAR)** and the **lower reference nutrient intake (LRNI)**, the estimated requirement of people with a particularly low need for the nutrient. Where data are limited, a **safe intake** is given.

Discretionary salt – salt that is added during home cooking of food or at the table.

Double-blind trial – a clinical trial using real and placebo treatments where neither the subject nor operator knows which is which until the trial is completed.

Doubly labelled water method – a method of estimating the long-term energy expenditure of free-living subjects. Subjects are given water labelled with both the heavy isotopes of oxygen and hydrogen. Labelled oxygen is lost as both CO_2 and water whereas hydrogen is lost only as water. The difference between the rate of loss of oxygen and hydrogen can thus be used to estimate CO_2 output and therefore energy expenditure.

Dual-centre hypothesis – the notion that feeding is regulated by two centres within the hypothalamus: a spontaneously active **feeding centre** in the lateral hypothalamus that is periodically inhibited by a **satiety centre** in the ventromedial hypothalamus.

Duplicate sample analysis – estimating nutrient intake by chemical analysis of duplicate samples of the food that has been eaten.

E numbers – the European system of designating food additives by number.

Eating disorders – a general term that encompasses **anorexia** and **bulimia nervosa** and the disorders of those people who are similarly affected but do not meet the strict diagnostic criteria for these conditions.

Eicosanoids – a group of locally acting, regulatory molecules synthesized from essential fatty acids, e.g. **prostaglandins, thromboxanes** and **prostacyclins**.

Eicosapentaenoic acid, $20:5_{\omega\text{-}3}$ (EPA) – fatty acid of the ω-3 or n-3 series. Together with **docosahexaenoic, $22:6_{\omega\text{-}3}$** (DHA), the 'active ingredients' of fish oils.

Elemental diet – a diet composed of purified nutrients, e.g. in the diagnosis of food allergy.

EDNOS (eating disorder not otherwise specified) – people with some of the signs and symptoms of anorexia nervosa or bulimia nervosa but who do not meet the formal diagnostic criteria for these conditions.

Endergonic reaction – a chemical reaction that absorbs energy.

Energy balance – see Balance.

Energy density – the amount of energy per unit weight of food, e.g. kcal/g.

Energy equivalent of oxygen – the energy expended when 1 L of oxygen is consumed by a subject. It varies according to the mix of substrates being metabolized (around 4.8 kcal/L or 20 kJ/L).

Enteral feeding – feeding via the gut, e.g. using a nasogastric or a surgically placed tube.

Entero-hepatic circulation – reabsorption and return to the liver of substances secreted in the bile, e.g. bile acids.

Enzymes – proteins that speed up cellular reactions. All cellular reactions are 'catalysed' by specific enzymes.

Erythrocyte glutathione reductase activation coefficient (EGRAC) – a biochemical indicator of riboflavin status derived from one of the erythrocyte enzyme activation tests used to assess vitamin status. The extent to which the enzyme is activated by addition of an excess of vitamin-derived coenzyme is inversely related to the vitamin status of the donor.

Essential amino acids – those amino acids that are essential in the diet because they cannot be made by transamination.

Essential fatty acids – polyunsaturated fatty acids that must be provided in the diet. They serve structural functions and are the precursors of the **eicosanoids**.

Estimated average requirement (EAR) – see Dietary reference values.

Ethnocentrism – the tendency to regard one's own cultural practices as the norm and those of others as inferior or wrong.

Exergonic reaction – a chemical reaction that releases energy.

Factorial calculation – an apparently logical prediction of, say, nutrient needs by taking into account a series of factors, e.g. predicting the additional calcium needs of pregnant women from the rate of calcium accumulation during pregnancy and the assumed efficiency of calcium absorption in the gut.

Familial hypercholesteraemia – an inherited condition characterized by very high serum LDL-cholesterol (type IIa). The defect is in the **LDL receptor** and is associated with increased risk of heart disease.

Fat-cell theory – the proposal that overfeeding in childhood permanently increases susceptibility to obesity by increasing the number of fat cells.

Fat-soluble vitamins – the lipid-soluble vitamins, i.e. A, D, E and K.

Fatty acids – the major components of fats. They are made up of a hydrocarbon chain and a terminal **carboxyl** or acid group (COOH): if there are no double bonds in the hydrocarbon chain – **saturated;** one double bond – **monounsaturated;** more than one – **polyunsaturated.** In **ω-3/n-3 polyunsaturated fatty acids**, the first double bond is between carbons 3 and 4 (prominent in fish oils). In **ω-6/n-6 polyunsaturated fatty acids**, the first double bond is between carbons 6 and 7 (the predominant polyunsaturates in most vegetable oils).

Favism – a haemolytic anaemia that may result from eating broad beans. Around 30 per cent of Mediterranean people and 10 per cent of black Americans may be susceptible.

Fenfluramine and dexfenfluramine – appetite-suppressant drugs that mimic the actions of 5-hydroxytryptamine in the brain. They were withdrawn from sale in 1996.

Ferritin – an iron–protein complex, the principal storage form of iron in the body.

Fetal alcohol syndrome – a syndrome of children born to women who consume excess alcohol during pregnancy.

First-class proteins (complete proteins) – proteins with good amounts of all the essential amino acids, e.g. most animal and legume proteins.

Fitness – conditioning brought about by exercise. It is often defined as aerobic capacity, but could include all physical and mental effects of training.

Flavin adenine dinucleotide (FAD) and **flavin mononucleotide (FMN)** – prosthetic groups derived from riboflavin; important as hydrogen acceptors/ donators in several cellular oxidation/ reduction reactions.

Food additives – chemicals deliberately added to food, e.g. preservatives, colours, flavourings, etc.

Food Advisory Committee (FAC) – the UK committee that advises upon the necessity for food additives.

Food allergy – intolerance to a food that involves an abnormal immunological reaction.

Food and Drug Administration (FDA) – the US department responsible for food and drug regulation.

Food and Expenditure Survey – *see* National Food Survey.

Food balance sheets – a population method of estimating food intake. The food available for human consumption is estimated and then expressed on a *per capita* basis.

Foodborne disease – a disease that can be transmitted via food, including both classic food poisoning and diseases such as typhoid and cholera, for which there is no need for the organism to grow in the food.

Food groups – dividing foods up into groups or categories according to their nutrient contents. Selecting from each group should ensure nutritional adequacy, e.g. the **four food group plan**: the meat group; the fruit and vegetable group; the milk group; and the cereal group.

Food guide plate – a visual guide to food selection used in the UK. A development of the four food group plan, which indicates the relative proportions of foods that should come from the four groups plus fats and sweets.

Food guide pyramid – a visual guide to food selection. A development of the four food group plan but it additionally indicates the ideal proportions from the different groups to meet current dietary guidelines.

Food intolerance – 'a reproducible, unpleasant (i.e. adverse) reaction to a specific food or ingredient which is not psychologically based'.

Food poisoning – classic food poisoning is an illness, usually acute gastro-enteritis, caused by ingestion of food in which there has been active growth of bacteria. In current usage, it includes other food-borne illnesses caused by bacteria and viruses that have not actively grown in food.

Food Standards Agency – a new and independent body set up to oversee and advise on food safety issues in the UK.

Fractional catabolic rate – the proportion of the total body pool of a nutrient that is catabolized each day, e.g. around 3 per cent of body vitamin C is broken down each day.

Free radicals – highly reactive chemical species produced as a by-product of oxidative processes in cells. Free-radical damage has been implicated in the aetiology of many diseases, including cancer and atherosclerosis.

Functional foods – foods that have components or ingredients incorporated into them to give a specific medical or physiological benefit in addition to their purely nutritional value.

Galactosaemia – an inherited condition in which galactose cannot be metabolized and accumulates in the blood. Sufferers must avoid lactose, milk sugar.

Gastric bypass – a surgical treatment for obesity in which a small pouch is created at the base of the oesophagus and then linked directly to the jejunum. The stomach and duodenum are by-passed.

Gastric stapling – a surgical treatment for obesity. The capacity of the stomach is reduced by surgically stapling off a large part of it.

Gatekeeper – someone who effectively controls the food choices of others. Wives and mothers have traditionally been family gatekeepers, but it also describes catering managers in institutions.

Generally recognized as safe (GRAS) – a list of permitted food additives whose use became widespread before current regulatory procedures were established.

Ghrelin – a recently discovered peptide hormone that is released from the stomach when it is empty and which has a stimulating effect on appetite.

Gingivitis – an inflammation of the gums that is caused by plaque bacteria and is responsible for most tooth loss in older people.

Gluconeogenesis – the synthesis of glucose, e.g. from amino acids.

Glucosamine – a natural metabolite synthesized by substituting an amino group for the hydroxyl group on carbon 2 of glucose. It is a major component of cartilage and so despite endogenous synthesis is widely taken as a dietary supplement in the belief that it might accelerate cartilage synthesis and thus aid in joint maintenance and repair, especially in osteoarthritis.

Glucostat theory – the notion that sensors (e.g. in the ventromedial hypothalamus) modulate the feeding drive in response to blood glucose concentration or rate of glucose utilization.

Glutathione peroxidase – a selenium-containing enzyme involved in free-radical disposal.

Glutathione reductase – a flavoprotein enzyme involved in free-radical disposal.

Gluten – a protein in wheat.

Glycaemic index – the rise in blood glucose induced by the test food expressed as a percentage of that induced by the same amount of pure glucose (the areas under the blood glucose–time curves are compared). Carbohydrate foods that are rapidly digested and absorbed have a high glycaemic index and cause steep rises in blood glucose and insulin release.

Glycogen – a form of starch stored in the liver and muscles of animals.

Glycosylated – (as in glycosylated haemoglobin) having reacted abnormally with glucose. Proteins become glycosylated due to hyperglycaemia in diabetics. Glycosylation may cause some of the long-term problems of diabetes, e.g. diabetic retinopathy and nephropathy.

Goitre – swelling of the thyroid gland, e.g. due to lack of dietary iodine.

Gold thioglucose – a chemical that produces permanent obesity in mice by damaging the ventromedial region of the hypothalamus.

Guideline daily amounts – these are based on the adult **dietary reference values** for energy, fat, saturated fat, sugar and the recommended maximum daily intake of salt. They are used on food labels to indicate to consumers what proportion of the total guideline intake of these nutrients is provided by a portion of the food.

Haemagglutinin – a substance that causes red blood cells to clump together. It is found in red kidney beans and causes vomiting and diarrhoea if undercooked beans are eaten.

Haemoglobin – an iron-containing pigment in blood that transports oxygen.

Hartnup disease – a rare inherited disorder with symptoms of pellagra. It is caused by failure to absorb tryptophan and responds to niacin therapy.

Hazard – 'being likely to produce injury under the circumstances of exposure', e.g. as in food (*cf.* **toxic**).

Heat stroke – a combination of hyperthermia and dehydration that may affect endurance athletes.

Hexose – a six-carbon sugar, e.g. glucose, fructose or galactose.

High-density lipoprotein (HDL) – a blood lipoprotein. It carries cholesterol from the tissues to the liver; anti-atherogenic.

High temperature–short time – a modern method of pasteurization that exposes food to a higher temperature than traditional pasteurization but for a much shorter time.

HMG CoA reductase – a rate-limiting enzyme in cholesterol biosynthesis that is inhibited by the **statin** group of cholesterol-lowering drugs.

Hormone replacement therapy (HRT) – oestrogen administered to post-menopausal women when the natural production of sex hormones ceases.

Hot and cold – a traditional food classification system, widely used in China, India and South America.

Hunger – the physiological drive or need to eat.

Hydrogenated vegetable oils – most margarine and solid vegetable-based shortening; vegetable oil that has been treated with hydrogen to solidify it.

Hydroxyapatite – the crystalline, calcium phosphate material of bones. In the presence of fluoride, **fluorapatite** is formed.

5-Hydroxytryptamine (5-HT) or serotonin – a nerve transmitter in the brain.

Hydroxyl radical – a free radical.

Hypernatraemic dehydration – literally, dehydration with high blood sodium concentration. It was associated with high-sodium infant formulae prior to 1976 in the UK.

Hypertension – high blood pressure.

Immediate hypersensitivity reactions – these are allergic reactions mediated by **IgE** where the symptoms occur very soon after exposure to the allergen.

Immunoglobulin (Ig) – antibodies. **IgA** protects mucosal surfaces, **IgG** is the main circulating antibody and **IgE** the fraction associated with allergic responses.

Incidence – the number of new cases of a disease occurring within a specified time period.

Infective dose – the number of micro-organisms that must be ingested to provoke illness.

Intestinal bypass – a surgical treatment in which a large proportion of the small intestine is bypassed. It is used in the treatment of obesity.

Intrinsic sugars – sugars that are naturally present within the cell walls of plants.

Irradiation – of food: exposing food to ionizing radiation in order to delay ripening, inhibit sprouting, kill insect pests or kill spoilage and pathogenic organisms.

Isomers – chemicals that have the same set of atoms but whose spatial arrangement is different.

Jaw wiring – a surgical procedure used to restrict feeding and treat obesity.

Joule – the Standard International unit of energy: 'the energy expended when a mass of 1 kg is moved through a distance of 1 m by a force of 1 newton'.

Kilojoule (kJ) = 1000 joules; megajoule (MJ) = a million joules; 4.2 kJ = 1 kcal.

Keshan disease – a degeneration of heart muscle seen in parts of China and attributed to selenium deficiency.

Ketone bodies – substances produced from fatty acids and used as alternative brain substrates during starvation – β-hydroxybutyrate, acetoacetic acid and acetone.

Ketosis – toxic accumulation of ketone bodies, e.g. in diabetes.

Keys equation – one of a number of equations that seek to predict the change in plasma cholesterol in response to specified changes in the nature and amount of dietary fat.

Krebs cycle – the core pathway of oxidative metabolism in mitochondria. Activated acetate feeds in and carbon dioxide, ATP and reduced co-enzymes (e.g. $NADH_2$) are the products.

Kwashiorkor – one manifestation of protein energy malnutrition in children. There is oedema and a swollen liver, and some subcutaneous fat may still remain. It was traditionally attributed to primary protein deficiency, but is now widely considered to be a manifestation of simple starvation.

Lactose – milk sugar, disaccharide of glucose and galactose.

Lactose intolerance – an inability to digest lactose, found in many adult populations; milk consumption causes diarrhoea and gas production.

Lathyrism – a severe disease of the spinal cord caused by eating very large amounts of chickling peas (*Lathyrus sativa*).

LDL receptor – a receptor that binds to LDL and removes it from the blood; 75 per cent of LDL receptors are in the liver.

Leptin – a newly discovered protein hormone that is produced in adipose tissue. Its concentration in blood reflects the size of the body fat stores. It seems to have the characteristics of the 'satiety factor' that was postulated in the **lipostat theory** of body-weight regulation.

Limiting amino acid – the essential amino acid present in the lowest amount relative to requirement. It can limit the extent to which other amino acids can be used for protein synthesis.

Lipase – a fat-digesting enzyme, e.g. in pancreatic juice.

Lipid peroxyl radical – a free radical produced by oxidative damage to polyunsaturated fatty acid residues.

Lipoprotein lipase – an enzyme in capillaries that hydrolyses fat in lipoproteins prior to absorption into the cell.

Lipoproteins – lipid–protein complexes. Fats are attached to **apoproteins** and transported in blood as lipoproteins.

Lipostat theory – the notion that body fat level is regulated by a satiety factor (**leptin?**) released from adipose tissue in proportion to the amount of fat stored within it.

Liposuction – literally, sucking out adipose tissue. A surgical procedure used in the cosmetic treatment of obesity.

Listeriosis – foodborne disease caused by *Listeria monocytogenes*. It can cause miscarriage, stillbirth or neonatal death and is associated with chilled foods such as pâté, cheese made with raw milk and chilled ready meals.

Lower reference nutrient intake (LRNI) – *see* Dietary reference values.

Low birth weight (LBW) – of babies: birth weight less than 2.5 g. It is associated with increased risk of perinatal mortality and morbidity.

Low-density lipoprotein (LDL) – a blood lipoprotein that is rich in cholesterol and the form in which cholesterol is transported to the tissues; atherogenic.

Luxoskonsumption – an adaptive increase in metabolic rate in response to overfeeding – **adaptive thermogenesis.**

Marasmus – one manifestation of protein energy malnutrition in children. It is attributed to simple energy deficit.

Meta-analysis – a statistical technique used to combine the results of several clinical trials into a single large trial of greater statistical power.

Metabolic rate – the rate of body energy expenditure. It may be measured directly as the heat output in a **whole-body calorimeter** or indirectly from the rate of oxygen consumption or carbon dioxide production.

Metabolic response to injury – changes in metabolism that follow mechanical or disease 'injury'. A period of reduced metabolism, shock or **ebb**, is followed by a longer period of increased metabolism and protein breakdown, **flow**.

Metabolic syndrome – a syndrome associated with insulin resistance in people who are not diabetic characterized by high blood insulin levels, some glucose intolerance, hypertension, raised plasma triacylglycerol levels, lowered high-density lipoprotein (HDL) levels and high waist circumference.

Metabolizable energy – the 'available energy' from a food after allowing for faecal loss of unabsorbed material and urinary loss of nitrogenous compounds from incomplete oxidation of protein.

Micelles – minute aggregates of fat-digestion products with bile acids that effectively solubolize them and facilitate their absorption.

Mid-arm circumference (MAC) – the circumference of the mid part of the upper arm. It is an anthropometric indicator of nutritional status, used in children in developing countries and bedridden hospital patients who cannot be weighed.

Mid-arm muscle circumference (MAMC) – a measure of lean body mass = MAC – (π × triceps skinfold).

Mindex – body weight (kg) divided by demi-span. It is used as a measure of body fatness in the elderly.

Mitochondria – subcellular particles; the site of oxidative metabolism.

Mutual supplementation of proteins – compensation for deficit of an essential amino acid in one dietary protein by excess in another.

Mycotoxins – toxic substances produced by fungi or moulds, e.g. **aflatoxins** (mouldy nuts), **patulin** (apples or apple juice) and **ergot** (mouldy grain). Some are known carcinogens.

Myelin – the fatty sheath around many nerve fibres.

Myoglobin – a pigment similar to haemoglobin that is found in muscle.

N-terminal – the end of a protein with a free amino group.

NADP – a phosphorylated derivative of NAD that usually acts as a hydrogen donor, e.g. in fat synthesis.

National Food Survey (NFS) – an example of a **household survey**. It was an annual survey of the household food purchases of a representative sample of UK households that was undertaken annually for 60 years until replaced in 2001 by the **Food and Expenditure Survey**. It provides information about regional and class differences in food purchasing and national dietary trends.

National Research Council (NRC) – a group that has produced several important reports relating to food and nutrition in the USA; under the auspices of the National Academy of Sciences.

Net protein utilization (NPU) – a measure of protein quality. The percentage of nitrogen retained when a protein (or diet) is fed at amounts that do not satisfy an animal's total protein needs. Losses are corrected for those on a protein-free diet.

Neural tube defect (NTD) – a group of birth defects in which the brain, spinal cord, skull and/or vertebral column fail to develop properly in early embryonic life, e.g. spina bifida and anencephaly.

Niacin equivalents – a way of expressing the niacin content of food. It includes both pre-formed niacin in the diet and niacin that can be produced endogenously from dietary tryptophan.

Niacytin – the bound form of niacin in many cereals. In this form it is unavailable to humans.

Nicotine adenine dinucleotide (NAD) – a hydrogen acceptor molecule produced from niacin. A coenzyme in numerous oxidation/reduction reactions. Re-oxidation of reduced NAD in oxidative phosphorylation yields most of the ATP from the oxidation of foodstuffs.

Night blindness – impaired vision at low light intensity; an early sign of vitamin A deficiency.

Nitrogen balance – *see* Balance.

No observable effect level – the intake of an additive that produces no adverse effects in animal tests.

Non-milk extrinsic sugars – added dietary sugars, i.e. all the sugars other than those naturally in fruits, vegetables and milk.

Non-starch polysaccharide (NSP) – dietary polysaccharides other than starch. They are indigestible by human gut enzymes and thus make up the bulk of **dietary fibre**.

Normal distribution – even distribution of individual values for a variable around the mean value. Most individual values are close to the mean and the further away from the mean, the lower the frequency of individuals becomes. It results in a bell-shaped curve when a frequency distribution is plotted.

Nutrient density – the amount of a nutrient per kcal or per kJ. It indicates the value of a food or diet as a source of the nutrient.

Nutritional supplements – concentrated nutrient sources, usually given in liquid form to boost the intakes of patients.

ob/ob mouse – a genetically obese mouse that has a mutation in its **leptin** gene and so fails to produce functional leptin.

Obligatory nitrogen loss – the loss of nitrogen that still occurs after a few days' adaptation to a protein-free diet.

Odds ratio – an indirect measure of relative risk in case-control studies: the odds of case exposure divided by the odds of control exposure.

Oedema – swelling of tissues due to excess water content. It is a symptom of several diseases, local injury and severe malnutrition.

Oil of evening primrose – a source of γ-linolenic acid ($18:3_{\omega-6}$). It is widely taken as a dietary supplement.

Olestra – an artificial fat that is not digested. If added to food, it gives some of the palatability effects of fat without adding calories.

Orlistat – a drug that blocks fat digestion and so reduces its absorption from the gut.

Osteomalacia – a disease of adults caused by lack of vitamin D.

Osteoporosis – a progressive loss of bone matrix and mineral making bones liable to fracture, especially in post-menopausal women.

β-Oxidation pathway – the process by which fatty acids are metabolized to acetyl coenzyme A in the mitochondria.

Oxidative phosphorylation – the re-oxidation of reduced coenzymes in the mitochondria with oxygen. This process produces the bulk of the ATP in aerobic metabolism.

Parenteral feeding – intravenous feeding.

Pasteurization – mild heat treatment of foods that kills likely pathogens without impairing their palatability or nutrient content, e.g. pasteurized milk.

Peak bone mass (PBM) – the maximum bone mass reached by adults in their thirties. After this, bone mass starts to decline.

Pellagra – a deficiency disease due to a lack of niacin.

Pentose phosphate pathway – a metabolic pathway that produces ribose for nucleic acid synthesis and reduced NADP for processes such as fatty acid synthesis.

Peptidases – enzymes that digest proteins. **Endopeptidases** hydrolyse peptide bonds within the protein and break it up into small peptides. **Exopeptidases** hydrolyse the N-terminal (**aminopeptidases**) or C-terminal (**carboxypeptidases**) amino acid.

Peptide bond – a bond that links amino acids together in proteins. An amino group of one amino acid is linked to the carboxyl group of another.

Pernicious anaemia – an autoimmune disease; failure to produce **intrinsic factor** in the stomach necessary for vitamin B_{12} absorption. Symptoms are severe **megaloblastic anaemia** and **combined subacute degeneration of the spinal cord** leading to progressive paralysis.

Phenylketonuria (PKU) – an inherited disease in which there is inability to metabolize the amino acid phenylalanine to tyrosine. Intake of phenylalanine must be strictly controlled to avoid severe learning disabilities.

Phospholipids – lipids containing a phosphate moiety; important components of membranes.

Phylloquinone – the major dietary form of vitamin K.

Physical activity level (PAL) – when estimating energy expenditure, the number by which the **basal metabolic rate** is multiplied to allow for energy used in the day's activity. It ranges from around 1.3 (e.g. housebound, elderly person) to well over 2 (e.g. a serious athlete in training).

Phytochemicals – chemicals found in fruits and vegetables. Some may reduce the risk of chronic disease.

Placebo – a 'dummy' treatment that enables the psychological effects of treatment to be distinguished from the physiological effects.

Plant secondary metabolites – substances produced by plants that serve functions such as attractants for pollination or seed dispersal, repellants to prevent predation and protection against microbial or fungal attack. There are tens of thousands of these substances, many are bioactive in mammals and some are potent poisons or the basis of established drugs. Many of these metabolites are claimed to have health benefits when consumed in foods or natural extracts taken as dietary supplements.

Plaque – a sticky mixture of food residue, bacteria and bacterial polysaccharides that adheres to teeth.

Prebiotics – non-digestible food ingredients that selectively promote the growth of some bacteria within the gut and have effects similar to those of **probiotics**, e.g. the plant polysaccharide inulin.

Pre-eclampsia – hypertension of pregnancy.

Prevalence – the number of cases of a disease at any point in time; it depends on both the incidence and the duration of the illness.

Prions – the transmissible agents in spongiform encephalopathies; abnormally shaped brain proteins that, on contact with the normal brain proteins, cause them also to change configuration. Prions are very resistant to proteases, heat and irradiation and their accumulation in brain causes tissue destruction.

Probiotics – fermented dairy products that contain living cultures of lactobacilli that may improve the microbial balance in the intestine. They may reduce gastro-intestinal and perhaps vaginal infections.

Proline hydroxylase – a vitamin C-dependent enzyme vital for collagen formation.

Prostaglandins – *see* Eicosanoids.

Prosthetic group – a non-protein moiety that is tightly bound to an enzyme and is necessary for enzyme function.

Protein-energy malnutrition (PEM) – the general term used to cover undernutrition due to lack of energy or protein, or both. It encompasses **kwashiorkor** and **marasmus**.

Protein gap – the notional gap between world protein requirements and supplies that disappeared as estimates of human protein requirements were revised downwards.

Protein turnover – the total amount of protein broken down and re-synthesized in a day.

Prothrombin time – a functional test of the prothrombin level in blood that is used as a measure of vitamin K status.

P:S ratio – the ratio of polyunsaturated to saturated fatty acids in a fat or diet.

PWC_{170} – the work load at which the pulse rate reaches 170 beats per minute; a measure of aerobic fitness.

PWC_{max} – the work load at maximum heart rate; a measure of aerobic fitness.

Rebound hypoglycaemia – when rapidly absorbed carbohydrates are absorbed, the rapid rise in blood glucose stimulates large amounts of insulin release which causes blood glucose level to fall below the starting level.

Recommended dietary allowance (RDA) (USA) – the suggested average daily intake of a nutrient for healthy people in a population. It is equivalent to the UK RNI, and represents the estimated requirement of those people with a particularly high need for the nutrient. The energy RDA is the best estimate of average requirement.

Reference nutrient intake (RNI) – the estimated need of those people with a particularly high need for the nutrient. People consuming the RNI or above are practically assured of adequacy.

Relative risk – an epidemiological term: the ratio of the number of cases per 1000 in an exposed population, to those in an unexposed population, e.g. the ratio of deaths per 1000 in smokers versus non-smokers.

Reliability – the technical accuracy or repeatability of a measurement (*cf.* Validity).

Resistant starch – starch that resists digestion by α-amylase in the gut and so passes into the large intestine undigested. It behaves like a component of **non-starch polysaccharide**.

Respiratory quotient (RQ) – ratio of carbon dioxide produced to oxygen consumed. It varies according to the substrates being oxidized and can indicate the mix of substrates being oxidized by a subject.

Retinol – vitamin A.

Retinol-binding protein – a protein in plasma that binds to and transports retinol.

Retinol equivalents – the way of expressing vitamin A content: 1 μg retinol or 6 μg carotene = 1 μg retinol equivalents.

Retinopathy of prematurity – blindness in newborn babies caused by exposure to high oxygen concentrations. It is believed to result from free-radical damage.

Rhodopsin – a light-sensitive pigment in the rods of the retina. It contains a derivative of vitamin A, **11 *cis*-retinal**. All visual pigments are based on 11 *cis*-retinal.

Rickets – a disease of children caused by lack of vitamin D.

Rimonabant – an appetite suppressant drug that binds to endocannabinoid receptors and blocks the effect of endogenous cannabinoids and those taken in the form of cannabis.

Risk factors – factors such as high blood pressure, high blood cholesterol and low fruit and vegetable consumption that predict a higher risk of developing a particular disease.

Saccharide – a sugar. Note, **mono**saccharide (comprised of one sugar unit), **di**saccharide (two units), **oligo**saccharide (a few) and **poly**saccharide (many).

Satiety signals – physiological signals that induce satiation, e.g. high blood glucose and stomach fullness.

Saxitoxin – a plankton neurotoxin that may cause poisoning if mussels are eaten at times when this red plankton is abundant in the sea – 'red tides'.

Scombrotoxin – a toxin produced in spoiled fish by the action of bacteria on fish protein.

Scurvy – a deficiency disease due to lack of vitamin C.

Second-class (incomplete) protein – a dietary protein that is relatively deficient in one or more essential amino acids.

Sensory-specific satiety – the phenomenon whereby, during eating, one's appetite for a previously consumed food diminishes rapidly but one's appetite for other foods is much less affected. As a consequence, increased variety might lead to overeating.

Set point theory – the notion that body weight-control mechanisms operate to maintain a fixed level of body fatness; analogous to a thermostat set to maintain a fixed temperature.

Sibutramine – an appetite suppressant drug that has combined noradrenaline and serotonin effects.

Sitostanol – a plant sterol that is effective in lowering plasma cholesterol by inhibiting cholesterol absorption (and reabsorption) in the gut. Other plant sterols have a similar but lesser effect.

Skin sensitivity tests – used in the identification of (food) allergens: suspected allergens are injected into the skin and the extent of the skin reaction is used to indicate sensitivity.

Solanine – a poisonous alkaloid found in small amounts in potatoes.

Soluble fibre/non-starch polysaccharide (NSP) – that part of the dietary fibre that forms gums or gels when mixed with water; *cf.* **Insoluble fibre/NSP** – that part which is insoluble in water, e.g. cellulose.

Specific activity – the amount of activity per unit weight, e.g. the amount of radioactivity per milligram of labelled substance or the amount of enzyme activity per milligram of protein.

Spoilage – deterioration in the appearance or palatability of food caused by the action of spoilage bacteria.

Standard deviation (SD) – a statistical term that describes the distribution of individual values around the mean in a normal distribution. Approximately 95 per cent of individual values lie within two SD either side of the mean.

Standard mortality ratio (SMR) – a way of comparing death rates in populations of differing age structures: 'the ratio of actual deaths in a test population to those predicted assuming it had the same age-specific death rates as a reference population'.

Subjective norm – the behaviour that is perceived to be the normal option.

Sugar–fat seesaw – the tendency for fat and sugar intakes of affluent individuals to be inversely related, i.e. low-fat diets tend to be high-sugar diets, and vice versa. Part of a more general **carbohydrate–fat seesaw** that is almost inevitable as these are the two principal energy sources in most diets.

Superoxide dismutase – a zinc-containing enzyme that disposes of superoxide free radicals.

Superoxide radical – a free radical.

Syndrome X – *see* Metabolic syndrome.

Taurine – an amino acid. It is not used in protein synthesis and can be made from cysteine. It is present in large amounts in breast milk and may be essential for babies.

Teratogenic – causing birth defects.

Thermic effect of feeding/postprandial thermogenesis – a short-term increase in metabolic rate (thermogenesis) that follows feeding. It is due to energy expended in digestion, absorption, etc.

Thermogenesis – literally, heat generation. Metabolic heat generation may be increased by exercise

(exercise-induced thermogenesis), eating (**diet-induced thermogenesis**), drugs (**drug-induced thermogenesis**) and cold stress (either shivering or **non-shivering thermogenesis**).

Thiamin pyrophosphate – an important coenzyme produced from thiamin (vitamin B_1).

Thyrotrop(h)in – a pituitary hormone that stimulates the release of **thyroxine** and **triiodothyronine** from the thyroid gland.

α-Tocopherol – a major dietary form of vitamin E.

Total parenteral nutrition (TPN) – feeding that is wholly by infusion into a large vein.

Toxic – 'being inherently capable of producing injury when tested by itself'; cf. **Hazard**.

Trans fatty acids – isomeric forms of unsaturated fatty acids in which the hydrogen atoms around a double bond are on opposite sides; cf. most natural fatty acids where they are on the same side (*cis* isomer). The major sources are hydrogenated vegetable oils.

Transamination – the transfer of an amino group (NH_2) from one amino acid to produce another.

Transferrin – a protein in plasma that transports iron. The level of **transferrin saturation** with iron is a measure of iron status.

Transit time – the time taken for ingested material to pass through the gut. Fibre/NSP decreases the transit time.

Traveller's diarrhoea – gastro-enteritis experienced by travellers. It is often caused by *Escherichia coli* from contaminated water to which the traveller has low immunity.

Triacylglycerol/triglyceride (TAG) – the principal form of fat in the diet and adipose tissue. It is composed of glycerol and three fatty acids.

Tumour necrosis factor – a **cytokine**.

Twenty-four-hour recall – a retrospective method of estimating food intake. Subjects recall and quantify everything eaten and drunk in the previous 24 hours. Note also **diet histories**, in which an interviewer tries to obtain a detailed assessment of the subject's habitual intake, and self-administered **food frequency questionnaires**.

Tyramine – a substance found in some foods (e.g. cheese) that causes a dangerous rise in blood pressure in people taking certain antidepressant drugs.

Ultra high temperature (UHT) – sterilization by exposing food (e.g. milk) to very high temperatures for very short times; it induces much less chemical change than traditional methods.

Uraemia – high blood urea concentration, seen in renal failure. It leads to symptoms that include nausea, anorexia, headache and drowsiness.

USDA – United States Department of Agriculture.

Use by – the date marked on foods in the UK to indicate when they are likely to become microbiologically unsafe.

Validity – the likelihood that a measurement is a true measure of what one is intending to measure; cf. Reliability, e.g. a biochemical index of nutritional status could be very precise (high reliability) but not truly indicate nutritional status (low validity).

Vegetarian – one who eats only food of vegetable origin. A **vegan** avoids all animal foods. The prefixes **lacto-** (milk), **ovo-** (eggs) and **pesco-** (fish) are used if some animal foods are eaten.

Very low-density lipoprotein (VLDL) – a triacylglycerol-rich blood lipoprotein. It transports endogenously produced fat to adipose tissue.

Very-low-energy diets (VLEDs) – preparations designed to contain very few calories but adequate amounts of other nutrients; used in obesity treatment.

Verocytotoxin-producing *Escherichia coli* (VTEC) – this emerged as a cause of food poisoning in the early 1980s and accounts for more than 1000 cases per year. Some of those affected develop renal complications and some die from acute renal failure.

VO_{2max} – the oxygen uptake when exercising maximally; the capacity of the cardiopulmonary system to deliver oxygen tissues; one definition of fitness.

Waist-to-hip ratio – the ratio of waist circumference to that at the hip; an indicator of the level of health risk of obesity. A high value is considered undesirable.

(The) 'Wall' – the state of exhaustion in endurance athletes when muscle glycogen reserves are depleted.

Water activity – the availability of water to bacteria in food. Drying and high solute concentration reduce water activity, i.e. reduce its availability to bacteria.

Water-soluble vitamins – vitamins that are soluble in water, i.e. the B and C vitamins.

Weaning – the process of transferring infants from breast milk or infant formula to a solid diet.

Weighed inventory – a prospective method of measuring food intake. Subjects weigh and record everything consumed. Household measures rather than weighing may be used.

Weight cycling or yo-yo dieting – cycles of weight loss and regain.

Wernicke–Korsakoff syndrome – a neurological manifestation of thiamin deficiency; often associated with alcoholism.

Whey – a milk protein; the dominant protein in human milk.

Whey-dominant formula – an infant formula with whey as the major protein.

World Health Organization (WHO) – the 'health department' of the United Nations.

Xerophthalmia – literally, dry eyes. It covers all of the ocular manifestations of vitamin A deficiency, which range from drying and thickening of the conjunctiva through to ulceration/rupture of the cornea and permanent blindness.

References

ACSM, ADA and DC 2000 American College of Sports Medicine, American Dietetic Association, Dietitians of Canada. Joint position statement: nutrition and athletic performance. *Medical Science for Sports and Exercise* **32**, 2130–2145.

Ahluwalia, J, Tinker, A, Clapp, LH, *et al.* 2004 The large-conductance Ca^{2+}-activated K^+ channel is essential for innate immunity. *Nature* **427**, 853–859.

Ajzen, I and Fishbein, M 1980 *Understanding attitudes and predicting social behaviour.* Engelwood Cliffs, New Jersey: Prentice-Hall.

Akintonwa, A and Tunwashe, OL 1992 Fatal cyanide poisoning from cassava-based meal. *Human and Experimental Toxicology* **11**, 47–49.

Allied Dunbar National Fitness Survey 1992 *A report on activity patterns and fitness levels.* London: Sports Council.

Altschul, AM 1965 *Proteins, their chemistry and politics.* New York: Basic Books, Inc.

Andres, R, Elahi, D, Tobin, JD, Muller, DC and Brait, L 1985 Impact of age on weight goals. *Annals of Internal Medicine* **103**, 1030–1033.

Anon 1980 Preventing iron deficiency. *Lancet* **i**, 1117–1118.

Anon 1984 Marine oils and platelet function in man. *Nutrition Reviews* **42**, 189–191.

Appel, LJ Moore, TJ Obarzanek, E, *et al.* 1997 A clinical trial of the effects of dietary patterns on blood pressure. DASH Collaborative Research Group. *New England Journal of Medicine* **336**, 1117–1124.

Artaud-Wild, SM, Connor, SL, Sexton, G and Connor, W 1993 Differences in coronary mortality can be explained by differences in cholesterol and saturated fat intakes in 40 countries but not in France and Finland. *Circulation* **88**, 2771–2779.

Ashwell, M 1994 Obesity in men and women. *International Journal of Obesity* **18** (supplement) S1–S7.

Astrup, A, Grunwald, GK, Melanson, EL, *et al.* 2000 The role of low-fat diets in body weight control: a meta-analysis of ad libitum dietary intervention studies. *International Journal of Obesity and Related Metabolic Disorders* **24**, 1545–1552.

Bado, A, Levasseur, S, Attoub, S, *et al.* 1998 The stomach is a source of leptin. *Nature* **394**, 790–793.

Baker, EM, Hodges, RE, Hood, J, Saubelich, HE, March, SC and Canham, JE 1971 Metabolism of ^{14}C- and ^3H-labeled L-ascorbic acid in human scurvy. *American Journal of Clinical Nutrition* **24**, 444–454.

Ball, GFM 2004 *Vitamins: their role in the human body.* Oxford: Blackwell.

Barker, DJP, Cooper, C and Rose, G 1998 *Epidemiology in medical practice*, 5th edn. Edinburgh: Churchill Livingstone.

Barnes, J 2003 Herbal therapeutic: Women's Health. *Pharmaceutical Journal* **270**, 16–19, www.pharmj.com/pdf/cpd/pj_20030104_herbal9.pdf (accessed on 3 August 2007).

Bassey, EJ, Rothwell, MC, Littlewood, JJ and Pye, DW 1998 Pre- and postmenopausal women have different bone density responses to the same high-impact exercise. *Journal of Bone Mineral Research* **13**, 1793–1796.

Bassleer, C, Rovati, L and Franchimont, P 1998 Stimulation of proteoglycan production by glucosamine sulphate in chondrocytes isolated from human osteoarthritic articular cartilage in vitro. *Osteoarthritis Cartilage* **6**, 427–434.

Bastow, MD, Rawlings, J and Allison, SP 1983 Benefits of supplementary tube feeding after fractured neck of femur; a randomised controlled trial. *British Medical Journal* **287**, 1589–1592.

Bavly, S 1966 Changes in food habits in Israel. *Journal of the American Dietetic Association* **48**, 488–495.

Bebbington, AC 1988 The expectation of life without disability in England and Wales. *Social Science and Medicine* **27**, 321–326.

Becker, MH (Ed.) 1984 *The health belief model and personal health behaviour.* Thorofare, New Jersey: Charles B Slack.

Bender, DA 1983 Effects of a dietary excess of leucine on tryptophan metabolism in the rat: a mechanism for the pellagragenic action of leucine. *British Journal of Nutrition* **50**, 25–32.

Bennett, K and Morgan, K 1992 Activity and morale in later life: preliminary analyses from the Nottingham Longitudinal Study of Activity and Ageing. In: Norgan, NG (Ed.) *Nutrition and physical activity.* Cambridge: Cambridge University Press, pp. 129–142.

Bennett, N, Dodd, T, Flatley, J, Freeth, S and Bolling, K 1995 *Health Survey for England 1993.* London: HMSO.

Beral, V and the Million Women Study Collaborators 2003 Breast cancer and hormone-replacement therapy in the Million Women Study. *Lancet* **362**, 419–427.

Bingham, SA 1990 Mechanisms and experimental and epidemiological evidence relating dietary fibre (non starch polysaccharides) and starch to protection against large bowel cancer. *Proceedings of the Nutrition Society* **49**, 153–171.

Bingham, SA 1996 Epidemiology and mechanisms relating diet to risk of colorectal cancer. *Nutrition Research Reviews* **9**, 197–239.

Bingham, SA 2006 The fibre-folate debate in colo-rectal cancer. *Proceedings of the Nutrition Society* **65**, 19–23.

Bingham, SA, Day, NE, Luben, R, *et al.* 2003 Dietary fibre in food and protection against colorectal cancer in the European Prospective Investigation into Cancer and Nutrition (EPIC): an observational study. *Lancet* **361**, 1496–1501.

Binns, NM 1992 Sugar myths. In: Walker, AF and Rolls, BA (Eds) *Nutrition and the consumer.* London: Elsevier Applied Science, pp. 161–181.

Bistrian, BR, Blackburn, GL, Hallowell, E and Heddle, R 1974 Protein status of general surgical patients. *Journal of the American Medical Association* **230**, 858–860.

Blair, SN, Kohl, HW, Paffenbarger, RS, Clark, DG, Cooper, KH and Gibbons, LW 1989 Physical fitness and all cause mortality. A prospective study of healthy men and women. *Journal of the American Medical Association* **262**, 2395–2401.

Blot, WJ, Li, J-Y, Tosteson, TD, *et al.* 1993 Nutrition intervention trials in Linxian, China: supplementation with specific vitamin, mineral combinations, cancer incidence and disease-specific mortality in the general population. *Journal of the National Cancer Institute* **85**, 1483–1492.

Blundell, JE and Burley, VJ 1987 Satiation, satiety and the action of dietary fibre on food intake. *International Journal of Obesity* **11** (supplement 1), 9–25.

Board, RG 1983 *A modern introduction to food microbiology.* Oxford: Blackwell Scientific Publications.

Bolinder, J, Engfeldt, P, Ostman, J and Arner, P 1983 Site differences in insulin receptor binding and insulin action in subcutaneous fat of obese females. *Journal of Clinical Endocrinology and Metabolism* **57**, 455–461.

Bolton-Smith, C and Woodward, M 1994 Dietary composition and fat and sugar ratios in relation to obesity. *International Journal of Obesity* **18**, 820–828.

Botto, LD, Lisi, A, Robert-Gnansia, E, *et al.* 2005 International retrospective cohort study of neural tube defects in relation to folic acid recommendations: are the recommendations working? *British Medical Journal* **330**, 571–576.

Bowen, DJ, Fesinmeyer, MD, Yasui, Y, *et al.* 2006 Randomized trial of exercise in sedentary middle aged women: effects on quality of life. *International Journal of Behavioral Nutrition and Physical Activity* **3**, 34–44.

Branca, F 2003 Dietary phyto-oestrogens and bone health. *Proceedings of the Nutrition Society* **62**, 877–887.

Brobeck, JR 1974 Energy balance and food intake. In: Mountcastle, VB (Ed.) *Medical physiology*, 13th edn, vol. 2. Saint Louis: Mosby, pp. 1237–1272

Brown, MS and Goldstein, JL 1984 How LDL receptors influence cholesterol and atherosclerosis. *Scientific American* **251**, 52–60.

Bruckdorfer, R 1992 Sucrose revisited: is it atherogenic? *Biochemist* **June/July** 8–11.

Bryan, FL 1978 Factors that contribute to outbreaks of foodborne disease. *Journal of Food Protection*, **41**, 816–827.

Burdge, G 2004 Alpha-linolenic acid metabolism in men and women: nutritional and biological implications. *Current Opinion in Clinical Nutrition and Metabolic Care* **7**, 137–144.

Burkitt, DP 1971 Epidemiology of cancer of the colon and rectum. *Cancer* **28**, 3–13.

Burr, ML, Fehily, AM, Gilbert, JF, *et al.* 1989 Effects of changes in fat, fish and fibre intakes on death and myocardial infarction: diet and reinfarction trial (DART). *Lancet* **ii**, 757–761.

Bush, H, Williams, R, Sharma, S and Cruikshank, K 1997 Opportunities for and barriers to good nutritional health in minority ethnic groups. London: Health Education Authority.

Buttriss, J 1999 *n-3 Fatty acids and health*. British Nutrition Foundation briefing paper. London: BNF.

Byers, T 1995 Body weight and mortality. *New England Journal of Medicine*, **333**, 723–724.

Campbell, AJ, Spears, GFS, Brown, JS, Busby, WJ and Borrie, MJ 1990 Anthropometric measurements as predictors of mortality in a community aged 70 years and over. *Age and Ageing* **19**, 131–135.

Cappuccio, FP and Macgregor, GA 1991 Does potassium supplementation lower blood pressure? A meta-analysis of published trials. *Journal of Hypertension* **9**, 465–473.

Carlson, E, Kipps, M, Lockie, A and Thomson, J 1985 A comparative evaluation of vegan, vegetarian and omnivore diets. *Journal of Plant Foods* **6**, 89–100.

CWT 1995 Caroline Walker Trust. *Eating well for older people: practical and nutritional guidelines for food in residential and nursing homes and for community meals*. London: Caroline Walker Trust.

Carpenter, KJ 1994 *Protein and energy: a study of changing ideas in nutrition*. Cambridge: Cambridge University Press.

Castilla, EE, Orioli, IM, Lopez-Camelo, JS, *et al.* 2003 Preliminary data on changes in neural tube defect prevalence rates after folic acid supplementation in South America. *American Journal of Medical Genetics* **123 A**, 123–128.

Chan, JM, Rimm, EB, Colditz, GA, Stampfer, MJ and Willett, WC 1994 Obesity, fat distribution and weight gain as risk factors for clinical diabetes in men. *Diabetes Care*, **17**, 961–969.

Chandra, RK 1985 Nutrition-immunity-infection interactions in old age. In: Chandra, RK (Ed.) *Nutrition, immunity and illness in the elderly*. New York: Pergamon Press, pp. 87–96.

Chandra, RK 1992 Effect of vitamin and trace element supplementation on immune responses and infection in elderly subjects. *Lancet* **340**, 1124–1126.

Chandra, RK 1993 Nutrition and the immune system. *Proceedings of the Nutrition Society* **52**, 77–84.

Chandra, RK 2004 Impact of nutritional status and nutrient supplements on immune responses and incidence of infection in older individuals. *Ageing Research Reviews* **3**, 91–104.

Chapuy, MC, Arlot, ME, Delmas, PD and Meunier, PJ 1994 Effects of calcium and cholecalciferol treatment for three years on hip fractures in elderly women. *British Medical Journal* **308**, 1081–1082.

Charlton, J and Quaife, K 1997 Trends in diet 1841–1993. In: Charlton, J and Murphy, M (Eds) *The health of adult Britain 1841–1994*. Volume 1. London: The Stationery Office, pp. 93–113.

Chen, A and Rogan, WJ 2004 Breastfeeding and the risk of postneonatal death in the United States. *Pediatrics* **113**, 435–439.

Chesher, 1990 Changes in the nutritional content of household food supplies during the 1980s. In: *Household food consumption and expenditure*. Annual report of the National Food Survey Committee. London: HMSO.

Chubak, J, McTiernan, A, Sorensen, B, *et al.* 2006 Moderate intensity exercise reduces the incidence of colds among postmenopausal women. *American Journal of Medicine* **119**, 937–942.

Church, M 1979 Dietary factors in malnutrition: quality and quantity of diet in relation to child development. *Proceedings of the Nutrition Society* **38**, 41–49.

Clement, K, Vaisse, C, Lahlous, N, *et al.* 1998 A mutation in the human leptin receptor gene causes obesity and pituitary dysfunction. *Nature* **392**, 398–401.

Cole, TJ, Bellizzi, MC, Flegal, KM and Dietz, WH 2000 Establishing a standard definition for child overweight and obesity worldwide: international survey. *British Medical Journal* **320**, 1240–1243.

Coleman, DL 1978 Obese and diabetes: two mutant genes causing diabetes-obesity syndromes in mice. *Diabetologia* **14**, 141–148.

COMA 1988 Committee on Medical Aspects of Food Policy. *Present day practice in infant feeding: third report.* Report on health and social subjects No. 32. London: HMSO.

COMA 1989a Committee on Medical Aspects of Food Policy. *Report of the panel on dietary sugars and human disease.* Report on health and social subjects No. 37. London: HMSO.

COMA 1989b Committee on Medical Aspects of Food Policy. *The diets of British schoolchildren.* Report on health and social subjects No. 36. London: HMSO.

COMA 1991 Committee on Medical Aspects of Food Policy. *Dietary reference values for food energy and nutrients for the United Kingdom.* Report on health and social subjects, No. 41. London: HMSO.

COMA 1992 Committee on Medical Aspects of Food Policy. *The nutrition of elderly people.* Report on health and social subjects, No. 43. London: HMSO.

COMA 1994a Committee on Medical Aspects of Food Policy. *Nutritional aspects of cardiovascular disease.* Report on health and social subjects, No. 46. London: HMSO.

COMA 1994b Committee on Medical Aspects of Food Policy. *Weaning and the weaning diet.* Report on health and social subjects, No. 45. London: HMSO.

COMA 1998 Committee on Medical Aspects of Food and Nutrition Policy. *Nutritional aspects of the development of cancer.* Report on health and social subjects, No. 48. London: The Stationery Office.

COMA 2000 Committee on Medical Aspects of Food and Nutrition Policy. *Folic acid and the prevention of disease.* London: The Stationery Office.

Cook, GC 1998 Diarrhoeal disease: a worldwide problem. *Journal of the Royal Society of Medicine* **91**, 192–194.

Cooper, C and Eastell, R 1993 Bone gain and loss in premenopausal women. *British Medical Journal* **306**, 1357–1358.

Corder, R, Mullen, W, Khan, NQ, *et al.* 2006 Oenology: red wine procyanidins and vascular health. *Nature* **444**, 566.

COT 2002 Draft report of the Committee on Toxicology on Phytoestrogens. Food Standards Agency. www.foodstandards.gov.uk/multimedia/webpage/phytoreportworddocs (accessed on 3 August 2007).

Coughlin, JW and Guarda, AS 2006 Behavioural disorders affecting food intake: eating disorders and other psychiatric conditions. In: Shils, ME, *et al.* (Eds) *Modern nutrition in health and disease, 10th edn.* Philadelphia: Lippincott, Williams and Wilkins, pp. 1353–1361.

Coulter, I, Hardy, M, Shekelle, P, *et al.* 2003 *Effect of the Supplemental Use of Antioxidants Vitamin C, Vitamin E, and the Coenzyme Q10 for the Prevention and Treatment of Cancer.* Summary, Evidence Report/Technology Assessment: Number 75. AHRQ Publication Number 04 - E002, October 2003. Rockville, MD: Agency for Healthcare Research and Quality. www.ahrq.gov/clinic/epcsums/aoxcansum.htm (accessed on 3 August 2007).

Coupland, CA, Cliffe, SJ, Bassey, EJ, *et al.* 1999 Habitual physical activity and bone mineral density in postmenopausal women in England. *International Journal of Epidemiology* **28**, 241–246.

CPPIH 2006 Commission for Patient and Public Involvement in Health. Press release, October 2006 Hospital food, could you stomach it? www.cppih.org/press_releases.html (accessed on 3 August 2007).

Cramer, DM, Harlow, BL, Willett, WC, *et al.* 1989 Galactose consumption and metabolism in relation to risk of ovarian cancer. *Lancet* **ii**, 66–71.

Crimmins, EM, Saito, Y and Ingegneri, D 1989 Changes in life expectancy and disability-free life expectancy in the United States. *Population and Development Review* **15**, 235–267.

Crouse, JR 1989 Gender, lipoproteins, diet, and cardiovascular risk. *Lancet* **i**, 318–320.

Crozier, A 2003 Classification and biosynthesis of secondary plant products: an overview. In: Goldberg, G (Ed.) *Plants: diet and health. Report of the British Nutrition Task Force*. Blackwell: Oxford, pp. 27–48.

Cummings, SR, Kelsey, JL, Nevitt, MC and O'Dowd, KJ 1985 Epidemiology of osteoporosis and osteoporotic fractures. *Epidemiological Reviews* **7**, 178–208.

Cuthbertson, DP 1980 Historical approach. (Introduction to a symposium on surgery and nutrition.) *Proceedings of the Nutrition Society* **39**, 101–105.

Czeizel, AF and Dudas, I 1992 Prevention of first occurrence of neural tube defects by periconceptual vitamin supplementation. *New England Journal of Medicine* **327**, 1832–1835.

Davey Smith, G, Chaturvedi, N, Harding, S, Nazroo, J, *et al.* 2000 Ethnic inequalities in health: a review of UK epidemiological evidence. *Critical Public Health* **10**, 397–408.

Davies, JNP 1964 The decline of pellagra in the United States. *Lancet* **ii**, 195–196.

Davies, J and Dickerson, JWT 1991 *Nutrient content of food portions*. Cambridge: Royal Society of Chemistry.

DCCT, The Diabetes Control and Complications Trial Research Group 1993 The effect of intensive treatment of diabetes on the development and progression of long term complications in insulin-dependent diabetes mellitus. *New England Journal of Medicine* **329**, 977–986.

Debenham, K 1992 Nutrition for specific disease conditions. In: Walker, AF and Rolls, BA (Eds) *Nutrition and the consumer*. London: Elsevier Applied Science, pp. 249–270.

Debons, AF, Krimsky, I, Maayan, MI, Fani, K and Jimenez, LA 1977 The goldthioglucose obesity syndrome. *Federation Proceedings of the Federation of American Societies for Experimental Biology* **36**, 143–147.

DEFRA, 2003–2006 Department for Environment, Food and Rural Affairs. *Family Food (annual reports)*. London: The Stationery Office.

Delmi, M, Rapin, C-H, Delmas, PD, Vasey, H and Bonjour, J-P 1990 Dietary supplementation in elderly patients with fractured neck of the femur. *Lancet* **335**, 1013–1016.

Denton, D, Weisinger, R, Mundy, NI, *et al.* 1995 The effect of increased salt intake on the blood pressure of chimpanzees. *Nature Medicine* **i**, 1009–1016.

DH 1992 Department of Health. *The health of the nation. A strategy for health in England*. London: HMSO.

DH 1993 Department of Health. *Report of the Chief Medical Officer's Expert Group on the sleeping position of infants and cot death*. London: HMSO.

DH 1995 Department of Health. *Sensible drinking. The report of an inter-departmental working group*. London: Department of Health. www.dh.gov.uk/en/Publicationsandstatistics/ Publications/PublicationsPolicyAndGuidance/ DH_4084701 (accessed on 3 August 2007).

DH 2000 Department of Health. *New advice on St John's wort*. www.dh.gov.uk/en/Publications andstatistics/Pressreleases/DH_4002579 (accessed on 3 August 2007).

DH/BHF 2004 Department of Health/ British Heart Foundation. *Heart disease and South Asians*. Department of Health Publications: London.

DHSS 1972 Department of Health and Social Security. *A nutrition survey of the elderly*. Report on health and social subjects, No. 3. London: HMSO.

DHSS 1979 Department of Health and Social Security. *Nutrition and health in old age*. Report on health and social subjects, No. 16. London: HMSO.

DHSS 1988 Department of Health and Social Security. *Present day practice in infant feeding*. Report on health and social subjects, No. 32. London: HMSO.

DHHS 1992 Department of Health and Human Services. *Healthy people 2000*. Boston: Jones and Bartlett Publishers, Inc.

DHHS 2000 Department of Health and Human Services. *Healthy people 2010*. Boston: Jones and Bartlett Publishers, Inc.

DHHS/USDA (2005) Department of Health and Human Services/US Department of Agriculture *Dietary guidelines for Americans 2005*. www.health.gov/dietaryguidelines/dga2005/recommendations.htm (accessed on 3 August 2007).

Diamond, J 1999 War babies. In: Cecci, SJ and Williams, WM (Eds) *The nature–nurture debate: the essential reading*. Oxford: Blackwell Publishing Company, pp. 4–12.

Dietz, WH 2006 Childhood obesity. In: Shils, ME, *et al*. (Ed.) *Modern nutrition in health and disease*, 10th edn. Lippincott, Williams and Wilkins: Philadelphia, pp. 979–990.

Dietz, WH and Gortmaker, SL 1985 Do we fatten our children at the television set? Obesity and television viewing in children and adolescents. *Pediatrics*, **75**, 807–812.

Dobson, B, Beardsworth, A, Keil, T and Walker, R 1994 *Diet, choice and poverty*. London: Family Policy Studies Centre.

Dodge, JA 1992 Nutrition in cystic fibrosis: a historical overview. *Proceedings of the Nutrition Society* **51**, 225–235.

Dodge, JA, Morrison, S, Lewis, PA, *et al*. 1997 Incidence, population and survival of cystic fibrosis in the UK 1968–1995. *Archives of Diseases in Childhood* **77**, 493–496.

Douglas, RM, Hemila, H, D'Souza, R, Chalker, EB and Treacy, B 2004 Vitamin C for preventing and treating the common cold. *Cochrane Database of Systematic Reviews* CD000980. (An update of a review in conducted in 2000.)

Drenick, EJ, Bale, GS, Seltzer, F and Johnson, DG 1980 Excessive mortality and causes of death and morbidly obese men. *Journal of the American Medical Association*, **243**, 443–445.

Druce, MR, Small, CJ and Bloom, SR 2004 Minireview: gut peptides regulating satiety. *Endocrinology* **145**, 2660–2665.

D'Souza AL, Rajkumar C, Cooke J and Bulpitt CJ 2002 Probiotics in prevention of antibiotic associated diarrhoea: meta-analysis. *British Medical Journal* **324**, 1361–1366.

http://bmj.bmjjournals.com/cgi/content/full/324/7350/1361 (accessed on 3 August 2007).

Dunnigan, MG 1993 The problem with cholesterol. *British Medical Journal* **306**, 1355–1356.

Durnin, JVGA 1992 In: Norgan, NG (Ed.) *Nutrition and physical activity*. Cambridge: Cambridge University Press, pp. 20–27.

Durnin, JVGA and Womersley, J 1974 Body fat assessed from total body density and its estimation from skinfold thickness: measurements on 481 men and women aged 16 to 72 years. *British Journal of Nutrition* **32**, 77–97.

Dyerberg, J and Bang, HO 1979 Haemostatic function and platelet polyunsaturated fatty acids in Eskimos. *Lancet* **ii**, 433–435.

Eastwood, M and Eastwood, M 1988 Nutrition and diets for endurance runners. *British Nutrition Foundation Nutrition Bulletin* **13**, 93–100.

Easterbrook, PJ, Berlin, JA, Gopalan, R and Matthews, DR 1992 Publication bias in clinical research. *Lancet* **337**, 867–872.

Eklund, H, Finnstrom, O, Gunnarskog, J, Kallen, B and Larsson, Y 1993 Administration of vitamin K to newborn infants and childhood cancer. *British Medical Journal* **307**, 89–91.

Elia, M, Stratton, R, Russel, C, Green C and Pan, F 2003 *The cost of disease-related malnutrition in the UK and economic considerations for the use of oral nutritional supplements (ONS) in adults*. Redditch, Surrey: BAPEN (British Association for Parenteral and Enteral Nutrition (www.bapen.org.uk).

Elsas, LJ and Acosta, PB 1999 Nutritional support of inherited metabolic disease. In: Shils, ME, *et al*. (Eds) *Modern nutrition in health and disease*, 9th edn. Lippincott, Williams and Wilkins: Philadelphia, pp. 1003–1056.

Elsas, LJ and Acosta, PB 2006 Inherited metabolic diseases: amino acids, organic acids and galactose. In: Shils, ME, *et al*. (Eds) *Modern nutrition in health and disease*, 10th edn. Philadelphia: Lippincott, Williams and Wilkins, pp. 909–959.

Enerback, S, Jacobsson, A, Simpson, EM, *et al*. 1997 Mice lacking mitochondrial uncoupling protein are cold-sensitive but not obese. *Nature* **387**, 90–97.

Englyst, HN and Kingman, SM 1993 Carbohydrates. In: Garrow JS and James WPT (Eds) *Human nutrition and dietetics*, 9th edn. Edinburgh: Churchill Livingstone, pp. 38–55.

Eskes, TKAB 1998 Neural tube defects, vitamins and homocysteine. *European Journal of Pediatrics* **157** (supplement 2), S139–S141.

FAO 1996 Food and Agriculture Organization. *World food summit. Food for all.* www.fao.org/docrep/x0262e/x0262e00.HTM (accessed 6 August 2007).

Farouhi, NG, Sattar, N, Tillin, T, *et al.* 2006 Do known risk factors explain the higher coronary heart disease mortality in South Asian compared with European men? Prospective follow-up of the Southall and Brent studies, UK. *Diabetologia* **49**, 2580–2588.

FDA 1992 Food and Drug Administration. The new food label. *FDA Backgrounder* **92–4**, 1–9.

Fentem, PH 1992 Exercise in prevention of disease. *British Medical Bulletin*, **48**, 630–650.

Fiatarone, MA, O'Neill, EF, Ryan, ND, *et al.* 1994 Exercise training and nutritional supplementation for physical frailty in very elderly people. *New England Journal of Medicine* **330**, 1769–1775.

Fieldhouse, P 1998 *Food and nutrition: customs and culture*, 2nd edn. London: Stanley Thornas.

Filteau, S and Tomkins, A 1994 Infant feeding and infectious disease. In: Walker AF and Rolls BA (Eds) *Infant nutrition*. London: Chapman and Hall, pp. 143–162.

Finch, S, Doyle, W, Lowe, C, *et al.* 1998 *National diet and nutrition survey: people aged 65 years and over.* London: The Stationery Office.

Fischbacher, CM, Hunt, S and Alexander, L 2004 How physically active are South Asians in the United Kingdom? A literature review. *Journal of Public Health (Oxford)* **26**, 250–258.

Fisher, KD, Yetley, EA and Taylor, CL 2006 Nutritional labelling of foods and dietary supplements. In: Shils, ME, *et al.* (Eds) *Modern nutrition in health and disease*, 10th edn. Lippincott, Williams and Wilkins: Philadelphia. 1827–1838.

Flegal, KM, Carroll, MD, Ogden, CL and Johnson, CL 2006 Prevalence and trends in obesity among US adults. *Journal of the American Medical Association* **288**, 1723–1727.

Fleury, C, Neverova, M, Collins, S, *et al.* 1997 Uncoupling protein 2: a novel gene linked to obesity and hyperinsulinaemia. *Nature Genetics* **15**, 269–273.

Forte, JG, Miguel, JM, Miguel, MJ, de Pyadua, F and Rose, G (1989) Salt and blood pressure: a community trial. *Journal of Human Hypertension* **3**, 179–184.

Foster, K, Lader, D and Cheesbrough, S 1997 *Infant feeding.* London: The Stationery Office.

Frantz, ID and Moore, RB 1969 The sterol hypothesis in atherogenesis. *American Journal of Medicine* **46**, 684–690.

Fraser, GE 1988 Determinants of ischemic heart disease in Seventh-day Adventists: a review. *American Journal of Clinical Nutrition* **48**, 833–836.

Friedman, J and Halaas, JL 1998 Leptin and the regulation of body weight in mammals. *Nature* **395**, 763–770.

Frost, CD, Law, MR and Wald, NJ 1991 By how much does dietary salt reduction lower blood pressure? II – Analysis of observational data within populations. *British Medical Journal* **302**, 815–818.

FSA 2003 Food Standards Agency. *Safe upper levels for vitamins and minerals. Report of the Expert Group on vitamins and minerals.* The Stationery Office: London. Available free online at www.food.gov.uk/multimedia/pdfs/vitmin2003.pdf (accessed on 3 August 2007).

FSA 2007 Food Standards Agency. Irradiated food. www.food.gov.uk/safereating/rad_in_food/irradfoodqa/ (accessed on 3 August 2007).

FSID 2007 The Foundation for the Study of Infant Deaths. www.fsid.org.uk (accessed on 3 August 2007).

Fujita, Y 1992 Nutritional requirements of the elderly: a Japanese view. *Nutrition Reviews* **50**, 449–453.

Garrow, JS 1992 The management of obesity. Another view. *International Journal of Obesity* **16** (supplement 2), S59–S63.

Gaullier, JM, Halse, J, Hoye, K, *et al.* 2004 Conjugated linoleic acid supplementation for 1 year reduces body fat mass in healthy overweight humans. *American Journal of Clinical Nutrition* **79**, 1118–1125.

Geissler, C and Powers H 2005 *Human nutrition and dietetics*, 11th edn. Edinburgh: Churchill Livingstone.

Gey, KF, Puska, P, Jordan, P and Moser, UK 1991 Inverse correlation between plasma vitamin E and mortality from ischemic heart disease in cross-cultural epidemiology. *American Journal of Clinical Nutrition* **53**, 326S–334S.

Ghani, AC, Donnelly, CA, Ferguson, NM and Anderson, RM 2003 Updated projections of future vCJD deaths in the UK. *BMC Infectious Diseases* **3**, 4.

Gibbs, WW 1996 Gaining on fat. *Scientific American* **August**, 70–76.

Gibson, GR 1998 Dietary modulation of the human gut microflora using prebiotics. *British Journal of Nutrition* **80**, S209–S212.

Gibson, GR, Beatty, EB, Wang, X and Cummings, JH 1995 Selective stimulation of bifidobacteria in the human colon by oligofructose and inulin. *Gastroenterology* **108**, 975–982.

Gilbert, S 1986 *Pathology of eating. Psychology and treatment.* London: Routledge and Kegan Paul.

GISSI Prevenzione Investigators 1999 Dietary supplementation with n-3 polyunsaturated fatty acids and vitamin E after myocardial infarction: results of the GISSI-Prevenzione trial. *Lancet* **354**, 447–455.

Gleibermann, L 1973 Blood pressure and dietary salt in human populations. *Ecology of Food and Nutrition* **2**, 143–156.

Goldin, BR 1998 Health benefits of probiotics. *British Journal of Nutrition* **80**, S203–S207.

Golding, J, Greenwood, R, Birmingham, K and Mott, M 1992 Childhood cancer: intramuscular vitamin K, and pethidine given during labour. *British Medical Journal* **305**, 341–345.

Gortmaker, SL, Must, A, Perrin, JM, Sobol, AM and Dietz, WH 1993 Social and economic consequences of overweight in adolescence. *New England Journal of Medicine* **329**, 1008–1012.

Gounelle de Pontanel, H 1972 Chairman's opening address. In: De Pontanel, H and Gounelle, H (Eds) *Proteins from hydrocarbons. The proceedings of the 1972 symposium at Aix-en-Provence.* London: Academic Press, pp. 1–2.

Gregory, J, Foster, K, Tyler, H and Wiseman, M 1990 *The dietary and nutritional survey of British adults.* London: HMSO.

Gregory, J, Lowe, S, Bates, CJ, *et al.* 2000 *National Diet and Nutrition Survey: young people aged 4 to 18 years.* Volume 1: *Findings.* London: The Stationery Office.

Gregory, JR, Collins, DL, Davies, PDW, Hughes, JM and Clarke, PC 1995 *National diet and nutrition survey: children aged 1½ to 4½ years.* Volume 1. London: HMSO.

Gronbaek, M, Deis, A, Sorensen, TIA, *et al.* 1994 Influence of sex, age, body mass index, and smoking on alcohol intake and mortality. *British Medical Journal* **308**, 302–306.

Groom, H 1993 What price a healthy diet? *British Nutrition Foundation Nutrition Bulletin* **18**, 104–109.

Gropper, SS, Smith, JL and Groff JL 2004 *Advanced nutrition and human metabolism*, 4th edn. Florence, Kentucky: Wadsworth Publishing Company.

Group 1994 The Alpha-Tocopherol, Beta Carotene Cancer Prevention Study Group. The effect of vitamin E and beta carotene on the incidence of lung cancer and other cancer in male smokers. *New England Journal of Medicine* **330**, 1029–1035.

Group 2002 Heart Protection Study Collaborative Group. MRC/BHF Heart Protection Study of cholesterol lowering with simvastatin in 20,536 high-risk individuals: a randomised placebo-controlled trial. *Lancet* **360**, 7–22.

Grundy, SM 1987 Monounsaturated fatty acids, plasma cholesterol, and coronary heart disease *American Journal of Clinical Nutrition* **45**, 1168–1175.

Grundy, SM 1998 Hypertriglyceridemia, atherogenic dyslipidemia and the metabolic syndrome. *American Journal of Cardiology* **81**, 18B–25B.

Halliday, A and Ashwell, M 1991a *Non-starch polysaccharides. Briefing paper 22.* London: British Nutrition Foundation.

Halliday, A and Ashwell, M 1991b *Calcium. Briefing paper 24*. London: British Nutrition Foundation.

Hamilton, EMN, Whitney, EN, and Sizer, FS 1991 *Nutrition. Concepts and controversies*, 5th edn. St. Paul, MN: West Publishing Company.

Hamlyn, B, Brooker, S, Oleinikova, K and Wands, S 2002 *Infant feeding 2002*. London: The Stationery Office.

Hancox, RJ, Milne, BJ and Poulton, R 2004 Association between child and adolescent television viewing and adult health: a longitudinal birth cohort study. *Lancet* **364**, 226–227.

Hardy, M, Coulter, I, Morton, SC, *et al*. 2002 *S-adenosyl-l-methionine for treatment of depression, osteoarthritis, and liver disease*. Evidence Report/Technology Assessment Number 64. AHRQ Publication No. 02-E034 Rockville, MD: Agency for Healthcare Research and Quality. www.ncbi.nlm.nih.gov/books/bv.fcgi?rid=hstat1a chapter.2159 (accessed on 3 August 2007).

Harper, AE 1999 Defining the essentiality of nutrients. In: Shils, ME, *et al*. (Eds) *Modern nutrition in health and disease*, 9th edn. Philadelphia: Lippincott, Williams and Wilkins, pp. 3–10.

Harris, MB 1983 Eating habits, restraint, knowledge and attitudes toward obesity. *International Journal of Obesity* **7**, 271–286.

Harris, WS 1989 Fish oils and plasma lipid and lipoprotein metabolism in humans: a critical review. *Journal of Lipid Research*, **30**, 785–807.

Hawthorn, J 1989 Safety and wholesomeness of irradiated foods. *British Nutrition Foundation Nutrition Bulletin* **14**, 150–162.

Hayden, RM and Allen, GJ 1984 Relationship between aerobic exercise, anxiety, and depression: convergent validation by knowledgeable informants. *Journal of Sports Medicine* **24**, 69–74.

Hazel, T and Southgate, DAT 1985 Trends in the consumption of red meat and poultry – nutritional implications. *British Nutrition Foundation Nutrition Bulletin* **10**, 104–117.

HEA 1994 Health Education Authority. *The balance of good health. The national food guide*. London: Health Education Authority.

Hegsted, DM 1986 Calcium and osteoporosis. *Journal of Nutrition*, **116**, 2316–2319.

Henderson, L, Irving, K, Gregory, J, *et al*. 2003 *The National Diet and Nutrition Survey: adults aged 19 to 64 years*. Volume 3. *Vitamin and mineral intakes and urinary analytes*. London: The Stationery Office. www.food.gov.uk/ multimedia/pdfs/ndnsv3.pdf (accessed on 3 August 2007).

Hennekens, CH, Buring, JF, Manson, JF, *et al*. 1996 Lack of effect of long-term supplementation with beta-carotene on the incidence of malignant neoplasms and cardiovascular disease. *New England Journal of Medicine* **334**, 1145–1149.

Henson, S 1992 From high street to hypermarket. Food retailing in the 1990s. In: National Consumer Council (Ed.) *Your food: whose choice?* London: HMSO, pp. 95–115.

Hetzel, BS and Clugston, GA 1999 Iodine. In: Shils, ME, *et al*. (Eds) *Modern nutrition in health and disease*, 9th edn. Philadelphia: Lippincott, Williams and Wilkins, pp. 253–264.

Heymsfield, SB and Baumgartner, RW 2006 Body composition and anthropometry. In: Shils, ME, *et al*. (Eds) *Modern nutrition in health and disease*, 10th edn. Philadelphia: Lippincott, Williams and Wilkins, pp. 751–770.

Hibbard, ED and Smithells, RW 1965 Folic acid metabolism and human embryopathy. *Lancet* **i**, 1254.

Higgins, JP and Flicker, L 2003 Lecithin for dementia and cognitive impairment. *Cochrane Database of Systematic Reviews* CD001015.

Hill, GL, Blackett, RL, Pickford, I, *et al*. 1977 Malnutrition in surgical patients. An unrecognised problem. *Lancet* **i**, 689–692.

Hill, JO, Catenacci, VA and Wyatt, HR 2006 Obesity: etiology. In: Shils, ME, *et al*. (Eds) *Modern nutrition in health and disease*, 10th edn. Philadelphia: Lippincott, Williams and Wilkins, pp. 1013–1028.

Hirsch, J 1997 Some heat but not enough light. *Nature* **387**, 27–28.

Hirsch, J and Han, PW 1969 Cellularity of rat adipose tissue: effects of growth, starvation and obesity. *Journal of Lipid Research* **10**, 77–82.

HMSO 2003 Food Supplements (England) Regulations 2003 www.legislation.hmso.gov.uk/si/si2003/20031387.htm (accessed on 3 August 2007).

Hoare, J, Henderson, L, Bates, CJ, *et al.* 2004 *National Diet and Nutrition Survey: adults aged 19 to 64 years.* Volume 5: *Summary report.* London: The Stationery Office.

Hobbs, BC and Roberts, D 1993 *Food poisoning and food hygiene,* 6th edn. London: Edward Arnold.

Hodge, AM, Dowse, GK, Poelupe, P, Collins, VR, Imo, T and Zimmet, PZ 1994 Dramatic increases in the prevalence of obesity in Western Samoa over the 13 year period 1978–1991. *International Journal of Obesity* 18, 419–428.

Honein, MA, Paolozzi, LJ, Mathews, TJ *et al.* 2001 Impact of folic acid fortification of the US food supply on the occurrence of neural tube defects. *Journal of the American Medical Association* 285, 2981–2986.

Hooper, L, Bartlett, C, Davey Smith, G and Ebrahim, S 2002 Systematic review of long term effects of advice to reduce dietary salt in adults. *British Medical Journal* 325, 628 www.bmj.com/cgi/content/full/325/7365/628 (accessed on 3 August 2007).

Hubley, J 1993 *Communicating Health – an action guide to health education and health promotion.* London: Macmillan.

Hulley, SB, Walsh, JMB and Newman, TB 1992 Health policy on blood cholesterol time to change directions. *Circulation* 86, 1026–1029.

Hunt, P, Gatenby, S and Rayner, M 1995 The format for the national food guide: Performance and preference studies. *Journal of Human Nutrition and Dietetics* 8, 335–351.

IFPRI 1996 International Food Policy Research Institute. *Key trends in feeding the world.* www.cgiar.org/ifpri/2020/synth/trends.htm (accessed on 3 August 2007).

IFT 1975 A report by the Institute of Food Technologists' Expert Panel on Food Safety and Nutrition and the Committee on Public Information. Naturally occurring toxicants in foods. *Food Technology* 29, 67–72.

IGD 2006 *Best practice guidance on the presentation of guideline daily amounts.*

IGD: Watford, Herts UK (www.igd.com). (accessed on 4 october 2007)

Inoue, K, Shone, T, Toyokawa, S and Kawakami, M 2006 Body mass index as a predictor of mortality in community-dwelling seniors. *Aging Clinical Experimental Research* 18, 205–210.

IOTF 2004 International Task Force on Obesity, press release. www.iotf.org/media/iotfchildhoodUK.pdf (accessed on 3 August 2007).

Iribarren, C, Sharp, DS, Burchfiel, CM and Petrovich, H 1995 Association of weight loss and weight fluctuation with mortality among Japanese American men. *New England Journal of Medicine* 333, 686–692.

Jackson, J 2003 Potential mechanisms of action of bioactive substances found in plants. In: Goldberg, G (Ed.) *Plants: Diet and Health. Report of the British Nutrition Task Force.* Blackwell: Oxford, pp. 65–75.

Jacob, M 1993 Legislation. In: Hobbs, BC and Roberts, D (Eds) *Food poisoning and food hygiene,* 6th edn. London: Edward Arnold, pp. 280–302.

Jacobsen, MS 1987 Cholesterol oxides in Indian Ghee: possible cause of unexplained high risk of atherosclerosis in Indian immigrant populations. *Lancet* ii, 656–658.

Jago, R, Baranowski, T, Baranowski, JC, *et al.* 2005 BMI from 3–6 y of age is predicted by TV viewing and activity, not diet. *International Journal of Obesity* 29, 557–564.

James, WP, Astrup, A, Finer, N, *et al.* 2000 Effect of sibutramine on weight maintenance after weight loss: a randomised trial. STORM study group. Sibutramine trial of obesity reduction and maintenance. *Lancet* 356, 2119–2125.

James, WPT, Ralph, A and Sanchez-Castillo, CP 1987 The dominance of salt in manufactured food in the sodium intake of affluent societies. *Lancet* i, 426–428.

Janssen, I, Katzmarzyk, PT and Ross, R 2005 Body mass index is inversely related to mortality in older people after adjustment for waist circumference. *Journal of the American Geriatric Society* 53, 2112–2118.

Jarjou, LMA, Prentice, A, Sawo, Y, *et al.* 1994 Changes in the diet of Mandinka women in The

Gambia between 1978–79 and 1990–91: consequences for calcium intakes. *Proceedings of the Nutrition Society* **53**, 258A.

Jebb, SA, Goldberg, GR, Coward, WA, Murgatroyd, PR and Prentice, AM 1991 Effects of weight cycling caused by intermittent dieting on metabolic rate and body composition in obese women. *International Journal of Obesity* **15**, 367–374.

Jelliffe, DB 1967 Parallel food classifications in developing and industrialised countries. *American Journal of Clinical Nutrition* **20**, 279–281.

Jenkins, DJA and Wolever, TMS 1981 Slow release carbohydrate and the treatment of diabetics. *Proceedings of the Nutrition Society* **40**, 227–236.

Johnell, O and the MEDOS study group 1992 The apparent incidence of hip fracture in Europe: a study of national register sources. *Osteoporosis International* **2**, 298–302.

Johnstone, PK and Sabate, J 2006 Nutritional implications of vegetarian diets. In: Shils, ME, *et al.* (Eds) *Modern nutrition in health and disease*, 10th edn. Philadelphia: Lippincott, Williams and Wilkins, pp. 1638–1654.

Jones, A 1974 *World protein resources*. Lancaster, England: Medical and Technical Publishing Company.

Jones, E, Hughes, R and Davies, H 1988 Intake of vitamin C and other nutrients by elderly patients receiving a hospital diet. *Journal of Human Nutrition and Dietetics* **1**, 347–353.

Joossens, JV and Geboers, J 1981 Nutrition and gastric cancer. *Proceedings of the Nutrition Society* **40**, 37–46.

Joossens, JV, Hill, MJ, Elliott, P, *et al.* 1996 On behalf of the European Cancer Prevention (ECP) and the Intersalt Cooperative Research Group: dietary salt, nitrate and stomach cancer mortality in 24 countries. *International Journal of Epidemiology* **25**, 494–504.

Kalliomaki, M, Salminen, S, Arvilommi, H, *et al.* 2001 Probiotics in the primary prevention of atopic disease: a randomised placebo-controlled trial. *Lancet* **357**, 1076–1079.

Kanarek, RB and Hirsch, E 1977 Dietary-induced overeating in experimental animals. *Federation Proceedings of the American Society for Experimental Biology* **36**, 154–158.

Kanis, JA 1993 The incidence of hip fracture in Europe. *Osteoporosis International* **3** (supplement 1), s10–s15.

Keen, H and Thomas, B 1988 Diabetes mellitus. In: Dickerson, JWT and Lee, HA (Eds) *Nutrition in the clinical management of disease*. London: Edward Arnold, pp. 167–190.

Kennedy, GC 1966 Food intake, energy balance and growth. *British Medical Bulletin* **22**, 216–220.

Keys, A, Anderson, JT and Grande, F 1959 Serum cholesterol in man: diet fat and intrinsic responsiveness. *Circulation* **19**, 201–204.

Keys, A, Anderson, JT and Grande, F 1965 Serum cholesterol responses to changes in the diet. II. The effect of cholesterol in the diet. *Metabolism* **14**, 759.

Keys, A, Brozek, J, Henschel, A, Mickelson, O and Taylor, HL 1950 *The biology of human starvation*. Minneapolis: University of Minnesota Press.

KFC 1992 King's Fund Centre *A positive approach to nutrition as treatment*. London: King's Fund Centre.

King, J and Ashworth, A 1994 Patterns and determinants of infant feeding practices worldwide. In: Walker, AF and Rolls, BA (Eds) *Infant nutrition*. London: Chapman and Hall, pp. 61–91.

Kittaka-Katsura, H, Fujita, T, Watanabe, F and Nakano, Y 2002 Purification and characterization of a corrinoid compound from Chlorella tablets as an algal health food. *Journal of Agricultural and Food Chemistry* **50**, 4994–4997.

Klahr, S, Levey, AS, Beck, GJ, *et al.* 1994 The effects of dietary protein restriction on the progression of chronic renal disease. *New England Journal of Medicine* **330**, 877–884.

Klatsky, AL, Armstrong, MA and Friedman, JD 1992 Alcohol and mortality. *Annals of Internal Medicine* **117**, 646–654.

Kremer, JM, Bigauoette, J, Mickalek, AV, *et al.* 1985 Effects of manipulation of dietary fatty acids on clinical manifestation of rheumatoid arthritis. *Lancet* **i**, 184–187.

Kromhout, D 1990 n-3 fatty acids and coronary heart disease: epidemiology from Eskimos to

Western populations. *British Nutrition Foundation Nutrition Bulletin* **15**, 93–102.

Kune, GA, Kune, S and Watson, LF 1993 Perceived religiousness is protective for colorectal cancer: data from the Melbourne Colorectal Cancer Study. *Journal of the Royal Society of Medicine* **86**, 645–647.

Larsson, J, Unosson, N, Ek, AC, Nisson, L, Thorslund, S and Bjurulf, P 1990 Effect of dietary supplement on nutritional status and clinical outcome in 501 geriatric patients – a randomised study. *Clinical Nutrition* **9**, 179–184.

Laurent, C 1993 Private function? *Nursing Times* **89**, 14–15.

Law, M 2000 Plant sterol and stanol margarines and health. *British Medical Journal* **320**, 861–864. www.bmj.bmjjournals.com/cgi/content/full/320 /7238/861 (accessed on 3 August 2007).

Law, MR, Frost, CD and Wald, NJ 1991a By how much does dietary salt reduction lower blood pressure? I – Analysis of observational data among populations. *British Medical Journal* **302**, 811–815.

Law, MR, Frost, CD and Wald, NJ 1991b By how much does dietary salt reduction lower blood pressure? III – Analysis of data from trials of salt reduction. *British Medical Journal* **302**, 819–824.

Leather, S 1992 Less money, less choice. Poverty and diet in the UK today. In: National Consumer Council (Eds) *Your food: whose choice?* London: HMSO, pp. 72–94.

Lee, CD, Jackson, AS and Blair, SN 1998 US weight guidelines, is it important to consider cardiopulmonary fitness. *International Journal of Obesity* **22** (supplement 2), 52–57.

Lee, I-M, Cook, NR, Gaziano, JM, *et al.* 2005 Vitamin E in the primary prevention of cardiovascular disease and cancer. *Journal of the American Medical Association* **294**, 56–65.

Leeds, AR 1979 The dietary management of diabetes in adults. *Proceedings of the Nutrition Society* **38**, 365–371.

Leeds, AR, Brand Miller, J, Foster-Powell, K and Colagiuri, S 1998 *The glucose revolution.* Australia: Hodder & Stoughton.

Lehmann, AB 1991 Nutrition in old age: an update and questions for future research: part 1. *Reviews in Clinical Gerontology* **1**, 135–145.

Lennard, TWJ and Browell, DA 1993 The immunological effects of trauma. *Proceedings of the Nutrition Society* **52**, 85–90.

Leichter, I, Margulies, JY, Weinreb, A, *et al.* 1982 The relationship between bone density, mineral content, and mechanical strength in the femoral neck. *Clinical Orthopaedics and Related Research* **163**, 272–281.

Leon, DA 1985 Physical activity levels and coronary heart disease: analysis of epidemiologic and supporting studies. *Medical Clinics of North America* **69**, 3–19.

Leon, DA 1991 Influence of birth weight on differences in infant mortality by social class and legitimacy. *British Medical Journal* **303**, 964–967.

Leon, DA 1993 Failed or misleading adjustment for confounding. *Lancet* **342**, 479–481.

Limer, JL and Speirs, V 2004 Phyto-oestrogens and breast cancer chemoprevention. *Breast Cancer Research* **6**, 119–127.

Lissner, L, Heitmann, BL and Bengtsson, C 2000 Population studies of diet and obesity. *British Journal of Nutrition* **83** (supplement 1), S21–S24.

Livingstone, B 1996 More ins than outs of energy balance. *British Nutrition Foundation Nutrition Bulletin* **21** (supplement), 6–15.

Locatelli, F, Alberti, D, Graziani, G, *et al.* 1991 Prospective, randomised, multicentre trial of the effect of protein restriction on progression of chronic renal insufficiency. *Lancet* **337**, 1299–1304.

Lock, S 1977 Iron deficiency anaemia in the UK. In: *Getting the most out of food, No. 12.* London: Van den Berghs and Jurgens Ltd.

McColl, K 1988 The sugar-fat 'seesaw'. *British Nutrition Foundation Nutrition Bulletin* **13**, 114–118.

McCormick, J and Skrabanek, P 1988 Coronary heart disease is not preventable by population interventions. *Lancet* **i**, 839–841.

McCrory, MA, Fuss, PJ, McCallum, JE, *et al.* 1999 Dietary variety within food groups: association with energy intake and body fatness in men and women. *American Journal of Clinical Nutrition* **69**, 440–447.

McGill, HC 1979 The relationship of dietary cholesterol to serum cholesterol concentration and to atherosclerosis in man. *American Journal of Clinical Nutrition* **32**, 2664–2702.

MacGregor, GA and de Wardener, HE 1998 *Salt, diet and health*. Cambridge: Cambridge University Press.

MacGregor, GA, Markandu, N, Best, F, *et al.* 1982 Double-blind random crossover of moderate sodium restriction in essential hypertension. *Lancet* i, 351–355.

McKeigue, PM, Marmot, MG, Adelstein, AM, *et al.* 1985 Diet and risk factors for coronary heart disease in Asians in northwest London. *Lancet* ii, 1086–1089.

McKeigue, PM, Shah, B and Marmot, MG 1991 Relation of central obesity and insulin resistance with high diabetes prevalence and cardiovascular risk in South Asians. *Lancet* **337**, 382–386.

McLaren, DS 1974 The great protein fiasco. *Lancet* ii, 93–96.

Macnair, AL 1994 Physical activity, not diet, should be the focus of measures for the primary prevention of cardiovascular disease. *Nutrition Research Reviews* **7**, 43–65.

McNutt, K 1998 Sugar replacers. A new consumer education challenge. *British Nutrition Foundation Nutrition Bulletin* **23**, 216–223.

McWhirter, JP and Pennington, CR 1994 Incidence and recognition of malnutrition in hospital. *British Medical Journal* **308**, 945–948.

MAFF 1991 Ministry of Agriculture Fisheries and Food. Slater, JM (Ed.) *Fifty years of the National Food Survey 1940–1990*. London: HMSO.

MAFF 1993 Ministry of Agriculture Fisheries and Food *The National Food Survey 1992*. Annual report of the National Food Survey committee. London: HMSO.

MAFF 1997 Ministry of Agriculture Fisheries and Food *The National Food Survey 1996*. Annual report of the National Food Survey committee. London: HMSO.

Mangiapane, EH and Salter, AM 1999 *Diet, lipoproteins and coronary heart disease. A biochemical perspective*. Nottingham: Nottingham University Press.

Manson, JE, Colditz, GA, Stampfer, MJ, *et al.* 1990 A prospective study of obesity and coronary heart disease in women. *New England Journal of Medicine* **322**, 882–889.

Manson, JE, Willett, WC, Stampfer, MJ, *et al.* 1995 Body weight and mortality among women. *New England Journal of Medicine* **333**, 677–685.

Manson, JJ and Rahman, A 2004 This house believes that we should advise our patients with osteoarthritis of the knee to take glucosamine. *Rheumatology* **43**, 100–101.

Maslow, AH 1943 A theory of human motivation. *Psychological Reviews* **50**, 370–396.

Mathews, F 1996 Antioxidant nutrients in pregnancy; a systematic review of the literature. *Nutrition Research Reviews* **9**, 175–195.

Mattila, K, Haavisto, M and Rajala, S 1986 Body mass index and mortality in the elderly. *British Medical Journal* **292**, 867–868.

Mattson, FH and Grundy, SM 1985 Comparison of effects of dietary saturated, monounsaturated and polyunsaturated fatty acids on plasma lipids and lipoproteins in man. *Journal of Lipid Research* **26**, 194–202.

Maughan, RJ 1994 Nutritional aspects of endurance exercise in humans. *Proceedings of the Nutrition Society* **53**, 181–188.

Mayer, J 1956 Appetite and obesity. *Scientific American* **195**, 108–116.

Mayer, J 1968 *Overweight: causes, cost and control*. Engelwood Cliffs, New Jersey: Prentice Hall.

Mela, DJ 1997 Fat and sugar substitutes: implications for dietary intakes and energy balance, *Proceedings of the Nutrition Society* **56**, 820–828.

Mensink, RP and Katan, MJ 1990 Effect of dietary trans fatty acids on high-density and low-density lipoprotein cholesterol levels in healthy subjects. *New England Journal of Medicine* **323**, 439–445.

Miettinen, TA, Puska, P, Gylling, H, Vanhanen, H and Vartiainen, E 1995 Reduction of serum cholesterol with sitostanol-ester margarine in a mildly hypercholesteremic population. *New England Journal of Medicine* **333**, 1308–1312.

Miller, DS 1979 Non-genetic models of obesity. In: Festing, MWF (Ed.) *Animal models of obesity*. London: Macmillan, pp. 131–140.

Miller, DS and Payne, PR 1969 Assessment of protein requirements by nitrogen balance. *Proceedings of the Nutrition Society* **28**, 225–234.

Mills, A and Patel, S 1994 *Food portion sizes,* 2nd edn. London: HMSO.

Millstone, E 1985 Food additive regulation in the UK. *Food Policy* **10**, 237–252.

Mitchell, EB 1988 Food intolerance. In: Dickerson, JWT and Lee, HA (Eds) *Nutrition in the clinical management of disease.* London: Edward Arnold, pp. 374–391.

Molarius, A, Seidell, JC, Sans, S, *et al.* 2000 Educational level, relative body weight, and changes in their association over 10 years: an international perspective from the WHO MONICA project. *American Journal of Public Health* **90**, 1260–1268.

Montague. CT, Farooq, IS, Whitehead, JP, *et al.* 1997 Congenital leptin deficiency is associated with severe early-onset obesity in humans. *Nature* **387**, 903–908.

Morgan, JB 1988 Nutrition for and during pregnancy. In: Dickerson, JWT and Lee, HA (Eds) *Nutrition in the clinical management of disease,* 2nd edn. London: Edward Arnold, pp. 1–29.

Morgan, JB 1998 Weaning: when and what. *British Nutrition Foundation Nutrition Bulletin* **23** (supplement 1), 35–45.

Moro, G, Arslanoglu, S, Stahl, B, *et al.* 2006 A mixture of prebiotic oligosaccharides reduces the incidence of atopic dermatitis during the first six months of age. *Archives of Diseases in Childhood* **91**, 814–819.

Morris, JN, Everitt, MG, Pollard, R, Chave, SPW and Semmence, AM 1980 Vigorous exercise in leisure-time: protection against coronary heart disease. *Lancet* **ii**, 1207–1210.

Mowe, M, Bohmer, T and Kindt, E 1994 Reduced nutritional status in elderly people is probable before disease and probably contributes to the development of disease. *American Journal of Clinical Nutrition* **59**, 317–324.

Moynihan, PJ 1995 The relationship between diet, nutrition and dental health: an overview and update for the 90s. *Nutrition Research Reviews* **8**, 193–224.

MRC 1991 The MRC Vitamin Study Group. Prevention of neural tube defects: results of the Medical Research Council Vitamin Study. *Lancet* **338**, 131–137.

MRFIT 1982 Multiple Risk Factor Intervention Trial Research Group. Multiple risk factor intervention trial. *Journal of the American Medical Association* **248**, 1465–1477.

Mulrow, C, Lawrence, V, Ackerman, R, *et al.* 2000 *Garlic: effects on cardiovascular risks and disease, protective effects against cancer, and clinical adverse effects.* Evidence report/ technology assessment number 20. AHRQ publication N. 01-E022. Rockville MD: Agency for Healthcare Research and Quality. www.ncbi.nlm.nih.gov/books/bv.fcgi?rid=hstat1. chapter.28361 (accessed 6 August 2007).

Murphy, KG and Bloom, SR 2004 Gut hormones in the control of appetite. *Experimental Physiology* **89**, 507–516.

NACNE 1983 The National Advisory Committee on Nutrition Education. *A discussion paper on proposals for nutritional guidelines for health education in Britain.* London: Health Education Council.

Naismith, DJ 1980 Maternal nutrition and the outcome of pregnancy – a critical appraisal. *Proceedings of the Nutrition Society* **39**, 1–11.

NAS 2004 National Academy of Sciences. Dietary Reference Intakes (DRIs). Food and Nutrition Board, Institute of Medicine, National Academy of Sciences. http://iom.edu/ Object.File/Master/21/372/0.pdf (accessed on 3 August 2007).

Naylor, CD 1997 Meta analysis and the meta-epidemiology of clinical research. *British Medical Journal* **315**, 617–619.

Nelson, HD, Humphrey, LL, Nygren, P, *et al.* 2002 Postmenopausal hormone replacement therapy. *Journal of the American Medical Association* **288**, 872–881.

Nelson, M, Atkinson, M and Meyer, J 1997 *Food portion sizes. A photographic atlas.* London: MAFF Publications.

Nicolaas, G 1995 *Cooking: attitudes and behaviour.* London: HMSO.

NRC 1943 National Research Council. *Recommended dietary allowances*, 1st edn. Washington DC: National Academy of Sciences.

NRC 1989a. *Recommended dietary allowances*, 10th edn. Washington DC: National Academy of Sciences.

NRC 1989b National Research Council. Diet and health: implications for reducing chronic disease risk. *Nutrition Reviews* **47**, 142–149.

Ogden, CL, Flegal, KM, Carroll, MD and Johnson, CL 2002 Prevalence and trends in overweight among US children and adolescents, 1999–2000. *Journal of the American Medical Association* **2888**, 1728–1732.

Oguma, Y, Sesso, HD, Paffenbarger, RS and Lee, I-M 2002 Physical activity and all cause mortality in women: a review of the evidence. *British Journal of Sports Medicine* **36**, 162–172.

Oliver, MF 1981 Diet and coronary heart disease. *British Medical Bulletin* **37**, 49–58.

Oliver, MF 1991 Might treatment of hypercholesteraemia increase non-cardiac mortality. *Lancet* **337**, 1529–1531.

Omenn, GS, Goodman, GE, Thornquist, MD, *et al.* 1996 Combination of beta-carotene and vitamin A on lung cancer and cardiovascular disease. *New England Journal of Medicine* **334**, 1150–1155.

Oosthuizen, W, Virster, HH, Vermaak, WJ, *et al.* 1998 Lecithin has no effect on serum lipoprotein, plasma fibrinogen and macro molecular protein complex levels in hyperlipidaemic men in a double-blind controlled study. *European Journal of Clinical Nutrition* **52**, 419–424.

Paffenbarger, RS, Hyde, RT, Wing, AL, Hsieh, C-C 1986 Physical activity, all-cause mortality, and longevity of college alumni. *New England Journal of Medicine* **314**, 605–613.

Paolini, M, Cantelli-Forti, G, Perocco, P, Pedulli, GF, Abdel-Rahman, SZ and Legator, MS 1999 Co-carcinogenic effect of β-carotene. *Nature* **398**, 760–761.

Passim, H and Bennett, JW 1943 *Social progress and dietary change.* National Research Council Bulletin 108. Washington DC: National Research Council.

Passmore, R and Eastwood, MA 1986 *Human nutrition and dietetics*, 8th edn. Edinburgh: Churchill Livingstone.

Paterakis, SE and Nelson, M 2003 A comparison between the National Food Survey and the Family Expenditure Survey food expenditure data. *Public Health Nutrition* **6**, 571–580.

Pauling, L 1972 *Vitamin C and the common cold.* London: Ballantine Books.

Penicaud, L, Leloup, C, Lorsignol, A, Alquier, T and Guillod, E 2002 Brain glucose sensing mechanism and glucose homeostasis. *Current Opinions in Clinical Nutrition and Metabolic Care* **5**, 539–543.

Pennington, CR 1997 Disease and malnutrition in British hospitals. *Proceedings of the Nutrition Society* **56**, 393–407.

Peto, R, Doll, R, Buckley, JD and Sporn, MB 1981 Can dietary beta-carotene materially reduce human cancer rates? *Nature* **290**, 201–208.

Phillips, F 2003 *Diet and Bone Health.* Flair-Flow 4 synthesis report. INRA: Paris.

Picciano, MF and McDonald, SS 2006 Lactation. In: Shils, ME, *et al.* (Eds) *Modern nutrition in health and disease.* Philadelphia: Lippincott, Williams and Wilkins, pp. 784–96.

Pocock, NA, Eisman, JA, Yeates, MG, Sambrook, PN and Ebert, S 1986 Physical fitness is a major determinant of femoral neck and lumbar spine bone mineral density. *Journal of Clinical Investigation* **78**, 618–621.

Pohlel, K, Grow, P, Helmy, T and Wenger, NK 2006 Treating dyslipidaemia in the elderly. *Current Opinions in Lipidology* **17**, 54–57.

Poleman, TT 1975 World food: a perspective. *Science* **188**, 510–518.

Pomrehn, PR, Wallace, RB and Burmeister, LF 1982 Ischemic heart disease mortality in Iowa farmers. *Journal of the American Medical Association* **248**, 1073–1076.

Pond, C 1987 Fat and figures. *New Scientist* **4 June**, 62–66.

Poskitt, EME 1988 Childhood. In: Dickerson, JWT and Lee, HA (Eds) *Nutrition in the clinical management of disease.* London: Edward Arnold, pp. 30–68.

Poskitt, EME 1998 Infant nutrition: lessons from the third world. *British Nutrition Foundation Nutrition Bulletin* **23** (supplement 1), 12–22.

Poston, L, Briley, AL, Seed, PT, Kelly, FJ and Shennan, AH 2006 Vitamin C and vitamin E in pregnant women at risk for pre-eclampsia (VIP trial): randomised placebo-controlled trial. *Lancet* **367**, 1145–1154.

Powell-Tuck, J 1997 Penalties of hospital undernutrition. *Journal of the Royal Society of Medicine* **90**, 8–11.

Powers, SK and Howley, ET 1990 *Exercise physiology.* Dubuque, Iowa: WC Brown.

Prentice, A 1997 Is nutrition important in osteoporosis? *Proceedings of the Nutrition Society* **56**, 357–367.

Prentice, A, Laskey, MA, Shaw, J, *et al.* 1993 The calcium and phosphorus intakes of rural Gambian women during pregnancy and lactation. *British Journal of Nutrition* **69**, 885–896.

Prentice, AM 1989 Energy expenditure in human pregnancy. *British Nutrition Foundation Nutrition Bulletin* **14**, 9–22.

Prentice, AM and Jebb, SA 1995 Obesity in Britain: gluttony or sloth? *British Medical Journal* **311**, 437–439.

Prentice, AM, Black, AE, Murgatroyd, PR, *et al.* 1989 Metabolism or appetite: questions of energy balance with particular reference to obesity. *Journal of Human Nutrition and Dietetics* **2**, 95–104.

Prentice, AM, Goldberg, GR, Jebb, SA, Black, AE, Murgatroyd, PR and Diaz, EO 1991 Physiological responses to slimming. *Proceedings of the Nutrition Society* **50**, 441–458.

Prescott-Clarke, P and Primatesta, P 1998 *Health survey for England 1996.* London: The Stationery Office.

Prusiner, SB 1995 The prion diseases. *Scientific American* January **1995**, 30–37.

Rapala, JM, Virtamo, J, Ripatti, S, *et al.* 1997 Randomised trial of alpha-tocopherol and beta-carotene supplements on incidence of major coronary events in men with previous myocardial infarction. *Lancet* **349**, 1715–1720.

Ravnskov, U 1992 Cholesterol lowering trials in coronary heart disease: frequency of citation and outcome. *British Medical Journal* **305**, 15–19.

Ray, JG, Meier, C, Vermeulen, MJ, *et al.* 2002 Association of neural tube defects and folic acid food fortification in Canada. *Lancet* **360**, 2047–2048.

RCN 1993 Royal College of Nursing *Nutrition standards and the older adult.* Dynamic Quality Improvement Programme. London: RCN.

RECORD trial group 2005 Oral vitamin D3 and calcium for secondary prevention of low-trauma fractures in elderly people (Randomised Evaluation of Calcium Or Vitamin D, RECORD): a randomised placebo-controlled trial. *Lancet* **365**, 1621–1628.

Reaven, GM 2006 Metabolic syndrome: definition, relationship to insulin resistance and clinical utility. In: Shils, ME, *et al.* (Eds) *Modern nutrition in health and disease*, 10th edn. Philadelphia: Lippincott, Williams and Wilkins, pp. 1004–1012.

Reddy, BS 1998 Prevention of colon cancer by pre- and probiotics: evidence from laboratory studies. *British Journal of Nutrition* **80**, S219–S223.

Reid, G, Burton, J and Devillard, E 2004 The rationale for probiotics in female urogenital healthcare. *Medscape General Medicine* **6**, 49.

Renaud, S and de Lorgeril, M 1992 Wine, alcohol, platelets and the French paradox for coronary heart disease. *Lancet* **339**, 1523–1526.

Report 1992 *Folic acid and the prevention of neural tube defects.* Report from an expert advisory group. London: Department of Health.

Richards, JR 1980 Current concepts in the metabolic responses to injury, infection and starvation. *Proceedings of the Nutrition Society* **39**, 113–123.

Riemersma, RA, Wood, DA, Macintyre, CCA, Elton, RA, Fey, KF and Oliver, MF 1991 Risk of angina pectoris and plasma concentrations of vitamins A, C, and E and carotene. *Lancet* **337**, 1–5.

Rimm, EB, Giovannucci, EL, Willett, WC, *et al.* 1991 Prospective study of alcohol consumption and risk of coronary disease in men. *Lancet* **338**, 464–468.

Rimm, EB, Stampfer, MJ, Ascheirio, A, Giovannucci, EL, Colditz, GA and Willett, WC 1993 Vitamin E consumption and the risk of coronary heart disease in men. *New England Journal of Medicine* **328**, 1450–1455.

Rissanen, A, Heliovaara, M, Knekt, P, Reunanen, A, Aromaa, A and Maatela, J 1990 Risk of disability and mortality due to overweight in a Finnish population. *British Medical Journal*, **301**, 835–837.

Rivers, JPW and Frankel, TL 1981 Essential fatty acid deficiency. *British Medical Bulletin* **37**, 59–64.

Roberts, D 1982 Factors contributing to outbreaks of food poisoning in England and Wales 1970–1979. *Journal of Hygiene* **89**, 491–498.

Robertson, I, Glekin, BM, Henderson, JB, Lakhani, A and Dunnigan, MG 1982 Nutritional deficiencies amongst ethnic minorities in the United Kingdom. *Proceedings of the Nutrition Society* **41**, 243–256.

Roche, HM, Noone, E, Nugent, A and Gibney, MJ 2001 Conjugated linoleic acid; a novel therapeutic nutrient? *Nutrition Research Reviews* **14**, 173–187.

Rolls, BA 1992 Calcium nutrition. In: Walker, AF and Rolls, BA (Eds) *Nutrition and the consumer.* London: Elsevier Appied Science, pp. 69–95.

Rolls, BJ 1993 Appetite, hunger and satiety in the elderly. *Critical Reviews in Food Science and Nutrition* **33**, 39–44.

Rolls, BJ and Phillips, PA 1990 Aging and disturbances of thirst and fluid balance. *Nutrition Reviews* **48**, 137–144.

Rolls, BJ, Rowe, EA and Rolls, ET 1982 How flavour and appearance affect human feeding. *Proceedings of the Nutrition Society* **41**, 109–117.

Rosado, JL 1997 Lactose digestion and maldigestion: implications for dietary habits in developing countries. *Nutrition Research Reviews* **10**, 137–149.

Rothwell, NJ and Stock, MJ 1979 A role for brown adipose tissue in diet thermogenesis. *Nature* **281**, 31–35.

Rudman, D 1988 Kidney senescence; a model for ageing. *Nutrition Reviews* **46**, 209.

Ryan, YM, Gibney, MJ and Flynn, MAT 1998 The pursuit of thinness: A study of Dublin schoolgirls aged 15y. *International Journal of Obesity* **22**, 485–487.

Saavedra, JM, Abi-Hanna, A, Moore, N and Yolke, RH 2004 Long term consumption of infant formula containing live probiotic bacteria: tolerance and safety. *American Journal of Clinical Nutrition* **79**, 261–267.

Sacks, FM, Willet, WC, Smith A, *et al.* 1998 Effect on blood pressure of potassium, calcium and magnesium in women with low habitual intake. *Hypertension* **31**, 131–138.

SACN 2003 Scientific Advisory Committee on Nutrition. *Salt and health.* London: The Stationery Office.

Sadler, M 1994 *Nutrition in pregnancy.* London: British Nutrition Foundation.

Samaras, K and Campbell, LV 1997 The non-genetic determinants of central adiposity. *International Journal of Obesity* **21**, 839–845.

Sanderson, FH 1975 The great food fumble. *Science* **188**, 503–509.

Sanders, TAB 1985 Influence of fish-oil supplements on man. *Proceedings of the Nutrition Society* **44**, 391–397.

Sanders, TAB 1988 Growth and development of British vegan children. *American Journal of Clinical Nutrition* **48**, 822–825.

Sanders, TAB, Mistry, M and Naismith, DJ 1984 The influence of a maternal diet rich in linoleic acid on brain and retinal docosahexaenoic acid in the rat. *British Journal of Nutrition* **51**, 57–66.

Schachter, S 1968 Obesity and eating. *Science* **161**, 751–756.

Schachter, S and Rodin, J 1974 *Obese humans and rats.* New York: Halstead Press.

Schrauwen, PS, Walder, K and Ravussin, E 1999 Role of uncoupling proteins in energy balance. In: Westerterp-Plantenga, MS, Steffens, AB and Tremblay, A (Eds) *Regulation of food intake and energy expenditure.* Milan: EDRA, pp. 415–428.

Schroll, M, Jorgensen, L, Osler, M and Davidsen, M 1993 Chronic undernutrition and the aged. *Proceedings of the Nutrition Society* **52**, 29–37.

Schutz, HG, Rucker, MH and Russell, GF 1975 Food and food-use classification systems. *Food Technology* **29**, 50–64.

Schutz, Y, Flatt, JP and Jequier, E 1989 Failure of dietary fat intake to promote fat oxidation is a factor favouring the development of obesity. *American Journal of Clinical Nutrition* **50**, 307–314.

Seidell, JC 2000 Obesity, insulin resistance and diabetes – a worldwide perspective. *British Journal of Nutrition* **83** (supplement 1), S5–S8.

Sever, PS, Dahlof, B and Poulter, NR 2003 Prevention of coronary and stroke events with atorvastatin in hypertensive patients who have average or lower-than-average cholesterol concentrations, in the Anglo-Scandinavian Cardiac Outcomes Trial – Lipid Lowering Arm (ASCOT-LLA): A multicentre randomised controlled trial. *Lancet* **361**, 1149–1158.

Shekelle P, Morton, S and Hardy, M 2003 *Effect of supplemental antioxidants vitamin C, vitamin E, and coenzyme Q$_{10}$ for the prevention and treatment of cardiovascular disease*. Evidence report/technology assessment No.83. Rockville MD: Agency for Health care Research and Quality. Available free online at www.ncbi.nlm.nih.gov/books/bv.fcgi?rid=hstat1a.chapter.16082 (accessed on 3 August 2007).

Shepherd, J 2004 A prospective study of pravastatin in the elderly at risk: a new hope for older persons. *American Journal of Geriatric Cardiology* **13**, 17–24.

Shepherd, J, Cobbe, SM, Forde, I, *et al.* 1995 Prevention of coronary heart disease with pravastatin in men with hypercholesteremia. *New England Journal of Medicine* **333**, 130–137.

Shils, ME, Shike, M, Ross, AC, Caballero, B and Cousins, RJ (Eds) *Modern nutrition in health and disease*, 10th edn. Philadelphia: Lippincott, Williams and Wilkins.

Shipley, MJ, Pocock, SJ and Marmot, MG 1991 Does plasma cholesterol concentration predict mortality from coronary heart disease in elderly people? 18 year follow up in the Whitehall study. *British Medical Journal* **303**, 89–92.

Simopolous, AP 1991 Omega 3 fatty acids in health and disease and in growth and development. *American Journal of Clinical Nutrition* **54**, 438–463.

Sims, EAH, Danforth, E Jr, Horton, ES, Bray, GA, Glennon, JA and Salans, LB 1973 Endocrine and metabolic effects of experimental obesity in man. *Recent Progress in Hormone Research* **29**, 457–496.

Smith, GD, Song, F and Sheldon, TA 1993 Cholesterol lowering and mortality: the importance of considering initial level of risk. *British Medical Journal* **306**, 1367–1373.

Smith, R 1987 Osteoporosis: cause and management. *British Medical Journal* **294**, 329–332.

Sobal, J and Stunkard, AJ 1989 Socioeconomic status and obesity: a review of the literature. *Psychological Bulletin* **105**, 260–275.

Sorensen, LB, Moller, P, Flint, A, *et al.* 2003 Effect of sensory perception of foods on appetite and food intake: a review of studies on humans. *International Journal of Obesity and Related Metabolic Disorders* **27**, 1152–1166.

Sorensen, TIA 1992 Genetic aspects of obesity. *International Journal of Obesity* **16** (supplement 2), S27–S29.

Sorensen, TIA, Echwald, SM and Holm, J-C 1996 Leptin in obesity. *British Medical Journal* **313**, 953–954.

Spector, TD, Cooper, C and Fenton Lewis, A 1990 Trends in admissions for hip fracture in England and Wales 1968–1985. *British Medical Journal* **300**, 1173–1174.

Sproston, K and Primatesta, P 2004 *Health Survey for England 2003*. London: The Stationery Office.

SSSS group 1994 Scandinavian Simvastatin Survival Study Group 1994 Randomised trial of cholesterol lowering in 4444 patients with coronary heart disease: the Scandinavian Simvastatin Survival Study (4S). *Lancet* **344**, 1383–1389.

Stampfer, MJ, Hennekens, CH, Manson, JE, Colditz, GA, Rosner, B and Willett, WC 1993 Vitamin E consumption and the risk of coronary disease in women. *New England Journal of Medicine* **328**, 1444–1449.

Steinberg, D, Parthasarathy, S, Carew, TE, Khoo, JC and Witztum, JC 1989 Beyond cholesterol: modifications of low-density lipoprotein that increase its atherogenicity. *New England Journal of Medicine* **320**, 915–924.

Stephens, NG, Parsons, A, Schofield, PM, *et al.* 1996 Randomised controlled trial of vitamin E in patients with coronary disease: Cambridge Heart Antioxidant Study {CHAOS}. *Lancet* **347**, 781–786.

Stratton, IM, Adler, AI, Weil, HAW, *et al.* 2000 Association of glycaemia with macrovascular and microvascular complications of type 2 diabetes (UKPDS 35): prospective observational study. *British Medical Journal* **321**, 405–412.

Stratton, RJ 2005 Should food or supplements be used in the community for the treatment of disease-related malnutrition? *Proceedings of the Nutrition Society* **64**, 325–333.

Symonds, ME and Clarke, L 1996 Nutrition–environment interactions in pregnancy. *Nutrition Research Reviews* **9**, 135–148.

Szajewska, H and Mrukowicz, JZ 2001 Probiotics in the treatment and prevention of acute infectious diarrhoea in infants and children: a systematic review of published randomized, double-blind, placebo-controlled trials. *Journal of Pediatric Gastroenterology and Nutrition* **33** (supplement), S17–25.

Tartaglia, LA, Dembski, M, Weng, X, *et al.* 1995 Identification and expression cloning of a leptin receptor OB-R. *Cell* **83**, 1263–1271.

Taylor, GR and Williams, CM 1998 Effects of probiotics and prebiotics on blood lipids. *British Journal of Nutrition* **80**, S225–S230.

Taylor, SL 2006 Food additives, contaminants and natural toxicants and their risk assessment. In: Shils, ME, *et al.* (Eds) *Modern nutrition in health and disease*, 10th edn. Philadelphia: Lippincott, Williams and Wilkins, pp. 1809–1826.

Thane, CW, Bates, CJ and Prentice, A 2003 Risk factors for low iron intake and poor iron status in a national sample of British young people aged 4–18 years. *Public Health Nutrition* **6**, 485–496.

Thomson, CD and Robinson, MF 1980 Selenium in human health and disease with emphasis on those aspects peculiar to New Zealand. *American Journal of Clinical Nutrition* **33**, 303–323.

Thorogood, M 1995 The epidemiology of vegetarianism and health. *Nutrition Research Reviews* **8**, 179–192.

Tisdale, MJ 1997 Isolation of a novel cachectic factor. *Proceedings of the Nutrition Society* **56**, 777–783.

Tobian, L 1979 Dietary salt (sodium) and hypertension. *American Journal of Clinical Nutrition* **32**, 2659–2662.

Todd, E 1991 Epidemiology of foodborne illness: North America. In: Waites, WM and Arbuthnott, JP (Eds) *Foodborne illness. A* Lancet *review.* London: Edward Arnold, pp. 9–15.

Tompson, P, Salsbury, PA, Adams, C and Archer, DL 1991 US food legislation. In: Waites, WM and Arbuthnott, JP (Eds) *Foodborne illness. A Lancet review.* London: Edward Arnold, pp. 38–43.

Trowell, HC 1954 Kwashiorkor. *Scientific American* **191**, 46–50.

Truswell, AS 1999 Dietary goals and guidelines: National and international perspectives. In: Shils, ME, *et al.* (Eds) *Modern nutrition in health and disease*, 9th edn. Philadelphia: Lippincott, Williams and Wilkins, pp. 1727–1742.

UK National Case Control Study Group 1993 Breast feeding and risk of breast cancer in young women. *British Medical Journal* **307**, 17–20.

UN 2005 United Nations. Press release POP/918. www.un.org/News/Press/docs/2005/pop918.doc.htm (accessed on 3 August 2007).

UNICEF 2004 UNICEF statistics. Breast feeding and complementary feeding available online at www.childinfo.org/areas/breastfeeding/patterns.php (accessed on 3 August 2007).

USDA 1992 United States Department of Agriculture. *The food guide pyramid.* Home and garden bulletin number 252. Washington DC: United States Department of Agriculture.

van Asp, N-G, Amelsvoort, JMM and Hautvast, JGAJ 1996 Nutritional implications of resistant starch. *Nutrition Research Reviews* **9**, 1–31.

Villamor, E and Cnattingius, S 2006 Interpregnancy weight change and risk of adverse pregnancy outcomes: a population-based study. *Lancet* **368**, 1164–1170.

Vincent, A and Fitzpatrick, LA 2000 Soy isoflavones: are they useful in menopause? *Mayo Clinic Proceedings* **75**, 1174–1184.

Viner, RM and Cole, TJ 2005 Television viewing in early childhood predicts adult body mass index. *Journal of Pediatrics* **147**, 429–435.

Vivekanathan, DP, Penn, MS, Sapp, SK, Hsu, A and Topol, EJ 2003 Use of antioxidant vitamins for the prevention of cardiovascular disease: meta-analysis of randomised trials. *Lancet* **361**, 2017–2023.

von Braun, J 2005 The world food situation an overview. Washington: International Food Policy Research Institute. www.ifpri.org/pubs/agm05/-jvbagm2005.asp#read (accessed on 3 August 2007).

Wadden, TA and Stunkard, AJ 1985 Social and psychological consequences of obesity. *Annals of Internal Medicine* **103**, 1062–1067.

Wadden, TA, Byrne, KJ and Krauthamer-Ewing, S 2006 Obesity: management. In: Shils, ME, *et al.* (Eds) *Modern nutrition in health and disease*, 10th edn. Philadelphia: Lippincott, Williams and Wilkins, pp. 1029–1042.

Wald, N, Idle, M, Boreham, J and Bailey, A 1980 Low serum-vitamin-A and subsequent risk of cancer. *Lancet* **ii**, 813–815.

Walker, AF 1990 The contribution of weaning foods to protein-energy malnutrition. *Nutrition Research Reviews* **3**, 25–47.

Wang, C, Chung, M, Lichtenstein, A, *et al.* 2004 *Effects of omega-3 fatty acids on cardiovascular disease*. Evidence report/technology assessment No. 94. AHRQ Publication No. 04-E009–2. Rockville, MD: Agency for Healthcare Research and Quality. www.ncbi.nlm.nih.gov/books/bv.fcgi?rid=hstat1a.chapter.38290 (accessed on 3 August 2007).

Wang, XD, Liu, C, Bronson, RT, *et al.* 1999 Retinoid signalling and activator protein-1 expression in ferrets given beta-carotene supplements and exposed to tobacco smoke. *Journal of the National Cancer Institute* **91**, 7–9.

Watanabe, F, Katsura, H, Takenaka, S, *et al.* 1999 Pseudovitamin B_{12} is the predominant cobalamin of an algal health food, Spirulina tablets. *Journal of Agricultural and Food Chemistry* **47**, 4736–4741.

Waterlow, JC 1979 Childhood malnutrition – the global problem. *Proceedings of the Nutrition Society* **38**, 1–9.

Waterlow, JC and Payne, PR 1975 The protein gap. *Nature* **258**, 113–117.

Waterlow, JC, Cravioto, J and Stephen, JML 1960 Protein malnutrition in man. *Advances in Protein Chemistry* **15**, 131–238.

Watts, G 1998 Avoiding action. *New Scientist* 28 November, p. 53.

Webb, GP 1989 The significance of protein in human nutrition. *Journal of Biological Education* **23**, 119–124.

Webb, GP 1990 A selective critique of animal experiments in human-orientated biological research. *Journal of Biological Education* **24**, 191–197.

Webb, GP 1992a A critical survey of methods used to investigate links between diet and disease. *Journal of Biological Education*, **26**, 263–271.

Webb, GP 1992b Viewpoint II: Small animals as models for studies on human nutrition. In: Walker, AF and Rolls, BA (Eds) *Nutrition and the consumer*. London: Elsevier Applied Science, pp. 279–297.

Webb, GP 1994 A survey of fifty years of dietary standards 1943–1993. *Journal of Biological Education* **28**, 101–108.

Webb, GP 1995 Sleeping position and cot death: does health promotion always promote health? *Journal of Biological Education* **29**, 279–285.

Webb, GP 1998 *Teach yourself weight control through diet and exercise*. London: Hodder and Stoughton.

Webb, GP 2006 *Dietary supplements and functional foods*. Oxford: Blackwell.

Webb, GP 2007 Nutritional supplements and conventional medicine; what should the physician know? *Proceedings of the Nutrition Society* **66**, 471–478.

Webb, GP and Copeman, J 1996 *The nutrition of older adults*. London: Arnold.

Webb, GP and Jakobson, ME 1980 Body fat of mice and men: a class exercise in theory or practice. *Journal of Biological Education* **14**, 318–324.

Webb, GP, Jagot, SA and Jakobson, ME 1982 Fasting induced torpor in *Mus musculus* and its implications in the use of murine models for human obesity studies. *Comparative Physiology and Biochemistry* **72A**, 211–219.

Wenham, NS and Wolff, RJ 1970 A half century of changing food habits among Japanese in Hawaii. *Journal of the American Dietetic Association* **57**, 29–32.

Wharton, B 1998 Nutrition in infancy. *British Nutrition Foundation Nutrition Bulletin* **23**, supplement 1.

Wheeler, E 1992 What determines food choice, and what does food choice determine? *The British Nutrition Foundation Nutrition Bulletin* 17(supplement 1), 65–73.

Wheeler, E and Tan, SP 1983 From concept to practice: food behaviour of Chinese immigrants in London. *Ecology of Food and Nutrition* **13**, 51–57.

White, A, Freeth, S and O'Brien, M 1992 *Infant feeding 1990*. London: HMSO.

White, A, Nicolaas, G, Foster, K, Browne, F and Carey, S 1993 *Health survey for England 1991* London: HMSO.

WHO 1990 *Diet, nutrition and the prevention of chronic diseases*. Geneva: World Health Organization.

WHO 2000 Effect of breastfeeding on infant and child mortality due to infectious diseases in less developed countries: a pooled analysis. WHO Collaborative Study Team on the Role Breastfeeding in the Prevention of Infant Mortality. *Lancet* **355**, 451–455.

WHO 2006 Obesity and overweight. World Health Organization. http://www.who.int/dietphysicalactivity/publications/facts/obesity/en/print.html, (accessed 4 October 2007).

Wickham, CAC, Walsh, K, Barker, DJP, Margetts, BM, Morris, J and Bruce, SA 1989 Dietary calcium, physical activity, and risk of hip fracture: a prospective study. *British Medical Bulletin* **299**, 889–892.

Wilcox, AJ, Lie, RT, Solvoll, K, *et al.* 2007 Folic acid supplements and risk of facial clefts: national

population based case-control study. *British Medical Journal* **334**, 433–434.

Willett, WC, Stampfer, MJ, Colditz, GA, Rosner, BA and Speizer, FE 1990 Relation of meat, fat and fiber intake to the risk of colon cancer in a prospective study among women. *The New England Journal of Medicine* **323**, 1664–1672.

Willett, WC, Stampfer, MJ, Manson, JE, *et al.* 1993 Intake of *trans* fatty acids and risk of coronary heart disease among women. *Lancet* **341**, 581–585.

Williams, CA and Qureshi, B 1988 Nutritional aspects of different dietary practices. In: Dickerson, JWT and Lee, HA (Eds) *Nutrition in the clinical management of disease*. London: Edward Arnold, pp. 422–439.

Williams, MH 2006 Sports nutrition. In: Shils, ME, *et al.* (Eds) *Modern nutrition in health and disease*, 10th edn. Philadelphia: Lippincott, Williams and Wilkins, pp. 1723–1740.

Wilson, JH 1994 Nutrition, physical activity and bone health in women. *Nutrition Research Reviews* **7**, 67–91.

Woo, J, Ho, SC, Mak, YT, Law, LK and Cheung, A 1994 Nutritional status of elderly people during recovery from chest infection and the role of nutritional supplementation assessed by a prospective randomised single-blind control trial. *Age and Ageing* **23**, 40–48.

Wortman, S 1976 Food and agriculture. *Scientific American* **235**, 31–39.

WRI 1997 World Resources Institute. Sustainable agriculture. http://pubs.wri.org/pubs_content_text.cfm?ContentID=2712 (accessed 6 August 2007).

Wynne, K, Park, AJ, Small, CJ, *et al.* 2006 Oxyntomodulin increases energy expenditure in addition to decreasing energy intake in overweight and obese humans: a randomised controlled trial. *International Journal of Obesity* **30**, 1729–1736.

Yeung, DL, Cheung, LWY and Sabrey, JH 1973 The hot-cold food concept in Chinese culture and its application in a Canadian-Chinese community. *Journal of the Canadian Dietetic Association* **34**, 197–203.

Yu, S, Derr, J, Etherton, TD and Kris Etherton, PM 1995 Plasma cholesterol-predictive equations demonstrate that stearic acid is neutral and monounsaturated fatty acids are hypocholesteraemic. *American Journal of Clinical Nutrition* **61**, 1129–1139.

Yudkin, J 1958 *This slimming business.* London: MacGibbon and Kee.

Zhang, Y and Scarpace, PJ 2006 The role of leptin in leptin resistance and obesity. *Physiology and Behaviour* **88**, 249–256.

Zhang, Y, Proenca, R, Maffei, M, Barone, M, Leopold, L and Friedman, JM 1994 Positional cloning of the mouse *obese* gene and its human homologue. *Nature* **372**, 425–432.

Ziegler, D, Reljanovic, M, Mehnert, H and Gries, FA 1999 Alpha-lipoic acid in the treatment of diabetic neuropathy in Germany: current evidence from clinical trials. *Experimental and Clinical Endocrinology and Diabetes* **107**, 421–430.

Ziegler, RG 1991 Vegetables, fruits and carotenoids and the risk of cancer. *American Journal of Clinical Nutrition* **53**, 251S–259S.

Zimmerman, M and Delange, F 2004 Iodine supplements of pregnant women in Europe: a review and recommendations. *European Journal of Clinical Nutrition* **58**, 979–984.

Zimmet, P, Hodge, A, Nicolson, M, *et al.* 1996 Serum leptin concentration, obesity, and insulin resistance in Western Samoa: cross sectional study. *British Medical Journal* **313**, 965–969.

Zipitis, CS, Markides, GA and Swann, IL 2006 Vitamin D deficiency: prevention or treatment? *Archives of Disease in Childhood* **91**, 1011–1014.

Index

Abbreviation 'PUFAs' means polyunsaturated fatty acids.
References to boxes, figures and tables are indicated by the suffixes b, f and t respectively.